VITAMINS
AND
HORMONES

VOLUME 74

INTERLEUKINS

VITAMINS AND HORMONES
ADVANCES IN RESEARCH AND APPLICATIONS

Editor-in-Chief

GERALD LITWACK

Former Professor and Chair
Department of Biochemistry and Molecular Pharmacology
Thomas Jefferson University Medical College
Philadelphia, Pennsylvania
Former Visiting Scholar
Department of Biological Chemistry
David Geffen School of Medicine at UCLA
Toluca Lake, California

VOLUME 74

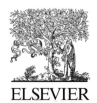

AMSTERDAM • BOSTON • HEIDELBERG • LONDON
NEW YORK • OXFORD • PARIS • SAN DIEGO
SAN FRANCISCO • SINGAPORE • SYDNEY • TOKYO
Academic Press is an imprint of Elsevier

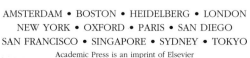

ELSEVIER

Academic Press is an imprint of Elsevier
525 B Street, Suite 1900, San Diego, California 92101-4495, USA
84 Theobald's Road, London WC1X 8RR, UK

This book is printed on acid-free paper.

For information on all Elsevier Academic Press publications
visit our Web site at www.books.elsevier.com

ISBN-13: 978-0-12-709874-6
ISBN-10: 0-12-709874-7

PRINTED IN THE UNITED STATES OF AMERICA
06 07 08 09 9 8 7 6 5 4 3 2 1

Former Editors

CONTENTS

1

IL-3, IL-5, AND GM-CSF SIGNALING: CRYSTAL STRUCTURE OF THE HUMAN BETA-COMMON RECEPTOR

JAMES M. MURPHY AND IAN G. YOUNG

2

CRYSTAL STRUCTURES AND INHIBITORS OF PROTEINS INVOLVED IN IL-2 RELEASE AND T CELL SIGNALING

KIERON BROWN AND GRAHAM M. T. CHEETHAM

3

STRUCTURAL STUDIES OF THE INTERLEUKIN-19 SUBFAMILY OF CYTOKINES

ALEXANDER ZDANOV

4

INTERLEUKIN-22 AND ITS CRYSTAL STRUCTURE

RONALDO ALVES PINTO NAGEM, JOSÉ RIBAMAR FERREIRA JÚNIOR, LAURE DUMOUTIER, JEAN-CHRISTOPHE RENAULD, AND IGOR POLIKARPOV

5

CONTROL OF INTERLEUKIN-2 GENE TRANSCRIPTION: A PARADIGM FOR INDUCIBLE, TISSUE-SPECIFIC GENE EXPRESSION

KAREN BUNTING, JUN WANG, AND M. FRANCES SHANNON

6

TRANSCRIPTION FACTORS MEDIATING INTERLEUKIN-3 SURVIVAL SIGNALS

JEFFREY JONG-YOUNG YEN AND HSIN-FANG YANG-YEN

7

INTERLEUKINS AND STAT SIGNALING

S. JAHARUL HAQUE AND PANKAJ SHARMA

8

THE NEWEST INTERLEUKINS: RECENT ADDITIONS TO THE EVER-GROWING CYTOKINE FAMILY

QIAN CHEN, HELEN P. CARROLL, AND MASSIMO GADINA

9

THE INTERLEUKIN-1 RECEPTOR FAMILY

DIANA BORASCHI AND ALDO TAGLIABUE

10

THE IL-17 CYTOKINE FAMILY

SARAH L. GAFFEN, JILL M. KRAMER, JEFFREY J. YU, AND FANG SHEN

11

NF-κB AND CYTOKINES

DAGMAR KULMS AND THOMAS SCHWARZ

12

IκB-ζ: AN INDUCIBLE REGULATOR OF NUCLEAR FACTOR-κB

TATSUSHI MUTA

13

THE INHIBITORY EFFECTS OF INTERLEUKIN-1 ON GROWTH HORMONE ACTION DURING CATABOLIC ILLNESS

ROBERT N. COONEY AND MARGARET SHUMATE

14

THE ROLE OF THE INTERLEUKIN-6/GP130 SIGNALING PATHWAY IN BONE METABOLISM

XIN-HUA LIU, ALEXANDER KIRSCHENBAUM, SHEN YAO, AND ALICE C. LEVINE

15

REGULATION OF OSTEOCLAST DIFFERENTIATION AND FUNCTION BY INTERLEUKIN-1

ICHIRO NAKAMURA AND EIJIRO JIMI

16

THE ROLE OF IL-1 AND IL-1RA IN JOINT INFLAMMATION AND CARTILAGE DEGRADATION

CLAIRE JACQUES, MARJOLAINE GOSSET, FRANCIS BERENBAUM, AND CEM GABAY

17

CYTOKINES IN TYPE 2 DIABETES

DANIEL R. JOHNSON, JASON C. O'CONNOR, ANSUMAN SATPATHY,
AND GREGORY G. FREUND

18

RELEASE OF INTERLEUKINS AND OTHER INFLAMMATORY CYTOKINES BY HUMAN ADIPOSE TISSUE IS ENHANCED IN OBESITY AND PRIMARILY DUE TO THE NONFAT CELLS

JOHN N. FAIN

19

ROLE OF INTERLEUKIN-13 IN CANCER, PULMONARY FIBROSIS, AND OTHER T$_H$2-TYPE DISEASES

BHARAT H. JOSHI, CORY HOGABOAM, PAMELA DOVER, SYED R. HUSAIN, AND RAJ K. PURI

20

INTERLEUKINS, INFLAMMATION, AND MECHANISMS OF ALZHEIMER'S DISEASE

DAVID WEISMAN, EDWIN HAKIMIAN, AND GILBERT J. HO

21

INTERLEUKIN-2: FROM T CELL GROWTH AND HOMEOSTASIS TO IMMUNE RECONSTITUTION OF HIV PATIENTS

MARKO KRYWORUCHKO AND JACQUES THÈZE

CONTRIBUTORS

Numbers in parentheses indicate the pages on which the authors' contributions begin.

Francis Berenbaum (371) UMR 7079 CNRS, Physiology and Physiopathology Laboratory, University Paris 6, Paris, 75252 Cedex 5, France; Department of Rheumatology, APHP Saint-Antoine Hospital, 75012 Paris, France.

Diana Boraschi (229) Institute of Biomedical Technologies, National Research Council, Pisa, Italy.

Kieron Brown (31) Vertex Pharmaceuticals (Europe) Ltd., Abingdon, Oxfordshire OX14 4RY, United Kingdom.

Karen Bunting (105) Division of Molecular Bioscience, John Curtin School of Medical Research, Australian National University, Canberra, ACT, Australia.

Helen P. Carroll (207) Division of Infection and Immunity, Centre for Cancer Research and Cell Biology, Queen's University Belfast, Belfast, United Kingdom.

Graham M. T. Cheetham (31) Vertex Pharmaceuticals (Europe) Ltd., Abingdon, Oxfordshire OX14 4RY, United Kingdom.

Qian Chen (207) Division of Infection and Immunity, Centre for Cancer Research and Cell Biology, Queen's University Belfast, Belfast, United Kingdom.

Robert N. Cooney (317) Department of Surgery and Department of Cellular and Molecular Physiology, The Pennsylvania State University–College of Medicine, Hershey, Pennsylvania 17033.

Pamela Dover (479) Tumor Vaccines and Biotechnology Branch, Division of Cellular and Gene Therapies, Center for Biologics Evaluation and Research, Food and Drug Administration, Bethesda, Maryland 20892.

Laure Dumoutier (77) Ludwig Institute for Cancer Research, Brussels Branch, The Experimental Medicine Unit, Christian de Duve Institute of Cellular Pathology, Université de Louvain, Brussels, Belgium.

John N. Fain (443) Department of Molecular Sciences, College of Medicine, University of Tennessee Health Science Center, Memphis, Tennessee 38163.

José Ribamar Ferreira Júnior (77) Instituto de Física de São Carlos, Universidade de São Paulo, Avenida Trabalhador Sãocarlense, 400 CEP 13560–970, São Carlos, São Paulo, Brazil.

Gregory G. Freund (405) Department of Animal Sciences and Department of Pathology, University of Illinois, Urbana, Illinois 61801.

Cem Gabay (371) Division of Rheumatology, University Hospital of Geneva, Geneva 14, Switzerland.

Massimo Gadina (207) Division of Infection and Immunity, Centre for Cancer Research and Cell Biology, Queen's University Belfast, Belfast, United Kingdom.

Sarah L. Gaffen (255) Department of Oral Biology, School of Dental Medicine, and Department of Microbiology and Immunology, School of Medicine and Biomedical Sciences, University at Buffalo, SUNY, Buffalo, New York 14214.

Marjolaine Gosset (371) UMR 7079 CNRS, Physiology and Physiopathology Laboratory, University Paris 6, Paris, 75252 Cedex 5, France.

Edwin Hakimian (505) Department of Neurosciences and the Alzheimer's Disease Research Center, University of California, San Diego, California 92093.

S. Jaharul Haque (165) Department of Cancer Biology, Lerner Research Institute, and Department of Pulmonary, Allergy, and Critical Care Medicine, and Brain Tumor Institute, Cleveland Clinic Foundation, Cleveland, Ohio 44195.

Gilbert J. Ho (505) Department of Neurosciences and the Alzheimer's Disease Research Center, University of California, San Diego, California 92093; Neurology Service, Department of Veterans Affairs Medical Center, San Diego, California 92161.

Cory Hogaboam (479) Department of Pathology, University of Michigan Medical School, Ann Arbor, Michigan 48109.

Syed R. Husain (479) Tumor Vaccines and Biotechnology Branch, Division of Cellular and Gene Therapies, Center for Biologics Evaluation and Research, Food and Drug Administration, Bethesda, Maryland 20892.

Claire Jacques (371) UMR 7079 CNRS, Physiology and Physiopathology Laboratory, University Paris 6, Paris, 75252 Cedex 5, France.

Eijiro Jimi (357) Department of Bioscience, Division of Molecular Biochemistry, Kyushu Dental College, Kita-Kyushu, Fukuoka 803-8580, Japan.

Daniel R. Johnson (405) Department of Animal Sciences and Department of Pathology, University of Illinois, Urbana, Illinois 61801.

Jeffrey Jong-Young Yen (147) Institute of Biomedical Sciences, Academia Sinica, Taipei 11529, Taiwan.

Bharat H. Joshi (479) Tumor Vaccines and Biotechnology Branch, Division of Cellular and Gene Therapies, Center for Biologics Evaluation and Research, Food and Drug Administration, Bethesda, Maryland 20892.

Alexander Kirschenbaum (341) Department of Urology, Mount Sinai School of Medicine, New York, New York 10029.

Jill M. Kramer (255) Department of Oral Biology, School of Dental Medicine, University at Buffalo, SUNY, Buffalo, New York 14214.

Marko Kryworuchko (531) Infectious Disease and Vaccine Research Centre, and Division of Virology, Children's Hospital of Eastern Ontario, Ottawa, Canada.

Dagmar Kulms (283) Department of Cell Biology and Immunology, University of Stuttgart, D-70569 Stuttgart, Germany.

Alice C. Levine (341) Department of Medicine, Division of Endocrinology, Diabetes and Bone Diseases, Mount Sinai School of Medicine, New York, New York 10029.

Xin-Hua Liu (341) Department of Medicine, Division of Endocrinology, Diabetes and Bone Diseases, Mount Sinai School of Medicine, New York, New York 10029.

James M. Murphy (1) Division of Molecular Bioscience, John Curtin School of Medical Research, Australian National University, Acton, ACT, Australia 0200.

Tatsushi Muta (301) Department of Molecular and Cellular Biochemistry, Graduate School of Medical Sciences, Kyushu University, Fukuoka 812-8582, Japan.

Ichiro Nakamura (357) Department of Rheumatology, Yugawara Kosei-Nenkin Hospital, Ashigara-shimo, Kanagawa 259-0314, Japan.

Jason C. O'Connor (405) Division of Nutritional Sciences, University of Illinois, Urbana, Illinois 61801.

Ronaldo Alves Pinto Nagem (77) Departamento de Bioquímica e Imunologia, Instituto de Ciências Biológicas, Universidade Federal de Minas Gerais, Avenida Antônio Carlos, 6627 CEP 31270910, Belo Horizonte, MG, Brazil.

Igor Polikarpov (77) Instituto de Física de São Carlos, Universidade de São Paulo, Avenida Trabalhador Sãocarlense, 400 CEP 13560–970, São Carlos, São Paulo, Brazil.

Raj K. Puri (479) Tumor Vaccines and Biotechnology Branch, Division of Cellular and Gene Therapies, Center for Biologics Evaluation and Research, Food and Drug Administration, Bethesda, Maryland 20892.

Jean-Christophe Renauld (77) Ludwig Institute for Cancer Research, Brussels Branch, The Experimental Medicine Unit, Christian de Duve Institute of Cellular Pathology, Université de Louvain, Brussels, Belgium.

Ansuman Satpathy (405) Department of Pathology, University of Illinois, Urbana, Illinois 61801.

Thomas Schwarz (283) Department of Dermatology, University of Kiel, D-24105 Kiel, Germany.

M. Frances Shannon (105) Division of Molecular Bioscience, John Curtin School of Medical Research, Australian National University, Canberra, ACT, Australia.

Pankaj Sharma (165) Department of Cancer Biology, Lerner Research Institute, and Department of Pulmonary, Allergy, and Critical Care Medicine, Cleveland Clinic Foundation, Cleveland, Ohio 44195.

Fang Shen (255) Department of Oral Biology, School of Dental Medicine, University at Buffalo, SUNY, Buffalo, New York 14214.

Margaret Shumate (317) Department of Surgery, The Pennsylvania State University–College of Medicine, Hershey, Pennsylvania 17033.

Aldo Tagliabue (229) ALTA S.r.l., Siena, Italy.

Jacques Thèze (531) ImmunoGénétique Cellulaire, Institut Pasteur, Paris, France.

Jun Wang (105) Division of Molecular Bioscience, John Curtin School of Medical Research, Australian National University, Canberra, ACT, Australia.

David Weisman (505) Department of Neurosciences and the Alzheimer's Disease Research Center, University of California, San Diego, California 92093; Neurology Service, Department of Veterans Affairs Medical Center, San Diego, California 92161.

Hsin-Fang Yang-Yen (147) Institute of Molecular Biology, Academia Sinica, Taipei 11529, Taiwan.

Shen Yao (341) Department of Medicine, Division of Endocrinology, Diabetes and Bone Diseases, Mount Sinai School of Medicine, New York, New York 10029.

Ian G. Young (1) Division of Molecular Bioscience, John Curtin School of Medical Research, Australian National University, Acton, ACT, Australia 0200.

Jeffrey J. Yu (255) Department of Microbiology and Immunology, School of Medicine and Biomedical Sciences, University at Buffalo, SUNY, Buffalo, New York 14214.

Alexander Zdanov (61) Macromolecular Crystallography Laboratory, Center for Cancer Research, National Cancer Institute at Frederick, Frederick, Maryland 21702.

PREFACE

This volume is an up-to-date coverage of the important topic of the interleukins. These regulators have gained great prominence in a wide number of biochemical mechanisms. This volume is arranged so that structural information appears first, then chapters on transcriptional and signaling aspects, followed by discussions on interleukin families. Next come two chapters related to nuclear factor-κB and finally a number of contributions relating interleukins to important diseases.

The specific articles follow. J. M. Murphy and I. G. Young contribute a chapter on "IL-3, IL-5, and GM-CSF Signaling: Crystal Structure of the Human Beta-Common Receptor." A contribution on "Crystal Structures and Inhibitors of Proteins Involved in IL-2 Release and T-Cell Signaling" is the work of K. Brown and G. M. T. Cheetham. A. Zdanov reviews "Structural Studies of the Interleukin-19 Subfamily of Cytokines" and "Interleukin-22 and Its Crystal Structure" is contributed by R. A. P. Nagem, J. R. Ferreira Junior, L. Dumoutier, J.-C. Renauld, and I. Polikarpov, K. Bunting, J. Wang, and M. F. Shannon describe the "Control of Interleukin-2 Gene Transcription: A Paradigm for Inducible, Tissue-Specific Gene Expression." "Transcription Factors Mediating Interleukin-3 Survival Signals" is offered by J. J.-Y. Yen and H.-F. Yang-Yen, and S. J. Haque and P. Sharma describe "Interleukins and STAT Signaling." Updating the newest interleukins, Q. Chen, H. P. Carroll and M. Gadina review "The Newest Interleukins: Recent Additions to the Ever-Growing Cytokine Family." D. Boraschi and A. Tagliabue offer "The Interleukin-1 Receptor Family." "The IL-17 Cytokine Family" is covered by S. L. Gaffen, J. M. Kramer, J. J. Yu, and F. Shen. "NF-κB and Cytokines" is contributed by D. Kulms and T. Schwarz and T. Muta describes "IκBξ: An Inducible Regulator of Nuclear Factor-κB."

In the final section, R.N. Cooney and M. Shumate write on "The Inhibitory Effects of Interleukin-1 on Growth Hormone Action During Catabolic Illness." "The Role of the Interleukin-6/gp130 Signaling Pathway in Bone Metabolism" was prepared by X.-H. Liu, A. Kirschenbaum, S. Yao, and A. C. Levine. I. Nakamura and E. Jimi review "Regulation of Osteoclast Differentiation and Function by Interleukin-1." "The Role of IL-1 and IL-1Ra in Joint Inflammation and Cartilage Degradation" was written by C. Jacques, M. Gosset, F. Berenbaum, and C. Gabay. "Cytokines in Type 2 Diabetes" is reviewed by D. R. Johnson, J. C. O'Connor, A. Satpathy, and G. G. Freund. J. N. Fain summarizes "Release of Interleukins and Other Inflammatory Cytokines by Human Adipose Tissue Is Enhanced in Obesity and Primarily Due to the Nonfat Cells." "Role of Interleukin-13 in Cancer, Pulmonary Fibrosis, and other T_H2-Type Diseases" was prepared by B. H. Joshi, C. Hogaboom, P. Dover, S. R. Husain, and R. K. Puri. The last two chapters are "Interleukins, Inflammation, and Mechanisms of Alzheimer's Disease" by D. Weisman, E. Hakimian, and G. J. Ho, and "Interleukin-2: From T-Cell Growth and Homeostases to Immune Reconstitution of HIV Patients" by M. Kryworuchko and J. Thèze.

The cover picture is a reproduction of the structure of interleukin-5 from Fig. 3 of the first chapter by J. M. Murphy and I. G. Young.

As always, Academic Press/Elsevier Science cooperates in rapid production of the volumes in this Serial and in the costly reproduction of color figures where these are warranted.

Gerald Litwack
Toluca Lake, California
March, 2006

1

IL-3, IL-5, AND GM-CSF SIGNALING: CRYSTAL STRUCTURE OF THE HUMAN BETA-COMMON RECEPTOR

JAMES M. MURPHY AND IAN G. YOUNG

*Division of Molecular Bioscience, John Curtin School of Medical Research
Australian National University, Acton, ACT, Australia 0200*

The cytokines, interleukin-3 (IL-3), interleukin-5 (IL-5), and granulocyte-macrophage colony stimulating factor (GM-CSF), are polypeptide growth factors that exhibit overlapping activities in the regulation of hematopoietic cells. They appear to be primarily involved in inducible

0083-6729/06 $35.00
DOI: 10.1016/S0083-6729(06)74001-8

hematopoiesis in response to infections and are involved in the pathogenesis of allergic and inflammatory diseases and possibly in leukemia. The X-ray structure of the beta common (βc) receptor ectodomain has given new insights into the structural biology of signaling by IL-3, IL-5, and GM-CSF. This receptor is shared between the three ligands and functions together with three ligand-specific α-subunits. The structure shows βc is an intertwined homodimer in which each chain contains four domains with approximate fibronectin type-III topology. The two βc-subunits that compose the homodimer are interlocked by virtue of the swapping of β-strands between domain 1 of one subunit and domain 3 of the other subunit. Site-directed mutagenesis has shown that the interface between domains 1 and 4 in this unique structure forms the functional epitope. This epitope is similar to those of other members of the cytokine class I receptor family but is novel in that it is formed by two different receptor chains. The chapter also reviews knowledge on the closely related mouse β_{IL-3} receptor and on the α-subunit–ligand interactions. The knowledge on the two β receptors is placed in context with advances in understanding of the structural biology of other members of the cytokine class I receptor family. © 2006 Elsevier Inc.

I. BACKGROUND

The cytokines, interleukin-3 (IL-3), IL-5, and granulocyte-macrophage colony stimulating factor (GM-CSF), are polypeptide growth factors that exhibit overlapping activities in the regulation of hematopoietic cells (Metcalf, 1993). These cytokines are produced mainly by activated T cells during immune responses to infections and their major role appears to be in the regulation of inducible hematopoiesis rather than in steady state production of blood cells. IL-3 has a broad spectrum of activities on myeloid cells and shares activities with GM-CSF, whereas IL-5 is more specific with its major activity on the eosinophil lineage. The three cytokines are involved in the pathogenesis of allergic and inflammatory diseases, such as asthma and arthritis, and IL-3 and GM-CSF may also be involved in leukemia. In addition, recombinant human GM-CSF is used clinically to reduce the severity of chemotherapy-induced neutropenia and accelerate hematopoietic recovery after the bone marrow transplantation (Armitage, 1998; Cebon and Lieschke, 1994). Therefore, understanding the molecular mechanisms by which these cytokines bind and activate their receptors is an important goal and may lead to the development of new drugs that modulate receptor function.

II. THE RECEPTOR SYSTEM FOR IL-3, IL-5, AND GM-CSF

IL-3, IL-5, and GM-CSF exert their effects on target cells via receptor systems composed of cytokine-specific α-subunits (Gearing *et al.*, 1989; Kitamura *et al.*, 1991; Murata *et al.*, 1992; Takaki *et al.*, 1993; Tavernier *et al.*, 1991) and βc-subunit (Hayashida *et al.*, 1990). Both the α- and βc-subunits are members of the class I cytokine receptor superfamily, a family of receptors characterized by ectodomains, which contain a functional unit known as the cytokine-receptor homology module (CRM). The CRM is formed by two barrel-like domains, each composed of seven β-strands, with approximate fibronectin type-III topology. The hallmark of the class I cytokine receptors' CRM is a conserved arrangement of disulfide bonds in the N-terminal fibronectin type-III domain and the conserved WSXWS motif (where, W = tryptophan, S = serine, and X = any amino acid) in the C-terminal domain. On the basis of these conserved sequence elements in receptor ectodomains, Bazan (1990) described the superfamily of class I cytokine receptors or hematopoietin receptors (Fig. 1). Notably, the cytoplasmic domains of these receptors lack any catalytic activity (Sakamaki *et al.*, 1992), but when the cytokine ligands bind to the oligomeric receptor, the receptor subunits are orientated so that the Janus Kinases (JAKs) that are constitutively associated with the receptor cytoplasmic domains are able to transactivate one another and initiate signaling. The signaling pathways that may be initiated in this manner are extensive and include the Ras/MAPK (mitogen-activated protein kinase), PI-3K (phosphatidylinositol-3-kinase), and JAK/STAT (signal transducers and activators of transcription) pathways (De Groot *et al.*, 1998).

III. STRUCTURAL FEATURES OF CLASS I CYTOKINE RECEPTORS

One of the simplest and best-studied members of this family is the growth hormone receptor. In 1992, De Vos *et al.* reported the crystal structure of the two human growth hormone receptor ectodomain molecules in complex with growth hormone (Fig. 2A), representing the first structure of a class I cytokine receptor. This structure confirmed Bazan's prediction (1990) that the two fibronectin type-III domains in the class I cytokine receptor CRM adopt a nearly orthogonal conformation, and in this structure the "elbow" between the domains was shown to serve as an interface for ligand binding. The binding of growth hormone to the elbow region of its receptor results in the burying of a large surface area, 1230 Å^2, a binding footprint known as the "structural epitope" (De Vos *et al.*, 1992). Extensive mutagenesis of the

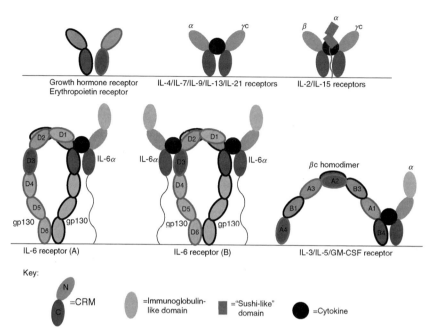

FIGURE 1. Representative members of the class I cytokine receptor superfamily. Cytokine-receptor homology *m*odules (CRMs) are composed of two fibronectin type-III domains: in this figure, the N-terminal fibronectin type-III domain is colored green and the C-terminal domain, red. This figure demonstrates the recurring role of the CRM as a cytokine-binding motif. In the depictions of the growth hormone and erythropoietin receptors, the two identical receptor subunits are distinguished by the blue and black outlines of the component domains. Likewise, the two identical gp130 and *β*c-subunits that form part of the IL-6 and IL-3/IL-5/GM-CSF receptors, respectively, are distinguished by blue and black outlines. The structure of the IL-2:IL-2α complex revealed that the IL-2α-subunit ligand-binding domain is composed of two "sushi-like" domains (Rickert *et al.*, 2005). The IL-6 receptor complex is depicted as (A) the 2 gp130:1 IL-6:1 IL-6α stoichiometry proposed by Grotzinger and colleagues (see Section XI) and (B) the 2:2:2 stoichiometry of the complex crystal structure (Boulanger *et al.*, 2003). (See Color Insert.)

growth hormone receptor has shown that only a small subset of the residues that form the structural epitope are energetically important for ligand binding (Bass *et al.*, 1991; Clackson and Wells, 1995). These residues, Trp104, Trp169, and six surrounding residues, of the growth hormone receptor were estimated to contribute ~85% of the ligand-binding energy and comprise what is referred to as the "functional epitope" (Clackson and Wells, 1995). The term "binding hot spot" was coined to describe the occurrence of ligand-binding residues in a highly localized cluster. These principles of ligand binding are preserved throughout the class I cytokine receptor superfamily. Other class I cytokine receptors, such as the erythropoietin receptor and IL-4α receptor, bind to their cytokine ligands via functional epitopes

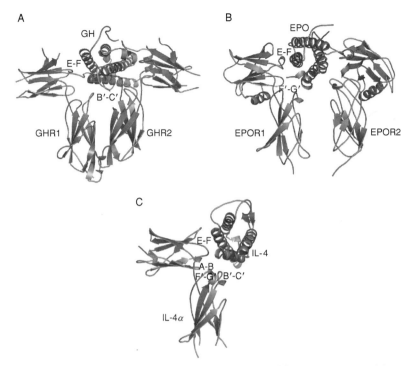

FIGURE 2. Receptor:ligand complexes for class I cytokine receptors containing two fibronectin type-III domains. Structures of the growth hormone (GH) in complex with two GH receptor (GHR) subunits (A); erythropoietin (EPO) in complex with two EPO receptor (EPOR) subunits (B); and the IL-4α receptor in complex with IL-4 (C). Receptor subunits and ligands are colored orange and blue, respectively. The receptor loops implicated in ligand binding are labeled. Coordinates for the GH, EPO, and IL-4 complex structures were taken from the Protein Data Bank files, 3HHR, 1CN4, and 1IAR, respectively. Figures were drawn using PyMOL (www.pymol.org). (See Color Insert.)

formed by residues in the loops in the elbow region between the two fibronectin type-III domains of the CRM (Fig. 2B and C). A combination of residues in the E-F and A-B loops of the membrane-distal fibronectin type-III domain and the B'-C' and F'-G' loops of the membrane-proximal fibronectin type-III domain compose the functional epitopes for all class I cytokine receptors characterized to date.[1]

---

[1]By convention, the loops are named for the β-strands that they connect (e.g., the loop between A and B strands is known as the A-B loop). A further convention in the loop nomenclature is that loops in the membrane-proximal fibronectin-III domain of a CRM are signified by an apostrophe (e.g., A'-B' loop is membrane-proximal while the A-B loop is membrane distal).

The growth hormone receptor structure has served as a paradigm for ligand binding and activation of class I cytokine receptors, despite this structure representing the simplest type of class I cytokine receptor, where receptor activation results from a one CRM receptor homodimer binding to a cytokine ligand. However, as depicted in Fig. 1, class I cytokine receptors exhibit enormous diversity in their domain compositions (such as the number of CRMs, the presence of immunoglobulin-like domains) and the mode of oligomerization required for receptor activation (such as homo- or heterodimerization or oligomerization). This chapter will detail how determination of the structure of the human βc receptor has provided insights into its activation by the three cytokines, IL-3, IL-5, and GM-CSF. Although the receptors for IL-3, IL-5, and GM-CSF are considerably more complicated than the growth hormone receptor, the principles of receptor activation established for this receptor have proved to be relevant to the IL-3/IL-5/GM-CSF system.

IV. THE LIGANDS: IL-3, IL-5, AND GM-CSF

IL-3, IL-5, and GM-CSF are members of the four-helical bundle family of cytokines which includes other cytokines, such as growth hormone, erythropoietin, and IL-4 (Mott and Campbell, 1995). The structures of IL-5 (Milburn et al., 1993) and GM-CSF (Diederichs et al., 1991) were determined by X-ray crystallography, while the structure of a functional analog of IL-3 was determined using NMR spectroscopy (Feng et al., 1996) (Fig. 3). The fold of these proteins consists of four α-helices arranged as two sets of antiparallel α-helices in an "up-up-down-down" topology (Abdel-Meguid et al., 1987). Although IL-5 shares this fold, IL-5 differs from other cytokines by virtue of the swapping of the D-helix and β-strand 2 between the two IL-5 monomers yielding an interdigitated homodimer (Milburn et al., 1993). IL-5 exists solely as a dimer due to a shortened hinge loop between helices C and D that prevents formation of a monomeric species. Extending the hinge loop of IL-5 with residues from the analogous loop in GM-CSF resulted in the generation of a monomer with biological activity (Dickason and Huston, 1996). Despite considerable differences in the primary amino acid sequences of GM-CSF, IL-3, and IL-5, their three-dimensional structures show remarkable similarity (Fig. 3). Only minor variations in topology are observed between these cytokines, as exemplified in the structure of the IL-3 analog by the helix A' rather than short sequences of β-structure found in equivalent regions of GM-CSF and IL-5 (Feng et al., 1996). The similar topologies of GM-CSF, IL-3, and IL-5 suggest the possibility of a common mechanism of activation in their receptors on target cells.

Extensive mutagenesis of IL-3, IL-5, and GM-CSF has been performed to determine the epitopes that mediate binding to (a) their respective α-subunits

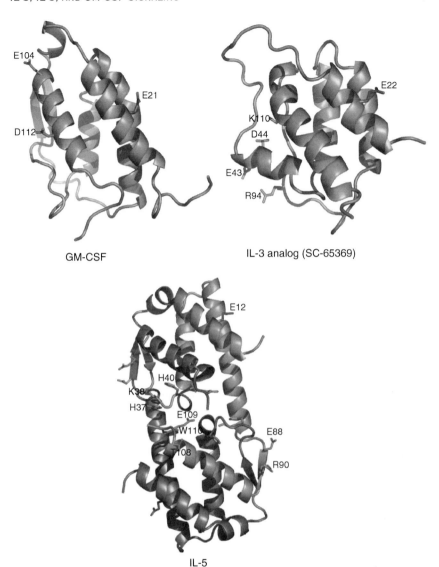

GM-CSF   IL-3 analog (SC-65369)

IL-5

FIGURE 3. Comparison of the structures and receptor-binding epitopes of human GM-CSF, IL-3, and IL-5. The side chains implicated in α-subunit binding are shown as green sticks. The conserved glutamic acid residues implicated in βc binding are shown as red sticks. Only residues in the orange chain of the IL-5 homodimer are labeled. The IL-3 analog used for structure determination contains 14 amino acid substitutions that improve solubility and do not compromise bioactivity (Feng *et al.*, 1996). The coordinates for GM-CSF, IL-3, and IL-5 were taken from the Protein Data Bank files, 2GMF, 1JLI, and 1HUL, respectively. Figures were drawn using PyMOL (www.pymol.org). (See Color Insert.)

and (b) the βc-subunit. These cytokines bind with low affinity to their respective α-subunits ($K_d < 1$ nM for IL-5; $K_d \sim$20–100 nM for IL-3; $K_d \sim$ 10 nM for GM-CSF). In the presence of both the βc- and α-subunits, high-affinity binding is observed: $K_d \sim$600 pM for IL-5; $K_d \sim$100 pM for IL-3; and $K_d \sim$60 pM for GM-CSF. Notably, these ligands do not detectably bind to the βc-subunit in the absence of their respective α-subunits. Consequently, the epitopes for βc binding must be inferred from mutations that do not disrupt α-subunit binding but prevent high-affinity binding in the presence of the βc-subunit. Using this approach, two distinct epitopes were identified on each of these cytokines (Fig. 3). Like the structural topologies of IL-3, IL-5, and GM-CSF, the epitopes for receptor binding are well conserved. A conserved glutamate residue in the A-helix of these cytokines is essential for βc-subunit interaction (Barry et al., 1994; Graber et al., 1995; Lopez et al., 1992; Olins et al., 1995; Tavernier et al., 1995). Additionally, these residues, Glu12 of human IL-5, Glu22 of human IL-3, and Glu21 of human GM-CSF, are absolutely conserved throughout species (Klein et al., 1997). Mutagenesis of these cytokines also identified a distinct epitope that is required for binding to their respective α-subunits (Fig. 3). The residues, Glu104 and Asp112, located on the D-helix of GM-CSF are necessary for binding to the cognate α-subunit (Hercus et al., 1994). IL-3 binding to its α-subunit requires Glu43 and Glu44 located in helix-A', Arg94 in the loop between the C- and D-helices, and Lys110 of the D-helix (Olins et al., 1995). The D-helix residues of IL-5, Thr108, Glu109, Trp110, and Ile112 are required for IL-5 binding to its α-subunit, as well as His37, Lys38, and His40 of the loop between β-strand 1 and helix-B, and the β-strand 2 residues Glu88 and Arg90 (Graber et al., 1995; Tavernier et al., 1995).

V. THE STRUCTURE OF THE HUMAN βc RECEPTOR

The growth hormone receptor ectodomain structure has served as a paradigm for class I cytokine receptors that contain one CRM. This paradigm has even been applicable to receptors containing complicated extracellular domains, such as the gp130 receptor (Boulanger et al., 2003), where the single CRM in the ectodomain serves as a ligand-binding interface analogous to that of the growth hormone receptor. The human βc receptor extracellular domain was predicted to be composed of two CRMs based on a number of conserved amino acid features, including the presence of conserved cysteine residues in domains 1 and 3 (Sato and Miyajima, 1994).[2] By analogy with the growth hormone receptor, the membrane-proximal

---

[2]By convention, the four fibronectin-III domains of the βc ectodomain are labeled from the membrane-distal (domain 1) to membrane-proximal domain (domain 4).

CRM (domains 3 and 4) would be expected to serve as the ligand-binding interface. Site-directed mutagenesis and ligand-binding studies successfully identified residues in domain 4 that are critical for formation of high-affinity IL-3, IL-5, and GM-CSF complexes (Lock et al., 1994; Woodcock et al., 1994, 1996) although no critical residues were identified in domain 3 (Mulhern et al., 2000). This finding was puzzling since all other class I cytokine receptors studied were found to engage their ligands via an elbow interface where ligand-binding residues are contributed by two contiguous fibronectin type-III domains. Further mutagenesis studies focused on a homologous murine receptor, β_{IL-3}, a receptor that, unlike βc, can bind murine IL-3 (mIL-3) directly with a dissociation constant of $\sim$20 nM (Wang et al., 1992). Wang et al. found that deleting either of the N- or C-terminal CRMs generated mutant β_{IL-3} receptors that were unable to bind mIL-3. Furthermore cysteine residues in domain 1 of βc have been implicated in the formation of disulfide cross-links with the respective α-subunits in the high-affinity complexes with IL-3, IL-5, and GM-CSF (Stomski et al., 1996, 1998). These findings clearly implicated the N-terminal CRM of the βc-subunit in ligand binding and receptor activation, although until the structure of the βc extracellular domain was solved, a mechanism by which the N-terminal CRM could participate in ligand binding and receptor activation could not be rationalized.

In 2001, we reported the X-ray structure of the human βc receptor ectodomain (Carr et al., 2001) (Fig. 4). βc was found to exist as an intertwined homodimer in which each chain contains four domains with approximate fibronectin type-III topology. The intertwining of the two βc-subunits results in the formation of an arch-like structure in which domain 4 of each subunit is positioned adjacent to the membrane. The two domains 4 are $\sim$100 Å apart and are positioned at an angle of $\sim$60° to the cell membrane. The two βc-subunits that compose the homodimer are interlocked by virtue of the swapping of β-strands between domain 1 of one subunit and domain 3 of the other subunit.

In agreement with the prediction that βc is composed of two CRMs, only domains 1 and 3 contained disulfide bonds: three were present in domain 1 and two in domain 3 in the crystal structure. Although domains 1 and 3 exhibit fibronectin type-III topology, the β-strand D is extended and forms part of both β-sheets as is observed in the h-type topological class of the immunoglobulin fold (Bork et al., 1994). A remarkable feature of domains 1 and 3 is that β-strand G extends away from its parent domain and forms the G-strand of a fibronectin type-III domain in the other protein chain. Therefore, the G-strand of domain 1 of one βc monomer forms the G-strand of domain 3 of the symmetry-related protein chain in the βc homodimer. As a consequence of this highly unusual fold, βc would be expected to exist as a very stable intertwined homodimer in solution and this has been confirmed by a variety of studies (see Section VI). Domains 2 and 4 of the human βc

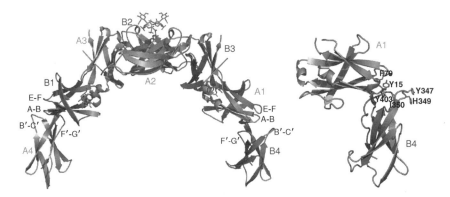

FIGURE 4. The structure of the human βc ectodomain. Left panel: the intertwined chains of the βc homodimer are colored orange ("A" chain) and blue ("B" chain) and the component domains of each chain are labeled in orange or blue text, respectively. N-linked glycosylation chains are shown as sticks at N34 and N167 (carbons are colored green; nitrogens, blue; and oxygens are colored red). The loops that contribute residues to the functional epitope for IL-3, IL-5, and GM-CSF binding are labeled in black text. Right panel: expanded view of the domain B1-A4 interface. The color scheme is as for the left panel, except the side chains of the functional epitopes residues are shown in green and are labeled with black text. The coordinates for βc are available from the Protein Data Bank (accession 1GH7). These figures were drawn using PyMOL (www.pymol.org). (See Color Insert.)

ectodomain are classical fibronectin type-III domains consisting of two anti-parallel β-sheets composed of the A, B, and E strands and the G, F, C, and D strands packed together via multiple hydrophobic interactions. As described earlier, domains 2 and 4 contain no disulfide bonds, a feature consistent with these domains each serving as the carboxy-terminal fibronectin type-III domain in a CRM.

The arrangement of β-strands in domains 1 and 3 of βc is similar to that observed in the N-terminal fibronectin type-III domain of the growth hormone receptor. Likewise, domains 2 and 4 of βc exhibit a similar topology to the growth hormone receptor C-terminal fibronectin type-III domain. In contrast to the well-conserved arrangement of β-strands between receptors of the class I cytokine superfamily, there is considerable variation in loop structure in each of the domains. Variation in loop structure is typical of class I cytokine receptors and reflects the differing contributions of residues in each loop to receptor function. For example, residues located in the E-F, A-B, B'-C', and F'-G' loops of CRMs contribute to ligand binding to different extents in each of the class I cytokine receptors characterized to date, including the growth hormone receptor (Clackson and Wells, 1995), erythropoietin receptor (Middleton *et al.*, 1996, 1999), and IL-4 α-subunit (Zhang *et al.*, 2002) (summarized in Table I). It has been postulated that these loops may exhibit some structural plasticity in order to adjust the positions of ligand-binding residues to accommodate different ligands and

TABLE I. Comparison of the Functional Epitopes of Class I Cytokine Receptors

		Growth hormone receptor[a]	Erythropoietin receptor[b]	Human IL-4α: IL-4 binding[c]	Human βc: GM-CSF binding[d]	β_{IL-3} direct mIL-3 binding[e]
Membrane-distal	E-F	Trp104	Phe93	Asp72	Phe79	Phe85
	A-B	Arg43		Tyr13	Tyr15	Tyr21
Membrane-proximal	B'-C'	Trp169		Tyr127	Tyr347, His349, Ile350	Tyr348
	F'-G'		Phe205	Tyr183	Tyr403	Tyr401

[a]Clackson and Wells, 1995.
[b]Middleton et al., 1996, 1999.
[c]Zhang et al., 2002.
[d]Lock et al., 1994; Murphy et al., 2003; Woodcock et al., 1994, 1996.
[e]Murphy et al., 2004; Wang et al., 1992.
Alanine mutants of the listed receptor residues resulted in impaired ligand binding. Phenylalanine substitution of the underlined Tyr residues yielded receptors with impaired ligand binding.

improve contacts with the ligand (Wilson and Jolliffe, 1999). However, this does not appear to be a commonly used mechanism as with the growth hormone receptor (Brown *et al.*, 2005; De Vos *et al.*, 1992) and the gp130 receptor (Boulanger *et al.*, 2003; Bravo *et al.*, 1998; Chow *et al.*, 2001) comparison of crystal structures in the presence and absence of their ligands demonstrates that only small changes occur in ligand-binding loops of the receptor upon ligand engagement.

VI. FORMATION AND BIOLOGICAL RELEVANCE OF THE βc HOMODIMER

The swapping of G-strands between domains 1 of one protein chain and domain 3 of the symmetry-related chain revealed the molecular basis for the existence of the βc receptor as a stable homodimer. This strand swapping also positions domain 1 of one protein chain adjacent to the membrane-proximal domain 4 of the symmetry-related protein chain, thereby rationalizing the importance of the N-terminal CRM for receptor function. The swapping of G-strands between domains 1 and 3 of symmetry-related βc chains resembles three-dimensional domain swapping (Schlunegger *et al.*, 1997), where an intertwined dimer is formed from the swapping of an element of secondary structure or a whole domain between identical protein chains. However, the swapping of β-strands in the βc homodimer differs from *bona fide* examples of three-dimensional domain swapping, such as the CD2 protein (Murray *et al.*, 1995), for two reasons: (1) no closed monomer form was detected when the purified βc ectodomain was subjected to chemical cross-linking (Carr *et al.*, 2001) or analyzed by analytical ultra-centrifugation (Murphy *et al.*, 2004); and (2) the G-strands of domains 1 and 3 differ in amino acid sequence and, therefore, the swapped domains do not make identical noncovalent bonds. This strand swapping closely mimics three-dimensional domain swapping as domains 1 and 3 of βc are the N-terminal fibronectin type-III domains of their respective CRMs and are highly homologous. Further examination of the G-strand residues and their neighboring atoms in βc did not reveal any interactions that would preclude the G-strands forming part of their parent domains (Carr *et al.*, 2001). However, the nature of the hinge loop, but not the swapped domain, is the critical determinant in three-dimensional domain-swapping events (Schlunegger *et al.*, 1997). We believe that the proline-containing, very short F-G loops of domains 1 and 3 predispose βc to dimer formation. These loops may be derived from evolutionary selection in a fashion analogous to IL-5, where the D-helix and strand 2 have undergone an ancestral domain-swapping event and a shortened hinge loop precludes the existence of a stable monomer (Dickason and Huston, 1996; Milburn *et al.*, 1993). The swapping of G-strands between domains 1 and 3 in the βc homodimer represents the first example of domain swapping within the class I cytokine receptor superfamily. The crystal structure of the IL-2 α-subunit was determined, revealing an example of a domain-swapping event analogous to that observed in the βc receptor (Rickert *et al.*, 2005).

Extensive evidence has accumulated that confirms that the βc receptor is homodimeric in nature. First, the crystal structure of the βc receptor ectodomain contains an elaborate intertwining where intricate noncovalent interactions generate a homodimer (described in Section V). Dimerization of the human βc ectodomain is therefore not a consequence of crystal packing where weak interactions between monomers would form during the crystallization process that are not representative of stoichiometry in solution. Furthermore, analytical ultracentrifugation and native gel electrophoresis studies using recombinant human βc ectodomain expressed and purified from insect cells demonstrated that βc was exclusively dimeric while no monomer was detected (Murphy *et al.*, 2004). These studies illustrate unambiguously that the soluble ectodomain form of βc is homodimeric. Chemical cross-linking studies demonstrated that the full-length βc receptor expressed in the cell membrane of insect cells (Carr *et al.*, 2001) and the murine lymphoid cell line, CTLL-2, (I. Walker and I. G. Young, unpublished data) exists entirely as a preformed dimer. A prior study detected a homodimeric form of the βc-subunit expressed in Ba/F3 cells (Muto *et al.*, 1996), although complete cross-linking was not achieved in this study. Muto *et al.* (1996) observed that the βc dimer was present in the cell membrane prior to the addition of GM-CSF, and upon addition of GM-CSF, the βc dimer formed a complex with the α-subunit and became phosphorylated. Taken together, these experiments confirm that the βc receptor is present on the cell membrane as a homodimer in the absence of cytokine ligand and can participate in normal receptor activation.

VII. ELUCIDATION OF THE βc FUNCTIONAL EPITOPE

As described in Section V , receptors of the class I superfamily studied to date possess a conserved cytokine binding motif, involving residues from a combination of the E-F and A-B loops of the membrane-distal fibronectin type-III domain and B'-C' and F'-G' loops of the membrane-proximal domain (summarized in Table I). Earlier studies of the βc receptor had assumed that fibronectin type-III domains 3 and 4 (the predicted C-terminal CRM) would form an elbow interface that would serve as a ligand-binding interface. While mutagenesis of the domain 4 identified residues in the B'-C' loop, Tyr347, His349, and Ile350 (Lock *et al.*, 1994; Woodcock *et al.*, 1994), and F'-G' loop, Tyr403 (Woodcock *et al.*, 1996), no residues in the predicted E-F and A-B loops of domain 3 were found to be necessary for ligand binding

(Mulhern *et al.*, 2000). The reason for this finding became apparent from the crystal structure of the βc-subunit. As can be seen in Fig. 4, fibronectin type-III domain 1 of one subunit and domain 4 of the other subunit form a membrane-proximal elbow that is analogous to that of the growth hormone receptor and other characterized class I cytokine receptors. This led us to probe the possibility that the novel, noncontiguous domain 1–domain 4 interface could serve as the ligand-binding site of βc. Residues in the domain 1 loops were mutated and the effect of these amino acid changes on the capacity of βc to bind GM-CSF or IL-3 in the presence of their cognate α-subunits was examined (Murphy *et al.*, 2003, 2004). Our binding studies did not include IL-5 since it is difficult to accurately assess the loss of IL-5 binding using these assays due to the IL-5 α-subunit K_d for IL-5 being $\sim$800 pM compared to the high-affinity binding by the βc:α-subunit complex having a K_d of $\sim$500 pM (Murphy *et al.*, 2003). In comparison, the GM-CSF and IL-3 α-subunits bind their ligands with nanomolar dissociation constants, whereas in the presence of the βc-subunit the K_d values are in the picomolar range. Phe79 in the E-F loop and Tyr15 in the A-B loop of domain 1 of βc were found to be absolutely required for high-affinity GM-CSF binding since individual mutation of these amino acids to alanine abolished detectable GM-CSF binding (Murphy *et al.*, 2003). Mutation of Tyr15 to phenylalanine resulted in wild-type binding, indicating that the hydrophobic character of Tyr15 rather than the phenyl hydroxyl moiety is critical for ligand binding. The *F79A* and *Y15A* mutant βc receptors coexpressed with the human IL-3 α-subunit were subsequently found to be unable to bind IL-3 with high affinity—demonstrating that the functional epitopes for GM-CSF and IL-3 binding overlap (Murphy *et al.*, 2004). Previous studies had demonstrated the involvement of Tyr347, His349, and Ile350 in the B′-C′ loop of domain 4 of βc (Lock *et al.*, 1994; Woodcock *et al.*, 1994). Lock *et al.* (1994) found that Tyr347 could be substituted with phenylalanine without a loss of high-affinity GM-CSF binding. The domain 4 F′-G′ loop residue, Tyr401, was also found to be a critical residue for GM-CSF, IL-3, and IL-5 binding (Woodcock *et al.*, 1996). We found that mutation of this residue to phenylalanine prevented high-affinity binding of GM-CSF, indicating that the phenolic hydroxyl moiety of this residue is the critical binding determinant (Murphy *et al.*, 2003).

The biological effects of reduced ligand binding by mutant βc-subunits were assessed using a growth response assay. Mutant βc-subunits that showed reduced GM-CSF or IL-3 binding were expressed in the growth factor–dependent CTLL-2 cell line together with either the GM-CSF, IL-3, or IL-5 α-subunits, and their growth responses to GM-CSF, IL-3, and IL-5, respectively, were determined. Cell lines coexpressing the *Y15A* and *F79A* mutant βc-subunits and either the GM-CSF, IL-3, and IL-5 α-subunits exhibited greatly reduced responsiveness to GM-CSF, IL-3, and IL-5 (Murphy *et al.*, 2003, 2004). In all cases, the *Y15A* mutant βc was found to be less responsive to cytokine than the *F79A* mutant βc.

   Collectively these studies have defined the βc functional epitope for
GM-CSF, IL-3, and IL-5 binding (depicted in Fig. 4). The position of
Tyr403 in the original structure was somewhat ambiguous with two possible
positions for this residue in the electron density. Recent data (Carr et al.,
2006) has given an unambiguous position for this residue in a more contiguous position with the other residues in the functional epitope making it more
compact. The data on the functional epitope for βc are summarized in
Table I alongside the functional epitopes that have been defined for the
growth hormone receptor, the erythropoietin receptor, and the IL-4 α-sub-
unit. One notable characteristic of these functional epitopes is the widespread involvement of aromatic residues. Such residues often contain
heteroatoms in their side chains that can form hydrogen bonds to mediate
ligand interactions. The involvement of residues located in each of the E-F
and A-B loops of the membrane-distal fibronectin type-III domain and the B'-
C' and F'-G' loops of the membrane-proximal domain of the IL-4 α-subunit
are analogous to residues in βc that are required for ligand binding. The
crystal structure of the IL-4:IL-4α receptor complex revealed that three
tyrosine residues, Tyr13 of the A-B loop, Tyr127 of the B'-C' loop, and
Tyr183 of the F'-G' loop, are involved in contacts with IL-4 (Hage et al.,
1999). Subsequent mutagenesis and binding studies revealed that Tyr13 and
Tyr183 hydroxyl moieties are required for hydrogen bonding the critical Glu9
in helix A of IL-4, while the Tyr127 hydrophobic character, and not the
phenolic hydroxyl group, is critical for IL-4 binding (Zhang et al., 2002).
However, there are obvious differences that indicate that IL-4α is not a
suitable model for the mechanism of βc ligand binding. First, the binding of
IL-4 by IL-4α is dependent on a critical charged-pair interaction between
Asp72 of the E-F loop of IL-4α and Arg88 of IL-4. Our studies have demonstrated that the analog of Asp72 in IL-4α in the human βc-subunit, Asp83, can
be replaced with alanine without perturbing high-affinity GM-CSF binding
(Murphy et al., 2003). This obvious difference may in part account for how the
IL-4α receptor can bind IL-4 directly with high affinity, whereas the βc-
subunit does not detectably bind its ligands in the absence of cytokine-specific
α-subunits; a characteristic critical to βc serving as a shared receptor. Second,
like IL-4, GM-CSF, IL-3, and IL-5 all possess a spatially conserved Glu in
helix A, but unlike the IL-4α receptor, the βc-subunit does not appear to
hydrogen bond the conserved glutamic acid residue in its ligands via its
functional epitope tyrosine hydroxyl moieties.

VIII. INTERACTION OF α-SUBUNITS WITH
GM-CSF, IL-3, AND IL-5

   To date, no structures have been reported for the GM-CSF, IL-3, or IL-5
α-subunits. Each of these α-subunits share the same predicted domain

architecture: an N-terminal immunoglobulin-like domain and a membrane-proximal, single CRM (Cosman *et al.*, 1990) (Fig. 1). The structure of the GM-CSF, IL-3, and IL-5 α-subunits is expected to be analogous to the IL-6 α-subunit (Varghese *et al.*, 2002), a receptor that facilitates IL-6 binding to the gp130 subunit to initiate gp130 dimerization and activation (Boulanger *et al.*, 2003). Several studies have demonstrated that the immunoglobulin-like domain of the IL-6 α-subunit can be deleted without compromising high-affinity IL-6 binding or gp130 signaling (Vollmer *et al.*, 1999; Yawata *et al.*, 1993). Analogous studies of the IL-3 α-subunit have shown that deletion of the N-terminal immunoglobulin domain reduces high-affinity IL-3 binding and increases the concentration of ligand required to activate the receptor (Barry *et al.*, 1997). This suggests a minor involvement of domain 1 in ligand interaction. Mutagenesis studies that have focused on the CRM of the GM-CSF, IL-3, and IL-5 α-subunits indicate that ligand binding follows the principles established by the growth hormone receptor paradigm. Arg188 in the predicted E-F loop of the IL-5 α-subunit CRM was found to be necessary for IL-5 binding (Cornelis *et al.*, 1995a). Similarly, Tyr226 in the predicted B′-C′ loop and Arg280 in the predicted F′-G′ loop of the GM-CSF α-subunit CRM were identified as GM-CSF binding residues by analogy with the growth hormone receptor paradigm (Haman *et al.*, 1999; Rajotte *et al.*, 1997). In the case of the IL-5 α-subunit, alanine sub-stitutions of Asp55, Asp56, and Tyr57 in the C-D loop of the human IL-5 α-subunit immunoglobulin-like domain ablated IL-5 binding (Cornelis *et al.*, 1995a). A role for the N-terminal immunoglobulin-like domain in IL-5 binding is supported by studies that show an IL-5-mimetic peptide competes with IL-5 for binding to the IL-5 α-subunit via an epitope that includes Asp55 and additional CRM residues (Ishino *et al.*, 2005).

IX. INTERACTION OF α-SUBUNITS WITH βc

Examination of cysteine residues located in the D-E loop of domain 1 of human βc unveiled a role for Cys62 and Cys67 in receptor activation (Stomski *et al.*, 1998). These residues form a disulfide bond in the βc structure that results in the D-E loop of domain 1 forming a "finger" pointed toward the interior of the archlike structure (Fig. 4). Stomski *et al.* (1998) found that mutation of these cysteines to alanine prevented receptor activa-tion but did not abrogate high-affinity ligand binding. The capacity of the mutant βc receptors to engage their ligand suggests that it is not a structural distortion that results in a loss of receptor activation, but instead the inability of the α-subunit to form a covalent cross-link with the βc receptor that prevents productive positioning of the two subunits for the initiation of signaling. The cysteine residues on the α-subunits involved in the cross-link with the βc receptor have not yet been identified and the mechanism of intersubunit disulfide cross-link formation is unresolved.

We have sought to better define determinants in the D-E loop of domain 1 in βc that govern disulfide cross-linking with the α-subunits. Notably, the βc D-E loop contains a sequence of positive charge (His64 and Arg66 in human βc) that is conserved throughout species and paralogous receptors. By making alanine substitutions in the human βc receptor, we were able to determine whether the D-E loop positive residues, His64 and Arg66, played a role in α-subunit recognition and receptor activation. The *H64A* and *R66A* βc-subunits were installed into the factor-dependent CTLL-2 cell line coexpressing the GM-CSF, IL-3, or IL-5 α-subunit. Each of these cell lines exhibited a wild-type growth response to GM-CSF, IL-3, or IL-5, respectively, whereas analogous cell lines expressing the *C67A* mutant βc did not detectably respond to GM-CSF, IL-3, or IL-5 (J. M. Murphy and I. G. Young, unpublished data). These findings strongly suggest that the critical role of the βc domain 1 D-E loop is in mediating the cross-linking of the βc- and α-subunits via Cys62 and Cys67, and that the positive residues of the D-E loop do not form a secondary interaction site for the α-subunits.

X. THE MURINE $\beta_{\text{IL-3}}$ RECEPTOR BINDS IL-3 VIA A FUNCTIONAL EPITOPE ANALOGOUS TO THAT OF βc

Like humans, mice possess a βc-subunit that is shared by the GM-CSF, IL-3, and IL-5 receptors which is unable to detectably bind GM-CSF, IL-3, or IL-5 in the absence of cytokine-specific α-subunits (Gorman *et al.*, 1990). Unlike humans, mice also possess a β-receptor that can specifically bind IL-3, known as $\beta_{\text{IL-3}}$ (Itoh *et al.*, 1990). $\beta_{\text{IL-3}}$ is able to bind mIL-3 directly with low affinity (Itoh *et al.*, 1990), although the presence of the IL-3 α-subunit is absolutely required for signaling to occur upon stimulation with mIL-3 (Hara and Miyajima, 1992).

The $\beta_{\text{IL-3}}$ and human βc receptors are 58% identical at the amino acid level suggesting that $\beta_{\text{IL-3}}$ is structurally homologous to βc (Murphy *et al.*, 2004). In addition, our analytical ultracentrifugation and chemical cross-linking studies have confirmed that $\beta_{\text{IL-3}}$ is a homodimer. Structural homology between βc and $\beta_{\text{IL-3}}$ implies that $\beta_{\text{IL-3}}$ will contain a membrane-proximal functional epitope composed of fibronectin type-III domains 1 and 4—contributed by symmetry-related chains in the $\beta_{\text{IL-3}}$ homodimer—as observed for βc. The mutagenesis studies performed on $\beta_{\text{IL-3}}$ to date are consistent with this hypothesis. Initial studies performed by Miyajima and colleagues sought to define the residues in $\beta_{\text{IL-3}}$ that facilitate direct binding of mIL-3 by replacing either domains or residues with their counterparts from βc, a receptor that does not bind mIL-3 directly. Wang et $al.$ (1992) individually deleted each of the two CRMs of $\beta_{IL\text{-}3}$ and found that in either case the resulting receptors were unable to detectably bind mIL-3, demonstrating an obligatory role for the N-terminal CRM in ligand binding. Replacement of the N-terminal CRM of $\beta_{IL\text{-}3}$ with its counterpart from murine βc yielded a chimera capable of wild-type direct mIL-3 binding, whereas replacement of the C-terminal CRM abolished direct mIL-3 binding (Wang et $al.$, 1992). These findings indicate that the C-terminal CRM of $\beta_{IL\text{-}3}$ makes a unique contribution to direct mIL-3 binding, whereas ligand-binding determinants in the N-terminal CRM are common to the $\beta_{IL\text{-}3}$ and βc receptors. Replacement of the $\beta_{IL\text{-}3}$ domain 4 B'-C' loop with the analogous loop of mouse βc generated a receptor that, when coexpressed with the mIL-5 α-subunit in factor-dependent cell lines, was able to respond to mIL-5 at about 20% the response of wild-type βc (Czabotar et $al.$, 1999). In comparison, cell lines coexpressing wild-type $\beta_{IL\text{-}3}$ and mIL-5 α-subunits did not measurably respond to mIL-5. This study suggests that while the domain 4 B'-C' loop of $\beta_{IL\text{-}3}$ plays a critical role in mIL-3 binding, there must be further determinants of whether a β-subunit behaves as a common or IL-3-specific subunit.

In light of the crystal structure of human βc and mutagenesis studies defining the functional epitope for GM-CSF, IL-3, and IL-5 binding, we sought to determine whether an analogous interface is utilized by $\beta_{IL\text{-}3}$. The properties of the $\beta_{IL\text{-}3}$ receptor allowed studies of both direct binding in the absence of the mIL-3 α-subunit and high-affinity mIL-3 binding in the presence of the mIL-3 α-subunit. These studies showed that Tyr21 of the A-B loop and Phe85 of the E-F loop in domain 1 of $\beta_{IL\text{-}3}$ were required for direct mIL-3 binding (Murphy et $al.$, 2004). Additionally, alanine substitution mutagenesis of B'-C' and F'-G' loop residues in domain 4 of $\beta_{IL\text{-}3}$ demonstrated an obligatory role for Tyr348 and Tyr401 in mIL-3 binding (Murphy et $al.$, 2004). The findings of these experiments are summarized in Table I. These experiments demonstrated that $\beta_{IL\text{-}3}$ directly engages mIL-3 via an interface formed between domains 1 and 4. This provides evidence that the residues in the domain 1–domain 4 interface of βc that were required for high-affinity GM-CSF, IL-3, and IL-5 binding by the βc:α complex play a role in ligand interaction in the high-affinity complex rather than α-subunit interactions.

When any of the $\beta_{IL\text{-}3}$ mutants unable to bind IL-3 directly were coexpressed with the wild-type mIL-3 α-subunit, high-affinity mIL-3 binding was still observed (Murphy et $al.$, 2004). Although completely unexpected, this indicates that the $\beta_{IL\text{-}3}$ receptor is activated by a different mechanism to that of the human βc receptor and that the residues involved in direct IL-3 binding are not required for the high-affinity complex. It leaves open the question of whether there is an alternative mechanism for the activation of this receptor which involves the IL-3 binding site.

XI. A MODEL FOR βc RECEPTOR ACTIVATION

Before discussing βc receptor activation, it is useful to briefly summarize what is known about the activation of other members of the class I receptor family. Mutagenesis studies of growth hormone established that growth hormone possesses two epitopes for receptor interaction, namely site I and site II (Cunningham and Wells, 1989). The classical view of growth hormone receptor activation follows from the biochemical and structural studies of the complex with growth hormone (Cunningham *et al.*, 1991; De Vos *et al.*, 1992). This complex was proposed to form sequentially by site I of growth hormone binding one receptor subunit, followed by the 1:1 complex recruiting a second receptor subunit via site II of growth hormone. The ligand-mediated homodimerization of the growth hormone receptor was thought to bring the growth hormone receptor subunits into proximity to enable JAKs that are constitutively associated with the intracellular portion of the receptor subunits to interact and transphosphorylate one another—leading to their activation and the initiation of downstream signaling pathways (Carter-Su and Smit, 1998). However, biochemical evidence argues that in fact the growth hormone receptor preexists as a homodimer, and growth hormone binding serves to reorientate the two receptor subunits so that the intracellular portions are positioned correctly for productive signaling (Brown *et al.*, 2005). Dimerization in the absence of growth hormone was found to be predominantly mediated by the transmembrane domain and insertion of four alanine residues into the transmembrane domain (rotation of ~400°) led to constitutive activation.

Analogous studies were performed on the erythropoietin receptor. The erythropoietin receptor has been shown to form homodimers and in fact crystallized as a homodimer in the absence of ligand (Livnah *et al.*, 1999). Other crystal structures of the erythropoietin receptor ectodomain in complex with an erythropoietin peptide mimetic that leads to receptor activation (Livnah *et al.*, 1996), an erythropoietin antagonistic peptide (Livnah *et al.*, 1998) and erythropoietin (Syed *et al.*, 1998) demonstrate that it is the orientation of the receptor subunits and not simply their dimerization that is central to activating intracellular signaling programs. These crystal structures represent a spectrum of relative receptor orientations. When viewed perpendicular to the membrane plane, the N-terminal fibronectin type-III domains of the two receptor subunits are ~180° relative to one another in the agonist peptide complex (Livnah *et al.*, 1996), whereas in the antagonist peptide complex and in the erythropoietin complex the two receptor N-terminal domains form angles of ~165° and ~120°, respectively (Livnah *et al.*, 1998; Syed *et al.*, 1998). The orientation of receptor subunits in the erythropoietin complex represents the active conformation, while the agonist peptide gives rise to only ~5% of the potency of erythropoietin (this structure therefore represents a partially active conformation of receptor subunits), and the antagonist peptide does not have any biological activity (therefore representing a biologically inactive conformation of the erythropoietin receptor). The biological relevance of the crystallized form of the unliganded erythropoietin receptor structure (Livnah *et al.*, 1999) remains unclear since the ligand-binding interface in the elbow region between the two domains is obscured by the dimer interface. Biochemical studies of the conformation change induced by erythropoietin binding to its receptor have established a model for receptor activation where erythropoietin binding results in a very precise orientation of receptor subunit ectodomains and consequently the juxtamembrane and transmembrane regions (Constantinescu *et al.*, 2001). The juxtamembrane and transmembrane segments appear to be helical (Kubatzky *et al.*, 2005). The disruption of the α-helical juxtamembrane or transmembrane domains by a single alanine insertion leads to the loss of JAK2 transactivation and subsequent downstream signaling, whereas an insertion of a further two alanines was found to restore normal transactivation and signaling—presumably by restoring the helical phase of the juxtamembrane segment to enable the productive interaction between the receptor-associated JAK2 molecules (Constantinescu *et al.*, 2001). Further work by Constantinescu's group has elaborated the role of the helical transmembrane–juxtamembrane segment in erythropoietin receptor activation. Cysteine-scanning mutagenesis of the transmembrane–juxtamembrane portion of the receptor yielded three mutants that were capable of ligand-independent activation (Kubatzky *et al.*, 2005). The introduced cysteine residues were shown to mediate covalent dimerization between two erythropoietin receptor subunits, leading to the receptors being locked into a constitutively active conformation where the JAK2 kinases associated with the intracellular portions could interact with to initiate signaling without erythropoietin stimulation. Consequently, the juxtamembrane–transmembrane segments of the two receptor monomers must be in close proximity, even in the absence of erythropoietin, for the cysteines to be near enough in space for a disulfide bond to form. These findings certainly cast a shadow of doubt over whether the crystal structure of the unliganded erythropoietin receptor dimer is representative of the physiological form of the receptor, since in this structure the juxtamembrane segments are estimated to be positioned ∼70 Å apart, and based on studies of the growth hormone receptor, it is possible that the transmembrane domain plays a key role in its homodimerization.

    Although studies have advanced our understanding of the activation of the erythropoietin and growth hormone receptors, there is on-going debate regarding the activation mechanisms of the more complicated class I cytokine receptors in which the receptor systems contain a shared receptor subunit. Examples include the gp130 subunit of the IL-6, IL-11, leukemia inhibitory factor, and oncostatin M receptors; and the βc-subunit of the IL-3, IL-5, and GM-CSF receptor. In the case of gp130, the crystal structure of the 2:2:2

hexameric complex of the gp130 N-terminal immunoglobulin-like domain and CRM, the CRM of the IL-6 α-subunit and IL-6 was solved (Boulanger *et al.*, 2003). The model of receptor activation most consistent with this structure is that a 1:1:1 gp130:IL-6 α:IL-6 complex forms in a sequential process where IL-6 is bound by the α-subunit CRM and gp130 is able to engage this complex via interaction of the CRM with IL-6. Subsequently, two 1:1:1 complexes are thought to form a hexameric complex where the N-terminal immunoglobulin-like domain of gp130 binds to a distinct epitope on IL-6 (known as "site III") within a second 1:1:1 complex. A second model is that at physiological IL-6: IL-6 α concentrations a tetrameric complex consisting of two gp130 subunits, one α-subunit, and one IL-6 molecule (Pflanz *et al.*, 2000) is more likely. Consistent with this model is the finding that coexpression of a gp130 subunit containing a mutated immunoglobulin-like domain epitope and another with a mutated CRM gave signaling for cell proliferation, whereas these mutant gp130 subunits individually were biologically inactive (Pflanz *et al.*, 2000). Grotzinger and colleagues have proposed that gp130 forms a preformed dimer and have reconstituted a soluble receptor complex between a soluble IL-6 α-subunit fused to IL-6 and a gp130 ectodomain-Fc fusion which constitutively forms a homodimer (Schroers *et al.*, 2005). The homodimeric gp130 fusion was found to bind the soluble IL-6 α:IL-6 fusion with a K_d ~60 pM, a dissociation constant that is akin to that for human cells that express the IL-6 receptor (Yamasaki *et al.*, 1988; Zohlnhöfer *et al.*, 1992). Further investigation will be required to resolve the debate over the stoichiometry of the activated gp130 complex and whether gp130:IL-6 α:IL-6 are present in a 2:1:1 tetramer or a 2:2:2 hexamer.

The structure of the human βc receptor for IL-3, IL-5, and GM-CSF (described in Section V) has provided a valuable starting point for understanding the mechanism of receptor activation. The intertwined nature of the βc homodimer was not predicted with reference to the growth hormone receptor paradigm or other structures of class I cytokine receptors. The domain swapping of the G-strands between fibronectin type-III domain 1 of one βc monomer and domain 3 of a second βc monomer within the βc homodimer facilitates the formation of a novel conformation (Carr *et al.*, 2001). Other data, which were summarized in Section VI, support the homodimer as the biologically relevant form of βc *in vivo*. Additionally, the structure of the βc homodimer revealed that the membrane-proximal CRM is actually a composite of domain 1 from one subunit and domain 4 from the other monomer in the βc dimer. Consequently, domains 1 and 4 form an approximately orthogonal elbow interface that was postulated to serve as the epitope for interaction with the ligands, IL-3, IL-5, and GM-CSF. Residues in the domain 4 B'-C' loop and F'-G' loop were previously identified as functional epitope residues in mutagenesis studies performed on the basis of the growth hormone receptor paradigm (Lock *et al.*, 1994; Woodcock *et al.*, 1994, 1996). Alanine-scanning mutagenesis was performed in light of the structure of the βc-subunit, identifying an additional two key residues in domain 1 that are critical for ligand binding and receptor activation (Murphy *et al.*, 2003). The identification of the functional epitope residues, Tyr15 of the A-B loop and Phe79 of the E-F loop, in domain 1 of βc provides further evidence for the biological relevance of the βc homodimer, since previous studies had failed to identify functional epitope residues in domain 3: the fibronectin type-III domain originally thought to form the membrane-proximal CRM with domain 4 (Mulhern *et al.*, 2000). These structure-function studies revealed the first case of a noncontiguous CRM—where a functional epitope conforming to the growth hormone receptor paradigm for ligand binding was composed of two fibronectin type-III domains that are nonsequential in their primary sequence.

Another interesting facet of the βc homodimer structure is that the two membrane-proximal fibronectin type-III domains (domains 4) in the dimer which would represent the point of insertion in the cell membrane are separated by $\sim$100 Å, a distance thought to be too great to allow the interaction of the intracellular portions of the βc receptor. This observation has important implications for the mechanism of activation of the βc receptor. There are several conceivable models for how the βc receptor may be activated upon ligand:α-subunit binding: (1) the formation of the activation complex may result in a total reorganization of the receptor to bring βc transmembrane domains and the intracellular portions into proximity for signaling; (2) the α-subunits may enable βc oligomers to form, where one "arm" of a βc homodimer is brought into proximity with that of another βc homodimer to enable intracellular signaling; or (3) the ligand is bound at the elbow interface between domains 1 and 4 of βc, and in the presence of the α-subunit, the βc- and α-subunit cytoplasmic portions are correctly positioned to enable the JAK2 kinases associated with each the βc- and α-subunit intracellular juxtamembrane regions to transactivate and commence signaling. Of these models, model (3) is certainly the most likely. From the structure of the βc homodimer, it is apparent that model (1) is unlikely due to the rigidity of the homodimeric structure imparted by the interlocking of the two subunits and a major reorganization is unlikely since no monomer form of the βc-subunit was detected (Carr *et al.*, 2001; Murphy *et al.*, 2004). Model (2) is similarly unlikely since no compelling biochemical evidence has been reported to favor higher oligomers of βc. In fact, work in our lab has demonstrated a 2:2:2 stoichiometry of β_{IL-3} ectodomain:mIL-3 α ectodomain:mIL-3 for the complex of the related β_{IL-3} receptor reconstituted *in vitro* using purified recombinant proteins (P. Fineran and I. G. Young, unpublished data).

By drawing upon the lessons learned for the activation of the growth hormone receptor, erythropoietin receptor and gp130 (described earlier), it is possible to infer a model for βc activation. First, it is important to appreciate the essential nature of the α-subunits for the activation of βc. The α-subunits are critical for enabling the βc-subunit to engage its cytokine ligands and their cytoplasmic domains are central to receptor activation. Unlike gp130 activation, where a soluble IL-6 α:IL-6 complex can activate the receptor, a naturally occurring splice variant of the GM-CSF α-subunit, that lacks the transmembrane and intracellular segments, is unable to bind to and activate βc-subunits on the surface of baby hamster kidney (BHK) cells when added exogeneously in the presence of GM-CSF (Murray *et al.*, 1996). Further studies have demonstrated roles for the cytoplasmic portions of the IL-5 and GM-CSF α-subunits. Coexpression of a deletion mutant of the human IL-5 α cytoplasmic portion with the wild-type human βc-subunit in the factor-dependent mouse cell line FDC-P1 resulted in receptors able to bind IL-5 with high affinity but unable to generate a biological signal (Cornelis *et al.*, 1995b; Takaki *et al.*, 1994). Similar studies using deletion mutants of the human GM-CSF α-subunit illustrated that the cytoplasmic domain of the GM-CSF α-subunit is essential for GM-CSF stimulation of cell proliferation and differentiation (Matsuguchi *et al.*, 1997). So what is the likely role of the α-subunits' cytoplasmic domains? Studies by Ogata *et al.* (1998) and Stafford *et al.* (2002) have demonstrated that the kinase, JAK2, is constitutively associated with the cytoplasmic domain of the IL-5 α-subunit, although JAK2 has not been shown to be constitutively associated with the IL-3 or GM-CSF α-subunits. Several studies have found that the βc receptor is also constitutively associated with JAK2 via a conserved motif in the membrane-proximal region of the cytoplasmic domain known as Box 1 (Muto *et al.*, 1995; Quelle *et al.*, 1994; Watanabe *et al.*, 1996). One study, however, found that JAK1, rather than JAK2, was constitutively associated with the βc receptor (Ogata *et al.*, 1998). High-affinity ligand binding by the GM-CSF, IL-3, or IL-5 receptors is believed to result in the cytoplasmic domains of the α- and βc-subunits being brought into close proximity, and in an appropriate orientation for the activation of the associated JAK2 molecules to occur (Kouro *et al.*, 1996). By replacing the ectodomains of the GM-CSF α- and the βc-subunits with the leucine zipper domain of Fos or Jun and installing these chimeras in the factor-dependent Ba/F3 cell line, Patel *et al.* (1996) demonstrated that the forced heterodimerization of the GM-CSFα and βc gave rise to constitutive signaling and cell proliferation in the absence of factor. Additional evidence for the importance of the α:βc interaction for receptor activation comes from the *C62A* and *C67A* βc mutants (described in Section IX). Mutation of either cysteine in the βc domain 1 D-E loop renders the βc receptor unable to form a disulfide cross-link with the α-subunit and as a result cannot be activated by IL-3, IL-5, or GM-CSF, even though the receptor is able to bind its ligands with wild-type affinity (Stomski *et al.*, 1998).

The aforementioned studies provide evidence that an α:βc complex is required for receptor activation in the presence of IL-3, IL-5, or GM-CSF. Additional reports indicate that when the α- and βc-subunits are coexpressed in cells, a complex is formed even in the absence of ligand. This has been clearly shown for the human βc and GM-CSFα complex. Murray *et al.* (1996) found that a splice variant of human GM-CSFα, known as soluble GM-CSFα (described earlier), was expressed as a preformed complex with the full-length βc receptor in BHK cells that was capable of binding GM-CSF with high affinity, while exogenously added soluble GM-CSF α-subunit:GM-CSF complex was unable to bind BHK cells expressing the βc-subunit. Woodcock *et al.* (1997) showed that the GM-CSF α-subunit and βc-subunit could be coimmunoprecipitated from primary myeloid cells and transfected cells using antibodies specific for either the GM-CSF α- or βc-subunits in the absence of GM-CSF. Additionally, work in our lab has shown that the IL-3 α-subunit and βc exist in a preformed complex in the absence of ligand (T. Soboleva and I. G. Young, unpublished data). The preformed GM-CSFα:βc complex parallels the preformed dimers of the growth hormone receptor, erythropoietin receptor, and gp130 (described earlier) and allows an analogous model for receptor activation to be inferred. It appears that the βc- and α-subunits need to be coexpressed in cells for preformed heterodimers to be observed, as studies of the purified βc and GM-CSFα ectodomains provide no evidence for a direct interaction in solution in the absence of GM-CSF (McClure *et al.*, 2003). Overall, this suggests that the transmembrane domains are likely to be central to the α:βc interaction as required for the growth hormone receptor to adopt a preformed homodimer (Brown *et al.*, 2005). Although there is some evidence for preformed α:βc complexes, a sequential model for receptor activation is also possible. This model would entail ligand being bound by the cognate α-subunit which in turn would engage the βc homodimer to form an activation complex.

Further progress in understanding the activation of the human βc receptor is dependent on elucidation of the crystal structures of the α receptors and the ligand receptor complexes. Judging from the unusual structure of the βc receptor, major surprises may be in store with the activation of this receptor system.

ACKNOWLEDGMENTS

J. M. M. is a C. J. Martin (Biomedical) fellow of the National Health and Medical Research Council of Australia (NH&MRC). I. G. Y. is the recipient of a NH&MRC program grant.

REFERENCES

Abdel-Meguid, S. S., Shieh, H. S., Smith, W. W., Dayringer, H. E., Violand, B. N., and Bentle, L. A. (1987). Three-dimensional structure of a genetically engineered variant of porcine growth hormone. *Proc. Natl. Acad. Sci. USA* **84,** 6434–6437.

Armitage, J. O. (1998). Emerging applications of recombinant human granulocyte-macrophage colony-stimulating factor. *Blood* **92,** 4491–4508.

Barry, S. C., Bagley, C. J., Phillips, J., Dottore, M., Cambareri, B., Moretti, P., D'Andrea, R., Goodall, G. J., Shannon, M. F., Vada, M. A., and Lopez, A. F. (1994). Two contiguous residues in human interleukin-3, Asp21 and Glu22, selectively interact with the α and β chains of its receptor and participate in function. *J. Biol. Chem.* **269,** 8488–8492.

Barry, S. C., Korpelainen, E., Sun, Q., Stomski, F. C., Moretti, P. A. B., Wakao, H., D'Andrea, R. J., Vadas, M. J., Lopez, A. F., and Goodall, G. J. (1997). Roles of the N and C terminal domains of the interleukin-3 α chain in receptor function. *Blood* **89,** 842–852.

Bass, S. H., Mulkerrin, M. G., and Wells, J. A. (1991). A systematic mutational analysis of hormone-binding determinants in the human growth hormone receptor. *Proc. Natl. Acad. Sci. USA* **88,** 4498–4502.

Bazan, J. F. (1990). Structural design and molecular evolution of a cytokine receptor superfamily. *Proc. Natl. Acad. Sci. USA* **87,** 6934–6938.

Bork, P., Holm, L., and Sander, C. (1994). The immunoglobulin fold. Structural classification, sequence patterns and common core. *J. Mol. Biol.* **242,** 309–320.

Boulanger, M. J., Chow, D.-C., Brevnova, E. E., and Garcia, K. C. (2003). Hexameric structure and assembly of the interleukin-6/IL-6 α-receptor/gp130 complex. *Science* **300,** 2101–2104.

Bravo, J., Staunton, D., Heath, J. K., and Jones, E. Y. (1998). Crystal structure of a cytokine-binding region of gp130. *EMBO J.* **17,** 1665–1674.

Brown, R. J., Adams, J. J., Pelekanos, R. A., Wan, Y., McKinstry, W. J., Palethorpe, K., Seeber, R. M., Monks, T. A., Eidne, K. A., Parker, M. W., and Waters, M. J. (2005). Model for growth hormone receptor activation based on subunit rotation within a receptor dimer. *Nat. Struct. Mol. Biol.* **12,** 814–821.

Carr, P. D., Gustin, S. E., Church, A. P., Murphy, J. M., Ford, S. C., Mann, D. A., Woltring, D. M., Walker, I., Ollis, D. L., and Young, I. G. (2001). Structure of the complete extracellular domain of the common β-subunit of the human GM-CSF, IL-3 and IL-5 receptors reveals a novel dimer configuration. *Cell* **104,** 291–300.

Carr, P. D., Conlan, F., Ford, S., Ollis, D. L., and Young, I. G. (2006). An improved resolution structure of the human beta common receptor involved in IL-3, IL-5 and GM-CSF signalling which gives better definition of the high-affinity binding epitope. *Acta Cryst. Sect. F-Struct. Biol. Cryst. Commun.* **62,** 509–513.

Carter-Su, C., and Smit, L. S. (1998). Signaling via JAK tyrosine kinases: Growth hormone receptor as a model system. *Recent Prog. Horm. Res.* **53,** 61–83.

Cebon, J. S., and Lieschke, G. J. (1994). Granulocyte-macrophage colony-stimulating factor for cancer treatment. *Oncology* **51,** 177–188.

Chow, D., He, X., Snow, A. L., Rose-John, S., and Garcia, K. L. (2001). Structure of an extracellular gp130 cytokine receptor signalling complex. *Science* **291,** 2150–2155.

Clackson, T., and Wells, J. A. (1995). A hot spot of binding energy in a hormone-receptor interface. *Science* **267,** 383–386.

Constantinescu, S. N., Huang, L. J., Nam, H., and Lodish, H. F. (2001). The erythropoietin receptor cytosolic juxtamembrane domain contains an essential, precisely oriented, hydrophobic motif. *Mol. Cell.* **7,** 377–385.

Cornelis, S., Plaetinck, G., Devos, R., Van der Heyden, J., Tavernier, J., Sanderson, C. J., Guisez, Y., and Fiers, W. (1995a). Detailed analysis of the IL-5-IL-5Rα interaction: Characterization of crucial residues on the ligand and the receptor. *EMBO J.* **14,** 3395–3402.

Cornelis, S., Fache, I., Van der Heyden, J., Guisez, Y., Tavernier, J., Devos, R., Fiers, W., and Plaetinck, G. (1995b). Characterization of critical residues in the cytoplasmic domain of the human interleukin-5 receptor α chain required for growth signal transduction. *Eur. J. Immunol.* **25,** 1857–1864.

Cosman, D., Lyman, S. D., Idzerda, R. L., Beckmann, M. P., Park, L. S., Goodwin, R. G., and March, C. J. (1990). A new cytokine receptor superfamily. *Trends Biochem. Sci.* **15**, 265–270.

Cunningham, B. C., and Wells, J. A. (1989). High-resolution epitope mapping of hGH-receptor interactions by alanine-scanning mutagenesis. *Science* **244**, 1081–1085.

Cunningham, B. C., Ultsch, M., De Vos, A. M., Mulkerrin, M. G., Clauser, K. R., and Wells, J. A. (1991). Dimerization of the extracellular domain of the human growth hormone receptor by a single hormone molecule. *Science* **254**, 821–825.

Czabotar, P. E., Holland, J., and Sanderson, C. J. (1999). Identification of residues involved in binding of IL-5 to βcom using β_{IL-3} and βcom chimeras. *FEBS Lett.* **460**, 99–102.

De Groot, R. P., Koffer, P. J., and Koenderman, L. (1998). Regulation of proliferation, differentiation and survival by the IL-3/IL-5/GM-CSF receptor family. *Cell Signal* **10**, 619–628.

De Vos, A. M., Ultsch, M., and Kossiakoff, A. A. (1992). Human growth hormone and extracellular domain of its receptor: Crystal structure of the complex. *Science* **255**, 306–312.

Dickason, R. R., and Huston, D. P. (1996). Creation of biologically active interleukin-5 monomer. *Nature* **379**, 652–655.

Diederichs, K., Boone, T., and Karplus, P. A. (1991). Novel fold and putative receptor binding sites of granulocyte-macrophage colony-stimulating factor. *Science* **254**, 1779–1782.

Feng, Y., Klein, B. K., and McWherter, C. A. (1996). Three-dimensional solution structure and backbone dynamics of a variant of human interleukin-3. *J. Mol. Biol.* **259**, 524–541.

Gearing, D. P., King, J. A., Gough, N. M., and Nicola, N. A. (1989). Expression cloning of a receptor for human granulocyte-macrophage colony-stimulating factor. *EMBO J.* **8**, 3667–3676.

Gorman, D. M., Itoh, N., Kitamura, T., Schreurs, J., Yonehara, S., Yahara, I., Arai, K., and Miyajima, A. (1990). Cloning and expression of a gene encoding and interleukin-3 receptor-like protein: Identification of another member of the cytokine receptor gene family. *Proc. Natl. Acad. Sci. USA* **87**, 5459–5463.

Graber, P., Proudfoot, A. E. I., Talabot, F., Bernard, A., McKinnon, M., Banks, M., Fattah, D., Solari, R., Peitsch, M. C., and Wells, T. N. C. (1995). Identification of key charged residues of human interleukin-5 in receptor binding and cellular activation. *J. Biol. Chem.* **270**, 15762–15769.

Hage, T., Sebald, W., and Reinemer, P. (1999). Crystal structure of the interleukin-4/receptor α chain complex reveals a mosaic binding interface. *Cell* **97**, 271–281.

Haman, A., Cadieux, C., Wilkes, B., Hercus, T., Lopez, A., Clark, S., and Hoang, T. (1999). Molecular determinants of the granulocyte-macrophage colony-stimulating factor receptor complex assembly. *J. Biol. Chem.* **274**, 34155–34163.

Hara, T., and Miyajima, A. (1992). Two distinct functional high-affinity receptors for mouse interleukin-3 (IL-3). *EMBO J.* **11**, 1875–1884.

Hayashida, K., Kitamura, T., Gorman, D. M., Arai, K., Yokota, T., and Miyajima, A. (1990). Molecular cloning of a second subunit of the receptor for human granulocyte-macrophage colony-stimulating factor (GM-CSF): Reconstitution of a high-affinity GM-CSF receptor. *Proc. Natl. Acad. Sci. USA* **87**, 9655–9659.

Hercus, T. R., Cambareri, B., Dottore, M., Woodcock, J., Bagley, C. J., Vadas, M. A., Shannon, M. F., and Lopez, A. F. (1994). Identification of residues in the first and fourth helices of human granulocyte-macrophage colony-stimulating factor involved in biologic activity and in binding to the α- and β-chains of its receptor. *Blood* **83**, 3500–3508.

Ishino, T., Urbina, C., Bhattacharya, M., Panarello, D., and Chaiken, I. (2005). Receptor epitope usage by an interleukin-5 mimetic peptide. *J. Biol. Chem.* **280**, 22951–22961.

Itoh, N., Yonehara, S., Schreurs, J., Gorman, D. M., Maruyama, K., Ishii, A., Yahara, I., Arai, K., and Miyajima, A. (1990). Cloning of an interleukin-3 receptor gene: A member of a distinct receptor gene family. *Science* **247**, 324–327.

Kitamura, T., Sato, N., Arai, K., and Miyajima, A. (1991). Expression cloning of the human IL-3 receptor cDNA reveals a shared β subunit for the human IL-3 and GM-CSF receptors. *Cell* **66**, 1165–1174.

Klein, B. K., Feng, Y. Q., McWherter, C. A., Hood, W. F., Paik, K., and McKearn, J. P. (1997). The receptor binding site of human interleukin-3 defined by mutagenesis and molecular modeling. *J. Biol. Chem.* **272**, 22630–22641.

Kouro, T., Kikuchi, Y., Kanazawa, H., Hirokawa, K., Harada, N., Shiiba, M., Wakao, H., Takaki, S., and Takatsu, K. (1996). Critical proline residues of the cytoplasmic domain of the IL-5 receptor α chain and its function in IL-5-mediated activation of JAK kinase and STAT5. *Int. Immunol.* **8**, 237–245.

Kubatzky, K. F., Liu, W., Goldgraben, K., Simmerling, C., Smith, S. O., and Constantinescu, S. N. (2005). Structural requirements of the extracellular to transmembrane domain junction for erythropoietin receptor function. *J. Biol. Chem.* **280**, 14844–14854.

Livnah, O., Stura, E. A., Johnson, D. L., Middleton, S. A., Mulcahy, L. S., Wrighton, N. C., Dower, W. J., Jolliffe, L. K., and Wilson, I. A. (1996). Functional mimicry of a protein hormone by a peptide agonist: The EPO receptor complex at 2.8Å. *Science* **273**, 464–471.

Livnah, O., Johnson, D. L., Stura, E. A., Farrell, F. X., Barbone, F. P., You, Y., Liu, K. D., Goldsmith, M. A., He, W., Krause, C. D., Pestka, S., Jolliffe, L. K., *et al.* (1998). An antagonist peptide-EPO receptor complex suggests that receptor dimerization is not sufficient for activation. *Nat. Struct. Biol.* **5**, 993–1004.

Livnah, O., Stura, E. A., Middleton, S. A., Johnson, D. L., Jolliffe, L. K., and Wilson, I. A. (1999). Crystallographic evidence for preformed dimers of erythropoietin receptor before ligand activation. *Science* **283**, 987–990.

Lock, P., Metcalf, D., and Nicola, N. A. (1994). Histidine-367 of the human common β-chain of the receptor is critical for high-affinity binding of human granulocyte-macrophage colony-stimulating factor. *Proc. Natl. Acad. Sci. USA* **91**, 252–256.

Lopez, A. F., Shannon, M. F., Hercus, T., Nicola, N. A., Cambareri, B., Dottore, M., Layton, M. J., Eglinton, L., and Vadas, M. A. (1992). Residue-21 of human granulocyte-macrophage colony-stimulating factor is critical for biological-activity and for high but not low affinity binding. *EMBO J.* **11**, 909–916.

Matsuguchi, T., Zhao, Y., Lilly, M. B., and Kraft, A. S. (1997). The cytoplasmic domain of granulocyte-macrophage colony-stimulating factor (GM-CSF) receptor α subunit is essential for both GM-CSF-mediated growth and differentiation. *J. Biol. Chem.* **272**, 17450–17459.

McClure, B. J., Hercus, T. R., Cambareri, B. A., Woodcock, J. M., Bagley, C. J., Howlett, G. J., and Lopez, A. F. (2003). Molecular assembly of the ternary granulocyte-macrophage colony-stimulating factor receptor complex. *Blood* **101**, 1308–1315.

Metcalf, D. (1993). Hematopoietic regulators: Redundancy or subtlety? *Blood* **82**, 3515–3523.

Middleton, S. A., Johnson, D. L., Jin, R., McMahon, F. J., Collins, A., Tullai, J., Gruninger, R. H., Jolliffe, L. K., and Mulcahy, L. S. (1996). Identification of a critical ligand binding determinant of the human erythropoietin receptor. Evidence for common ligand binding motifs in the cytokine receptor family. *J. Biol. Chem.* **271**, 14045–14054.

Middleton, S. A., Barbone, F. P., Johnson, D. L., Thurmond, R. L., You, Y., McMahon, F. J., Jin, R., Livnah, O., Tullai, J., Farrell, F. X., Goldsmith, M. A., Wilson, I. A., *et al.* (1999). Shared and unique determinants of the erythropoietin (EPO) receptor are important for binding EPO and EPO mimetic peptide. *J. Biol. Chem.* **274**, 14163–14169.

Milburn, M. V., Hassell, A. M., Lambert, M. H., Jordan, S. R., Proudfoot, A. E., Graber, P., and Wells, T. N. (1993). A novel dimer configuration revealed by the crystal structure at 2.4Å resolution of human interleukin-5. *Nature* **363**, 172–176.

Mott, H. R., and Campbell, I. D. (1995). Four-helix bundle growth factors and their receptors: Protein-protein interactions. *Curr. Opin. Struct. Biol.* **5**, 114–121.

Mulhern, T. D., Lopez, A. F., D'Andrea, R. J., Gaunt, C., Vandeleur, L., Vadas, M. A., Booker, G. J., and Bagley, C. J. (2000). The solution structure of the cytokine-binding domain of the common β-chain of the receptors for granulocyte-macrophage colony-stimulating factor, interleukin-3 and interleukin-5. *J. Mol. Biol.* **297**, 989–1001.

Murata, Y., Takaki, S., Migita, M., Kikuchi, Y., Tominaga, A., and Takatsu, K. (1992). Molecular cloning and expression of the human interleukin-5 receptor. *J. Exp. Med.* **175**, 341–351.

Murphy, J. M., Ford, S. C., Wiedemann, U. M., Carr, P. D., Ollis, D. L., and Young, I. G. (2003). A novel functional epitope formed by domains 1 and 4 of the human common β-subunit is involved in receptor activation by granulocyte-macrophage colony-stimulating factor and interleukin-5. *J. Biol. Chem.* **278**, 10572–10577.

Murphy, J. M., Ford, S. C., Olsen, J. E., Gustin, S. E., Jeffrey, P. D., Ollis, D. L., and Young, I. G. (2004). Interleukin-3 binding to the murine $β_{IL-3}$ and human βc receptors involves functional epitopes formed by domains 1 and 4 of different protein chains. *J. Biol. Chem.* **279**, 26500–26508.

Murray, A. J., Lewis, S. J., Barclay, A. N., and Brady, R. L. (1995). One sequence, two folds: A metastable structure of CD2. *Proc. Natl. Acad. Sci. USA* **92**, 7337–7341.

Murray, E. W., Pihl, C., Morcos, A., and Brown, C. B. (1996). Ligand-independent cell surface expression of the human soluble granulocyte-macrophage colony-stimulating factor receptor α-subunit depends on co-expression of the membrane-associated receptor β subunit. *J. Biol. Chem.* **271**, 15330–15335.

Muto, A., Watanabe, S., Itoh, T., Miyajima, A., Yokota, T., and Arai, K. (1995). Roles of the cytoplasmic domains of the α and β subunits of the human granulocyte-macrophage colony-stimulating factor receptor. *J. Allergy Clin. Immunol.* **96**, 1100–1114.

Muto, A., Watanabe, S., Miyajima, A., Yokota, T., and Arai, K. (1996). The β subunit of human granulocyte-macrophage colony-stimulating factor receptor forms a homodimer and is activated via association with the α receptor. *J. Exp. Med.* **183**, 1911–1916.

Ogata, N., Kouro, T., Yamada, A., Koike, M., Hanai, N., Ishikawa, T., and Takatsu, K. (1998). JAK2 and JAK1 Constitutively associate with an interleukin-5 (IL-5) receptor α and βc subunit, respectively, and are activated upon IL-5 stimulation. *Blood* **91**, 2264–2271.

Olins, P. O., Bauer, S. C., Braford-Goldberg, S., Sterbenz, K., Polazzi, J. O., Caparon, M. H., Klein, B. K., Easton, A. M., Paik, K., Klover, J. A., Thiele, B. R., and McKearn, J. P. (1995). Saturation mutagenesis of human interleukin-3. *J. Biol. Chem.* **270**, 23754–23760.

Patel, N., Herrman, J. M., Timans, J. C., and Kastelein, R. A. (1996). Functional replacement of cytokine receptor extracellular domains by leucine zippers. *J. Biol. Chem.* **271**, 30386–30391.

Pflanz, S., Kurth, I., Grotzinger, J., Heinrich, P. C., and Muller-Newen, G. (2000). Two different epitopes of the signal transducer gp130 sequentially cooperate on IL-6-induced receptor activation. *J. Immunol.* **165**, 7042–7049.

Quelle, F. W., Sato, N., Witthuhn, B. A., Inhorn, R. C., Eder, M., Miyajima, A., Griffin, J. D., and Ihle, J. N. (1994). JAK2 associates with the βc chain of the receptor for granulocyte-macrophage colony-stimulating factor, and its activation requires the membrane-proximal region. *Mol. Cell. Biol.* **14**, 4335–4341.

Rajotte, D., Cadieux, C., Haman, A., Wilkes, B. C., Clark, S. C., Hercus, T., Woodcock, J. A., Lopez, A., and Hoang, T. (1997). Crucial role of the residue R280 at the F′-G′ loop of the human granulocyte/macrophage colony-stimulating factor receptor α chain for ligand recognition. *J. Exp. Med.* **185**, 1939–1950.

Rickert, M., Wang, X., Boulanger, M., Goriatcheva, N., and Garcia, K. C. (2005). The structure of interleukin-2 complexed with its α receptor. *Science* **308**, 1477–1480.

Sakamaki, K., Miyajima, I., Kitamura, T., and Miyajima, A. (1992). Critical cytoplasmic domains of the common β subunit of the human GM-CSF, IL-3 and IL-5 receptors for growth signal transduction and tyrosine phosphorylation. *EMBO J.* **11**, 3541–3549.

Sato, N., and Miyajima, A. (1994). Multimeric cytokine receptors: Common versus specific functions. *Curr. Opin. Cell. Biol.* **6**, 174–179.

Schlunegger, M. P., Bennett, M. J., and Eisenberg, D. (1997). Oligomer formation by 3D domain swapping: A model for protein assembly and misassembly. *Adv. Prot. Chem.* **50**, 61–122.

Schroers, A., Hecht, O., Kallen, K. J., Pachta, M., Rose-John, S., and Grotzinger, J. (2005). Dynamics of the gp130 cytokine complex: A model for assembly on the cellular membrane. *Protein Sci.* **14**, 783–790.

Stafford, S., Lowell, C., Sur, S., and Alam, R. (2002). Lyn tyrosine kinase is important for IL-5-stimulated eosinophil differentiation. *J. Immunol.* **168**, 1978–1983.

Stomski, F., Sun, Q., Bagley, C., Woodcock, J., Goodall, G., Andrews, R., Berndt, M., and Lopez, A. (1996). Human interleukin-3 (IL-3) induces disulfide-linked IL-3 receptor α- and β-chain heterodimerization, which is required for receptor activation but not high-affinity binding. *Mol. Cell. Biol.* **16**, 3035–3046.

Stomski, F. C., Woodcock, J. M., Zacharakis, B., Bagley, C. J., Sun, Q., and Lopez, A. F. (1998). Identification of a Cys motif in the common β-chain of the interleukin-3, granulocyte-macrophage colony-stimulating factor, and interleukin-5 receptors essential for disulfide-linked receptor heterodimerization and activation of all three receptors. *J. Biol. Chem.* **273**, 1192–1199.

Syed, R. S., Reid, S. W., Li, C., Cheetham, J. C., Aoki, K. H., Liu, B., Zhan, H., Ossland, T. D., Chirino, A. J., Zhang, J., Finer-Moore, J., Elliot, S., *et al.* (1998). Efficiency of signalling through cytokine receptors depends critically on receptor orientation. *Nature* **395**, 511–516.

Takaki, S., Murata, Y., Kitamura, T., Miyajima, A., Tominaga, A., and Takatsu, K. (1993). Reconstitution of the functional receptors for murine and human interleukin-5. *J. Exp. Med.* **177**, 1523–1529.

Takaki, S., Kanazawa, H., Shiiba, M., and Takatsu, K. (1994). A critical cytoplasmic domain of the interleukin-5 (IL-5) receptor α chain and its function in IL-5-mediated growth signal transduction. *Mol. Cell. Biol.* **14**, 7404–7413.

Tavernier, J., Devos, R., Cornelis, S., Tuypens, T., Van der Heyden, J., Fiers, W., and Plaetinck, G. (1991). A human high affinity interleukin-5 receptor (IL-5R) is composed of an IL-5-specific α chain and a β chain shared with the receptor for GM-CSF. *Cell.* **66**, 1175–1184.

Tavernier, J., Tuypens, T., Verhee, A., Plaetinck, G., Devos, R., Van der Heyden, J., Guisez, Y., and Oefner, C. (1995). Identification of receptor-binding domains on human interleukin-5 and design of an interleukin 5-derived receptor antagonist. *Proc. Natl. Acad. Sci. USA* **92**, 5194–5198.

Varghese, J. N., Moritz, R. L., Lou, M. Z., van Donkelaar, A., Ji, H., Ivancic, N., Branson, K. M., Hall, N. E., and Simpson, R. J. (2002). Structure of the extracellular domain of the human interleukin-6 receptor α-chain. *Proc. Natl. Acad. Sci. USA* **99**, 15959–15964.

Vollmer, P., Oppmann, B., Voltz, N., Fischer, M., and Rose-John, S. (1999). A role for the immunoglobulin-like domain of the human IL-6 receptor. Intracellular protein transport and shedding. *Eur. J. Biochem.* **263**, 438–446.

Wang, H., Ogorochi, T., Arai, K., and Miyajima, A. (1992). Structure of mouse interleukin-3 (IL-3) binding protein (AIC2A). Amino acid residues critical for IL-3 binding. *J. Biol. Chem.* **267**, 979–983.

Watanabe, S., Itoh, T., and Arai, K. (1996). JAK2 is essential for activation of c-fos and c-myc promoters and cell proliferation through the human granulocyte-macrophage colony-stimulating factor receptor in BA/F3 cells. *J. Biol. Chem.* **271**, 12681–12686.

Wilson, I. A., and Jolliffe, L. K. (1999). The structure, organization, activation and plasticity of the erythropoietin receptor. *Curr. Opin. Struct. Biol.* **9**, 696–704.

Woodcock, J. M., Zacharakis, B., Plaetinck, G., Bagley, C. J., Qiyu, S., Hercus, T. R., and Lopez, A. F. (1994). Three residues in the common β chain of the human GM-CSF, IL-3 and IL-5 receptors are essential for GM-CSF and IL-5 but not IL-3 high-affinity binding and interact with Glu21 of GM-CSF. *EMBO J.* **13**, 5176–5185.

Woodcock, J. M., Bagley, C. J., Zacharakis, B., and Lopez, A. F. (1996). A single tyrosine residue in the membrane-proximal domain of the granulocyte-macrophage colony-stimulating factor, interleukin (IL)-3, and IL-5 receptor common β-chain is necessary and sufficient for high affinity binding and signaling by all three ligands. *J. Biol. Chem.* **271**, 25999–26006.

Woodcock, J. M., McClure, B. J., Stomski, F. C., Elliott, M. J., Bagley, C. J., and Lopez, A. F. (1997). The human granulocyte-macrophage colony-stimulating factor (GM-CSF) receptor exists as a preformed receptor complex that can be activated by GM-CSF, interleukin-3, or interleukin-5. *Blood* **90**, 3005–3017.

Yamasaki, K., Taga, T., Hirata, Y., Yawata, H., Kawanishi, Y., Seed, B., Taniguchi, T., Hirano, T., and Kishimoto, T. (1988). Cloning and expression of the human interleukin-6 (BSF-2/IFN beta 2) receptor. *Science* **241**, 825–828.

Yawata, H., Yasukawa, K., Natsuka, S., Murakami, M., Yamasaki, K., Hibi, M., Taga, T., and Kishimoto, T. (1993). Structure-function analysis of human IL-6 receptor: Dissociation of amino acid residues required for IL-6-binding and for IL-6 signal transduction through gp130. *EMBO J.* **12**, 1705–1712.

Zhang, J. L., Simeonowa, I., Wang, Y., and Sebald, W. (2002). The high-affinity interaction of human IL-4 and the receptor α chain is constituted by two independent binding clusters. *J. Mol. Biol.* **315**, 399–407.

Zohlnhöfer, D., Graeve, L., Rose-John, S., Schooltink, H., Dittrich, E., and Heinrich, P. C. (1992). The hepatic interleukin-6 receptor. Down-regulation of the interleukin-6 binding subunit (gp80) by its ligand. *FEBS Lett.* **306**, 219–222.

2

CRYSTAL STRUCTURES AND INHIBITORS OF PROTEINS INVOLVED IN IL-2 RELEASE AND T CELL SIGNALING

KIERON BROWN AND GRAHAM M. T. CHEETHAM

Vertex Pharmaceuticals (Europe) Ltd., Abingdon
Oxfordshire OX14 4RY, United Kingdom

Vitamins and Hormones, Volume 74
0083-6729/06 $35.00
DOI: 10.1016/S0083-6729(06)74002-X

I. OVERVIEW

Ligation of the T cell receptor (TCR) by major histocompatibility complex (MHC) initiates a cascade of complex molecular events leading to T cell activation, proliferation, and release of important cytokines. While these events are an important and normal action of the immune system following infection, several human diseases are associated with inappropriate activation of the T cell response. Consequently, identifying inhibitors of TCR signaling and IL-2 production has been a high priority in the pharmaceutical industry for many years, and offers an attractive route for designing immunosuppressive and cancer therapeutics.

A number of natural products or small molecules that inhibit IL-2 release from T cells (and also release of several other cytokines) have been identified. Most importantly, Cyclosporin and FK-560 (also called Tacrolimus) are potent immunosuppressive agents. Despite being discovered more than 20 years ago, they are still the drug of choice for preventing organ rejection following transplantation. Several inhibitors of *de novo* synthesis of nucleotides or signal transduction in lymphocytes have established uses in treating immune disease. These inhibitors include mycophenolate mofetil, mizoribine, brequinar, and leflunomide. Mycophenolate mofetil and mizoribine act by inhibiting inosine monophosphate dehydrogenase (IMPDH).

Significantly, in the last few years, several new X-ray and NMR structures of protein kinases that play important roles in TCR signaling pathways have been solved. The crystal structure of Interleukin-2 tyrosine kinase (Itk) is the most recent of these and a number of potent inhibitors of its catalytic activity have already been reported. This chapter will provide a structural overview of several important enzymes involved in T cell signaling and IL-2 release and a summary of potential opportunities for the design of inhibitors that might improve upon Cyclosporin and FK-506.

II. IMPORTANCE OF IL-2 RELEASE BY T CELLS AND ITS ROLE IN HUMAN DISEASE

The adaptive immune response is mediated by two types of lymphocyte, B cells and T cells, and is characterized by high specificity and memory for antigen. A subset of T cells referred to as helper T cells, or Th cells, can be identified by expression of CD4 coreceptors on their cell surface. The function of Th cells differs from cytotoxic T cells (Tc), which express CD8 coreceptors (Fig. 1).

An important function of $CD4^+T$ cells function in the immune system is to recognize antigen in association with MHC Class II molecules and respond by producing cytokines, including IL-2. Production of cytokines

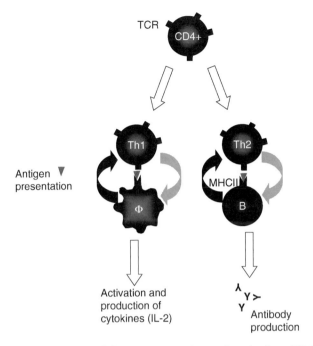

FIGURE 1.   The role of Th cells in response to antigen and production of IL-2. (See Color Insert.)

helps trigger the immune response by enhancing the function of other cells in the immune system. IL-2 is one of the first cytokines identified and is a member of the four-helix bundle cytokine superfamily. It is a potent T cell growth factor and an essential component of T cell function, stimulating growth and differentiation and thereby amplifying immune response. The biological activity of IL-2 is mediated by an autocrine interaction to its membrane receptor, IL-2R, which is expressed exclusively on activated T cells. A crystal structure of IL-2 bound to the alpha (IL-2Rα) chain of its receptor has recently been solved.

The absolute requirement for IL-2 in immune signaling has been studied *in vivo* using IL-2 deficient mice. Mice homozygous for the IL-2 gene mutation are normal with regard to thymotcyte and peripheral T cell composition during the first 3–4 weeks of age. However, a dysregulation of the immune system is manifested by reduced polyclonal *in vitro* T cell responses and by dramatic changes in the isotype levels of serum immunoglobulins. Furthermore, IL-2-deficient mice have been shown to develop an inflammatory bowel disease, similar to ulcerative colitis in humans. Subsequently, a number of diseases have been specifically associated with the aberrant expression of IL-2 or IL-2 receptors, including Hodgkin's disease, multiple sclerosis, rheumatoid arthritis, type-1 diabetes, and immunodeficiency syndrome.

III. A PARADIGM FOR BLOCKING IL-2 RELEASE *IN VIVO:* INHIBITION OF CALCINEURIN ACTIVITY BY CYCLOSPORIN AND FK-506

It was first demonstrated in the 1970s and 1980s through discovery of two natural products, Cyclosporin and FK-560, that the inhibition of IL-2 release would be a useful mechanism to treat human disease. Cyclosporin, a cyclic nonribosomal peptide of 11 amino acids (Pritard, 2005) and FK-506, a 23-membered macrolide lactone have distinct molecular targets in T cells (Fig. 2). However, both have profound immunosupressive properties, with FK-506 being the more potent suppressor of IL-2 secretion.

The molecular targets of Cyclosporin and FK-506 are the small, ubiquitous, cytosolic proteins cyclophilin and FKBP-12, respectively, which function enzymatically as *cis-trans* peptidylprolyl isomerases. Although both enzymes are strongly inhibited, this function is not sufficient in itself to block T cell signaling (Heitman *et al.*, 1991). Instead, the individual complexes cycophilin–cyclosporin and FKBP-12–FK-506 bind to calcineurin and inhibit its phosphatase activity. A consequence of calcineurin inhibition is

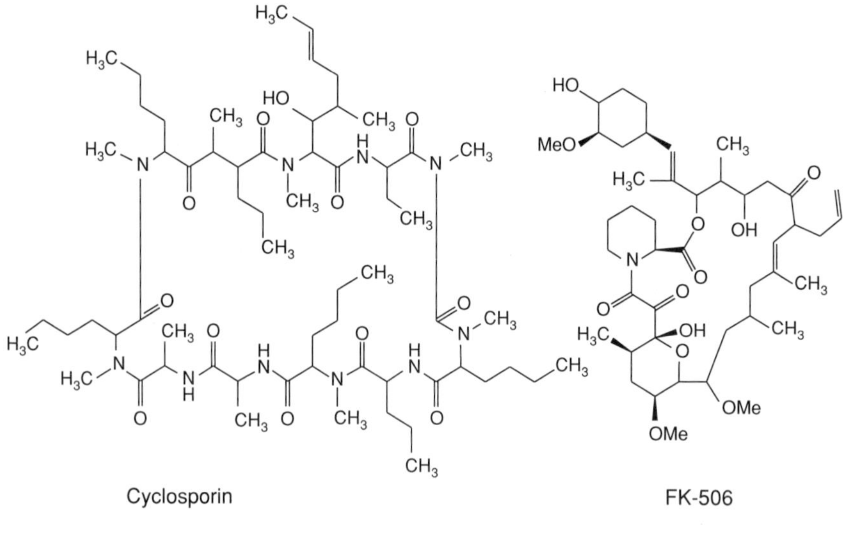

Cyclosporin   FK-506

FIGURE 2.   Inhibitors of calcineurin activity.

that nuclear factor of activated T cells (NF-AT), an important transcription factor, remains phosphorylated and inactive and the transcription of IL-2 is suppressed (Lui *et al.*, 1991). Calcineurin inhibition by FKBP-12–FK-506 or cyclophilin–cyclosporin correlates closely with inhibition of IL-2 production (Fruman *et al.*, 1992). The crystal structure of a calcineurin complex with FKBP-12 and FK-506 bound has been solved, and provides a useful framework for the coordination of information on this and related systems (Griffith *et al.*, 1995). The structure shows how the highly specific binding of the FK-506–FKBP-12 complex is mediated by a composite ligand-protein complementary surface that interacts with a matching surface on the calcineurin molecule. The crystal structure of calcineurin–cyclophilin–cyclosporin (Huai *et al.*, 2002) compared to the calcineurin–FKBP-12–FK-506 reveals that both bind to the same region of calcineurin and share major common recognition elements.

The structure-based design of novel urea-containing FKBP-12 inhibitors that target the same binding site as FK-506 have been described (Dragovich *et al.*, 1996). These compounds disrupt the *cis-trans* peptidylprolyl isomerase activity of FKBP-12 with K_i values equal to 100 nM. Crystal structures of these FKBP-12-urea complexes demonstrate that the inhibitors associate

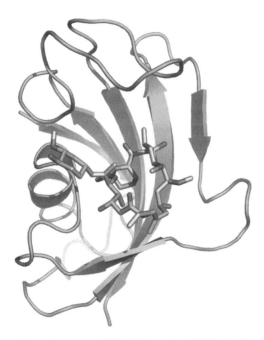

FIGURE 3.   Crystal structure of FK-506 bound to FKBP-12. (See Color Insert.)

with FKBP-12 in a manner that is significantly different from that observed for FK-506.

The association of cyclophilin with calcineurin has been of enormous interest for the design of novel immunosuppressant compounds. Cyclosporin is widely used in post allogenic organ transplant to reduce the activity of patients' immune system (which would normally be stimulated by IL-2 release) and thus the risk of organ rejection. However, such potent *in vivo* inhibition of IL-2 activity by targeting calcineurin comes at the price of mechanism-related toxicities. Treatment with Cyclosporine or FK-506 has a number of serious side effects and the potential for adverse interactions with a wide variety of other drugs. Side effects can include gum hyperplasia, convulsions, peptic ulcers, pancreatitis, fever, vomiting, diarrhea, pruritits, kidney and liver disfunction, hyperkalemia, hepatotoxicity, nephrotoxicity, and an increased vulnerability to opportunistic fungal and viral infections. Although studies have shown that the incidence of acute rejections was reduced by the use of FK-506 compared to Cyclosporin, severe side effects including blurred vision, liver and kidney problems, seizures, hypertension, hypomagnesemia, diabetes mellitus, hyperkalemia, and hyperglycemia are observed.

Therefore, identification of alternative targets in the TCR signaling pathway that may afford equally potent inhibition of IL-2 production, but with significantly reduced toxicities is an extremely important route to find improved drugs for immunosression.

IV. MOLECULAR SIGNALING IN T CELLS: MULTIPLE OPPORTUNITIES FOR THERAPEUTIC INTERVENTION

As depicted schematically in Fig. 4, the TCR is a multimeric complex composed of antigen recognition and signal-transducing components. While $\alpha\beta$ heterodimer (or in 5% of T cells $\gamma\delta$ heterodimers) recognizes processed peptide antigen, in association with MHC molecules, noncovalently associated CD3 and ζ chains are responsible for transmitting these signals to the intracellular compartment.

Downstream of the TCR, T cell activation and subsequent release of IL-2 results from the integration of multiple signal-transduction pathways (Alberola-Ita *et al.*, 1997; Qian and Weiss, 1997). Precisely how TCR signaling regulates Th cell differentiation remains poorly understood, however signaling molecules, especially protein kinases including Lck, Itk, ERK, JNK, and PKC-ω, plus TCR-ligation induced transcription factors (including NFAT and API) have been strongly implicated in the regulation of T cell differentiation (Mowen and Glimcher, 2004). Lymphocyte specific kinase (Lck) binds directly to the TCR to achieve full activation. Activated Lck is

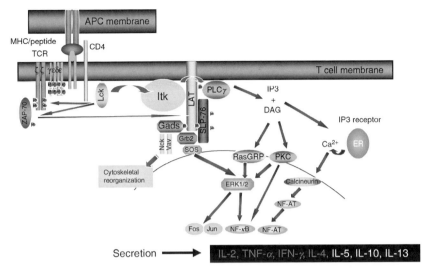

FIGURE 4. The T cell signaling cascade, showing the kinase Lck, ZAP-70, and Itk proximal to the T cell receptor. (See Color Insert.)

then able phosphorylate a number of downstream substrates to propagate the signal (van Oers et al., 1996). These substrates include the immunoreceptor tyrosine kinase-based activation motifs (ITAMs) in CD3 and ζ chains (Barber et al., 1989; Thome et al., 1996; van Oers et al., 1996). The purpose of phosphorylated ITAMs is to serve as high-affinity docking sites for the recruitment of additional signaling factors, including ζ-chain associated protein kinase of 70 kDa (ZAP-70) (Straus and Weiss, 1993; Wange et al., 1992) via its SH2 domain. In this way, Lck facilitates the activation and subsequent autophosphorylation of ZAP-70 (Chan and Kurosaki, 1995; LoGrasso et al., 1996; Neumeister et al., 1995; Wange et al., 1995; Watts et al., 1994).

ZAP-70 then phosphorylates the adaptors linker of activation of T cells (LAT) and SH2 domain containing leukocyte protein 76 kDa (SLP-76), which act together as a platform for the assembly of several key signaling molecules, including Itk and phospholipase C-gamma (PLKγ) (Rudd, 1999; Straus and Weiss, 1992). PLCγ catalyzes the hydrolysis of phosphatidylinositol-4,5-bisphosphate [PtdIns(4,5)P2] (PIP2) to yield diacylglycerol (DAG) and inositol-3,4,5-triphosphate (IP3). While DAG activates members of the PKC family, IP3 signals the release of Ca^{2+} from intracellular stores. This results in the downstream activation of mitogen-activated protein kinases, such as JUN amino-terminal kinase (JNK), extracellular signal-regulated kinase 1 (ERK1) and ERK2, as well as other effectors that direct gene expression.

Many of the effects of the Ca^{2+} released from intracellular stores are mediated by the Ca^{2+}-binding protein calmodulin, which is activated by Ca^{2+} binding. Ca^{2+}/calmodulin then binds to a variety of target proteins, including calcineurin, whose target in T cells is the nuclear factor of activated transcription (NFAT) (McCaffrey et al., 1993). After dephosphorylation by calcineurin, NFAT translocates from the cytoplasm to the nucleus where it binds to the promoter of the IL-2 gene and stimulates IL-2 expression.

The dependence of T cell signaling on multiple signaling pathways in addition to calcineurin provides a variety of opportunities for the development of immunosuppressive agents. These pathways involve signaling by protein kinases, making the rational design of small molecule inhibitors highly attractive as a route to effective immunosuppressive agents.

V. INHIBITION OF PROTEIN KINASES PROXIMAL TO THE TCR

Drug discovery based on targeting the protein kinase family is currently a hot topic in pharmaceutical research. Protein kinases play pivotal roles at numerous stages in multiple cellular events and are thus attractive targets for targeting cancer and immune disease. Compared to many other classes of enzyme, including transcription factor, such as NFAT, is has now been established that the ATP-binding site is a highly "drugable" site for small molecule inhibitors. However, designing inhibitors that are selective for the chosen kinase target remains a challenge. In an immunology setting, where one of the major goals is to improve upon mechanism-based toxicities associated with Cyclosporin and FK-506, it is postulated that potency against the target and inhibition of IL-2 secretion be combined with other enzymes and receptors that utilize ATP.

A. LCK: LYMPHOCYTE SPECIFIC KINASE

Several studies have implicated Lck as essential to TCR signaling. Most importantly, ablation of Lck expression in human Jurkat T cells results in a loss of signaling in response to TCR ligation. Expression of dominant negative genes in mice results in the early arrest of thymocyte maturation (Molina et al., 1992).

Lck is a modular protein consisting of a C-terminal catalytic kinase domain, a single SH2 and SH3 domain, and a unique N-terminal region. This N-terminal region is involved in anchoring Lck to CD4/8 through Zn^{2+} coordination via conserved cysteine residues present in both proteins (Huse et al., 1998; Lin et al., 1998). The catalytic activity of Lck is regulated by the autophosphorylation of Tyr394 located in the catalytic domain activation loop (Watts *et al.*, 1992) and by the phosphorylation of Tyr505 by C-terminal Src kinase (CSK) (Bougeret *et al.*, 1996; Gervais *et al.*, 1993; Jullien *et al.*, 1994). The SH2 and SH3 domains of Lck negatively regulate activity by forming intramolecular contacts that stabilize the catalytic domain in an inactive conformation (Reynolds *et al.*, 1992). The SH2 domain binds to phosphorylated Tyr505 and the SH3 domain associates with a proline-containing motif in a hinge region connecting the SH2 and catalytic domains (Sicheri *et al.*, 1997; Williams *et al.*, 1997; Xu *et al.*, 1997). Release of these intramolecular regulatory constraints by the dephosphorylation of Tyr505 (Mustelin and Altman, 1990) and/or the presence of competing SH3/SH2 ligands (Moarefi *et al.*, 1997) results in the autophosphorylation of Tyr394 in the activation loop and a catalytically active kinase (Watts *et al.*, 1994).

The design of ATP-competitive Lck inhibitors, with good selectivity over the other Src family members has been only recently been achieved. BMS-243117 and, more recently A-770041 (Fig. 5), demonstrate the potential benefit of targeting Lck for the treatment of immunological diseases (Burchat *et al.*, 2006; Das *et al.*, 2003). BMS-243117 belongs to a series of inhibitors based a benzothiazole core and is moderately selective over Src family members. It inhibits T cell proliferation with an IC50 value of 1.1 μM (Das *et al.*, 2003). The pyrazolo-pyrimidine A-770041 is the most selective Lck inhibitor described to date, displaying greater than 60-fold selectivity over other Src family members (Burchat *et al.*, 2006). Most importantly, A-770041 is also very potent at inhibiting the production of IL-2 in anti-CD3 stimulated human whole blood assays with an IC50 value of 80 nM. This value is comparable to reported values for FK-506 and Cyclosporine of 30 and 200 nM, respectively, in similar whole blood assays.

Several crystal structures of the catalytic kinase domain of Lck are available in the public domain (Yamaguchi and Hendrickson, 1996; Zhu *et al.*, 1999; Table I) and all share common feature in that the enzymes used for crystallization are phosphorylated, on Tyr394 in the activation loop. Their crystal structures correspond to an active conformation of the kinase domain. It is therefore interesting that the development of A-77041 appears to have exploited knowledge specifically derived from the binding affinities of inhibitors for the unphosphorylated or inactive kinase. It is not known whether targeting inactive Lck offers a better route to selectivity over other kinases or potent *in vivo* activity. It is tempting to suggest that inhibitors that specifically utilize the published crystal structure information will be forthcoming to test this hypothesis.

The SH2 domain of Lck binds a peptide substrate of sequence pTyr-Glu-Glu-Ile with high affinity (Kd ~140 nM for recombinant human p56Lck; Morelock *et al.*, 1995). Both X-ray crystallographic and NMR structures reveal the nature of this interaction (Schweimer *et al.*, 2002; Tong *et al.*, 1998) and have guided the design of potent phosphotyrosyl-containing

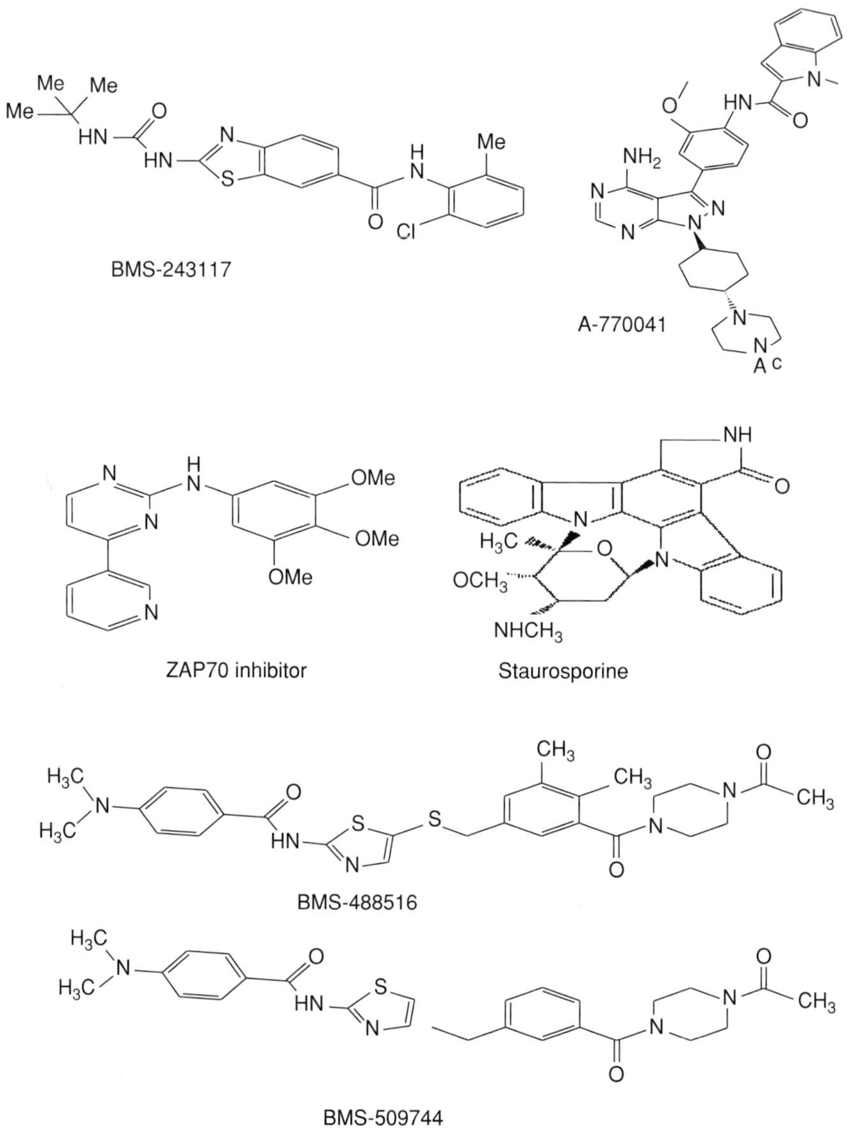

FIGURE 5. Protein kinase inhibitors of TCR signaling.

in vitro inhibitors of Lck. However, the major challenge for drug discovery has been to translate these inhibitors into successful therapeutic agents: the phosphate group is metabolically labile and prone to hydrolysis and its doubly negative charge at physiological pH significantly reduces cell permeability. Many attempts to replace the phosphate group with stable, less charged alternatives, including phosphonates (Mikol et al., 1995), difluorophosphonates (Charifson et al., 1997) and prodrugs have met with limited success. Although inhibitors with improved pharmacokinetic properties have been designed, their potency against Lck is typically reduced by more than 450-fold. In this instance, structural information has not facilitated rapid drug discovery as the SH2 domain appears to be a hard-to-drug site.

B. ZAP-70: ζ-CHAIN ASSOCIATED PROTEIN KINASE OF 70 KDA

ZAP-70 is a member of the Syk nonreceptor tyrosine family and contains two N-terminal Src homology domain 2 (SH2) domains and a C-terminal kinase domain. Lck is responsible for the phosphorylation of Tyr493 in the activation loop of the kinase domain, ZAP-70 subsequently phosphorylates itself on multiple tyrosine residues in the region between the SH2 domains and the kinase domain. The crystal structure of the ZAP-70 SH2 domains in complex with a TCR ζ-subunit peptide has been reported (Hatada et al., 1995), followed by a more recent report of the human form of the catalytic kinase domain (Jin et al., 2004).

Several reports point to an important role for ZAP-70 in T cell activation. First, a familial form of severe combined immunodeficiency in humans characterized by loss of functional ZAP-70 protein has been documented (Chan et al., 1994). Targeted disruption of the ZAP-70 gene in mice confirms this observation and leads to defects in thymic development and T cell activation (Negishi et al., 1995). Also, a T cell line (P116) lacking ZAP-70 displays severe defects in TCR induced signaling functions, including tyrosine phosphorylation, intracellular Ca^{2+} mobilization and, importantly, IL-2 transcription (Williams et al., 1998).

ZAP-70 belongs to the Syk family of tyrosine kinases, which includes Syk (spleen tyrosine kinase). Syk and ZAP-70 share similar functions in the transduction of immunoreceptor signals; Syk operates downstream of the B-cell receptor in B-cells, while ZAP-70 is found within T cells.

Importantly, ZAP-70 and Syk share a high degree of sequence similarity, in particular in the region of the ATP-binding site. This is perhaps one reason why the majority of drug discovery appears to have been directed toward the design of peptidic inhibitors that bind the SH2 domain of ZAP-70. However, ATP-competitive small molecules have now been identified (Moffat et al., 1999) and these are based upon a commonly utilized aminopyrimidine kinase pharmacophore (Fig. 3). Furthermore, the recent availability of a crystal structure of the ZAP-70 kinase domain (Jin et al., 2004) in complex with staurosporine has revealed a number of elements that maybe useful in improving the design of selective inhibitors. The presence of the ZAP-70 unique sequence motif -GPLHK-, adjacent to the kinase hinge region forms a surface

TABLE 1. Structures of Protein Kinases Involved in TCR Signaling and IL-2 Secretion

PDB ID	Description	References
LCK kinase		
1BHF 1BHH	Crystal structures of free and an inhibitor complex SH2 domain	(Tong et al., 1998)
1CWD 1CWE	Crystal structures of the SH2 domain complexed with phosphonopeptides	(Mikol et al., 1995)
1FBZ	Crystal structure of the SH2 domain complexed with a nonpeptide inhibitor	(Wulfing et al., 2000)
1H92	NMR structure of the SH3 domain	(Schweimer et al., 2002)
1IJR	Crystal structure of SH2 domain complexed with nonpeptide phosphotyrosine mimetic	Bioorg. Med. Chem. Lett. 11, 2319, 2001
1KIK	NMR structure of the SH3 domain	BMC Struct. Biol. 3, 3, 2003
1LCJ	Crystal structure of the SH2 domain complexed with a phosphopeptide	(Eck et al., 1993)
1LCK	Crystal structure of the SH3-SH2 domain fragment complexed with a phosphopeptide	Nature 368, 764, 1994
1LKK 1LKL	Crystal structures of the SH2 domain in complex with phosphopeptides	JMB 256, 601, 1996
1QPC 1QPD, 1QPE, 1QPJ	Crystal structures of kinase domain in complex with nonselective and Src family kinase inhibitors	(Zhu et al., 1999)

3LCK	Crystal structure of the activated catalytic kinase domain	(Yamaguchi and Hendrickson, 1996)
ZAP-70 kinase		
1M61	Crystal structure of the apo SH2 domains	Biochemistry 41, 14176, 2002
1U59	Crystal structure of the catalytic kinase domain in complex with staurosporine	(Brown et al., 2004)
TEC family kinases		
1AWX 1AWW	NMR structures of the SH3 domain from Btk	(Hansson et al., 1998)
1B55 1BWN	Wild-type and E41k mutant PH domain from Btk in complex with inositol 1,3,4,5-tetrakisphosphate	(Baraldi et al., 1999)
1Btk	PH domain and Btk motif of a Btk mutant, R28C	EMBO J. 16, 3396, 1997
1K2P	Crystal structure of the unphosphorylated Btk kinase domain	JBC 276, 41435, 2001
1QLY	NMR structure of the SH3 domain from Btk	J. Bio. NMR, 16, 303, 2000
1AWJ	NMR structure of the intramolecular Itk-proline complex	(Andreotti et al., 1997)
1LUI, 1LUK, 1LUM, 1LUN	NMR Structures of the Itk SH2 domain	(Mallis, 2002)
1SM2 1SNX, 1SNU	Crystal structures of the phosphorylated and unphosphorylated Itk catalytic domain	(Brown, 2004)

whose shape and electrostatic properties differ from those of Syk (where the histidine is replaced with an asparagine) and other members of the Syk family. The role of protein flexibility and dynamics in identifying differences between ZAP-70 and Syk, particularly in the Gly-rich loop, activation loop, and DFG motifs, have yet to be exploited.

C. TEC-FAMILY KINASES AND THE ROLE OF ITK IN T CELL SIGNALING

The Tec family of kinases comprises five homologous members: Itk, Rlk, Btk, Tec, and Bmx, however, only three of these are expressed in lymphocytes; Itk, Rlk, and Tec. While Btk appears to act independently of T cell signaling, and instead is essential for B cell development and activation, Itk is the most recent new target to emerge downstream of the TCR and Lck. Itk appears to function through two mechanisms: through its catalytic kinase activity and also forming a ternary complex with LAT, SLP-76, and PLCγ proteins (Bunnell et al., 2000; Ching et al., 2000; Shan and Wange, 1999; Su et al., 1999). As part of this large Itk/LAT/SLP-76 signalsome assembly, it is believed that Itk is not only responsible for the phosphorylation of PLCγ (Bunnell et al., 2000; Ching et al., 2000), but also contributes to TCR-induced rearrangement of the actin cytoskeleton (Grasis et al., 2003; Labno et al., 2003). This arises from the fact that the LAT/SLP-76 complex functions as a platform for the accumulation of molecules including VAV1 that regulate the polymerization of F-actin, which then controls TCR-mediated T cell proliferation adhesion and migration (Bustelo, 2000; Cannon and Burkhardt, 2002; Fischer et al., 1998; Holsinger et al., 1998; Tybulewicz et al., 2003; Wulfing et al., 2000).

A number of factors appear to support the importance of Itk in IL-2 production and immune disease. Itk mRNA and protein expression levels are increased during differentiation of T cells into Th2 cells compared with the levels in naïve T cells (Miller et al., 2004). The role that Itk might have in differentiation into Th2 cells is then provided from studies of Itk-deficient mice. Itk $^{-/-}$ mice show ineffective Th2 cell responses to infection with those pathogens used to evaluate Th2 cell differentiation (Fowell et al., 1999). In a mouse model of allergic asthma, Itk $^{-/-}$ mice have decreased IL-5 and IL-13 production as well as reduced mucus production and T cell infiltration in the lungs (Mueller and August, 2003). Consistent with these results, expression of Itk has been seen to be increased in peripheral-blood T cells from humans with atopic dermatitis (Matsumoto et al., 2002). Additionally, mice deficient in cyclophilin spontaneously develop allergic disease that is driven by Th2 cells, with corresponding increases in serum IgE levels and tissue infiltration by mast cells and eosinophils (Colgan et al., 2004). This provides further evidence that the overactivation of Itk might be associated with increased Th2 cell responses. Gene knockout studies have also revealed various degrees of immunodeficiency in mice lacking Lck, ZAP-70, and Itk (Liao and Littman, 1995; Molina *et al.*, 1992; Negishi *et al.*, 1995; Schaeffer *et al.*, 1999). Importantly, expression of Itk is induced upon T cell activation and treatment with IL-2 (Gibson *et al.*, 1993; Siliciano *et al.*, 1992; Tanaka *et al.*, 1993).

Although Itk is the main TEC-family kinase expressed by naïve mouse T cells, Rlk and Tec are present at 3-fold and 100-fold lower levels (Lucas *et al.*, 2003), respectively. Upon T cell activation, Itk expression is increased, most notably in Th2 cells, whereas Rlk expression drops, only to increase in Th1 cells (Miller *et al.*, 2004). Therefore, a major challenge for developing inhibitors of Itk is expected to be the requirement for selectivity over other TEC-family kinases. Because Itk, Rlk, and Tec have extremely homologous ATP-binding sites, crystal structures of these enzymes will be essential to identify unique pockets and features of Itk that facilitate the design of selective inhibitors.

VI. INTERLEUKIN-2 TYROSINE KINASE: A NOVEL DOWNSTREAM TARGET

A. A MOLECULAR DESCRIPTION

Itk has a complex domain structure composed of an amino-terminal phosphatidylinositol 3,4,5-trisphosphate PtdIns(3,4,5)P3-binding pleckstrin homology (PH) domain, a TEC-homology domain that contains one or two proline-rich regions (PRRs), an Src homology 3 (SH3) and SH2 domain, and a carboxy-terminal kinase domain (Fig. 6). This organization is shared with the other members of the Tec family.

Because of its ability to bind phosphoinositides, the PH domain of Itk is used for recruitment of the holo-enzyme to the plasma membrane. Phosphoinositides are produced by PI3K, which is activated upon TcR receptor stimulation, and this establishes a link between Itk and PI3K

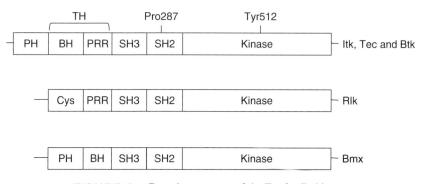

FIGURE 6.   Domain structures of the Tec-family kinases.

activity (August *et al.*, 1997; Lu *et al.*, 1998; Yang *et al.*, 2001). Localization of Itk to the plasma membrane is an essential first step for its subsequent phosphorylation and activation (Bunnell *et al.*, 2000; Ching *et al.*, 1999). Interestingly, the TEC family are the only tyrosine kinases to have PH domains, the homologous Src and Abl protein tyrosine families contain N-terminal lipid modulation signals instead. Itk lacking the PH domain and a portion of the TH domain has been shown to be less catalytically efficient (k_{cat}/K_m reduced by 4- to 29-fold) but had identical K_m values for ATP, indicating that removal of these N-terminal residues does not interfere with substrate interaction, but instead impairs the catalytic ability (Hawkins and Marcy, 2001). This hints at the critical role for the PH domain in Itk activity, beyond simple membrane recruitment. The regulatory role of the PH domain has been observed in non-TEC kinase family. In PKB, for example, the removal of the PH domain results in a 3-fold increase in activity (Sable *et al.*, 1998) and in protein kinase D, a 16-fold increase in activity is observed (Iglasias *et al.*, 1998).

The TH domain is unique to TEC kinases and is located downstream of the PH region. The proline-rich region found within the TH domain has been shown to participate in an intramolecular interaction with the downstream SH3 domain (Andreotti *et al.*, 1997) and that the formation of this complex with Itk regulates binding of other protein ligands, and may therefore control Itk activity (Andreotti *et al.*, 1997). Deletion of the TH domain in combination with the SH3 regions has been shown to affect the catalytic efficiency of the kinase, but not to ATP-binding affinity. Removal of the proline-rich sequence found in the TEC homology domain results in the two-fold reduction of basal activity of Itk (Hao and August, 2002). Furthermore, the Itk mutant containing an altered proline-rich region Itk P158A, P159A was significantly deficient in catalytic efficiency (k_{cat}/K_m decreased by 233- to 300-fold) and for the catalytic kinase domain alone, impaired even further (k_{cat}/K_m > 1000-fold decrease). In addition, it has been shown that the PRR regulates the ability of Lck to interact with and therefore activate Itk enzymatic activity. These results provide unambiguous evidence of the importance of the proline-rich region in the regulation of Itk activity.

The SH2 and SH3 domains play important roles in regulating intermolecular interactions. The SH2 has the important function of mediating the formation of the Itk-LAT complex (Ching *et al.*, 2000), which it achieves via the binding of a specific peptide motif containing a phosphorylated tyrosine residue. The SH3 domain binds to proline-rich sequences in the cytoplasmic domain of the T cell costimulatory receptor CD28 (Marengere *et al.*, 1997). Deletion of the SH3 and TH region has been shown to affect the catalytic efficiency of the kinase but not the ATP-binding affinity (Hawkins and Marcy, 2001) indicating a positive role for the SH3 function. Deletion of the SH3 domain in the homologous family member Tec, on the other hand, results in a constitutively active form of the kinase (Park *et al.*, 1996), consistent with a negative regulatory role for the SH3 domain (Yamashita et al., 1996).

Studies on the Itk SH2 domain (Mallis et al., 2002) reveal that it contains a conformationally heterogeneous proline residue. Cis-trans isomerization of this single prolyl imide bond causes a global conformational change in the SH2 domain structure and mediates conformer-specific ligand recognition; in the cis form, the SH2 domain interacts preferentially with the Itk SH3 domain, while in the trans form, the SH2 domain binds preferentially to phosphotyrosine-containing ligands, such as SLP-76 (Mallis et al., 2002). This conformational switch is also the key to the recognition of the Itk SH2 domain as a substrate for the petidylprolyl isomerase cyclophilin A (Brazin et al., 2002). In vitro and in vivo functional data reveals a stable CypA-Itk complex in T cells (Brazin et al., 2002).

Cyclophilin A has been shown to catalyze the cis-trans isomerization of the conformational heterogeneous proline residue in Itk and points to a role of CypA in repressing Itk kinase activity. Intriguingly, the proline involved in this conformational switch is unique to Itk and not conserved within the Tec kinase family (Mallis et al., 2002).

1. PH and SH Domains

PH domains have been found in nearly a hundred different eukaryotic proteins (Gibson et al., 1994). While the structure of the PH domain of Itk has yet to be solved, the three-dimensional structure of that in the TEC family member Btk is available (Baraldi et al., 1999) (Fig. 7A). This reveals that the PH domain is around 100 residues in length and consists of a seven-stranded bent β-sheet that packs against a C-terminal α-helix. The structure was solved in complex with Inositol (1,3,4,5) tetrakisphosphate, which binds in a site that is similar to the inositol 1,4,5-trisphosphate binding site in the PH domain of phospholipase Cδ (Ferguson et al., 1995). Intriguingly, in contrast to solution studies, the crystal structure suggests that the PH domain forms a stable dimer, which has been suggested to play a role in the activation mechanism of Btk (Baraldi et al., 1999). However, further studies will be necessary to establish whether a similar mechanism exists for Itk.

The solution structure of the Itk SH2 domain has been solved (Mallis et al., 2002) and adopts a fold typical of SH2 domains comprising a central three-stranded anti-parallel β-sheet flanked by two α-helices (Pawson et al., 2001) (Fig. 7B). The phosphotyrosine binding pocket closely resembles that of the Lck SH2 domain (Eck et al., 1993). The solution structure of the Itk SH3 domain is also available (Andreotti et al., 1997) and reveals that the SH3 domain has two triple-stranded anti-parallel β-sheets arranged in a β-sandwich with the two sheets at right angles to one another (Fig. 7C). These β-sheets create a binding pocket on the surface that recognizes proline-rich regions adopting a left-handed polyproline type II (PPII) helix conformation, containing either the sequence motif (R/K)xxPxxP or PxxPxR. This is

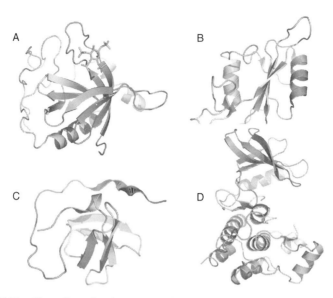

FIGURE 7.   Three-dimensional structures of the TEC-family domains: (A) Btk PH domain in complex with Inositol (1,3,4,5) tetrakis phosphate (PDB code 1B55); (B) energy minimized average NMR structure of the SH2 domain (PDB code ILUK); (C) minimized average NMR structure of the SH3 domain (PDB code IAWJ); and (D) the kinase domain (PD code ISNU). (See Color Insert.)

the same motif as the PRR of Itk and the solution structure of a fragment containing both the SH3 domain and adjacent PRR confirms that there is an intramolecular association between these two regions (Andreotti *et al.*, 1997). This association is believed to play a key role in the regulation of Itk activity. Recently, it has been demonstrated that a construct of Itk containing only the SH3 and SH2 domains dimerizes in an interaction involving the binding of the surface of the SH2 domain to the SH3 domain in the place of the polyproline motif (Brazin *et al.*, 2000). The structure of the Itk SH3 domain provides a better understanding of how displacement of the SH3-PRR interaction might depend upon the selection of the appropriate proline conformer in the SH2 domain, and reveals that cyclophilin which catalyses this *cis-trans* isomerization has a critical role to play in the Itk activation mechanism.

The structure of the full-length form of Btk, including PH, TH, SH2, SH3, and kinase domains, has been investigated using X-ray scatting in solution (Marquez *et al.*, 2003). This low-resolution data suggested that the domains are arranged in a linear arrangement, with few interdomain interactions. This is in contrast to Src and Abl, in which the SH3 and SH2 domains are assembled in a globular form in the inactive form and pack against the kinase domain (Nagar *et al.*, 2003; Sicheri *et al.*, 1997; Xu *et al.*, 1997). This globular form unravels in response to phosphorylation, and allows for the activation mechanism to proceed correctly. The linear nature of Btk and other TEC family members in solution suggests that a globular conformation is not required for the regulation of its activity in the same way as Src.

2. Catalytic Kinase Domain

The ATP-binding site of Itk is contained with the catalytic kinase domain, whose crystal structure has recently been reported (Brown *et al.*, 2004) (Fig. 7D). Structures of both the phosphorylated and unphosphorylated kinase domains bound to the broad-spectrum kinase inhibitor staurosporine were determined, as well as of the apo, unphosphorylated kinase domain (Brown *et al.*, 2004) (Figs. 7D and 8). Itk has a fold that is typical of other protein kinases. A small N-terminal lobe is connected to a large C-terminal lobe via a flexible hinge region. This hinge region is located in the cleft between the two lobes and forms part of the catalytic active site in which ATP binds. The N-terminal lobe is a five-stranded antiparallel β-sheet with a single α-helix (C helix) connecting two of the strands. The C-terminal lobe is mainly α-helical and contains the substrate-binding site, located in a groove on its surface, as well as the activation loop, in which the phosphorylation site Tyr504 is located.

The ability of protein kinases to alternate between catalytically active and inactive states in response to specific cellular signals underlies their use as

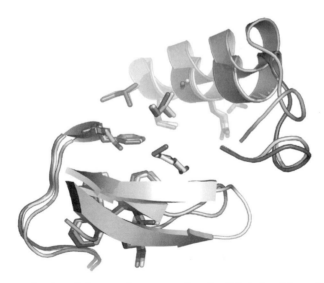

FIGURE 8. Overlay of the crystal structure of murine Btk (colored brown) (PDB code 1K2P) on the stauropsporine-bound unphosphorylated (colored white) and (phosphorylated colored blue) kinase structures of ITK in the region of the ATP-binding site. The Gly-rich loop of phosphorylated Itk is omitted for clarity. (See Color Insert.)

molecular switches. Structural studies have revealed that there are several key elements that play a role in the transition from one state to the other, which are found in the vicinity of the ATP-binding site. The activation loop is a region found in the C-lobe of the kinase domain and plays a central role in catalytic regulation; it is the phosphorylation of specific residues in this loop that is required for full activity of many kinases. Trans-phosphorylation of Itk on the activation loop tyrosine in the kinase domain leads to increased kinase activity *in vitro* and is critical for Itk mediated signal transduction in T cells (Chamorro *et al.*, 2001; Heyeck *et al.*, 1997). Unlike Src family tyrosine kinases, Itk does not autophosphorylate this tyrosine, instead Lck phosphorylates Tyr511 in Itk. Jurkat T cells lacking Lck show no TCR-induced tyrosine phosphorylation of Itk (Gibson *et al.*, 1996; Heyeck *et al.*, 1997), showing the critical role for Lck in Itk activation. Crystal structures of both active and inactive kinases have shown that this phosphorylation event often triggers dramatic conformational changes in the activation loop, which are necessary for a competent arrangement of catalytic residues. In the case of Itk, the majority of the activation loop is disordered, however, the DFG motif at the beginning of the activation loop, in both the unphosphorylated and phosphorylated inhibitor-bound structures are readily superimposed, suggesting that large conformational movements of the activation loop in Itk are not triggered upon phosphorylation. This surprising result brings into question the activating role of phosphorylation of Tyr512 in Itk.

The observed orientation of the αC-helix in the N-lobe reflects the catalytic state of the kinase. This helix carries a conserved glutamate residue, which in the active state interacts with the conserved active-site lysine, allowing the lysine side-chain to coordinate the α- and β-phosphate groups of ATP (Narayana *et al.*, 1997). However, in the inactive state, the αC-helix is displaced, and the interaction between the glutamate and lysine is lost, resulting in the nonproductive alignment of the ATP phosphate groups (Xu *et al.*, 1999). The crystal structures of staurosporine bound to Itk show that the αC-helix can be readily superimposed in both the unphosphorylated and phosphorylated states, and that its orientation resembles the active form of the kinase (Narayana *et al.*, 1997). Comparison of these structures with the apo, unphosphorylated structure suggested that this too resembles the active form. This contrasts to the situation in Btk, where the αC-helix resembles more closely the inactive structure of Src, and is consistent with the observation that Btk is catalytically inactive (Fig. 8). These results suggest that, in the absence of the neighboring regulatory domains, Itk is conformationally primed in the active state.

The active site of Itk is bounded by the glycine-rich loop, which contains the consensus kinase sequence Gly-X-Gly-X-X-Gly (residues 370–375), and the hinge region (residues 435–442). These regions determine the overall size and shape of the ATP-binding pocket. While the hinge is rigid in nature, the

Gly-rich loop is inherently flexible, a consequence of its amino-acid composition and its conformation might be influenced by the shape of bound inhibitors. For example, the Gly-rich loop in the staurosporine-bound forms of Itk are more open and extended compared to the apo structure of Btk, where the ATP-binding site appears occluded (Fig. 8).

The crystal structures of Itk reveal that the active-site residue Phe435 acts as a gatekeeper to an extensive hydrophobic pocket defined by Ala407, Met410, Leu421, Leu433, and Lys391 (Fig. 5). While the lipophilic residue at this position is unique to Itk (sequence alignments reveal that a Thr occupies this position in the other TEC family members) the hydrophoibic nature of the pocket lying behind it is conserved. Comparing the crystal structure of Itk and Btk reveals the contrast between electrostatic properties in this region of the ATP-binding site arising from the polar Thr and lipophilic Phe residue (Fig. 8).

B. INHIBITION OF ITK ACTIVITY

1. PH and SH Domain Inhibitors

The development of phosphatidylinositol analogues as inhibitors (with IC50s of approximately 4 μM (Castillo et al., 2004)) of PH domains has to date been restricted to the protein kinase B (PKB/Akt). PKB possesses an N-terminal PH domain, similar to Itk, which is responsible for the recruitment of PKB to the plasma membrane. As PH domain inhibitors have a potential to interfere with the function of other PH domain containing proteins, and in addition, phosphatidylinositol analogues commonly have problems with solubility, aggregation, pharmacokinetics, and potency there is an inherent limit their utility as small molecule drug leads.

An inhibitor targeted at the Itk SH2 domain would disrupt the protein–protein interaction with the LAT chains. There are no known inhibitors specifically for the Itk SH2 domain. However, the design of inhibitors of Grb2 and Src SH2 domains indicates that even small peptides can be sufficient to compete for large protein ligands (Garcia-Echeverria, 2001). Since pTyr pocket of the SH2 domain is extremely well conserved in three-dimensional structure, suggesting that any inhibitor with high affinity to this site is unlikely to be selective for a particular SH2 domain.

Due to the nature of the SH3-binding site, inhibitors reported to date have been peptide-like compounds based on proline or similar amino acids. These compounds have been difficult to use as therapeutic agents because they are generally unstable in blood, poorly absorbed when orally administered and often poorly absorbed by cells due to their high molecular weight. Recently, UCS15A was identified as a small molecule inhibitor of Src-signal transduction (Sharma et al., 2001). Studies have since revealed that UCS15A represented the first example of a nonpeptide, small molecule agent capable of disrupting SH3 mediated protein–protein interactions by interacting directly with proline-rich ligands in target proteins (Oneyama *et al.*, 2002). UCS15A is the first and only small molecule inhibitor of proline-rich ligand-mediated protein–protein interactions thus far identified, and therefore it represents a promising lead compound.

2. ATP-Binding Site Inhibitors

Staurosporine binds to the Itk kinase domain with a K_i of less than 10 nM. The crystal structure reveals that it binds at the interface of the N- and C-terminal lobes via hydrophobic interactions with Ile369, Val377, and Ala389 (N-terminal lobe), Phe435 and Tyr437 (hinge region), Leu489, and Cys442 (C-terminal lobe) all of which line the active site. Upon inhibitor binding, the gatekeeper residue, Phe435, makes a beneficial edge-face interaction with the conjugated ring system of staurosporine. In addition, the lactam group mimics the interactions of the adenine base in ATP with the hinge region of the protein backbone, where two conserved hydrogen bonds are formed between the lactam-nitrogen N19 and the lactam-oxygen O30 in staurosporine to the protein backbone.

The challenge for finding useful inhibitors of Itk is to identify a small molecule that binds to the ATP-site of with an equal potency but vastly improved cross-reactivity profile compared to staurosporine. The Itk inhibitors BMS 488516 and BMS 509744 (Fig. 5) have gone a long way to reach this goal. They have been shown to reduce TCR-induced function including PLCγ tyrosine phosphorylation, calcium mobilization, and T cell proliferation *in vitro*, in both human and mouse cells (Lin *et al.*, 2004). The inhibitors also suppress the production of IL-2 induced by anti-TCR antibody when given to mice. Both the compounds exhibited competitive kinetics with respect to ATP, confirming that they bind to the ATP-binding site of the Itk kinase domain. BMS 488516 and 509744 are both aminothiazoles, thio-linked to a phenyl ring. Interestingly, the length of the linker and the precise substitution pattern on the phenyl ring appear to be crucial in determining the selectivity profile of the inhibitors, both for a broad range of kinases and within the TEC family.

VII. CONCLUSIONS

In an earlier section it was described how potent inhibition of calcineurin readily translates into potent *in vivo* inhibition of IL-2 secretion and immunosupression. However, a major problem of using Cyclosporine and FK-506 for immunotherapy arises from the broad expression profile of their protein targets, causing numerous unpleasant side effects. A marker of this toxicity is the extreme potency of these agents at inhibiting the release of many other cytokines, including IL-4, IL-5, IL-10, IL-12, IL-13, and TNF-α. There has therefore been much effort in recent years to identify and exploit new targets on TCR/IL-2 signaling pathways. Determination of selective and potent inhibitors of these proteins, including the kinases Lck, Zap-70, and Itk, has been rapid and facilitated by many crystal structures as useful drug discovery tools.

Arguably the greatest success in targeting protein kinases with small molecule inhibitors aimed at ablation IL-2 secretion and immunosupression has been demonstrated for Lck by A-770041. This inhibitor is selective for its target enzyme, against many other kinases, and extremely potent at inhibiting cellular production of IL-2 at levels comparable with FK-506. Furthermore, good *in vivo* efficacy in survival models of transplantation has been reported. Thus, A-770041 validates an approach of targeting protein kinases in TCR-signaling and immune disease. The clinical status of this inhibitor has not been reported.

In this chapter, we have identified several other protein kinases that are implicated in signaling downstream of the TCR receptor and secretion of IL-2 by T cells. While Zap-70 is an established target for treating immune disease, the TEC-family kinases are new and promising targets for treating immune disease. Itk is the most recent of these to be highlighted and is located immediately downstream of Lck. It appears to be an attractive alternative to calcineurin as a therapeutic target, although inhibitors suitable for *in vivo* and clinical use have yet to be presented.

A rapid rise in the use of crystal structure information to drive drug discovery continues to reveal the molecular basis for signaling downstream of the TCR and this holds great promise for identifying novel and powerful agents for immunosupression.

REFERENCES

Alberola-Ita, J., Takaki, S., Kerner, J. D., and Perlmutter, R. M. (1997). Differential signalling by lymphocyte antigen receptors. *Annu. Rev. Immunol.* **15**, 125–154.

Andreotti, A. H., Bunnell, S. C., Feng, S, Berg, L. J., and Schreiber, S. L. (1997). Regulatory intramolecular association in a tyrosine kinase of the Tec family. *Nature* **385**, 93–97.

August, A., Sadra, A., Dupont, B., and Hanafusa, H. (1997). Src-induced activation of inducible T cell kinase (ITK) requires phosphatidylinositol 3-kinase activity and the Pleckstrin homology domain of inducible T cell kinase. *Proc. Natl. Acad. Sci. USA* **94**, 11227–11232.

Baraldi, E., Carugo, K. D., Hyvoenen, M., Surdo, P. L., Riley, A. M., Potter, B. V., O'Brien, R., Ladbury, J. E., and Saraste, M. (1999). Structure of the PH domain from Bruton's tyrosine kinase in complex with inositol 1,3,4,5-tetrakisphosphate. *Structure Fold Des.* **7**, 449–460.

Barber, E. K., Dasgupta, J. D., Schlossman, S. F., Trevillyan, J. M., and Rudd, C. E. (1989). The CD4 and CD8 antigens are coupled to a protein-tyrosine kinase (p56lck) that phosphorylates the CD3 complex. *Proc. Natl. Acad. Sci. USA* **86**, 3277–3281.

Bougeret, C., Delaunay, T., Romero, F., Jullien, P., Sabe, H., Hanafusa, H., Benarous, R., and Fischer, S. (1996). Detection of a physical and functional interaction between Csk and Lck which involves the SH2 domain of Csk and is mediated by autophosphorylation of Lck on tyrosine 394. *J. Biol. Chem.* **271**, 7465–7472.

Brazin, K. N., Fulton, D. B., and Andreotti, A. H. (2000). A specific intermolecular association between the regulatory domains of a Tec family kinase. *J. Mol. Biol.* **302**, 607–623.

Brazin, K. N., Mallis, R. J., Fulton, D. B., and Andreotti, A. H. (2002). Regulation of the tyrosine kinase Itk by the peptidyl-prolyl isomerase cyclophilin A. *Proc. Natl. Acad. Sci. USA* **99**, 1899–1904.

Brown, K., Long, J. M., Vial, S. C., Dedi, N., Dunster, N. J., Renwick, S. B., Tanner, A. J., Frantz, J. D., Fleming, M. A., and Cheetham, G. M. (2004). Crystal structures of interleukin-2 tyrosine kinase and their implications for the design of selective inhibitors. *J. Biol. Chem.* **279**, 18727–18732.

Bunnell, S. C., Diehn, M., Yaffe, M. B., Findell, P. R., Cantley, L. C., and Berg, L. J. (2000). Biochemical interactions integrating Itk with the T cell receptor-initiated signaling cascade. *J. Biol. Chem.* **275**, 2219–2230.

Burchat, A., Borhani, D. W., Calderwood, D. J., Hirst, G. C., Biqin, L., and Stachlewitz, R. F. (2006). Discovery of A-770041, a src-family selective orally active lck inhibitor that prevents organ allograft rejection. *Bio. Med. Chem. Lett.* **16**, 118–122.

Bustelo, X. R. (2000). Vav proteins, adaptors and cell signaling. *Oncogene* **20**, 6372–6381.

Cannon, J. L., and Burkhardt, J. K. (2002). The regulation of actin remodeling during T-cell-APC conjugate formation. *Immunol. Rev.* **186**, 90–99.

Castillo, S. S., Brognard, J., Petukhov, P. A., Zhang, C., Tsurutani, J., Granville, C. A., Li, M., Jung, M., West, K. A., Gills, J. G., Kozikowski, A. P., and Dennis, P. A. (2004). Preferential inhibition of Akt and killing of Akt-dependent cancer cells by rationally designed phosphatidylinositol ether lipid analogues. *Cancer Res.* **64**, 2782–2792.

Chamorro, M., Czar, M. J., Debnath, J., Cheng, G., Lenardo, M. J., Varmus, H. E., and Schwartzberg, P. L. (2001). Requirements for activation and RAFT localization of the T-lymphocyte kinase Rlk/Txk. *BMC Immunol.* **2**, 3.

Chan, A. C., and Kurosaki, T. (1995). Activation of ZAP-70 kinase activity by phosphorylation of tyrosine 493 is required for lymphocyte antigen receptor function. *EMBO J.* **14**, 24499–24508.

Chan, A. C., Kadlecek, T. A., Elder, M. E., Filipovich, A. H., Kuo, W. L., Iwashima, M., Parslow, T. G., and Weiss, A. (1994). ZAP-70 deficiency in an autosomal recessive form of severe combined immunodeficiency. *Science* **264**, 1599–1601.

Charifson, P., Shewchuk, L. M., Rocque, W., Hummel, C. W., Jordan, S. R., Mohr, C., Pacofsky, G. J., Peel, M. R., Rodriguez, M., Sternbach, D. D., and Consler, T. G. (1997). Peptide ligands of pp60(c-src) SH2 domains: A thermodynamic and structural study. *Biochemistry* **36**, 6283–6293.

Ching, K. A., Kawakami, Y., Kawakami, T., and Tsoukas, C. D. (1999). Emt/Itk associates with activated TCR complexes: Role of the pleckstrin homology domain. *J. Immunol.* **163**, 6006–6013.

Ching, K. A., Grasis, J. A., Tailor, P., Kawakami, Y., Kawakami, T., and Tsoukas, C. D. (2000). TCR/CD3-Induced activation and binding of Emt/Itk to linker of activated T cell complexes: Requirement for the Src homology 2 domain. *J. Immunol.* **165**, 256–262.

Colgan, J., Asmal, M., Neagu, M., Yu, B., Schneidkraut, J., Lee, Y., Sokolskaja, E., Andreotti, A., and Luban, J. (2004). Cyclophilin A regulates TCR signal strength in T cells via a proline-directed conformational switch in Itk. *Immunity* **21**, 189–201.

Das, J., Lin, J., Moquin, R. V., Shen, Z., Spergel, S. H., Wityak, J., Doweyko, A. M., DeFex, H. F., Fang, Q., Pang, S., Pitt, S., Shen, D. R., *et al.* (2003). Molecular design, synthesis, and structure-activity relationships leading to the potent and selective p56(lck) inhibitor BMS-243117. *Bioorg. Med. Chem. Lett.* **13**, 2145–2149.

Dragovich, P. S., Barker, J. E., French, J., Imbacuan, M., Kalish, V. J., Kissinger, C. R., Knighton, D. R., Lewis, C. T., Moomaw, E. W., Parge, H. E., Pelletier, L. A., Prins, T. J., et al. (1996). Structure-based design of novel, urea-containing FKBP12 inhibitors. *J. Med. Chem.* **39**, 1872–1884.

Eck, M. J., Shoelson, S. E., and Harrison, S. C. (1993). Recognition of a high-affinity phosphotyrosyl peptide by the Src homology-2 domain of p56lck. *Nature* **362**, 87–91.

Ferguson, K. M., Lemmon, M. A., Schlessinger, J., and Sigler, P. B. (1995). Structure of the high affinity complex of inositol trisphosphate with a phospholipase C pleckstrin homology domain. *Cell* **83**, 1037–1046.

Fischer, K. D., Kong, Y. Y., Nishina, H., Tedford, K., Mareng Åre, L. E., Kozieradzki, I., Sasaki, T., Starr, M., Chan, G., Gardener, S., Nghiem, M. P., Bouchard, D., et al. (1998). Vav is a regulator of cytoskeletal reorganization mediated by the T-cell receptor. *Curr. Biol.* **8**, 554–562.

Fowell, D. J., Shinkai, K., Liao, X. C., Beebe, A. M., Coffman, R. L., Littman, D. R., and Locksley, R. M. (1999). Impaired NFATc translocation and failure of Th2 development in Itk-deficient CD4$^+$T cells. *Immunity* **11**, 399–409.

Fruman, D. A., Klee, C. B., Bierer, B. E., and Burakoff, S. J. (1992). Calcineurin phosphatase activity in T lymphocytes is inhibited by FK506 and Cyclosporin A. *Proc. Natl. Acad. Sci. USA* **89**, 3686–3690.

Garcia-Echeverria, C. (2001). Antagonists of the Src homology 2 (SH2) domains of Grb2, Src, Lck and ZAP-70. *Curr. Med. Chem.* **8**, 1589–1604.

Gervais, F. G., Chow, L. M., Lee, J. M., Branton, P. E., and Veillette, A. (1993). The SH2 domain is required for stable phosphorylation of p56lck at tyrosine 505, the negative regulatory site. *Mol. Cell. Biol.* **13**, 7112–7121.

Gibson, S., Leung, B., Squire, J. A., Hill, M., Arima, M., et al. (1993). Identification, cloning and characteristaion of a novel human T-cell specific tyrosine kinase located at the hematopoietin complex on chromosome 5q. *Blood* **82**, 1561–1572.

Gibson, T. J., Hyvonen, M., Musacchio, A., Saraste, M., and Birney, E. (1994). P. H. domain: The first anniversary. *Trends. Biochem. Sci.* **19**, 349–353.

Gibson, S., August, A., Branch, D., Dupont, B., and Mills, G. (1996). Functional LCK Is required for optimal CD28-mediated activation of the TEC family tyrosine kinase EMT/ITK. *J. Biol. Chem.* **271**, 7079–7083.

Griffith, J. P., Kim, J. L., Kim, E. E., Sintchak, M. D., Thomson, J. A., Fitzgibbon, M. J., Fleming, M. A., Caron, P. R., Hsiao, K., and Navia, M. A. (1995). X-ray structure of calcineurin inhibited by the immunophilin-immunosuppreesant FKBP12-FK506 complex. *Cell* **82**, 507–522.

Grasis, J. A., Browne, C. D., and Tsoukas, C. D. (2003). Inducible T cell tyrosine kinase regulates actin-dependent cytoskeletal events induced by the T cell antigen receptor. *J. Immunol.* **170**, 3971–3976.

Hansson, H., Mattsson, P. T., Allard, P., Haapaniemi, P., Vihinen, M., Smith, C. I., and Hard, T. (1998). Solution structure of the SH3 domain from Bruton's tyrosine kinase. *Biochemistry* **37**, 2912–2924.

Hao, S., and August, A. (2002). The proline-rich region of the Tec homology domain of ITK regulates its activity. *FEBS Lett.* **525**, 53–58.

Hawkins, J., and Marcy, A. (2001). Characterization of Itk tyrosine kinase: Contribution of noncatalytic domains to enzymatic activity. *Prot. Expr. Purif.* **22**, 211–219.

Hatada, M. H., Lu, X., Laird, E. R., Green, J., Morgenstern, J. P., Lou, M., Marr, C. S., Phillips, T. B., Ram, M. K., Theriault, K., Zoller, M. J., and Karas, J. L. (1995). Molecular basis for interaction of the protein tyrosine kinase ZAP-70 with the T-Cell receptor. *Nature* **377**, 32–38.

Heitman, J., Movva, N. R., Hiestand, P. C., and Hall, M. N. (1991). The FK-506 binding protein proline rotamase is a target for the immunosuppressive agent FK506 in *Saccharomyces cerevisiae*. *Proc. Natl. Acad. Sci. USA* **88**, 1948–1952.

Heyeck, S. D., Wilcox, H. M., Bunnell, S. C., and Berg, L. J. (1997). Lck phosphorylates the activation loop tyrosine of the Itk kinase domain and activates Itk kinase activity. *J. Biol. Chem.* **272**, 25401–25408.

Holsinger, L. J., Graef, I. A., Swat, W., Chi, T., Bautista, D. M., Davidson, L., Lewis, R. S., Alt, F. W., and Crabtree, G. R. (1998). Defects in actin-cap formation in Vav-deficient mice implicate an actin requirement for lymphocyte signal transduction. *Curr. Biol.* **8**, 563–572.

Huai, Q., Kim, H. Y., Liu, Y., Zhao, Y., Mondragon, A., Liu, J. O., and Ke, H. (2002). Crystal structure of calcineurin-cyclophilin-cyclosporin shows common but distinct regognition of immunophilin-drug complexes. *Proc. Natl. Acad. Sci. USA* **99**, 12037–12042.

Huse, M., Eck, M. J., and Harrison, S. C. (1998). A Zn2+ ion links the cytoplasmic tail of CD4 and the N-terminal region of Lck. *J. Biol. Chem.* **273**, 18729–18733.

Jin, L., Pluskey, S., Petrella, E. C., Cantin, S. M., Gorga, J. C., Rynkiewicz, M. J., Pandey, P., Strickler, J. E., Babine, R. E., Weaver, D. T., and Seidl, K. J. (2004). The three-dimensional structure of the ZAP-70 kinase domain in complex with staurosporine: Implications for the design of selective inhibitors. *J. Biol. Chem.* **279**, 42818–42825.

Jullien, P., Bougeret, C., Camoin, L., Bodeus, M., Durand, H., Disanto, J. P., Fischer, S., and Benarous, R. (1994). Tyr394 and Tyr505 are autophosphorylated in recombinant Lck protein-tyrosine kinase expressed in *Escherichia coli*. *Eur. J. Biochem.* **224**, 589–596.

Labno, C. M., Lewis, C. M., You, D., Leung, D. W., Takesono, A., Kamberos, N., Seth, A., Finkelstein, L. D., Rosen, M. K., Schwartzberg, P. L., and Burkhardt, J. K. (2003). Itk functions to control actin polymerization at the immune synapse through localized activation of Cdc42 and WASP. *Curr. Biol.* **13**, 1619–1624.

Liao, X. C., and Littman, D. R. (1995). Altered T cell receptor signaling and disrupted T cell development in mice lacking Itk. *Immunity* **3**, 757–769.

Lin, R. S., Rodriguez, C., Veillette, A., and Lodish, H. F. (1998). Zinc is essential for binding of p56(lck) to CD4 and CD8α. *J. Biol. Chem.* **273**, 32878–32882.

Lin, T. A., McIntyre, K. W., Das, J., Liu, C., O'Day, K. D., Penhallow, B., Hung, C. Y., Whitney, G. S., Shuster, D. J., Yang, X., Townsend, R., Postelnek, J., *et al.* (2004). Selective Itk inhibitors block T-cell activation and murine lung inflammation. *Biochemistry* **43**, 11056–11062.

LoGrasso, P. V., Hawkins, J., Frank, L. J., Wisniewski, D., and Marcy, A. (1996). Mechanism of activation for ZAP-70 catalytic activity. *Proc. Natl. Acad. Sci. USA* **93**, 12165–12170.

Lu, Y., Cuevas, B., Gibson, S., Khan, H., LaPushin, R., Imboden, J., and Mills, G. B. (1998). Phosphatidylinositol 3-kinase is required for CD28 but not CD3 regulation of the TEC family tyrosine kinase EMT/ITK/TSK: Functional and physical interaction of EMT with phosphatidylinositol 3-kinase. *J. Immunol.* **161**, 5404–5412.

Lucas, J. A., Miller, A. T., Atherly, L. O., and Berg, L. J. (2003). The role of Tec family kinases in T-cell development and function. *Immunol. Rev.* **191**, 119–138.

Lui, J., Farmer, J. D., Jr., Lane, W. S., Friedman, J., Weissman, I., and Schreiber, S. L. (1991). Calcineurin is a common target of cyclophilin-cyclosporin A and FKBP-FK506 complexes. *Cell* **66**, 807–815.

Mallis, R. J., Brazin, K. N., Fulton, D. B., and Andreotti, A. H. (2002). Structural characterization of a proline-driven conformational switch within the Itk SH2 domain. *Nat. Struct. Biol.* **9**, 900–905.

Marengere, L. E., Okkenhaug, K., Clavreul, A., Couez, D., Gibson, S., Mills, G. B., Mak, T. W., and Rottapel, R. (1997). The SH3 domain of Itk/Emt binds to proline-rich sequences in the cytoplasmic domain of the T cell costimulatory receptor CD28. *J. Immunol.* **159**, 3220–3229.

Marquez, J. A., Smith, C. I., Petoukhov, M. V., Lo Surdo, P., Mattsson, P. T., Knekt, M., Westlund, A., Scheffzek, K., Saraste, M., and Svergun, D. I. (2003). Conformation of full-length Bruton tyrosine kinase (Btk) from synchrotron X-ray solution scattering. *EMBO J.* **22**, 4616–4624.

Matsumoto, Y., Oshida, T., Obayashi, I., Imai, Y., Matsui, K., Yoshida, N. L., Nagata, N., Ogawa, K., Obayashi, M., Kashiwabara, T., Gunji, S., Nagasu, S., *et al.* (2002). Identification of highly expressed genes in peripheral blood T cells from patients with atopic dermatitis. *Int. Arch. Allergy Immunol.* **129**, 327–340.

McCaffrey, P. G., Luo, C., Kerppola, T. K., Jain, J., Badalian, T. M., Ho, A. M., Burgeon, E., Lane, W. S., Lambert, J. N., Curran, T., *et al.* (1993). Isolation of the cyclosporin-sensitive T cell transcription factor NFATp. *Science* **262**, 750–754.

Mikol, V., Baumann, G., Keller, T. H., Manning, U., and Zurini, M. G. M. (1995). The crystal structures of the SH2 domain of p56lck complexed with two phosphonopeptides suggest a gated peptide binding site. *J. Mol. Biol.* **246**, 344–355.

Miller, A. T., Wilcox, H. M., Lai, Z., and Berg, L. J. (2004). Signalling through Itk promotes T helper 2 differentiation via negative regulation of T-bet. *Immunity* **21**, 67–80.

Moarefi, I., LaFevre-Bernt, M., Sicheri, F., Huse, M., Lee, C. H., Kuriyan, J., and Miller, W. T. (1997). Activation of the Src-family tyrosine kinase Hck by SH3 domain displacement. *Nature* **385**, 650–653.

Moffat, D., Davis, P., Hutchings, M., Davis, J., Berg, D., Batchelor, M., Johnson, J., O'Connell, J., Martin, R., Crabbe, T., Delgado, J., and Perry, M. (1999). 4-Pyridin-5-yl-2-(3,4,5-trimethoxyphenylamino)pyrimidines: Potent and selective inhibitors of ZAP 70. *Bioorg. Med. Chem. Lett.* **9**, 3351–3356.

Molina, T. J., Kishihara, K., Siderovski, D. P., van Ewijk, W., Narendran, A., Timms, E., Wakeham, A., Paige, C. J., Hartmann, K. U., and Veillette, A. (1992). Profound block in thymocyte development in mice lacking p56lck. *Nature* **357**, 161–164.

Morelock, M. M., Ingraham, R. H., Betageri, R., and Jakes, S. (1995). Determination of receptor-ligand kinetic and equilibrium binding constants using surface plasmon resonance: Application to the lck SH2 domain and phosphotyrosyl peptides. *J. Med. Chem.* **38**, 1309–1318.

Mowen, K. A., and Glimcher, L. H. (2004). Signalling Pathways in TH2 development. *Immunol. Rev.* **202**, 203–222.

Mueller, C., and August, A. (2003). Attenuation of immunological symptoms of allergic asthma in mice lacking the tyrosine kinase ITK. *J. Immunol.* **170**, 5056–5063.

Mustelin, T., and Altman, A. (1990). Dephosphorylation and activation of the T cell tyrosine kinase pp56lck by the leukocyte common antigen (CD45). *Oncogene* **5**, 809–813.

Nagar, B., Hantschel, O., Young, M. A., Scheffzek, K., Veach, D., Bornmann, W., Clarkson, B., Superti-Furga, G., and Kuriyan, J. (2003). Structural basis for the autoinhibition of c-Abl tyrosine kinase. *Cell* **112**, 859–871.

Narayana, N., Cox, S., Shaltiel, S., Taylor, S. S., and Xuong, N. (1997). Crystal structure of a polyhistidine-tagged recombinant catalytic subunit of cAMP-dependent protein kinase complexed with the peptide inhibitor PKI(5–24) and adenosine. *Biochemistry* **36**, 4438–4448.

Negishi, I., Motoyama, N., Nakayama, K., Nakayama, K., Senju, S., Hatakeyama, S., Zhang, Q., Chan, A. C., and Loh, D. Y. (1995). Essential role for ZAP-70 in both positive and negative selection of thymocytes. *Nature* **376**, 435–438.

Neumeister, E. N., Zhu, Y., Richard, S., Terhorst, C., Chan, A. C., and Shaw, A. S. (1995). Binding of ZAP-70 to phosphorylated T-cell receptor zeta and eta enhances its autophosphorylation and generates specific binding sites for SH2 domain-containing proteins. *Mol. Cell. Biol.* **15**, 3171–3178.

Oneyama, C., Nakano, H., and Sharma, S. V. (2002). UCS15A, a novel small molecule, SH3 domain-mediated protein-protein interaction blocking drug. *Oncogene* **21**, 2037–2050.

Park, H., Wahl, M. I., Afar, D. E., Turck, C. W., Rawlings, D. J., Tam, C., Scharenberg, A. M., Kinet, J. P., and Witte, O. N. (1996). Regulation of Btk function by a major autophosphorylation site within the SH3 domain. *Immunity* **4**, 515–525.

Pawson, T., Gish, G. D., and Nash, P. (2001). SH2 domains, interaction modules and cellular wiring. *Trends Cell. Biol.* **11**, 504–511.

Pritard, D. I. (2005). Sourcing a chemical successor of Cyclosporin from parasites and human pathogens. *Drug Discovery Today* **10**, 688–691.

Qian, D., and Weiss, A. (1997). Lymphocyte activation in health and disease. *Crit. Rev. Immunol.* **17**, 155–178.

Reynolds, P. J., Hurley, T. R., and Sefton, B. M. (1992). Functional analysis of the SH2 and SH3 domains of the lck tyrosine protein kinase. *Oncogene* **7**, 1949–1955.

Rudd, C. E. (1999). Adaptors and molecular scaffolds in immune cell signaling. *Cell* **96**, 5–8.

Sable, C. L., Filippa, N., Filloux, C., Hemmings, B. A., and Van Obberghen, E. (1998). Involvement of the pleckstrin homology domain in the insulin-stimulated activation of protein kinase, B. *J. Biol. Chem.* **273**, 29600–29606.

Schaeffer, E. M., Debnath, J., Yap, G., McVicar, D., Liao, X. C., Littman, D. R., Sher, A., Varmus, H. E., Lenardo, M. J., and Schwartzberg, P. L. (1999). Requirement for Tec kinases Rlk and Itk in T cell receptor signaling and immunity. *Science* **284**, 638–641.

Schweimer, K., Hoffmann, S., Bauer, F., Friedrich, U., Kardinal, C., Fcller, S. M., Biesinger, B., and Sticht, H. (2002). Structural investigation of the binding of a herpesviral protein to the SH3 domain of tyrosine kinase Lck. *Biochemistry* **41**, 5120–5130.

Sharma, S. V., Oneyama, C., Yamashita, Y., Nakano, H., Sugawara, K., Hamada, M., Kosaka, N., and Tamaoki, T. (2001). UCS15A, a non-kinase inhibitor of Src signal transduction. *Oncogene* **20**, 2068–2079.

Shan, X., and Wange, R. L. (1999). Itk/Emt/Tsk activation in response to CD3 cross-linking in Jurkat T cells requires ZAP-70 and Lat and is independent of membrane recruitment. *J. Biol. Chem.* **274**, 29323–29330.

Sicheri, F., Moarefi, I., and Kuriyan, J. (1997). Crystal structure of the Src family tyrosine kinase Hck. *Nature* **385**, 602–609.

Siciliano, J. D., Morrow, T. A., and Desiderio, S. V. (1992). Itk, a T-cell specific tyrosine kinase gene inducible by interleukin-2. *Proc. Natl. Acad. Sci. USA* **89**, 11194–11198.

Straus, D. B., and Weiss, A. (1992). Genetic evidence for the involvement of the Lck tyrosine kinase in signal transduction through the T cell antigen receptor. *Cell* **70**, 585–593.

Straus, D. B., and Weiss, A. (1993). The CD3 chains of the T cell antigen receptor associate with the ZAP-70 tyrosine kinase and are tyrosine phosphorylated after receptor stimulation. *J. Exp. Med.* **178**, 1523–1530.

Su, Y. W., Zhang, Y., Schweikert, J., Koretzky, G. A., Reth, M., and Wienands, J. (1999). Interaction of SLP adaptors with the SH2 domain of Tec family kinases. *Eur. J. Immunol.* **29**, 3702–3711.

Tanaka, N., Asao, H., Ohtani, K., Nakamura, M., and Sugamura, K. (1993). A novel human tyrosine kinase gene inducible in T cells by interluekin-2. *FEBS Lett.* **324**, 1–5.

Thome, M., Germain, V., DiSanto, J. P., and Acuto, O. (1996). The p56lck SH2 domain mediates recruitment of CD8/p56lck to the activated T cell receptor/CD3/zeta complex. *Eur. J. Immunol.* **26**, 2093–2100.

Tong, L., Warren, T. C., Lukas, S., Schembri-King, J., Betageri, R., Proudfoot, J. R., and Jakes, S. (1998). Carboxymethyl-phenylalanine as a replacement for phosphotyrosine in SH2 domain binding. *J. Biol. Chem.* **273**, 20238–20242.

Tybulewicz, V. L., Ardouin, L., Prisco, A., and Reynolds, L. F. (2003). Vav1: A key signal transducer downstream of the TCR. *Immunol. Rev.* **192**, 42–52.

van Oers, N. S., Killeen, N., and Weiss, A. (1996). Lck regulates the tyrosine phsophorylation of the T cell receptor subunits and ZAP-70 in murine thymocytes. *J. Exp. Med.* **183**, 1053–1062.

Wange, R. L., Kong, A. N., and Samelson, L. E. (1992). A tyrosine phosphorylated 70 kDa protein binds a photoaffinity analogue of ATP and associates with both the zeta chain and CD3 components of the activated T cell antigen receptor. *J. Biol. Chem.* **267**, 11685–11688.

Wange, R. L., Guitan, R., Isakov, N., Watts, J. D., Aebersold, R., and Samelson, L. E. (1995). Activating and inhibitory mutations in adjacent tyrosines in the kinase domain of ZAP-70. *J. Biol. Chem.* **270,** 18730–18733.

Watts, J. D., Wilson, G. M., Ettenhadieh, E., Clark-Lewis, I., Kubanek, C. A., Astell, C. R., Marth, J. D., and Aebersold, R. (1992). Purification and initial characterization of the lymphocyte-specific protein-tyrosyl kinase p56lck from a baculovirus expression system. *J. Biol. Chem.* **267,** 901–907.

Watts, J. D., Affolter, M., Krebs, D. L., Wange, R. L., Samelson, L. E., and Aebersold, R. (1994). Identification by electrospray ionisation mass spectrometry of the sites of tyrosine phosphorylation induced in activated Jurkat T cells on the protein tyrosine kinase ZAP-70. *J. Biol. Chem.* **269,** 29520–29529.

Williams, B. L., Schreiber, K. L., Zhang, W., Wange, R. L., Samelson, L. E., Leibson, P. J., and Abraham, R. T. (1998). Genetic evidence for differential coupling of Syk family kinases to the T-cell receptor: Reconstitution studies in a ZAP-70-deficient Jurkat T-cell line. *Mol. Cell. Biol.* **18,** 1388–1399.

Williams, J. C., Weijland, A., Gonfloni, S., Thompson, A., Courtneidge, S. A., Superti-Furga, G., and Wierenga, R. K. (1997). The 2.35 Å crystal structure of the inactivated form of chicken Src: A dynamic molecule with multiple regulatory interactions. *J. Mol. Biol.* **274,** 757–775.

Wulfing, C., Bauch, A., Crabtree, G. R., and Davis, M. M. (2000). The vav exchange factor is an essential regulator in actin-dependent receptor translocation to the lymphocyte-antigen-presenting cell interface. *Proc. Natl. Acad. Sci. USA* **97,** 10150–10155.

Xu, W., Harrison, S. C., and Eck, M. J. (1997). Three-dimensional structure of the tyrosine kinase c-Src. *Nature* **385,** 595–602.

Xu, W., Doshi, A., Lei, M., Eck, M. J., and Harrison, S. C. (1999). Crystal structures of c-Src reveal features of its autoinhibitory mechanism. *Mol. Cell* **3,** 629–638.

Yamaguchi, H., and Hendrickson, W. A. (1996). Structural basis for activation of human lymphocyte kinase Lck upon tyrosine phosphorylation. *Nature* **384,** 484–489.

Yamashita, Y., Miyazato, A., Ohya, K., Ikeda, U., Shimada, K., Miura, Y., Ozawa, K., and Mano, H. (1996). Deletion of Src homology 3 domain results in constitutive activation of Tec protein-tyrosine kinase. *Jpn. J. Cancer Res.* **87,** 1106–1110.

Yang, W. C., Ching, K. A., Tsoukas, C. D., and Berg, L. J. (2001). Tec kinase signaling in T cells is regulated by phosphatidylinositol 3-kinase and the Tec pleckstrin homology domain. *J. Immunol.* **166,** 387–395.

Zhu, X., Kim, J. L., Newcomb, J. R., Rose, P. E., Stover, D. R., Toledo, L. M., Zhao, H., and Morgenstern, K. A. (1999). Structural analysis of the lymphocyte-specific kinase Lck in complex with non-selective and Src family selective kinase inhibitors. *Struct. Fold Des.* **7,** 651–661.

3

STRUCTURAL STUDIES OF THE INTERLEUKIN-19 SUBFAMILY OF CYTOKINES

ALEXANDER ZDANOV

Macromolecular Crystallography Laboratory, Center for Cancer Research National Cancer Institute at Frederick, Frederick, Maryland 21702

The interleukin-19 (IL-19) subfamily of cytokines is part of a larger family of homologs of IL-10 that includes two groups of proteins: five viral cytokines, and eight cellular cytokines, having quite different biological activities. Among proteins of the latter group, IL-19, IL-20, IL-22, and IL-24 were suggested to form a structurally unique IL-19 subfamily characterized by their structural features and aggregation state as monomers. IFN-λ1, IFN-λ2, and IFN-λ3 are likely to belong to this subfamily, and it is still not clear whether IL-26 belongs to it or not. In spite of their differences in biological function, all cellular homologs of IL-10 used for signaling a set of five overlapping membrane-bound receptors: three long receptor chains (IL-20R1, IL-22R1, and IFN-λR) and two short receptor chains (IL-20R2 and IL-10R2). Signal transduction is

0083-6729/06 $35.00
DOI: 10.1016/S0083-6729(06)74003-1

initiated when a cytokine binds two receptor chains, one long and one short, forming a ternary complex. Crystal structures of IL-19 and IL-22 showed that these cytokines consist of seven amphipathic helices of different length organized in helical bundle, covering an extensive hydrophobic core. Based on the similarity of the structures with the structure of a single domain of IL-10, and with the crystal structure of a binary IL-10/IL-10R1 complex, putative receptor binding sites on the surface of IL-19 and IL-22 were identified. This chapter summarizes the available structural data on the IL-19 subfamily of cytokines and their putative ligand/receptor complexes.

I. INTRODUCTION

A. INTERLEUKIN-19 SUBFAMILY OF CYTOKINES

The interleukin-19 (IL-19) subfamily of cytokines was identified based on structural features of IL-19 (Chang et al., 2003) and IL-22 (Nagem et al., 2002a,b), as a group of proteins having structures topologically similar to IL-19 and belonging to a larger IL-10 (Moore et al., 2001; Pestka et al., 2004) family of cytokines. This family, in turn, is divided into two major groups of cellular and viral homologs of IL-10 (Dumoutier and Renauld, 2002; Fickenscher et al., 2002; Kotenko, 2002; Ozaki and Leonard, 2002; Renauld, 2003; Walter, 2004; Zdanov, 2004). The viral homologs were found in the Epstein-Barr virus (EBV) (Hsu et al., 1990; Moore et al., 1990; Vieira et al., 1991), equine herpesvirus type 2 (Rode et al., 1993), Orf parapoxvirus (Fleming et al., 1997, 2000), human and simian cytomegaloviruses (CMV) (Kotenko et al., 2000; Lockridge et al., 2000), and Yaba-like disease virus (Lee et al., 2001). Although the amino acid identity of these proteins with hIL-10 varies between 23% and 85%, they are all dimers having three-dimensional structures similar to IL-10 (Jones et al., 2002; Walter and Nagabhushan, 1995; Yoon et al., 2005; Zdanov et al., 1995, 1996, 1997). Since the viral homologs, except Yaba-like disease virus, which is a homolog of IL-24 (Bartlett et al., 2004; Renauld, 2003), imitate the biological function of IL-10, they use the IL-10 receptor system, although the affinity of the receptors toward a particular viral IL-10 may vary (Jones et al., 2002; Liu et al., 1997). Cellular homologs, including IL-19 (Gallagher et al., 2000), IL-20 (Blumberg et al., 2001), IL-22 (Dumoutier et al., 2000b; Xie et al., 2000), IL-24 (Jiang et al., 1996), IL-26 (Fickenscher and Pirzer, 2004; Igawa et al., 2005; Knappe et al., 2000), IFN-λ1, IFN-λ2, and IFN-λ3 (IL-29, IL-28A, IL-28B) (Kotenko et al., 2003; Sheppard et al., 2003), have much lower amino acid sequence similarity with hIL-10 and differ from both IL-10 and from each other in their biological functions. In spite of the differences, these cytokines have been suggested to belong to a unique IL-19 subfamily of cytokines because of the topological similarity of their structures and the mode of aggregation (Chang *et al.*, 2003). These proteins belong to the group of long-chain cytokines (Rozwarski *et al.*, 1994), having structures similar to the structure of the IL-10 domain in which the first helix A is substituted by two shorter helices connected by a short β-strand (Chang *et al.*, 2003; Nagem *et al.*, 2002b). Unlike IL-10, they are monomers in solution, the only exception being IL-26, which exists and is active both as a dimer (Fickenscher and Pirzer, 2004; Fickenscher *et al.*, 2002; Knappe *et al.*, 2000) and as a monomer.

All members of the IL-10 family of cytokines initiate signal transduction on binding to two membrane-bound receptor chains (Bach *et al.*, 1997; Kotenko, 2002; Kotenko and Pestka, 2000; Pestka *et al.*, 1997), for example, IL-10R1 (Liu *et al.*, 1994) and IL-10R2 (Kotenko *et al.*, 1997) in the case of IL-10, or IL-20R1 and IL-20R2 in the case of IL-20 (Dumoutier *et al.*, 2001a; Parrish-Novak *et al.*, 2002). Both chains consist of extracellular, transmembrane, and intracellular/cytoplasmic domains, and belong to the class II or interferon receptor family (Bazan, 1990; Ho *et al.*, 1993). The receptor chain having longer cytoplasmic domain is called chain 1, whereas the receptor chain having a short cytoplasmic domain is called chain 2 (Kotenko and Langer, 2004). The intracellular domain of chain 1 is associated with Janus tyrosine kinase 1 (JAK1), while that of chain 2 is associated with tyrosine kinase Tyk2. When a cytokine binds both receptor chains together, the signaling, ternary complex is formed and the tyrosine kinases cross-phosphorylate each other, bringing the signal transducers and activators of transcription (STAT) proteins to be recruited to the cytokine/receptor complex. After that, STATs are activated by JAK-mediated tyrosine phosphorylation, form corresponding homo- or heterodimers, dissociate from the receptor complex, and translocate to the nucleus, where, together with other factors, they initiate and modulate transcription of appropriate genes (Decker and Meinke, 1997; Schindler and Darnell, Jr., 1995). Which genes are transcribed is determined by specific DNA sequences to which STATs bind in the promoter region of the gene. Kinetic-binding data also showed that usually receptor chain 1 has much higher affinity toward the ligand than the chain 2 (Logsdon *et al.*, 2002), although this is not always the case (Pletnev *et al.*, 2003).

Cellular cytokines of the IL-10 family, including the subfamily of IL-19, signal through binding to two appropriate receptor chains: IL-20R1, IL-20R2 (Blumberg *et al.*, 2001; Dumoutier *et al.*, 2001a; Wang *et al.*, 2002), IL-22R1 (Kotenko *et al.*, 2001a; Xie *et al.*, 2000) and IFN-λR (Kotenko *et al.*, 2003; Sheppard *et al.*, 2003) which have been discovered, along with their ligands. Except for IL-20R2, all the other newly discovered receptors have long cytoplasmic domains. Thus nine cytokines, including IL-10, signal by using one of four first receptor chains (IL-10R1, IL-20R1, IL-22R1, IFN-λR) in combination with one of two second receptor chains (IL-20R2 or IL-10R2).

IL-22 also has a natural soluble receptor (called IL-22-binding protein, IL-22BP), which is also a type-II receptor, but lacks both the transmembrane and intracellular domains (Dumoutier *et al.*, 2001b; Kotenko *et al.*, 2001b; Xu *et al.*, 2001), and is capable of binding IL-22 on its own.

This chapter reviews the available structural data on the IL-19 subfamily of cytokines and their putative complexes with the corresponding receptors.

1. Interleukin-19

Biological function of IL-19, helical cytokine, which was discovered not long ago, still requires clarification, although it is known that IL-19 is expressed mostly by cells involved in immune system, monocytes, and B cells (Gallagher *et al.*, 2000; Wolk *et al.*, 2002). In monocytes, IL-19 is directly induced by lipopolysaccharides (LPS) and granulocyte-macrophage colony-stimulating factor (GM-CSF) and further upregulated by IL-4 and IL-13. It has been reported that IL-19 induces production of IL-10 in human periph-eral blood mononuclear cells (PBMC) (Jordan *et al.*, 2005) and also is able to induce its own expression, followed by IL-10 downregulation of this IL-19 autoinduction.

A molecule of IL-19 is a monomer, consisting of seven amphipathic helices A–G of different lengths (Fig. 1), forming a unique seven-helix bundle with an extensive internal hydrophobic core. Three disulfide bridges located on the top of the bundle make the polypeptide chain framework quite rigid. Helices B, D, E, and G form a four-helix bundle, which is a characteris-tic feature of all helical cytokines (Presnell and Cohen, 1989). The position

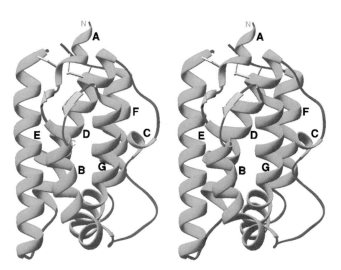

FIGURE 1. Stereo diagram of IL-19, (pdb code 1N1F), disulfide bonds shown in yellow. All figures were made with program RIBBONS (Carson, 1991). (See Color Insert.)

of helix A, covering the top of the molecule (Fig. 1), is stabilized by the disulfide bridge Cys10-Cys103, linking it covalently to the C terminus of helix E. The second and third disulfide bridges, Cys57-Cys109 and Cys58-Cys111, hold together the N terminus of helix D, interhelical loop EF, and the N terminus of helix F. The C-terminal strand 154–159 is bent along the surface of the molecule and makes hydrogen bonds with the short interhelical strand AB. These two parallel strands form a short β-sheet, never seen previously in helical cytokines (Fig. 1).

2. Interleukin-22

IL-22, also known as IL-10 related T cell–derived inducible factor (IL-TIF) was initially identified as a gene induced by IL-9 in mouse T cells, and mast cells (Dumoutier et al., 2000a). Human IL-22 was cloned and reported later based on its homology with murine ortholog (Dumoutier et al., 2000b; Xie et al., 2000). IL-22 mRNA expression can be induced by anti-CD-3 stimulation followed by upregulation with Con A and by LPS in vivo in a variety of organs including gut, thymus, spleen, lung, liver, kidney, stomach, and heart (Dumoutier et al., 2000b). It is accepted that IL-22 is involved in the inflammatory and probably in immune responses in various tissues (Kotenko, 2002).

The crystal structure of IL-22 was solved twice, first at resolution 2.0 Å (Nagem et al., 2002b) and later at 2.6 Å (Xu et al., 2005). The first time the protein was expressed in *Escherichia coli* (IL-22$_{EC}$) (Nagem et al., 2002a,b) and the second time in *Drosophila* S2 cells (IL-22$_{DS}$) (Xu et al., 2004, 2005) which means that IL-22$_{DS}$ was glycosylated in accordance with insect cells glycosylation pattern. Both structures were found to be very similar, indicating that glycosylation causes only minor structural changes to the protein. Although sequence similarity between IL-19 and IL-22 is only 36%, the structure of IL-22 is topologically very similar to that of IL-19 (Fig. 2). IL-22 also consists of seven α-helices A–G, which are packed as a seven-helix bundle covering an extensive hydrophobic core inside. The first helix A is also very short as in IL-19 and is connected with helix B by a short β-strand. A superposition of the structures of IL-19 and IL-22$_{EC}$ (Nagem et al., 2002b) results in root mean square (rms) deviation of 1.7 Å for 123 pairs of Cα-atoms. The main difference between IL-19 and IL-22 is that helixes of IL-19 are somewhat longer than that of IL-22, for example, helix E is seven turns long in IL-19 and only four in IL-22 (Figs. 1 and 2). There is also a difference in the position of the disulfide bridges and lengths of the interhelical loops. The first disulfide bridge, Cys10-Cys103 of IL-19 corresponds to Cys7-Cys99 of IL-22, although its position is not the same, rms deviations for the respective Cα coordinates are in the range 2.5–5.5 Å. In the second disulfide bridge, Cys57 of IL-19 is equivalent in sequence to Cys56 of IL-22; their Cα coordinates are only 3.3 Å apart, however, their disulfide partners are different: in IL-19, Cys57 makes a disulfide bond to Cys109 (loop EF); in

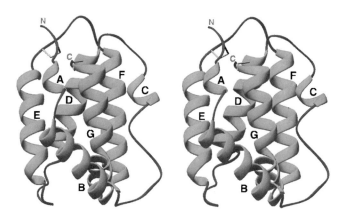

FIGURE 2.   Stereo diagram of IL-22$_{EC}$, (pdb code 1MR4). (See Color Insert.)

IL-22, Cys56 makes a bond to Cys145, which is the C terminus of helix G. A similar variability of the disulfides has previously been reported for short-chain helical cytokines (Rozwarski *et al.*, 1994). Therefore, in the IL-19 structure, the seven-helix bundle is stabilized by disulfides holding together the N terminus of helix A with the C terminus of helix E, the N terminus of helix D with both loop EF, and the N terminus of helix F; while in IL-22, the first disulfide similar to IL-19 also holds together the N terminus of helix A and the C terminus of helix E, but the second disulfide is between the N terminus of helix D and the C terminus of helix G. There are two molecules of IL-22$_{EC}$ forming a dimer and six molecules of IL-22$_{DS}$, which form three dimers similar to IL-22$_{EC}$ in the asymmetric part of their corresponding crystal form. Root mean square deviations between all independent molecules of IL-22$_{EC}$ and IL-22$_{DS}$ and between IL-22$_{EC}$ and IL-22$_{DS}$ themselves are better than 1.0 Å, although some pairs of IL-22$_{DS}$ showed even better similarity with rms deviation of 0.3–0.6 Å (Xu *et al.*, 2005).

B. COMPARISON OF THE CRYSTAL STRUCTURES OF IL-19 AND IL-22 WITH IL-10 DOMAIN

The superposition of IL-19 (Fig. 3) and IL-22$_{EC}$ with one domain of IL-10 gives an rms deviation between the positions of Cα atoms 1.7 Å and 1.9 Å (Nagem *et al.*, 2002b), respectively. The main differences are in the area of the first 21 residues of the IL-10 domain, helix C, interhelical loops, orientation of helix E (helix D of IL-10) relative to the rest of the helical bundle, with the rms deviation at its N terminus about 1 Å, increasing to 3.8 Å at the C terminus, and the C terminus of helix G (helix F of the IL-10). Therefore, the general architecture of these molecules is very much alike,

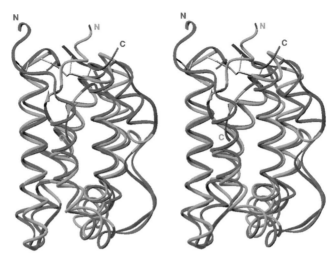

FIGURE 3. Stereo diagram of the superposition of IL-19 with IL-10 domain. IL-19 ribbons are shown in cyan, coils in brown, and β-strands in green. IL-10 domain is shown in pink. (See Color Insert.)

although the orientation of the new helix A and the short β-sheet in the IL-19 make the overall shape of the molecule more compact and smooth.

1. Interleukin-20

IL-20 was found to be important for regulation of development and proper functioning of the skin (Blumberg *et al.*, 2001). IL-20 initiates its signal through binding to two pairs of receptors IL-20R1/IL-20R2 and IL-22R1/IL-20R2 (Dumoutier *et al.*, 2001a; Parrish-Novak *et al.*, 2002). Comparison (Genetics Computer Group, 1994) of IL-19 and IL-20 amino acid sequences gives 44.1% identity and 52.4% similarity without any gaps or deletions, beginning in the sequence at the position corresponding to the N terminus of helix A of IL-19. The superposition of the sequences of IL-19, IL-20, and IL-10 shows a remarkable degree of similarity in the positions of hydrophobic residues and of the cysteines involved in the formation of the disulfide bridges. In fact, all three disulfide bonds present in IL-19 are also preserved in IL-20. Taken together, we may conclude that the three-dimensional structure of IL-20 is very similar to IL-19, and it is no surprise that these two cytokines share their receptors. The only obvious difference between IL-19 and IL-20, besides their N-termini, is expected at the C terminus, in the region of the C-terminal β-strand of IL-19. There is no such strand in IL-20 since Glu157, the last residue of IL-20, corresponds to His153 of IL-19, which is the last residue in the helix G.

2. Interleukin-24

IL-24 or melanoma differentiation-associated gene-7 (MDA-7) was the first cellular homolog of IL-10 reported in the literature (Jiang *et al.*, 1995, 1996) and identified as a novel protein, upregulated in terminal differentiation of human melanoma cells by interferon-β and the protein kinase C-activator mezerein (Jiang *et al.*, 1995). IL-24 was found to have two distinct functional activities, at low concentration it functions as a cytokine (Caudell *et al.*, 2002), but when it is overexpressed via an adenovirus-mediated gene delivery system, it selectively induces apoptosis in cancer cells but not in normal cells (Chada *et al.*, 2004a,b; Chen *et al.*, 2003; Cunningham *et al.*, 2005; Ekmekcioglu *et al.*, 2001; Huang *et al.*, 2001; Jiang *et al.*, 1996). Similar to IL-20, IL-24 initiates signaling through the binding to IL-20R1/IL-20R2 and IL-22R1/IL-20R2 receptors (Dumoutier *et al.*, 2001a; Parrish-Novak *et al.*, 2002; Wang *et al.*, 2002). Sequence identity between IL-19 and IL-24 is only 31%, with 40% similarity. However, allocation of similar and hydrophobic amino acid residues confirms that the three-dimensional structure of IL-24 is likely to be similar to that of IL-19. IL-24 has only two cysteines (Cys16 and Cys63), corresponding to Cys10 and Cys57 of IL-19. Since these two cysteines are involved in making separate disulfide bonds, and IL-24 is a monomer, this must indicate that the N terminus of IL-24 should have a unique conformation, which is likely to bring Cys16 into the proximity of Cys63 to form a disulfide bridge between them. Because of that, the position of short helix A relative to the rest of the helical bundle may be different and may also affect binding to the receptor. Another structural feature, which is highly conserved between these cytokines, is a salt bridge formed between Lys27 and Asp143 and located on the surface of the molecule. This bridge is strictly conserved in IL-19, IL-10, IL-22, and IL-24, with a mutation to Arg in IL-20.

3. Interleukin-26

IL-26, originally called as AK155, was identified as a protein expressed in human herpesvirus simiri (HVS) transformed T cells (Fickenscher and Pirzer, 2004; Knappe *et al.*, 2000). HVS is a tumor virus of neotropical squirrel monkeys. The fact that IL-26 was induced by viral infection indicates that this protein may play an important role in immune response, particularly as antiviral defense. IL-26 initiates signal transduction through the formation of the ternary complex with IL-20R1/IL-10R2 receptor pair (Hor *et al.*, 2004; Sheikh *et al.*, 2004), none of the other cellular homologs of IL-10 use this particular receptor pair. There are also unpublished data that IL-26 can bind IL-20R2 receptor chain, however, what could be the other chain is not clear yet. IL-26 appears to be the only cellular homolog of IL-10 which is active as a dimer (Fickenscher and Pirzer, 2004; Knappe *et al.*, 2000) and as a monomer. Amino acid sequence analysis (Genetics

Computer Group, 1994) of IL-26 gives 31% identity and 45% similarity with hIL-10, which is slightly higher than with IL-19 (27% and 35%), IL-22 (27% and 38%), or IL-24 (30% and 37%). It is likely that IL-26 structure should be similar to IL-10, however, it still remains to be seen to what degree. Another feature of IL-26 is that it has a very high isoelectric point of 10.8, which is quite unusual for the family of cellular homologs of IL-10, where they normally have isoelectric point in the range of 7–8. It is not clear why IL-26 needs to be positively charged. The question of whether or not IL-26 belongs to the IL-19 subfamily is still open.

II. INTERFERONS-λ 1,2,3 (IFN-λ1, IFN-λ2, AND IFN-λ3, OR IL-29, IL-28A, AND IL-28B)

IFN-λ1, IFN-λ2, and IFN-λ3 (IL-29, IL-28A, and IL-28B) are the latest discovered members of the class II cytokine family. They have quite low sequence identity with IL-10 (10–13%); nevertheless, all three were recognized perhaps to belong to the family of IL-10 homologs (Dumoutier et al., 2004; Kotenko et al., 2003; Sheppard et al., 2003). IFN-λs are expressed by PBMC and dendritic cells in response to a viral infection. Sequence identity between IFN-λ1 and IFN-λ2 is 81%, and between IFN-λ2 and IFN-λ3 is 96%. The proteins are monomers in solution (A. Zdanov, unpublished data) and initiate signal transduction through formation of ternary complex with receptor chains IFN-λR and IL-10R2 (Kotenko et al., 2003; Sheppard et al., 2003). It was also shown, that sequence identity between IFN-λs and IFN-α 2 is even slightly higher (Sheppard et al., 2003) than with IL-10, particularly in terms of the positions of cysteine residues, which implies that IFN-λ1, IFN-λ2, and IFN-λ3 may have the same disulfide bridges as IFN-α2 (IFN-α 2 and IFN-λ1 have five cysteines, IFN-λ2 and IFN-λ3 have seven). The three-dimensional structure of IFN-λ1, IFN-λ2, or IFN-λ3 has not yet been determined; however, it is possible that it will be similar to IL-19 subfamily, since the first helix of IFN-α2 (Radhakrishnan et al., 1996) is shorter than that of IL-10 and somewhat similar to helix B of IL-19.

III. CYTOKINE/RECEPTOR COMPLEXES

As it is already mentioned above, cellular cytokines, including the IL-19 subfamily, employ different from IL-10 receptor systems, although they very often overlap and IL-10R2 is sometimes utilized as the second receptor chain, IL-10R1 is never used.

It was shown that IL-19, IL-20, and IL-24 signal through the same two chains, IL-20R1 and IL-20R2 (Parrish-Novak et al., 2002; Pletnev et al., 2003); in addition, IL-20 and IL-24 signal through the pair IL-22R1/IL-20R2

(Dumoutier *et al.*, 2001a; Ramesh *et al.*, 2003; Wang *et al.*, 2002) and IL-22 uses IL-22R1 and IL-10R2 (Dumoutier *et al.*, 2000b; Kotenko *et al.*, 2001a). It was also shown that despite what had been commonly accepted, IL-20R2 is a high-affinity receptor chain in the case of IL-19 and IL-20. It binds the ligand first (Pletnev *et al.*, 2003), forming a binding site for the long receptor chain IL-20R1, which binds the second. It is very likely that IL-24 binds to IL-20R2 first too. In the receptor pair IL-20R1/IL-10R2 of IL-26 (Sheikh *et al.*, 2004), both receptor chains always play a role of low-affinity receptor chains in other complexes (Logsdon *et al.*, 2002, 2004; Pletnev *et al.*, 2003). Although IL-26 binds to soluble receptor/extracellular domain of IL-20R1, it still remains to be explored if there is a possibility for a new IL-26 receptor chain.

Since the three-dimensional structure of these cytokines is similar to the structure of one domain of IL-10 and all receptors belong to the same family, it is reasonable to assume that receptor-binding sites and general topology of the complexes should also be somewhat similar. The simple superposition of IL-19 onto one domain of IL-10 bound to sIL-10R1 (Josephson *et al.*, 2001) allowed to mark the IL-19 surface with amino acid residues which may potentially interact with the receptor (Chang *et al.*, 2003); these included helix B, loop BC, and helix G. No crystal structures of any of the IL-19 subfamily ligand/receptor complexes are available at present; however, a model of the complex of IL-22 with sIL-22R1, generated on the basis of the crystal structure of the complex of hIL-10/sIL-10R1, was published (Logsdon *et al.*, 2002). Not only was the sIL-22R1 structure generated in this model but IL-22 was modeled also, since no crystal structure of IL-22 was available at that time. Nevertheless, amino acid residues which might be involved in specific contacts with the receptor were identified and they were essentially the same as the ones found with the help of the crystal structure of IL-22$_{EC}$ (Nagem *et al.*, 2002b), and later IL-22$_{DS}$ (Xu *et al.*, 2005). It is to note that intermolecular interface in a dimer of IL-22 molecules in the asymmetric part of the crystal unit cell included a receptor-binding site with one of the arginines playing the role of Arg-96 of the receptor (Nagem *et al.*, 2002b; Xu *et al.*, 2005), making extensive hydrogen bonds similar to those found in the hIL-10/sIL-10R1 complex.

IV. CONCLUDING REMARKS

Most of the cellular members of the IL-10 family of cytokines also belong to the IL-19 subfamily, including IL-19, IL-20, IL-22, and IL-24. Even though the crystal structures of IFN-λ1, IFN-λ2, and IFN-λ3 have not been determined and amino acid sequence with IL-10 is quite low, it is likely that they also belong to the IL-19 subfamily. Classification for IL-26 is not clear because of its aggregation state; it is active in both monomer and dimer.

At the same time the receptor system for this cytokine overlaps with the members of IL-19 subfamily and this may indicate that the structure of the IL-26 is similar to other members of IL-19 subfamily. All eight members (excluding IL-10) of cellular homologs of IL-10 signal with the help of three long receptor chains (first receptors) IL-20R1, IL-22R1, and IFN-Rλ, and two short receptor chains (second receptors) IL-10R2 and IL-20R2, in addition, IL-20 and IL-24 each use two different combinations of these receptors. Since the biological functions of all these cytokines are different, an idea of tissue-specific expression of appropriate receptors and affinity modulation is quite plausible. It is known that the second receptor chain IL-10R2, for example, is constitutively expressed in a variety of cells (Gibbs and Pennica, 1997; Lutfalla *et al.*, 1993) and different levels of expression of the first receptor chain will certainly affect the formation of the signaling ternary complex depending on the affinity of the first chain toward corresponding cytokine. It is obvious that structural information on structure of the ternary complex similar to what has been obtained for signaling ternary complex of IL-6/IL-6R1/gp130 (Boulanger *et al.*, 2003) or quaternary complex of IL-2/IL-2R1/IL-2R2/IL-2R3 (Wang *et al.*, 2005) would be invaluable and likely to produce some answers on the issue of how different ligands initiate their signals by using overlapping receptor chains.

ACKNOWLEDGMENT

I would like to thank Dr. Alexander Wlodawer for critical reading of the chapter and helpful discussions. This research was supported by the Intramural Research Program of the NIH, National Cancer Institute, Center for Cancer Research.

REFERENCES

Bach, E. A., Aguet, M., and Schreiber, R. D. (1997). The IFN gamma receptor: A paradigm for cytokine receptor signaling. *Annu. Rev. Immunol.* **15**, 563–591.

Bartlett, N. W., Dumoutier, L., Renauld, J. C., Kotenko, S. V., McVey, C. E., Lee, H. J., and Smith, G. L. (2004). A new member of the interleukin 10-related cytokine family encoded by a poxvirus. *J. Gen. Virol.* **85**, 1401–1412.

Bazan, J. F. (1990). Structural design and molecular evolution of a cytokine receptor superfamily. *Proc. Natl. Acad. Sci. USA* **87**, 6934–6938.

Blumberg, H., Conklin, D., Xu, W. F., Grossmann, A., Brender, T., Carollo, S., Eagan, M., Foster, D., Haldeman, B. A., Hammond, A., Haugen, H., Jelinek, L., *et al.* (2001). Interleukin 20: Discovery, receptor identification, and role in epidermal function. *Cell* **104**, 9–19.

Boulanger, M. J., Chow, D. C., Brevnova, E. E., and Garcia, K. C. (2003). Hexameric structure and assembly of the interleukin-6/IL-6 alpha-receptor/gp130 complex. *Science* **300**, 2101–2104.

Carson, M. (1991). RIBBONS 4.0. *J. Appl. Crystallogr.* **24**, 958–961.

Caudell, E. G., Mumm, J. B., Poindexter, N., Ekmekcioglu, S., Mhashilkar, A. M., Yang, X. H., Retter, M. W., Hill, P., Chada, S., and Grimm, E. A. (2002). The protein product of the tumor suppressor gene, melanoma differentiation-associated gene 7, exhibits immunostimulatory activity and is designated IL-24. *J. Immunol.* **168,** 6041–6046.

Chada, S., Mhashilkar, A. M., Ramesh, R., Mumm, J. B., Sutton, R. B., Bocangel, D., Zheng, M., Grimm, E. A., and Ekmekcioglu, S. (2004a). Bystander activity of Ad-mda7: Human MDA-7 protein kills melanoma cells via an IL-20 receptor-dependent but STAT3-independent mechanism. *Mol. Ther.* **10,** 1085–1095.

Chada, S., Sutton, R. B., Ekmekcioglu, S., Ellerhorst, J., Mumm, J. B., Leitner, W. W., Yang, H. Y., Sahin, A. A., Hunt, K. K., Fuson, K. L., Poindexter, N., Roth, J. A., *et al.* (2004b). MDA-7/IL-24 is a unique cytokine-tumor suppressor in the IL-10 family. *Int. Immunopharmacol.* **4,** 649–667.

Chang, C., Magracheva, E., Kozlov, S., Fong, S., Tobin, G., Kotenko, S., Wlodawer, A., and Zdanov, A. (2003). Crystal structure of interleukin-19 defines a new subfamily of helical cytokines. *J. Biol. Chem.* **278,** 3308–3313.

Chen, J., Chada, S., Mhashilkar, A., and Miano, J. M. (2003). Tumor suppressor MDA-7/IL-24 selectively inhibits vascular smooth muscle cell growth and migration. *Mol. Ther.* **8,** 220–229.

Cunningham, C. C., Chada, S., Merritt, J. A., Tong, A., Senzer, N., Zhang, Y., Mhashilkar, A., Parker, K., Vukelja, S., Richards, D., Hood, J., Coffee, K., *et al.* (2005). Clinical and local biological effects of an intratumoral injection of mda-7 (IL24; INGN 241) in patients with advanced carcinoma: A phase I study. *Mol. Ther.* **11,** 149–159.

Decker, T., and Meinke, A. (1997). Jaks, Stats and the immune system. *Immunobiology* **198,** 99–111.

Dumoutier, L., and Renauld, J. C. (2002). Viral and cellular interleukin-10 (IL-10)-related cytokines: From structures to functions. *Eur. Cytokine Netw.* **13,** 5–15.

Dumoutier, L., Louahed, J., and Renauld, J. C. (2000a). Cloning and characterization of IL-10-related T cell-derived inducible factor (IL-TIF), a novel cytokine structurally related to IL-10 and inducible by IL-9. *J. Immunol.* **164,** 1814–1819.

Dumoutier, L., Van Roost, E., Colau, D., and Renauld, J. C. (2000b). Human interleukin-10-related T cell-derived inducible factor: Molecular cloning and functional characterization as an hepatocyte-stimulating factor. *Proc. Natl. Acad. Sci. USA* **97,** 10144–10149.

Dumoutier, L., Leemans, C., Lejeune, D., Kotenko, S. V., and Renauld, J. C. (2001a). Cutting edge: STAT activation by IL-19, IL-20 and mda-7 through IL-20 receptor complexes of two types. *J. Immunol.* **167,** 3545–3549.

Dumoutier, L., Lejeune, D., Colau, D., and Renauld, J. C. (2001b). Cloning and characterization of IL-22 binding protein, a natural antagonist of IL-10-related T cell-derived inducible factor/IL-22. *J. Immunol.* **166,** 7090–7095.

Dumoutier, L., Tounsi, A., Michiels, T., Sommereyns, C., Kotenko, S. V., and Renauld, J. C. (2004). Role of the interleukin (IL)-28 receptor tyrosine residues for antiviral and antiproliferative activity of IL-29/interferon-lambda 1: Similarities with type I interferon signaling. *J. Biol. Chem.* **279,** 32269–32274.

Ekmekcioglu, S., Ellerhorst, J., Mhashilkar, A. M., Sahin, A. A., Read, C. M., Prieto, V. G., Chada, S., and Grimm, E. A. (2001). Down-regulated melanoma differentiation associated gene (mda-7) expression in human melanomas. *Int. J. Cancer* **94,** 54–59.

Fickenscher, H., and Pirzer, H. (2004). Interleukin-26. *Int. Immunopharmacol.* **4,** 609–613.

Fickenscher, H., Hor, S., Kupers, H., Knappe, A., Wittmann, S., and Sticht, H. (2002). The interleukin-10 family of cytokines. *Trends Immunol.* **23,** 89–96.

Fleming, S. B., McCaughan, C. A., Andrews, A. E., Nash, A. D., and Mercer, A. A. (1997). A homolog of interleukin-10 is encoded by the poxvirus orf virus. *J. Virol.* **71,** 4857–4861.

Fleming, S. B., Haig, D. M., Nettleton, P., Reid, H. W., McCaughan, C. A., Wise, L. M., and Mercer, A. (2000). Sequence and functional analysis of a homolog of interleukin-10 encoded by the parapoxvirus orf virus. *Virus Genes* **21,** 85–95.

Gallagher, G., Dickensheets, H., Eskdale, J., Izotova, L. S., Mirochnitchenko, O. V., Peat, J. D., Vazquez, N., Pestka, S., Donnelly, R. P., and Kotenko, S. V. (2000). Cloning, expression and initial characterization of interleukin-19 (IL-19), a novel homologue of human interleukin-10 (IL-10). *Genes Immun.* **1**, 442–450.

Genetics Computer Group. (1994). *Program Manual for the GCG Package, Ver. 8.* Madison, WI.

Gibbs, V. C., and Pennica, D. (1997). CRF2–4: Isolation of cDNA clones encoding the human and mouse proteins. *Gene* **186**, 97–101.

Ho, A. S. Y., Liu, Y., Khan, T. A., Hsu, D.-H., Bazan, J. F., and Moore, K. W. (1993). A receptor for interleukin 10 is related to interferon receptors. *Proc. Natl. Acad. Sci. USA* **90**, 11267–11271.

Hor, S., Pirzer, H., Dumoutier, L., Bauer, F., Wittmann, S., Sticht, H., Renauld, J. C., de Waal, M. R., and Fickenscher, H. (2004). The T-cell lymphokine interleukin-26 targets epithelial cells through the interleukin-20 receptor 1 and interleukin-10 receptor 2 chains. *J. Biol. Chem.* **279**, 33343–33351.

Hsu, D. H., de Waal Malefyt, R., Fiorentino, D. F., Dang, M. N., Vieira, P., de Vries, J., Spits, H., Mosmann, T. R., and Moore, K. W. (1990). Expression of interleukin-10 activity by Epstein-Barr virus protein BCRF1. *Science* **250**, 830–832.

Huang, E. Y., Madireddi, M. T., Gopalkrishnan, R. V., Leszczyniecka, M., Su, Z., Lebedeva, I. V., Kang, D., Jiang, H., Lin, J. J., Alexandre, D., Chen, Y., Vozhilla, N., *et al.* (2001). Genomic structure, chromosomal localization and expression profile of a novel melanoma differentiation associated (mda-7) gene with cancer specific growth suppressing and apoptosis inducing properties. *Oncogene* **20**, 7051–7063.

Igawa, D., Sakai, M., and Savan, R. (2005). An unexpected discovery of two interferon gamma-like genes along with interleukin (IL)-22 and -26 from teleost: IL-22 and -26 genes have been described for the first time outside mammals. *Mol. Immunol.* **43**, 999–1009.

Jiang, H., Lin, J. J., Su, Z. Z., Goldstein, N. I., and Fisher, P. B. (1995). Subtraction hybridization identifies a novel melanoma differentiation associated gene, mda-7, modulated during human melanoma differentiation, growth and progression. *Oncogene* **11**, 2477–2486.

Jiang, H., Su, Z. Z., Lin, J. J., Goldstein, N. I., Young, C. S., and Fisher, P. B. (1996). The melanoma differentiation associated gene mda-7 suppresses cancer cell growth. *Proc. Natl. Acad. Sci. USA* **93**, 9160–9165.

Jones, B. C., Logsdon, N. J., Josephson, K., Cook, J., Barry, P. A., and Walter, M. R. (2002). Crystal structure of human cytomegalovirus IL-10 bound to soluble human IL-10R1. *Proc. Natl. Acad. Sci. USA* **99**, 9404–9409.

Jordan, W. J., Eskdale, J., Boniotto, M., Lennon, G. P., Peat, J., Campbell, J. D., and Gallagher, G. (2005). Human IL-19 regulates immunity through auto-induction of IL-19 and production of IL-10. *Eur. J. Immunol.* **35**, 1576–1582.

Josephson, K., Logsdon, N. J., and Walter, M. R. (2001). Crystal structure of the IL-10/IL-10R1 complex reveals a shared receptor binding site. *Immunity* **15**, 35–46.

Knappe, A., Hor, S., Wittmann, S., and Fickenscher, H. (2000). Induction of a novel cellular homolog of interleukin-10, AK155, by transformation of T lymphocytes with herpesvirus saimiri. *J. Virol.* **74**, 3881–3887.

Kotenko, S. V. (2002). The family of IL10 related cytokines and their receptors: Related, but to what extent? *Cytokine Growth Factor Rev.* **13**, 223–240.

Kotenko, S. V., and Langer, J. A. (2004). Full house: 12 receptors for 27 cytokines. *Int. Immunopharmacol.* **4**, 593–608.

Kotenko, S. V., and Pestka, S. (2000). Jak-Stat signal transduction pathway through the eyes of cytokine class II receptor complexes. *Oncogene* **19**, 2557–2565.

Kotenko, S. V., Krause, C. D., Izotova, L. S., Pollack, B. P., Wu, W., and Pestka, S. (1997). Identification and functional characterization of a second chain of the interleukin-10 receptor complex. *EMBO J.* **16**, 5894–5903.

Kotenko, S. V., Saccani, S., Izotova, L. S., Mirochnitchenko, O. V., and Pestka, S. (2000). Human cytomegalovirus harbors its own unique IL-10 homolog (cmvIL-10). *Proc. Natl. Acad. Sci. USA* **97**, 1695–1700.

Kotenko, S. V., Izotova, L. S., Mirochnitchenko, O. V., Esterova, E., Dickensheets, H., Donnelly, R. P., and Pestka, S. (2001a). Identification of the functional interleukin-22 (IL-22) receptor complex: The IL-10R2 chain (IL-10Rbeta) is a common chain of both the IL-10 and IL-22 (IL-10-related T cell-derived inducible factor, IL-TIF) receptor complexes. *J. Biol. Chem.* **276**, 2725–2732.

Kotenko, S. V., Izotova, L. S., Mirochnitchenko, O. V., Estcrova, E., Dickensheets, H., Donnelly, R. P., and Pestka, S. (2001b). Identification, cloning, and characterization of a novel soluble receptor that binds IL-22 and neutralizes its activity. *J. Immunol.* **166**, 7096–7103.

Kotenko, S. V., Gallagher, G., Baurin, V. V., Lewis-Antes, A., Shen, M., Shah, N. K., Langer, J. A., Sheikh, F., Dickensheets, H., and Donnelly, R. P. (2003). IFN-lambdas mediate antiviral protection through a distinct class II cytokine receptor complex. *Nat. Immunol.* **4**, 69–77.

Lee, H. J., Essani, K., and Smith, G. L. (2001). The genome sequence of Yaba-like disease virus, a yatapoxvirus. *Virology* **281**, 170–192.

Liu, Y., Wei, S. H. Y., Ho, A. S. Y., Malefyt, R. W., and Moore, K. W. (1994). Expression cloning and characterization of a human IL-10 receptor. *J. Immunol.* **152**, 1821–1829.

Liu, Y., de Waal Malefyt, R., Briere, F., Parham, C., Bridon, J. M., Banchereau, J., Moore, K. W., and Xu, J. (1997). The EBV IL-10 homolog is a selective agonist with impaired binding to the IL-10 receptor. *J. Immunol.* **158**, 605–613.

Lockridge, K. M., Zhou, S. S., Kravitz, R. H., Johnson, J. L., Sawai, E. T., Blewett, E. L., and Barry, P. A. (2000). Primate cytomegaloviruses encode and express an IL-10-like protein. *Virology* **268**, 272–280.

Logsdon, N. J., Jones, B. C., Josephson, K., Cook, J., and Walter, M. R. (2002). Comparison of interleukin-22 and interleukin-10 soluble receptor complexes. *J. Interferon Cytokine Res.* **22**, 1099–1112.

Logsdon, N. J., Jones, B. C., Allman, J. C., Izotova, L., Schwartz, B., Pestka, S., and Walter, M. R. (2004). The IL-10R2 binding hot spot on IL-22 is located on the N-terminal helix and is dependent on N-linked glycosylation. *J. Mol. Biol.* **342**, 503–514.

Lutfalla, G., Gardiner, K., and Uze, G. (1993). A new member of the cytokine receptor gene family maps on chromosome 21 at less than 35 kb from IFNAR. *Genomics* **16**, 366–373.

Moore, K. W., Vieira, P., Fiorentino, D. F., Trounstine, M. L., Khan, T. A., and Mosmann, T. R. (1990). Homology of cytokine synthesis inhibitory factor (IL-10) to the Epstein-Barr virus gene BCRFI. *Science* **248**, 1230–1234.

Moore, K. W., de Waal, M. R., Coffman, R. L., and O'Garra, A. (2001). Interleukin-10 and the interleukin-10 receptor. *Annu. Rev. Immunol.* **19**, 683–765.

Nagem, R. A., Lucchesi, K. W., Colau, D., Dumoutier, L., Renauld, J. C., and Polikarpov, I. (2002a). Crystallization and synchrotron X-ray diffraction studies of human interleukin-22. *Acta Crystallogr. D Biol. Crystallogr.* **58**, 529–530.

Nagem, R. A. P., Colau, D., Dumoutier, L., Renauld, J.-C., Ogata, C., and Polikarpov, I. (2002b). Crystal structure of recombinant human interleukin-22. *Structure* **10**, 1051–1062.

Ozaki, K., and Leonard, W. J. (2002). Cytokine and cytokine receptor pleiotropy and redundancy. *J. Biol. Chem.* **277**, 29355–29358.

Parrish-Novak, J., Xu, W., Brender, T., Yao, L., Jones, C., West, J., Brandt, C., Jelinek, L., Madden, K., McKernan, P. A., Foster, D. C., Jaspers, S., *et al.* (2002). Interleukins 19, 20, and 24 signal through two distinct receptor complexes. Differences in receptor-ligand interactions mediate unique biological functions. *J. Biol. Chem.* **277**, 47517–47523.

Pestka, S., Kotenko, S. V., Muthukumaran, G., Izotova, L. S., Cook, J. R., and Garotta, G. (1997). The interferon gamma (IFN-gamma) receptor: A paradigm for the multichain cytokine receptor. *Cytokine Growth Factor Rev.* **8**, 189–206.

Pestka, S., Krause, C. D., Sarkar, D., Walter, M. R., Shi, Y., and Fisher, P. B. (2004). Interleukin-10 and related cytokines and receptors. *Annu. Rev. Immunol.* **22,** 929–979.

Pletnev, S., Magracheva, E., Kozlov, S., Tobin, G., Kotenko, S. V., Wlodawer, A., and Zdanov, A. (2003). Characterization of the recombinant extracellular domains of human interleukin-20 receptors and their complexes with interleukin-19 and interleukin-20. *Biochemistry* **42,** 12617–12624.

Presnell, S. R., and Cohen, F. E. (1989). Topological distribution of four-α-helix bundles. *Proc. Natl. Acad. Sci. USA* **86,** 6592–6596.

Radhakrishnan, R., Walter, L. J., Hruza, A., Reichert, P., Trotta, P. P., Nagabhushan, T. L., and Walter, M. R. (1996). Zinc-mediated dimer of human interferon-alpha 2b revealed by X-ray crystallography. *Structure* **4,** 1453–1463.

Ramesh, R., Mhashilkar, A. M., Tanaka, F., Saito, Y., Branch, C. D., Sieger, K., Mumm, J. B., Stewart, A. L., Boquio, A., Dumoutier, L., Grimm, E. A., Renauld, J. C., *et al.* (2003). Melanoma differentiation-associated gene 7/interleukin (IL)-24 is a novel ligand that regulates angiogenesis via the IL-22 receptor. *Cancer Res.* **63,** 5105–5113.

Renauld, J. C. (2003). Class II cytokine receptors and their ligands: Key antiviral and inflammatory modulators. *Nat. Rev. Immunol.* **3,** 667–676.

Rode, H. J., Janssen, W., Rosen-Wolff, A., Bugert, J. J., Thein, P., Becker, Y., and Darai, G. (1993). The genome of equine herpesvirus type 2 harbors an interleukin 10 (IL10)-like gene. *Virus Genes* **7,** 111–116.

Rozwarski, D. A., Gronenborn, A. M., Clore, G. M., Bazan, J. F., Bohm, A., Wlodawer, A., Hatada, M., and Karplus, P. A. (1994). Structural comparisons among the short-chain helical cytokines. *Structure* **2,** 159–173.

Schindler, C., and Darnell, J. E., Jr. (1995). Transcriptional responses to polypeptide ligands: The JAK-STAT pathway. *Annu. Rev. Biochem.* **64,** 621–651.

Sheikh, F., Baurin, V. V., Lewis-Antes, A., Shah, N. K., Smirnov, S. V., Anantha, S., Dickensheets, H., Dumoutier, L., Renauld, J. C., Zdanov, A., Donnelly, R. P., and Kotenko, S. V. (2004). Cutting edge: IL-26 signals through a novel receptor complex composed of IL-20 receptor 1 and IL-10 receptor 2. *J. Immunol.* **172,** 2006–2010.

Sheppard, P., Kindsvogel, W., Xu, W., Henderson, K., Schlutsmeyer, S., Whitmore, T. E., Kuestner, R., Garrigues, U., Birks, C., Roraback, J., Ostrander, C., Dong, D., *et al.* (2003). IL-28, IL-29 and their class II cytokine receptor IL-28R. *Nat. Immunol.* **4,** 63–68.

Vieira, P., Malefyt, R. W., Dang, M.-N., Johnson, K. E., Kastelein, R., Fiorentino, D. F., DeVries, J. E., Roncarolo, M.-G., Mosmann, T. R., and Moore, K. W. (1991). Isolation and expression of human cytokine synthesis inhibitory factor cDNA clones: Homology to Epstein-Barr virus open reading frame BCRFI. *Proc. Natl. Acad. Sci. USA* **88,** 1172–1176.

Walter, M. R. (2004). Structural analysis of IL-10 and type I interferon family members and their complexes with receptor. *Adv. Protein Chem.* **68,** 171–223.

Walter, M. R., and Nagabhushan, T. L. (1995). Crystal structure of interleukin 10 reveals an interferon gamma-like fold. *Biochemistry* **34,** 12118–12125.

Wang, M., Tan, Z., Zhang, R., Kotenko, S. V., and Liang, P. (2002). Interleukin 24 (MDA-7/ MOB-5) signals through two heterodimeric receptors, IL-22R1/IL-20R2 and IL-20R1/ IL-20R2. *J. Biol. Chem.* **277,** 7341–7347.

Wang, X., Rickert, M., and Garcia, K. C. (2005). Structure of the quaternary complex of interleukin-2 with its alpha, beta, and gammac receptors. *Science* **310,** 1159–1163.

Wolk, K., Kunz, S., Asadullah, K., and Sabat, R. (2002). Cutting edge: Immune cells as sources and targets of the IL-10 family members? *J. Immunol.* **168,** 5397–5402.

Xie, M. H., Aggarwal, S., Ho, W. H., Foster, J., Zhang, Z., Stinson, J., Wood, W. I., Goddard, A. D., and Gurney, A. L. (2000). Interleukin (IL)-22, a novel human cytokine that signals through the interferon receptor-related proteins CRF2-4 and IL-22R. *J. Biol. Chem.* **275,** 31335–31339.

Xu, T., Logsdon, N. J., and Walter, M. R. (2004). Crystallization and X-ray diffraction analysis of insect-cell-derived IL-22. *Acta Crystallogr. D Biol. Crystallogr.* **60,** 1295–1298.

Xu, T., Logsdon, N. J., and Walter, M. R. (2005). Structure of insect-cell-derived IL-22. *Acta Crystallogr. D Biol. Crystallogr.* **61,** 942–950.

Xu, W., Presnell, S. R., Parrish-Novak, J., Kindsvogel, W., Jaspers, S., Chen, Z., Dillon, S. R., Gao, Z., Gilbert, T., Madden, K., Schlutsmeyer, S., Yao, L., *et al.* (2001). A soluble class II cytokine receptor, IL-22RA2, is a naturally occurring IL-22 antagonist. *Proc. Natl. Acad. Sci. USA* **98,** 9511–9516.

Yoon, S. I., Jones, B. C., Logsdon, N. J., and Walter, M. R. (2005). Same structure, different function crystal structure of the Epstein-Barr virus IL-10 bound to the soluble IL-10R1 chain. *Structure (Camb.)* **13,** 551–564.

Zdanov, A. (2004). Structural features of the interleukin-10 family of cytokines. *Curr. Pharm. Des.* **10,** 3873–3884.

Zdanov, A., Schalk-Hihi, C., Gustchina, A., Tsang, M., Weatherbee, J., and Wlodawer, A. (1995). Crystal structure of interleukin-10 reveals the functional dimer with an unexpected topological similarity to interferon γ. *Structure* **3,** 591–601.

Zdanov, A., Schalk-Hihi, C., and Wlodawer, A. (1996). Crystal structure of human interleukin-10 at 1.6 Å resolution and a model of a complex with its soluble receptor. *Protein Sci.* **5,** 1955–1962.

Zdanov, A., Schalk-Hihi, C., Menon, S., Moore, K. W., and Wlodawer, A. (1997). Crystal structure of Epstein-Barr virus protein BCRF1, a homolog of cellular interleukin-10. *J. Mol. Biol.* **268,** 460–467.

4

INTERLEUKIN-22 AND ITS CRYSTAL STRUCTURE

RONALDO ALVES PINTO NAGEM,* JOSÉ RIBAMAR
FERREIRA JÚNIOR,[†] LAURE DUMOUTIER,[‡]
JEAN-CHRISTOPHE RENAULD,[‡] AND
IGOR POLIKARPOV[†]

*Departamento de Bioquímica e Imunologia, Instituto de Ciências Biológicas
Universidade Federal de Minas Gerais, Avenida Antônio Carlos
6627 CEP 31270910, Belo Horizonte, MG, Brazil
[†]Instituto de Física de São Carlos, Universidade de São Paulo
Avenida Trabalhador Sãocarlense, 400 CEP 13560–970
São Carlos, São Paulo, Brazil
[‡]Ludwig Institute for Cancer Research, Brussels Branch
The Experimental Medicine Unit
Christian de Duve Institute of Cellular Pathology
Université de Louvain, Brussels, Belgium

Vitamins and Hormones, Volume 74
Copyright 2006, Elsevier Inc. All rights reserved.

0083-6729/06 $35.00
DOI: 10.1016/S0083-6729(06)74004-3

A. *Putative Structural Interactions between IL-22 and*
   Its Receptors Binary Complex
B. *Ternary Complex*
References

Interleukin-22 (IL-22) is a cytokine that regulates the production of acute phase proteins of the immunological response. On binding to its cognate receptor (IL-22R1), which is associated to the interleukin-10 receptor 2 (IL-10R2), IL-22 promotes activation of signal transducer and activator of transcription (STAT) pathway and several other cellular responses. A soluble receptor termed interleukin-22 binding protein (IL-22BP) is also able to bind to IL-22 as a natural protein antagonist, and probably provides systemic regulation of IL-22 activity. This inflammatory response system is analyzed here in terms of its molecular physiology and structural assembly. Three-dimensional (3D) model of IL-22 and structural basis of its interactions with the cognate receptors are discussed. © 2006 Elsevier Inc.

I. INTERLEUKIN-22 IDENTIFICATION AND GENE EXPRESSION

Interleukin-22 (IL-22) is a cytokine that was first identified by cDNA subtraction method in a screen for genes induced by IL-9 in BW5147 murine T lymphoma cells (Dumoutier *et al.*, 2000a). It encodes a glycosylated 179 amino acids long protein (NP_065386 Genbank entry), including a potential signal peptide, and bears 22% identity to IL-10, hence its original designation: IL-10-related T cell–derived inducible factor (IL-TIF). The expression of this protein is induced by IL-9 in thymic lymphomas, T helper cells and mast cells, or by ConA activated freshly isolated splenocytes, and its constitutive expression was detected in thymus and brain. A further step in the analysis of IL-22 was the identification of the human ortholog, which shares 79% amino acid identity with mouse IL-22 and 25% identity with human IL-10 (NP_000563 Genbank entry) (Dumoutier *et al.*, 2000c; Xie *et al.*, 2000). Recombinant IL-22 upregulates the production of acute phase reactants such as serum amyloid A, α1-antichymotrypsin, and haptoglobin in HepG2 human hepatoma cells (Dumoutier *et al.*, 2000c). Similar induction of acute phase reactants was also detected in mouse liver upon IL-22 injection, and the expression of this interleukin was induced after lipopolysaccharide (LPS) injection, indicating the involvement of IL-22 in the inflammatory response *in vivo*.

A. IL-22 GENOMIC ORGANIZATION

The mapping of the human IL-22 gene by fluorescent *in situ* hybridization (FISH) and by polymerase chain reaction (PCR) screening of the GeneBridge 4 radiation panel (Walter *et al.*, 1994) specified its location on chromosome 12q15, approximately 90 kb from interferon-γ (IFN-γ) and 30 kb from IL-26 genes (Dumoutier *et al.*, 2000b), and showed that these three genes are arranged in head to tail orientation. Human IL-22 is most probably a single copy gene and its genomic structure presents five introns and six exons, bearing similarity in size and organization to IL-10, except for a short noncoding exon, 24 nucleotides downstream a putative TATA box, which is not present in IL-10 and IL-26.

Murine IL-22 is very similar in genomic organization to the human counterpart. It is located on chromosome 10, also close to the *IFN-γ* gene, although the sequencing of the mouse genome has not been completed between these two genes. The gene is spreading over about 6 kb, and contains five introns and six exons, which are well conserved between the human and mouse (from 74% to 86% nucleotide identity), whereas the promoter region displays 77% nucleotide identity over 0.8 kb (Dumoutier *et al.*, 2000b). There is a single copy of the IL-22 gene in BALB/c and DBA/2 mice, but polymorphism analysis showed gene duplication in other strains, such as C57B1/6, FVB, and 129, and the two copies which show 98% nucleotide identity in the coding region were initially designated IL-TIFα and IL-TIFβ. Moreover, they differ by a 658 nucleotide deletion in IL-TIFβ, including the first noncoding exon and a 603 nucleotides segment from the putative promoter, suggesting that the IL-TIFβ gene is not functional.

B. IL-22 ORTHOLOGS

To date, complete amino acid sequences for human IL-22 orthologs have been identified in a few mammalian species such as dog (*Canis familiaris*, dogIL-22, XP_538274 Genbank entry), cow (*Bos Taurus*, cowIL-22, XP_584453 Genbank entry), and rat (*Rattus norvegicus*, ratIL-22, XP_576228 Ensembl entry). As alluded to an earlier discussion, in certain mouse strains, the IL-22 gene is found as a double copy gene such that in *Mus musculus* they have been also termed interleukin-22 alpha (mouIL-22α, NP_058667 Genbank entry) and beta (mouIL-22β, NP_473420 Genbank entry) (Dumoutier *et al.*, 2000b). In addition, incomplete amino acid sequences from pig (*Sus scrofa*, pigIL-22, AAX33671 Genbank entry) and chimpanzee (*Pan troglodytes*, chiIL-22, ENSPTRP00000008824, and ENSPTRP00000008825 Ensembl entries) as well as nonannotated genes in rhesus macaque (*Macaca mulatta*, rheIL-22, contig_76029 Ensembl entry) and elephant (*Loxodonta africana*, eleIL-22, contig_306674 Ensembl entry) indicate that IL-22 is also present in these mammalian species.

The use of comparative genomics allows one to suggest the existence of IL-22 orthologs in nonmammals such as in chicken (*Gallus gallus*, cckIL-22, XP_416079 Genbank entry). However, the fish interleukin-22 (*Danio rerio*, fisIL-22, truncated version of NP_001018628 Ensembl entry) was the first IL-22 ortholog to be discovered outside of realm of mammals (Igawa *et al.*, 2006).

Primary structure alignments of IL-22 orthologs (Fig. 1) indicate that among available mammalian cytokines the amino acid sequence is highly conserved with identity in the range of 60% (cowIL-22 and ratIL-22) to 95% (humIL-22 and rheIL-22). On the other hand, IL-22 amino acid sequences

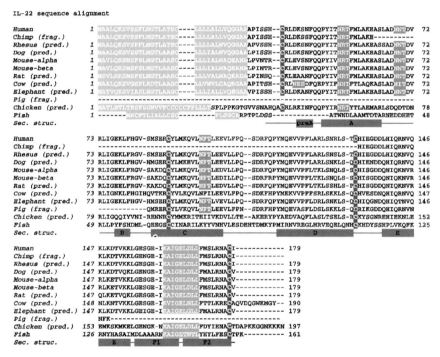

FIGURE 1. Amino acid sequence alignment of IL-22 orthologs. Amino acid sequences were retrieved from deposited Genbank and Ensembl entries reported in text. Predicted sequences (*pred.*) and partial sequences (*frag.*) are also shown. Predicted signal peptides are colored in cyan, potential glycosylation sites are colored in orange, and cysteine residues potentially involved in disulfide bridges are highlighted in green. Human interleukin-22 secondary structure elements (red for helices and blue for loops) are shown under the alignment. Box shaded in gray is the characteristic IL-10-family signature. Full-length amino acid sequences (signal peptides included) were considered for numbering. This and subsequent primary structure alignments were performed with ClustalW software (Thompson *et al.*, 1994) using the web interface (http://www.ebi.ac.uk/clustalw) at the European Bioinformatics Institute. (See Color Insert.)

from chicken and fish display limited similarity with mammal orthologs. Chicken interleukin-22 shares only 39% identity with rheIL-22 while fisIL-22 is only very distantly related to the closest ortholog, cowIL-22 (18% amino acid sequence identity).

Even though a number of differences are observed among primary structures of IL-22s, all of them have a molecular mass of 18–22 kDa, a predicted 19–33 amino acid long signal peptide (SignalP 3.0 Server at http://www.cbs.dtu.dk/services/SignalP/) (Bendtsen *et al.*, 2004) and the characteristic IL-10-family signature KAIGELDLL at the helix F (see in a later section). They also display a fairly conserved disulfide bridge pattern (Cys40-Cys132 and Cys89-Cys178; humIL-22 numbering) that may be directly involved in IL-22 folding (Nagem *et al.*, 2002). It might be important to mention that most of the available IL-22 sequences analyzed in this work have two inframe methionines but only the second one can be aligned with IL-10. As a result, we cannot be sure which one is the real initiation codon.

The humIL-22 amino acid sequence contains three N-linked glycosylation sites that are partially conserved among other mammalian orthologs (N54, N68, and N97). The IL-22 cytokine from *Bos taurus* appears to be an exception. It lacks the *N*-glycosylation site at position N97 but has an additional potential site at N43. The situation is, however, very different with chicken and fish IL-22. Only one potential N-linked glycosylation site is found in cckIL-22 (N54) and none in fisIL-22, which suggests that the putative physiological role of *N*-linked carbohydrates in IL-22 function must be somewhat different in cckIL-22 and nonexisting in fish. This fact makes them potentially interesting targets for structural and biochemical comparative analysis with their mammalian counterparts.

II. IL-22R1 IDENTIFICATION AND GENE EXPRESSION

It was experimentally determined that a functional IL-22 receptor complex, which consists of two receptor chains: IL-22R1 (CRF2–9, cytokine receptor family class 2 member 9) and IL-10R2 (CRF2–4, the second chain of the IL-10 receptor complex), is anchored to the cell surface (Kotenko *et al.*, 2001a; Xie *et al.*, 2000). This conclusion is based on the fact that monkey COS cells expressing IL-22R1 are sensitive to IL-22, whereas in Chinese hamster cells both chains IL-22R1 and IL-10R2 must be expressed to sustain IL-22 signaling through signal transducer and activator of transcription (STAT) activation (Kotenko *et al.*, 2001a). In addition, anti-IL-10R2 antibodies blocked IL-22 activity on hepatocytes (Dumoutier *et al.*, 2000c). This discovery suggested that other class 2 cytokine receptors may share the IL-10R2 chain with the IL-10 receptor complex. Later on, the involvement of IL-10R2 has been demonstrated, together with IL-20R1, in

IL-26 receptor complex (Hor *et al.*, 2004; Sheikh *et al.*, 2004), and, together with IL-28R in type 3 IFN receptors (Kotenko *et al.*, 2003; Sheppard *et al.*, 2003). Human IL-22R1 is located on the chromosome 1 and form a cytokine gene receptor cluster with interleukin-28 receptor (IL-28R1) in the chromosomal region 1p36, with both genes in head to tail orientation, and its genomic structure is composed of seven exons and six introns (obtained from http://www.ncbi.nlm.nih.gov).

Extensive database searches rewarded Tachiiri and co-workers (Tachiiri *et al.*, 2003) with the identification of the mouse IL-22R gene genomic sequence homologous to human IL-22R1. This gene, consisting of about 24 kb, was mapped to mouse chromosome 4 and its coding region is split in seven exons (Tachiiri *et al.*, 2003). Comparison of human and murine genes revealed their 71.9% identity at the amino acid level (78% and 66% for the extra- and intracellular domains, respectively). All three putative *N*-glycosylation sites in the extracellular region are also conserved between the two species as well as in the dog, rat, and bovine orthologs.

Expression of IL-22R1 is highly restricted whereas IL-10R2 expression is ubiquitous (Gurney, 2004). Northern blot analysis for IL-22R1 shows a very strong signal in pancreas and lower but detectable signals in tissues of the gastrointestinal tract, kidney, and liver (Aggarwal *et al.*, 2001). Other organs with detectable expression include the skin but not the hematopoietic organs (Gurney, 2004; Nagalakshmi *et al.*, 2004). The mouse IL-22R mRNA is constitutively expressed in organs, such as kidney, liver, and lung, but it is further upregulated in liver after LPS stimulation (Tachiiri *et al.*, 2003).

A. SIGNAL TRANSDUCTION

Cytokines activate signal transduction pathways within the cell by binding to their cognate receptors, which for most cases consist in a complex of two transmembrane proteins. All receptor complexes for IL-10-related cytokines include a long chain and a short chain, based on the length of the cytoplasmic domain of these transmembrane proteins. IL-22 signals through recognition of and binding to IL-22R1/IL-10R2 receptor complex and this binding is followed by rapid STAT pathway activation, observed in a variety of cell lines (Dumoutier *et al.*, 2000a,c; Kotenko *et al.*, 2001a; Xie *et al.*, 2000). IL-10R2 is a typical short-chain component, with only 76 amino acids in the cytoplasmic domain, whose main function seems to consist in recruiting the Tyk2 tyrosine kinase. By contrast, the longer cytoplasmic domain of IL-22R1 is responsible for the specificity of the cellular response because substitution of the intracellular domain of IL-22R1 by the similar domain of the *IFN-γR1* gene, expressed in COS cells as a chimera IL-22R1/γR1, rendered, upon IL-22 stimulation, a cellular response characteristic of IFN-γ signaling (Kotenko *et al.*, 2001a), and because truncation of the cytoplasmic

domain of IL-22R1 abolish signaling downstream activation of Janus kinases (JAKs) (Lejeune *et al.*, in preparation).

In the rat hepatoma cell line (H4IIE), IL-22 activates JAK1, Tyk2, and
STAT1, STAT3, and STAT5 inducing their phosphorylation. In addition
STAT3 S727A mutant overexpression showed that serine 727 phosphorylation is required for maximum STAT transactivation response upon IL-22
stimulation. Three major mitogen-activated protein kinase (MAPK) pathways were also activated as revealed by antibodies against the phosphorylated forms of MEK1/2, ERK1/2, p90RSK, JNK, and p38 kinase (Lejeune
et al., 2002).

III. PHYSIOLOGICAL ROLE OF IL-22

Although the conventional classification of cytokines into proinflammatory and anti-inflammatory cytokines falls short of matching the complexity
of cytokine biology, IL-10 has been shown to be one of the main anti-
inflammatory cytokines, exerting protective effects in various experimental
models of inflammation. By contrast, available data on IL-22 activities rather
point to a proinflammatory function. Both cytokines share the common
receptor chain IL-10R2 and they can be simultaneously produced in local
and systemic inflammation. This raises important questions on whether IL-10
can regulate IL-22 activity and vice versa but lack of concomitant expression
of both IL-10R1 and IL-22R1 in identical cells (Wolk *et al.*, 2005), and the
fact that both IL-10 and IL-22 have only a very low affinity for their common
IL-10R2 receptor chain (Kotenko *et al.*, 1997, 2000, 2001a), rule out this
possibility.

Two distinct approaches were used to unravel IL-22 biological targets:
screening various cell lines for STAT activation by IL-22 or screening for
IL-22R1 mRNA expression. The first approach led to the finding that IL-22
strongly activates STAT3 in hepatocytes (Dumoutier *et al.*, 2000c). In line with
the well-described roles of STAT3 in liver cells, IL-22 was thus demonstrated
to be able to induce production of acute phase response genes, such as serum
amyloid A protein, haptoglobin, and α1-antichymotrypsin (Dumoutier *et al.*,
2000c), and to have a protective effect in the ConA-induced hepatitis model by
promoting hepatocyte survival (Pan *et al.*, 2004; Radaeva *et al.*, 2004). Induction of acute phase response gene expression was further demonstrated in
pancreas cell lines (Aggarwal *et al.*, 2001).

Independently, detection of IL-22R1 receptor expression helped to identify other tissue contexts in which IL-22 is promoting cellular responses.
Besides the liver and gastrointestinal tract, IL-22 receptor complex
(IL-22R1/IL-10R2) is found in the cells of skin, digestive and respiratory
systems. In keratinocytes IL-22 stimulates the production of β-defensin
2 and 3 (Wolk *et al.*, 2004). These small cationic proteins kill bacteria, fungi,

and other viruses, and are expressed in skin and mucosal epithelia, where they create a protection wall against microbial infections (Lehrer and Ganz, 2002; Zasloff, 2002), supporting the hypothesis that on bacterial infection, IL-22 activation in skin and mucosal epithelia tissues initiates the immunoprotection of these barriers by stimulating the production of β-defensins that kill pathogens and activate local mast cells (Wolk et al., 2004). Therefore, IL-22 might play a role of a T cell mediator molecule directly promoting the innate nonspecific immunity.

In addition, IL-22 induces keratinocyte migration in an in vitro injury model, and downregulates the expression of genes associated with keratinocyte differentiation (Boniface et al., 2005). The same authors showed that IL-22 induces hyperplasia of reconstituted human epidermis in vitro, further pointing to a role for IL-22 in wound healing. Inhibition of keratinocyte differentiation and epidermis hyperplasia is also a characteristic of psoriatic lesion. Preliminary reports on IL-22 transgenic mice suggest that IL-22 constitutive expression in the skin disturbs the regulation of keratinocyte differentiation and proliferation, mimicking psoriasis in human. In line with these observations, IL-22 was shown to be expressed in skin samples from psoriasis patients but not control donors (Boniface et al., 2005; Wolk et al., 2004). Further studies are definitely required to confirm the hypothesis that IL-22, or IL-20 which can also activate the IL-22R receptor chain, plays a role in this disease, or in other inflammatory diseases, such as rheumatoid arthritis (RA), where IL-22 production was also reported (Ikeuchi et al., 2005).

IV. IL-22BP: A DECOY RECEPTOR THAT REGULATES IL-22

IL-22 binding protein (IL-22BP, also named CRF2-X, CRF2–10, IL-22-RA2, CRF2-s1) is encoded by a novel gene of the class 2 cytokine receptor family identified by screening genomic DNA databases for IL-22R1 homologues (Dumoutier et al., 2001; Gruenberg et al., 2001; Kotenko et al., 2001b; Xu et al., 2001). This soluble receptor, which lacks a hydrophobic transmembrane domain, encodes a 231 amino acids protein secreted as a 27 kDa polypeptide (Dumoutier et al., 2001; Kotenko et al., 2001b). IL-22BP contains five potential N-linked glycosylation sites and four of them are conserved in the mouse, rat, dog, and bovine species, suggesting that this protein is highly glycosylated. Comparison with other members of the family revealed that IL-22BP is 34% identical to IL-22R1 chain and 33% to the extracellular domain of IL-20R1 (subunit of IL-20R complex). IL-22BP is capable of binding IL-22 as indicated by cross-linking and direct binding experiments, and of preventing its association to the cell surface IL-22R complex, thereby inhibiting its activity in hepatocytes and intestinal or lung epithelial cells.

The human IL-22BP gene is composed of six exons spanning about 29 kb of genomic DNA. It is physically located on human chromosome 6, at about 24 kb from the *IFN-γR1* gene, and approximately 100 kb from the gene encoding the IL-20R1 (CRF2–8) (Dumoutier *et al.*, 2001; Kotenko *et al.*, 2001b; Xu *et al.*, 2001). This chromosome region is associated to neonatal, type II, and type I diabetes mellitus and with several other disorders (Arthur *et al.*, 1997).

The tissue distribution of IL-22BP mRNA was analyzed by reverse transcription-polymerase chain reaction (RT-PCR) and by Northern blot. The highest expression levels were observed in breast, placenta, skin; the expression was also high in spleen, gastrointestinal tract, and lungs, whereas somewhat lower levels were detected in brain, heart, thymus, pancreas, testis, and prostate (Dumoutier *et al.*, 2001; Xu *et al.*, 2001). Many tissues expressing IL-22BP, such as skin and lungs, show mRNA variants resulting from alternative splicing (Dumoutier *et al.*, 2001; Kotenko *et al.*, 2001b; Xu *et al.*, 2001). This might represent a posttranscriptional regulation of either IL-22BP production or a way of altering its activity. So far, none of these mRNA variants has been shown to encode a protein able to bind IL-22 or to have any other biological activity.

IL-22BP is clearly an IL-22 antagonist *in vitro* and may play a role in inflammatory, autoimmune, and cancer diseases. It could also be useful as a therapeutic agent for pathologies associated to IL-22 overproduction. Although precise physiological roles of IL-22BP still remain to be elucidated, it is most likely that a secretion of the soluble IL-22BP into the circulation would provide systemic inhibition of IL-22 activity. However, its inhibitory activity *in vivo* remains to be confirmed, and we cannot fully rule out the possibility that circulating IL-22BP may act as a carrier molecule form IL-22.

The murine IL-22 binding protein (mou-IL22BP) was identified by screening a mouse genomic library for a human IL-22BP homologue (Wei *et al.*, 2003; Weiss *et al.*, 2004). The mouIL-22BP gene contains five exons and four introns and the genomic structure of its coding region is similar to that of the human IL-22BP gene. Splicing variants were also detected in the lung tissue, similar to what was observed for its human counterpart, which suggests that both receptors are subject to the same regulatory mechanism.

The mouIL-22BP gene shares 67.1% amino acid sequence identity with human IL-22BP and encodes a protein of 230 amino acids, including a putative 18 amino acids hydrophobic signal peptide (Wei *et al.*, 2003; Weiss *et al.*, 2004). The predicted molecular mass of the mature protein is 24.6 kDa, but this polypeptide chain still contains six potential N-linked glycosylation sites. Murine IL-22BP production could be upregulated by LPS stimulation in mouse monocytes, suggesting a role in the immune response induced by infection. Incubation of mouIL-22BP with either mouse or human IL-22 before addition to cells neutralized STAT3 activation induced by both cytokines in human (HepG2) and rat (H4IIE) hepatoma cell lines.

V. IL-22 INFLAMMATORY SYSTEM
AND DISEASE

It has been suggested that IL-22 is involved in the regulation of inflammatory lung diseases, whose characteristic is the increase of inflammatory cells in the alveoli, even in the presence of IL-10 (Martinez et al., 1997). Supporting this hypothesis is the detection IL-22 mRNA in alveolar macrophages (AM), monocytes, and alveolar epithelial (AE) cells isolated from bronchoalveolar lavage fluid or lung tissue of patients with interstitial lung disease (ILD) (Whittington et al., 2004). In such patients, IL-22BP is expressed in AM, AE cells, and neutrophils whereas IL-22R1 is detected in only in AE. Moreover, Western blotting analysis showed that IL-22 is expressed in lower levels in patients with ILD, suggesting a role for the cytokine in the regulation of pulmonary inflammation.

Similar study examined the expression of IL-22 and IL-22R1 by RT-PCR, Western blot, and immunohistochemical analysis in RA patient's samples. IL-22 mRNA was detected in RA synovial fibroblasts and macrophages and significant levels of IL-22R1 mRNA were also expressed in RA synovial tissues (Ikeuchi et al., 2005). The presence of IL-22 and its cognate receptor may promote inflammatory responses in RA synovial tissues by inducing synovial fibroblast proliferation and production of chemokines. RA is a chronic inflammatory autoimmune disorder that causes progressive joint damage. It is elicited by inflammatory cytokines, including tumor necrosis factor-α (TNF-α—direct inducer of synovial fibroblast proliferation), IL-1β, and IL-6, which are mainly produced by macrophages (Choy and Panayi, 2001; Gitter et al., 1989), giving rise to synovitis. Neutralization of such cytokines has been proven effective in the treatment of RA; however, many patients do not respond to such therapy. It is possible that IL-22 is one member of the heterogeneous cytokine population produced by macrophages and inflammatory T cells in such cases. Therefore, inactivation studies of IL-22 with IL-22BP or any other IL-22 antagonist in animal models must be conducted to better understand the involvement of this cytokine in RA in order to design new therapy strategies.

A polymorphic intronic CA-repeat in the IFN-γ gene was reported to be associated with gender bias in susceptibility to multiple sclerosis (MS) in a Sardinian population (Goris et al., 1999; Vandenbroeck et al., 1998). Later, another linkage disequilibrium analysis of chromosome 12q14–15 delineated a 118-kb interval around IFN-γ that is involved in male versus female differential susceptibility to MS (Goris et al., 2002). However, the results of this study seems to exclude IL-22, indicating that most probably IFN-γ is the only gene (or a gene located in its immediate vicinity) linked to the susceptibility. Because IL-22 is an IFN-γ-cluster cytokine expressed in the brain (Dumoutier et al., 2000c; Xie et al., 2000) it may still have a role in neurobiology.

Finally, genetic data suggested links between the IL-22 locus and malaria (Koch *et al.*, 2005) and MS (Goris *et al.*, 2002). The genomic region linked to such diseases is the cytokine gene cluster composed of IFN-γ, IL-22, and IL-26 (IFN-γ cluster). In malaria, IFN-γ is believed to play both protective and pathological roles. Linkage disequilibrium analysis across 100 kb emcompassing the IFN-γ cluster identified several single nucleotide polymorphysms (SNP) and this variation was linked to susceptibility to disease. This analysis showed that, in particular, two IL-22 haplotypes are associated to resistance and susceptibility to severe malaria (Koch *et al.*, 2005).

VI. IL-22 TERTIARY AND QUATERNARY STRUCTURE ORGANIZATION

Although IL-22 genes have been identified in a number of organisms, only two three-dimensional (3D) crystal structures of IL-22 have been determined to date, both of a human protein. The first to be determined was the structure of recombinant human IL-22 expressed in *Escherichia coli* [humIL-22$_{Ec}$; 1M4R PDB entry (Nagem *et al.*, 2002)] while the second one was of the same human cytokine recombinantly produced in *Drosophila melanogaster* S2 cells [humIL-22$_{Dm}$; 1YKB PDB entry (Xu *et al.*, 2005)]. The crystallographic structures of humIL-22$_{Ec}$ and humIL-22$_{Dm}$ were determined at 2.0 and 2.6 Å of resolution, respectively. The 3D structure of humIL-22$_{Dm}$ is practically identical to humIL-22$_{Ec}$, set aside a bonus of additional information concerning the configuration of *N*-linked carbohydrates at the glycosylation sites (Xu *et al.*, 2005).

The crystallographic structures of humIL-22 revealed the presence of two IL-22 molecules in the humIL-22$_{Ec}$ asymmetric unit while six monomers were found in humIL-22$_{Dm}$. In both structures, the IL-22 molecules were assembled as noncovalent dimers. At a first glance this fact could indicate that the IL-22 dimer found in the crystal assymetric unit would represent the functional biological unit for this cytokine. One might expect this, given that the IL-10 forms tightly bound intertwined dimers composed of two separate IL-10 polypeptide chains (Walter and Nagabhushan, 1995; Zdanov *et al.*, 1995, 1996). However, additional structural analyses (Nagem *et al.*, 2002) and gel filtration chromatography experiments (Logsdon *et al.*, 2002) showed that IL-22 is a monomer at very low concentrations in solution and the IL-22 dimer found in crystal structure is most likely an artifact of the crystallization conditions. This notion, although *a priori* not ruling out other quaternary assemblies of IL-22, was further corroborated by the finding that IL-19, another IL-10 family member, also does not form stable intertwined dimers (Chang *et al.*, 2003) and that IL-19, together with IL-22, IL-20, and possibly IL-24, could be joined together in a subfamily of monomeric helical cytokines (Chang *et al.*, 2003; Zdanov, 2004).

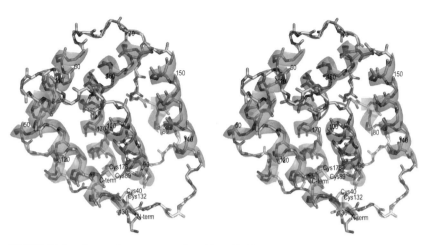

FIGURE 2.   Stereo view representation of humIL-22 monomer tertiary structure. Only main chain atoms (nitrogen in blue, carbon in orange, and oxygen in red) are represented as *stick* for clarity. Amino acid numbers are displayed in intervals of 10. Disulfide bridges (in green) and protein N- and C-terminus are also shown. Secondary structure elements are superimposed to main chain trace. Semitransparent red are used for helices and semitransparent blue for loops. The figure was created using the PyMOL molecular graphics system (DeLano, 2002). (See Color Insert.)

The humIL-22 monomer is an all-helical cytokine composed by six helices (A–F) assembled as a compact helix bundle (Fig. 2). A single turn N-terminal helix (residues 44–47), termed preA, precedes helix A and is oriented at approximately right angle with respect to helix A. Apart from helix F, all other helices (4–23 amino acids long) are practically straight. Characteristic bend of the class 2 alpha-helical cytokines (Walter, 2004), also observed in the structures of IFN-γ (Ealick *et al.*, 1991; Randal and Kossiakoff, 2000; Samudzi and Rubin, 1993; Samudzi *et al.*, 1991)?, IL-10 (Walter and Nagabhushan, 1995; Zdanov *et al.*, 1995, 1996), and IL-19 (Chang *et al.*, 2003), divides C-terminal helix F into parts F1 and F2. In humIL-22 this bend occurs precisely at the position of Glu166 which results in exposure of Glu166 and some other charged amino acid side chains to solvent and allowing for their putative interactions with the extracellular domains of IL-22 receptor chains IL-22R1 and IL-22BP.

It is worth pointing out that the kink in helix F drastically changes the orientation of its N-terminal part F1 in comparison to its C-terminal portion F2. At least in IL-22, this bend seems to be the result of a highly conserved disulfide bond between Cys89 and Cys178. However, this does not seem to be the only reason for this feature since the human IL-10, IL-19, and IFN-γ do not have a similar disulfide bridge.

In addition to Cys89-Cys178, humIL-22 has another disulfide bridge formed between Cys40 (N-terminal) and Cys132 (helix D). The presence of this single covalent bond before loop DE renders sufficient flexibility and extension to the loop allowing helices E and F to fold back into the cleft formed by helices A–D from the same polypeptide chain. In IL-10, the loop DE is more stiff which makes helices E and F to fold as a separate domain in the V-shaped monomer structure (Walter and Nagabhushan, 1995; Zdanov *et al.*, 1995, 1996). In IFN-γ, a short DE loop is the main reason for a similar structural architecture (Ealick *et al.*, 1991; Randal and Kossiakoff, 2000; Samudzi and Rubin, 1993; Samudzi *et al.*, 1991). Stabilization of IL-10 and IFN-γ monomers is accomplished by homodimerization in which helices E and F of one polypeptide chain dock to the cleft formed by helices A–D from the other polypeptide chain, thus assembling, in a cooperative fashion, a V-shaped homodimer. Given the fact that, opposite to IL-10, an IL-22 monomer folds in a compact structure, its dimerization observed in a crystal appears to be an electrostatic interaction effect that occurs at high protein concentrations under crystallization condition and that is mainly driven by charged surface amino acids. Quaternary arrangement in the form of intimate intertwined dimer is one of the main structural differences that separate IL-10 and IFN-γ from IL-22 (Nagem *et al.*, 2002).

To the best of our knowledge, the glycosylation state of native human IL-22 has never been determined. However, insect-cell-expressed human IL-22(humIL-22$_{Dm}$) provides an insight in its N-linked carbohydrate composition. Sodium dodecyl sulfate-polyacrylamide gel electrophoresis (SDS-PAGE) and mass-spectroscopy analysis revealed that the most abundant form of humIL-22$_{Dm}$ contains two or three N-linked glycans (hexa- and pentasaccharides) composed of N-acetyl glucosamine, mannose, and fucose chemical groups. Furthermore, heterogeneity in the glycans seems to be predominantly a result of the presence or absence of a fucose moiety (Xu *et al.*, 2004). These results were partially confirmed by the humIL-22$_{Dm}$ crystallographic structure. Because of the lack of a discernible electron density in certain glycans positions, only a few carbohydrate moieties could be modeled at N54 and N97 side chains. At N68 position, no glycans were modeled as a result of a high mobility of the loop AB and the absence of an interpretable electron density map for this part of the macromolecule (Xu *et al.*, 2005). Apart from a few side chain rearrangements and several additional hydrogen bonds between carbohydrate and protein atoms, the protein regions surrounding glycosylation sites are identical in the humIL-22$_{Dm}$ and humIL-22$_{Ec}$ structures.

VII. IL-22 SIGNALING COMPLEX

The assembly of the IL-22 ternary signaling complex is initiated by the IL-22 binding to the extracellular domain of its high-affinity receptor chain IL-22R1. There are indications that the IL-22/IL-22R1 binary complex may induce conformational changes both into IL-22 and IL-22R1 tertiary structures, creating a new surface-binding site for the interactions with the extracellular domain of the low-affinity receptor chain IL-10R2 (Li et al., 2004; Wolk et al., 2005). The conformational changes induced into both protein structures are consistent with the fact that IL-10R2 exhibits virtually no affinity to the native IL-22 or IL-22R1 alone but displays an increased affinity for the IL-22/IL-22R1 complex (Li et al., 2004; Logsdon et al., 2002). The engagement of the extracellular domain of the low-affinity receptor chain IL-10R2 stabilizes the IL-22 within the ternary complex and places the intracellular domain of both receptors in position for activation of JAK/STAT and MAP kinase signaling pathways (Lejeune et al., 2002).

The soluble IL-22 receptor, IL-22BP, displays around 35% identity (48% similarity) in amino acid composition as compared to the extracellular domain of IL-22R1 (Fig. 3) and it is believed that they have the same or overlapping binding sites on IL-22 surface. Binding of this naturally occurring IL-22 antagonist to IL-22 completely prevents the interactions between IL-22 and IL-22R1 (Li et al., 2004) and, most important, does not create a new binding site for IL-10R2 (Wolk et al., 2005). As a result, IL-22BP binding to IL-22 inhibits triggering of IL-22 signaling pathways.

A. PUTATIVE STRUCTURAL INTERACTIONS BETWEEN IL-22 AND ITS RECEPTORS BINARY COMPLEX

The lack of experimental 3D information about IL-22 binary complex impedes precise structural analyses of the molecular mechanism of ligand-receptors interactions. Nevertheless, 3D modeling using the IL-10/IL-10R1 complex and IL-22 crystallographic structures as templates [PDB entries 1J7V, 1LQS, 1M4R, and 1YKB (Jones et al., 2002; Josephson et al., 2001; Nagem et al., 2002; Xu et al., 2005)] and available biochemical evidence, greatly advanced our knowledge of important amino acids putatively involved in the IL-22:receptor complex formation. The similarities in the amino acid sequences of the extracellular domains of IL-10R1, IL-22R1, and IL-10R2 as well as IL-22BP allow one to contemplate that all these receptor chains will display a common fold, similar to other class 2 cytokine receptors. Their prototype 3D structure is formed by two fibronectin type-III (FBNIII) domains each one composed by seven β-strands (A, B, C, C', E, F, and G) as exemplified by tissue factor (TF) (Harlos et al., 1994; Muller et al., 1994), IFN-γRα (Thiel et al., 2000; Walter et al., 1995), and IL-10R1 (Jones et al., 2002; Josephson et al., 2001).

In humIL-10R1, strands C and C' from the first FBNIII domain (D1) are connected by a disulfide bridge between Cys56 and Cys75 (complete IL-10R1 numbering, signal peptide included). In IL-22R1, IL-22BP, and IL-10R2 the cysteine residue located on strand C' is conserved but Cys on the strand C is replaced by another Cys on the strand E. This exchange promotes formation of Cys71-Cys79 (humIL-22R1), Cys78-Cys86 (humIL-22BP),

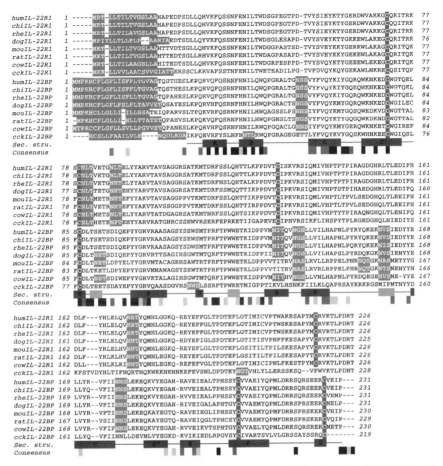

FIGURE 3. Primary structure alignment of the extracellular domain of IL-22R1 and IL-22BP orthologs. Amino acid sequences were obtained from the following entries: humIL-22R1 (NP_067081.2 Genbank), chiIL-22R1 (ENSPTRP00000000593 Ensembl), rheIL-22R1 (NP_067081.2 Ensembl), dogIL-22R1 (XP_855113.1 Genbank), mouIL-22R1 (NP_839988.1 Genbank), ratIL-22R1 (XP_342948.2 Ensembl), cowIL-22R1 (NP_001029483.1 Genbank), cckIL-22R1 (XP_417840.1 Genbank), humIL-22BP (NP_851826.1 Genbank), chiIL-22BP (ENSPTRP00000031824 Ensembl), rheIL-22BP (NM_181309.1 Ensembl), dogIL-22BP (ENSCAFP00000000373 Ensembl), mouIL-22BP (NP_839989.2 Genbank), ratIL-22BP (NP_001003404.1 Genbank), cowIL-22BP (ENSBTAP00000022606 Ensembl), and cckIL-22BP (ENSGALP00000022451 Ensembl). Predicted signal peptides are colored in cyan, potential glycosylation sites are colored in orange, and cysteine residues potentially involved in disulfide bridges are highlighted in green. The secondary structure elements (green for strands, red for helices, and blue for loops) were predicted by comparison with the available structure of human IL-10R1 [PDB entry 1J7V (Josephson et al., 2001)]. A consensus among amino acid sequences is displayed in shades of blue in the last line; the darker the color the highest the similarity. Full-length amino acid sequences (signal peptides included) were used for numbering. (See Color Insert.)

and Cys66-Cys74 (humIL-10R2) disulfide bridges (following complete IL-22R1, IL-22BP, and IL-10R2 numbering) which are structurally similar to the disulfide bond found in IFN-γhigh-affinity receptor (Walter *et al.*, 1995). The second humIL-10R1 disulfide bridge (Cys202-Cys223), connecting strands F and G, is located at FBNIII domain 2 (D2). This disulfide bond is structurally conserved in IL-22BP (Cys206-Cys227), IL-10R2 (Cys188-Cys209) and all other class 2 cytokine receptors, with an exception of IL-22R1. In the later, the second disulfide bridge is formed by Cys128 (strand A) and Cys217 (strand G) of the second FBNIII domain. By comparative analysis, this difference is likely to result in a subtle rearrangement of the strands A and G of the IL-22R1 structure but due to its location, it is difficult to predict the effect this rearrangement would have, if any, on creation of an IL-22R1-specific binding surface.

Based on the crystallographic structures of the IL-10/IL-10R1 binary complex and IL-22 structures as templates (Jones *et al.*, 2002; Josephson *et al.*, 2001; Nagem *et al.*, 2002; Xu *et al.*, 2005), the putative binding interface formed in IL-22/IL-22R1 and IL-22/IL-22BP complexes is likely to be composed of surface amino acids grouped in clusters. While these binding clusters are spread over amino acid sequences of two receptor domains (D1 and D2), their location at the ligand (IL-22) can be mapped to the protein N- and C-termini. A closer 3D analysis permits identification of several distinct groups of amino acid residues or "hot spots" that are strongly involved in the binary complex formation, as reported in Table I and Fig. 4.

The hot spot 1 (interactions 1 to 3 of the Table I and Fig. 4A and B) involves three different ligand residues and a single hydroxyl group in the receptor chain, which is donated by a conserved tyrosine residue (humIL-10R1 Tyr64, humIL-22R1 Tyr60, and humIL-22BP Tyr67). These interactions are among the most important for binary complex formation, and the hydrogen bond network formed by these atoms seems to be structurally conserved in IL-10/IL-10R1, IL-22/IL-22R1, and IL-22/IL-22BP complexes. In the IL-10/IL-10R1 complex, the three interacting atoms of the ligand (IL-10) are spatially disposed in the vertices of a triangle while the hydroxyl group from the receptor (IL-10R1) adopts a position above the triangle plane forming a pyramidal assembly of atoms connected by hydrogen bonds (Fig. 4A). The structure of native humIL-22 indicates no impediments to the conservation of this architecture in putative IL-22/receptor binary complexes. In humIL-22 structure (Nagem *et al.*, 2002), Val72-O, Lys162-NZ, and Glu166-OE2 atoms are spatially located in the vertices of a triangle and a well-defined water molecule (occupancy equal to 1.0 and B_{factor} equal to 21.8 $\overset{\circ}{A}{}^2$) occupies the position of the hydroxyl group (Fig. 4B). Binding of IL-22 to IL-22R1 or to IL-22BP would most probably cause displacement of this water molecule to allow a direct interaction between ligand and receptors, while causing little conformational changes to the rest of the binding cluster. Amino acid sequence comparisons among IL-22 orthologs demonstrate that Lys162 and Glu166 are highly conserved in all known sequences, indicating importance of this dimerization hot spot. The position of Val72, conserved in all mammalian IL-22 is mutated in cckIL-22 and fisIL-22, however, since only a main chain carbonyl group is involved in the hydrogen bond network of the cluster, amino acid replacement at this position is probably neutral to its function. An additional conserved charged amino acid from the ligand (humIL-22 Asp67) also probably makes part to this binding site cluster, contributing to the formation of a charged surface on IL-22.

Similarly to the previous group of interactions, we predict the second interaction hot spot between a single receptor amino acid residue and several residues of the ligand, IL-22. The interactions of a second hot spot are listed as numbers 4–8 in Table I and are shown in Fig. 4C and D. A conserved receptor arginine side chain (IL-10R1 Arg117, IL-22R1 Arg112, and IL-22BP Arg119) is involved in hydrogen bond interactions with ligand residues within the helix F and AB loop regions. It is likely that in IL-22/IL-22R1 and IL-22/IL-22BP complexes the correspondent Arg residue would probably interact with the Gly165 main chain carbonyl group and the carboxyl of the Asp168 side chain (humIL-22), both predominantly conserved in IL-22s. While in IL-10/IL-10R1 additional interactions are observed between the arginine residue (Arg117) and humIL-10 Gln56 (Fig. 4C), it is likely that in IL-22 binary complexes this interaction would not exist, due to the nonconservative substitution of Gln56 (IL-10) to Ser64 (IL-22). In the structure of humIL-22 a serine residue (Ser64) occupies the same spatial position adopted by Gln56 in humIL-10. A shorter Ser side chain impedes its direct interactions with the receptor arginine residue, but still allows for water-mediated contacts. In the structure of native humIL-22 this surface region is filled with ordered water molecules that could potentially be reorganized to participate in the ligand-receptor binding interface (Fig. 4D).

A third cluster of interactions (9–13, Table I) appears to be considerably different between IL-10/IL-10R1 and IL-22/IL-22R1 (or IL-22/IL-22BP) binary complexes. While in IL-10/IL-10R1 structure the positively charged Arg97 side chain of the IL-10R1 adopts two alternate conformations which allows its interaction with three different IL-10 amino acids (Gln56, Gln60, and Asp62), in the putative IL-22/IL-22R1 (or IL-22/IL-22BP) complex the equivalent receptor residue is substituted by a well-conserved tyrosine (humIL-22R1 Tyr93 and humIL-22BP Tyr100). Due to the extension and conformational mobility of the IL-10R1 arginine residue side chain, an extensive hydrogen bond network is formed between ligand and receptor atoms (Fig. 4E). The same does not seem to hold true in IL-22 binary complexes. Even though the tyrosine residue of the IL-22 receptors may point toward an equivalent region in IL-22, its side chain hydroxyl group seems to be too distant from any IL-22 amino acid residues to form a stable cluster of

TABLE 1. Binding Surface Composition and Specific Interactions on IL-10/IL-10R1, IL-22/IL-22R1, and IL-22/IL-22BP Binary Complexes

IL-10/IL-10R1 complex		IL-22/IL-22R1 (or IL-22BP) complexes		
Composition of binding surface		Potential composition of binding surface		
humIL-10	humIL-10R1	humIL-22	humIL-22R1	humIL-22BP
Pro38-Asp46	Leu62-Trp69	Ser45-Asn54	Lys58-Trp65	Lys65-Trp72
Lys52-Leu65	Asn94-Arg97	Lys61-Leu74	Glu90-Tyr93	Glu97-Tyr100
Lys156-Arg177	Val113-Glu122	Lys162-Ile179	Met109-His118	Met116-Glu125
	His163-Glu166		His161-Phe164	Ile163-Tyr166
	Ser208-Asn214		Cys204-Lys210	Tyr212-Arg218

	Observed crystallographic interactions			Potential interactions		
#	humIL-10	humIL-10R1	Distance (Å)	humIL-22	humIL-22R1	humIL-22BP
1	Asn63-O	Tyr64-OH	3.29	Val72	Tyr60	Tyr67
2	Lys156-NZ	Tyr64-OH	2.96	Lys162	Tyr60	Tyr67

3	Glu160-OE2	Tyr64-OH	2.75	Glu166	Tyr60	Tyr67
4	Gln56-OE1	Arg117-N	2.54	Ser64	Arg112	Arg119
5	Gln56-NE2	Arg117-NH1	3.23	Ser64	Arg112	Arg119
6	Ser159-O	Arg117-NH1	2.92	Gly165	Arg112	Arg119
7	Asp162-OD1	Arg117-NH2	2.46	Asp168	Arg112	Arg119
8	Asp162-OD2	Arg117-NH2	2.47	Asp168	Arg112	Arg119
9	Gln56-O	Arg97-NH2	2.74	Ser64	Tyr93	Tyr100
10	Gln60-NE2	Arg97-NH1	3.15	Asn68	Tyr93	Tyr100
11	Asp62-OD1	Arg97-NH2	2.55	Thr70	Tyr93	Tyr100
12	Asp62-OD1	Arg97-NE	2.94	Thr70	Tyr93	Tyr100
13	Asp62-OD2	Arg97-NH2	3.29	Thr70	Tyr93	Tyr100
14	Asp62-O	Gly65-N	2.74	Thr70	Gly61	Gly68
15	Glu169-OE2	Ser211-OG	3.10	Arg175	Thr207	Met215
16	Glu169-OE2	Arg212-NH1	3.02	Arg175	Trp208	Leu216
17	Arg42-N	Ser211-O	3.22	——	Thr207	Met215
18	Arg42-NE	Arg212-O	3.13	——	Trp208	Met216
19	Arg45-NE	Ser211-O	3.04	——	Thr207	Met215

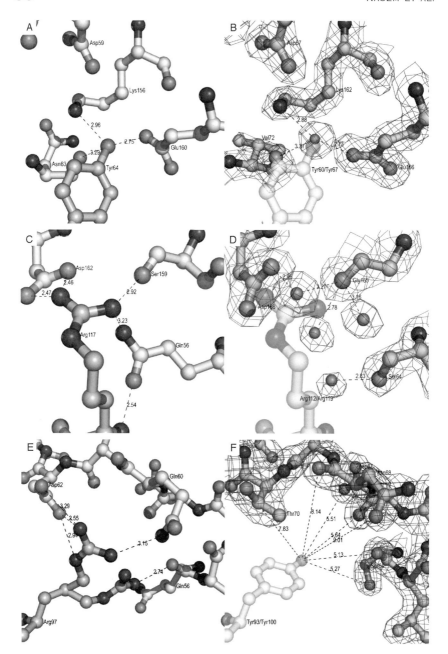

FIGURE 4. Ball and stick representation of binary complexes interactions listed on Table I. Interactions 1–3 (A, B), 4–8 (C, D), and 9–13 (E, F) in IL-10 (A, C, E) and IL-22 (B, D, F) complexes. Nitrogen and oxygen atoms are colored blue and red, respectively. Carbon atoms are colored according to the molecule which they belong: yellow for IL-10, orange for IL-10R1, cyan

interactions without requiring any additional conformational adaptations (Fig. 4F). Moreover, at least two other aspects may contribute to classify this cluster region as distinct between IL-10 and IL-22 binary complexes: (1) In addition to the amino acid substitution of the key receptor interacting residue (Arg to Tyr), an important subtitution also occurs for the ligand (humIL-10 Asp62 to humIL-22 Thr70; also involved in interaction number 14). (2) The IL-22 AB loop (humIL-22 Leu65 to humIL-22 Gly76) involved in this binding site is longer than its IL-10 counterpart (humIL-10 Met57 to humIL-10 Lys67) which results in a different main chain conformation, particularly in the region between humIL-22 Thr70 and Val72 as well as a potential rearrangement of the loop between strands C and C' from D1 of IL-22R1 or IL-22BP extracellular domains.

As evident from Table I that the last five interactions (15–19) of IL-10/IL-10R1 complex interface are the only contacts established by IL-10 with the second receptor FBNIII domain. Visual inspection of ligand-receptor complexes indicates that these interactions may be either very different or completely absent in IL-22 binary complexes. One of the reasons for this resides in the fact that Arg212, an important charged IL-10R1 residue, is substituted by nonpolar residues in IL-22 receptors (Trp208 in humIL-22R1 and Leu216 in humIL-22BP). In addition, there are two important changes in the respective ligand binding site: (1) in interactions 15 and 16 a positively charged humIL-22 residue (Arg175) is spatially superimposed with its negatively charged (Glu169) IL-10 counterpart; (2) due to the significant differences in main chain conformation between IL-10 and IL-22 N-termini, it is difficult to accurately assign the IL-22 amino acids that would be responsible for interactions 17–19.

In summary, potential IL-22/receptor interactions listed in Table I suggest that IL-22R1 and IL-22BP could display very similar IL-22 binding surface aside from a cluster of interactions with the second FBNIII domain (D2). Furthermore, the different disulfide bonds pattern observed for the second FBNIII domains of two receptors might indicate that the differences in these domains are responsible for creating a new binary complex binding surface that selects for the interaction with IL-10R2, the second IL-22 receptor chain. This hypothesis is consistent with the fact that primary structure similarity between IL-22R1 extracellular domain and IL-22BP is much higher between their first FBNIII domains than between their second domains (Fig. 3).

for IL-22, and green for IL-22R1 or IL-22BP. Nonbonded red spheres represent structurally defined water molecules. An experimental electron density map is shown around IL-22 atoms. Residues from IL-22 receptors are shown in semitransparent sticks to represent their potential location in the IL-22/receptor complex. The figure was created using the PyMOL molecular graphics system (DeLano, 2002). (See Color Insert.)

B. TERNARY COMPLEX

It is much harder to speculate about structural architecture of the IL-22/IL-22R1/IL-10R2 ternary complex. Due to the fact that very little is known about the structure and the interactions between ligands and low-affinity class 2 cytokine receptors, such as the IL-10R2, the location of the second receptor binding site on the body of IL-22 remained elusive. However, human IL-22 3D structure, IL-22/IL-22R1 model, and available biochemical evidence can help us to have a first idea about putative IL-10R2 binding site.

The identification of the human IL-22 amino acid residues that are specifically involved in IL-10R2 recognition was reported in the work of Logsdon and coworkers (2004). In this work, it was shown that the IL-10R2 binding site on human IL-22 includes one N-glycosylated residue (Asn54) and that the glycosylation itself has a five- to tenfold increasing effect on IL-22's affinity for IL-10R2. In addition, the site-directed mutagenesis experiments, guided by the humIL-22 crystal structure, allowed for the identification of Tyr51, Asn54, and Arg55 on N-terminus of helix A and Tyr114 and Glu117 on N-terminus of helix D as the main important residues involved in IL-10R2 binding. Based on protein–carbohydrate interactions studies, it has been also suggested the involvement of Pro50 in the binding surface. An amino acid sequence analysis indicates that apart from fish IL-22, all other IL-22 sequences have a high degree of conservation of these amino acid residues.

The group of Sabat used cellulose-bound IL-22-derived fragments to demonstrate that 15 amino acid long peptides from helices A (residues 44–58) and D (residues 116–136) region display measurable affinity for soluble IL-10R2 (Wolk *et al.*, 2005). This result reinforces the conclusions of Logsdon and coworkers (2004) and sustains the idea that conformational changes induced in IL-22 at the moment of IL-22/IL-22R1 complex creation promotes formation or exposure of an IL-10R2-specific binding site from the binary complex. The latter work also demonstrates that helices A and D are definitely involved in the binding interface between IL-22 and IL-10R2 and it is probable that additional amino acids from these regions are implicated in binding interactions.

Unfortunately, so far, no specific IL-10R2 residues involved in binding have been determined; this renders conjectures about the IL-10R2 position and orientation in the IL-22/IL-22R1/IL-10R2 ternary complex very imprecise. Nevertheless, it seems that both IL-22 receptor chains share the same side of the IL-22 molecule for binding (Fig. 5). While helices A, D, and F and a part of AB loop form the binding side of the protein, helices B, C, and E gather at the opposite side (nonbinding side) of the molecule. The helix A is located just ahead of and in between helices D and F at the binding side of the molecule and, upon IL-22R1 binding, helix F and parts of helix A and AB loop are covered by the receptor molecule. At the same time,

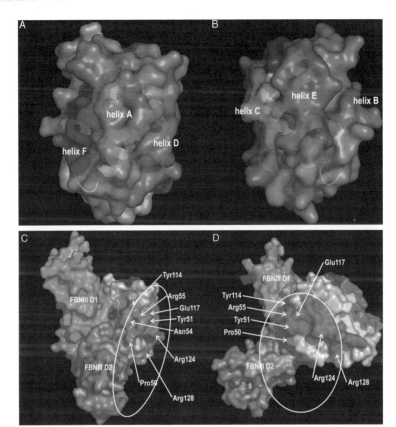

FIGURE 5.   Representation of IL-22 and IL-22/IL-22R1 surfaces. The IL-22 surface was divided in two sides: (A) the binding side composed by helices A (green), D (magenta), and F (blue); (B) the nonbinding side composed by helices B (orange), C (yellow), and E (red). The figure in (B) was obtained after rotation of figure in (A) by 180° around a vertical axis passing through the molecule. (C, D) IL-22/IL-22R1 surfaces are represented in two different orientations. The figure in (D) was obtained after rotation of the figure in (C) by 75° around a vertical axis passing through the molecules. Fibronectin type-III domains are shown in cyan (domain 1) and dark cyan (domain 2). The hypothetical location of IL-10R2 binding surface is marked with white ellipses. IL-22 amino acid residues involved in IL-10R2 recognition are marked and labeled in white. The figure was created using the PyMOL molecular graphics system (DeLano, 2002). (See Color Insert.)

helix D and a part of helix A continue to be solvent exposed in a putative IL-22/IL-22R1 complex (Fig. 5C and D). One, therefore, is free to hypothesize that parts of helices A and D and also, potentially, part of the IL-22R1, create the binding surface for IL-10R2. In addition to binding interactions between IL-22 and IL-10R2, one might suggest that potential interactions can occur between receptor's FBNIII second domains, which would contribute to the ternary IL-22/IL-22R1/IL-10R2 complex assembly.

REFERENCES

Aggarwal, S., Xie, M. H., Maruoka, M., Foster, J., and Gurney, A. L. (2001). Acinar cells of the pancreas are a target of interleukin-22. *J. Interferon Cytokine Res.* **21**, 1047–1053.

Arthur, E. I., Zlotogora, J., Lerer, I., Dagan, J., Marks, K., and Abeliovich, D. (1997). Transient neonatal diabetes mellitus in a child with invdup(6)(q22q23) of paternal origin. *Eur. J. Hum. Genet.* **5**, 417–419.

Bendtsen, J. D., Nielsen, H., von Heijne, G., and Brunak, S. (2004). Improved prediction of signal peptides: SignalP 3.0. *J. Mol. Biol.* **340**, 783–795.

Boniface, K., Bernard, F. X., Garcia, M., Gurney, A. L., Lecron, J. C., and Morel, F. (2005). IL-22 inhibits epidermal differentiation and induces proinflammatory gene expression and migration of human keratinocytes. *J. Immunol.* **174**, 3695–3702.

Chang, C., Magracheva, E., Kozlov, S., Fong, S., Tobin, G., Kotenko, S., Wlodawer, A., and Zdanov, A. (2003). Crystal structure of interleukin-19 defines a new subfamily of helical cytokines. *J. Biol. Chem.* **278**, 3308–3313.

Choy, E. H., and Panayi, G. S. (2001). Cytokine pathways and joint inflammation in rheumatoid arthritis. *N. Engl. J. Med.* **344**, 907–916.

DeLano, W. L. (2002). The PyMOL Molecular Graphics System. DeLano Scientific, San Carlos, CA, USA.

Dumoutier, L., Louahed, J., and Renauld, J. C. (2000a). Cloning and characterization of IL-10–related T cell-derived inducible factor (IL-TIF), a novel cytokine structurally related to IL-10 and inducible by IL-9. *J. Immunol.* **164**, 1814–1819.

Dumoutier, L., Van Roost, E., Ameye, G., Michaux, L., and Renauld, J. C. (2000b). IL-TIF/IL-22: Genomic organization and mapping of the human and mouse genes. *Genes Immun.* **1**, 488–494.

Dumoutier, L., Van Roost, E., Colau, D., and Renauld, J. C. (2000c). Human interleukin-10–related T cell-derived inducible factor: Molecular cloning and functional characterization as an hepatocyte-stimulating factor. *Proc. Natl. Acad. Sci. USA* **97**, 10144–10149.

Dumoutier, L., Lejeune, D., Colau, D., and Renauld, J. C. (2001). Cloning and characterization of IL-22 binding protein, a natural antagonist of IL-10–related T cell-derived inducible factor/IL-22. *J. Immunol.* **166**, 7090–7095.

Ealick, S. E., Cook, W. J., Vijay-Kumar, S., Carson, M., Nagabhushan, T. L., Trotta, P. P., and Bugg, C. E. (1991). Three-dimensional structure of recombinant human interferon-gamma. *Science* **252**, 698–702.

Gitter, B. D., Labus, J. M., Lees, S. L., and Scheetz, M. E. (1989). Characteristics of human synovial fibroblast activation by IL-1 beta and TNF alpha. *Immunology* **66**, 196–200.

Goris, A., Epplen, C., Fiten, P., Andersson, M., Murru, R., Sciacca, F. L., Ronsse, I., Jackel, S., Epplen, J. T., Marrosu, M. G., Olsson, T., Grimaldi, T., *et al.* (1999). Analysis of an IFN-gamma gene (IFNG) polymorphism in multiple sclerosis in Europe: Effect of population structure on association with disease. *J. Interferon Cytokine Res.* **19**, 1037–1046.

Goris, A., Heggarty, S., Marrosu, M. G., Graham, C., Billiau, A., and Vandenbroeck, K. (2002). Linkage disequilibrium analysis of chromosome 12q14–15 in multiple sclerosis: Delineation of a 118–kb interval around interferon-gamma (IFNG) that is involved in male versus female differential susceptibility. *Genes Immun.* **3**, 470–476.

Gruenberg, B. H., Schoenemeyer, A., Weiss, B., Toschi, L., Kunz, S., Wolk, K., Asadullah, K., and Sabat, R. (2001). A novel, soluble homologue of the human IL-10 receptor with preferential expression in placenta. *Genes Immun.* **2**, 329–334.

Gurney, A. L. (2004). IL-22, a Th1 cytokine that targets the pancreas and select other peripheral tissues. *Int. Immunopharmacol.* **4**, 669–677.

Harlos, K., Martin, D. M., O'Brien, D. P., Jones, E. Y., Stuart, D. I., Polikarpov, I., Miller, A., Tuddenham, E. G., and Boys, C. W. (1994). Crystal structure of the extracellular region of human tissue factor. *Nature* **370**, 662–666.

Hor, S., Pirzer, H., Dumoutier, L., Bauer, F., Wittmann, S., Sticht, H., Renauld, J. C., de Waal Malefyt, R., and Fickenscher, H. (2004). The T-cell lymphokine interleukin-26 targets epithelial cells through the interleukin-20 receptor 1 and interleukin-10 receptor 2 chains. *J. Biol. Chem.* **279,** 33343–33351.

Igawa, D., Sakai, M., and Savan, R. (2006). An unexpected discovery of two interferon gamma-like genes along with interleukin (IL)-22 and -26 from teleost: IL-22 and -26 genes have been described for the first time outside mammals. *Mol. Immunol.* **43,** 999–1009.

Ikeuchi, H., Kuroiwa, T., Hiramatsu, N., Kaneko, Y., Hiromura, K., Ueki, K., and Nojima, Y. (2005). Expression of interleukin-22 in rheumatoid arthritis: Potential role as a pro-inflammatory cytokine. *Arthritis Rheum.* **52,** 1037–1046.

Jones, B. C., Logsdon, N. J., Josephson, K., Cook, J., Barry, P. A., and Walter, M. R. (2002). Crystal structure of human cytomegalovirus IL-10 bound to soluble human IL-10R1. *Proc. Natl. Acad. Sci. USA* **99,** 9404–9409.

Josephson, K., Logsdon, N. J., and Walter, M. R. (2001). Crystal structure of the IL-10/IL-10R1 complex reveals a shared receptor binding site. *Immunity* **15,** 35–46.

Koch, O., Rockett, K., Jallow, M., Pinder, M., Sisay-Joof, F., and Kwiatkowski, D. (2005). Investigation of malaria susceptibility determinants in the IFNG/IL26/IL22 genomic region. *Genes Immun.* **6,** 312–318.

Kotenko, S. V., Krause, C. D., Izotova, L. S., Pollack, B. P., Wu, W., and Pestka, S. (1997). Identification and functional characterization of a second chain of the interleukin-10 receptor complex. *EMBO J.* **16,** 5894–5903.

Kotenko, S. V., Saccani, S., Izotova, L. S., Mirochnitchenko, O. V., and Pestka, S. (2000). Human cytomegalovirus harbors its own unique IL-10 homolog (cmvIL-10). *Proc. Natl. Acad. Sci. USA* **97,** 1695–1700.

Kotenko, S. V., Izotova, L. S., Mirochnitchenko, O. V., Esterova, E., Dickensheets, H., Donnelly, R. P., and Pestka, S. (2001a). Identification of the functional interleukin-22 (IL-22) receptor complex: The IL-10R2 chain (IL-10Rbeta) is a common chain of both the IL-10 and IL-22 (IL-10–related T cell-derived inducible factor, IL-TIF) receptor complexes. *J. Biol. Chem.* **276,** 2725–2732.

Kotenko, S. V., Izotova, L. S., Mirochnitchenko, O. V., Esterova, E., Dickensheets, H., Donnelly, R. P., and Pestka, S. (2001b). Identification, cloning, and characterization of a novel soluble receptor that binds IL-22 and neutralizes its activity. *J. Immunol.* **166,** 7096–7103.

Kotenko, S. V., Gallagher, G., Baurin, V. V., Lewis-Antes, A., Shen, M., Shah, N. K., Langer, J. A., Sheikh, F., Dickensheets, H., and Donnelly, R. P. (2003). IFN-lambdas mediate antiviral protection through a distinct class II cytokine receptor complex. *Nat. Immunol.* **4,** 69–77.

Lehrer, R. I., and Ganz, T. (2002). Defensins of vertebrate animals. *Curr. Opin. Immunol.* **14,** 96–102.

Lejeune, D., Dumoutier, L., Constantinescu, S., Kruijer, W., Schuringa, J. J., and Renauld, J. C. (2002). Interleukin-22 (IL-22) activates the JAK/STAT, ERK, JNK, and p38 MAP kinase pathways in a rat hepatoma cell line. Pathways that are shared with and distinct from IL-10. *J. Biol. Chem.* **277,** 33676–33682.

Li, J., Tomkinson, K. N., Tan, X. Y., Wu, P., Yan, G., Spaulding, V., Deng, B., Annis-Freeman, B., Heveron, K., Zollner, R., De Zutter, G., Wright, G., *et al.* (2004). Temporal associations between interleukin 22 and the extracellular domains of IL-22R and IL-10R2. *Int. Immunopharmacol.* **4,** 693–708.

Logsdon, N. J., Jones, B. C., Josephson, K., Cook, J., and Walter, M. R. (2002). Comparison of interleukin-22 and interleukin-10 soluble receptor complexes. *J. Interferon Cytokine Res.* **22,** 1099–1112.

Logsdon, N. J., Jones, B. C., Allman, J. C., Izotova, L., Schwartz, B., Pestka, S., and Walter, M. R. (2004). The IL-10R2 binding hot spot on IL-22 is located on the N-terminal helix and is dependent on N-linked glycosylation. *J. Mol. Biol.* **342,** 503–514.

Martinez, J. A., King, T. E. Jr., Brown, K., Jennings, C. A., Borish, L., Mortenson, R. L., Khan, T. Z., Bost, T. W., and Riches, D. W. (1997). Increased expression of the interleukin-10 gene by alveolar macrophages in interstitial lung disease. *Am. J. Physiol.* **273**, L676–L683.

Muller, Y. A., Ultsch, M. H., Kelley, R. F., and de Vos, A. M. (1994). Structure of the extracellular domain of human tissue factor: Location of the factor VIIa binding site. *Biochemistry* **33**, 10864–10870.

Nagalakshmi, M. L., Murphy, E., McClanahan, T., and de Waal Malefyt, R. (2004). Expression patterns of IL-10 ligand and receptor gene families provide leads for biological characterization. *Int. Immunopharmacol.* **4**, 577–592.

Nagem, R. A., Colau, D., Dumoutier, L., Renauld, J. C., Ogata, C., and Polikarpov, I. (2002). Crystal structure of recombinant human interleukin-22. *Structure* **10**, 1051–1062.

Pan, H., Hong, F., Radaeva, S., and Gao, B. (2004). Hydrodynamic gene delivery of interleukin-22 protects the mouse liver from concanavalin A-, carbon tetrachloride-, and Fas ligand-induced injury via activation of STAT3. *Cell Mol. Immunol.* **1**, 43–49.

Radaeva, S., Sun, R., Pan, H. N., Hong, F., and Gao, B. (2004). Interleukin 22 (IL-22) plays a protective role in T cell-mediated murine hepatitis: IL-22 is a survival factor for hepatocytes via STAT3 activation. *Hepatology* **39**, 1332–1342.

Randal, M., and Kossiakoff, A. A. (2000). The 2.0 A structure of bovine interferon-gamma; assessment of the structural differences between species. *Acta Crystallogr. D Biol. Crystallogr.* **56**(Pt. 1), 14–24.

Samudzi, C. T., and Rubin, J. R. (1993). Structure of recombinant bovine interferon-gamma at 3.0 A resolution. *Acta Crystallogr. D Biol. Crystallogr.* **49**, 513–521.

Samudzi, C. T., Burton, L. E., and Rubin, J. R. (1991). Crystal structure of recombinant rabbit interferon-gamma at 2.7–A resolution. *J. Biol. Chem.* **266**, 21791–21797.

Sheikh, F., Baurin, V. V., Lewis-Antes, A., Shah, N. K., Smirnov, S. V., Anantha, S., Dickensheets, H., Dumoutier, L., Renauld, J. C., Zdanov, A., Donnelly, R. P., and Kotenko, S. V. (2004). Cutting edge: IL-26 signals through a novel receptor complex composed of IL-20 receptor 1 and IL-10 receptor 2. *J. Immunol.* **172**, 2006–2010.

Sheppard, P., Kindsvogel, W., Xu, W., Henderson, K., Schlutsmeyer, S., Whitmore, T. E., Kuestner, R., Garrigues, U., Birks, C., Roraback, J., Ostrander, C., Dong, C., *et al.* (2003). IL-28, IL-29 and their class II cytokine receptor IL-28R. *Nat. Immunol.* **4**, 63–68.

Tachiiri, A., Imamura, R., Wang, Y., Fukui, M., Umemura, M., and Suda, T. (2003). Genomic structure and inducible expression of the IL-22 receptor alpha chain in mice. *Genes Immun.* **4**, 153–159.

Thiel, D. J., le Du, M. H., Walter, R. L., D'Arcy, A., Chene, C., Fountoulakis, M., Garotta, G., Winkler, F. K., and Ealick, S. E. (2000). Observation of an unexpected third receptor molecule in the crystal structure of human interferon-gamma receptor complex. *Structure* **8**, 927–936.

Thompson, J. D., Higgins, D. G., and Gibson, T. J. (1994). CLUSTAL W: Improving the sensitivity of progressive multiple sequence alignment through sequence weighting, position-specific gap penalties and weight matrix choice. *Nucleic Acids Res.* **22**, 4673–4680.

Vandenbroeck, K., Opdenakker, G., Goris, A., Murru, R., Billiau, A., and Marrosu, M. G. (1998). Interferon-gamma gene polymorphism-associated risk for multiple sclerosis in Sardinia. *Ann. Neurol.* **44**, 841–842.

Walter, M. A., Spillett, D. J., Thomas, P., Weissenbach, J., and Goodfellow, P. N. (1994). A method for constructing radiation hybrid maps of whole genomes. *Nat. Genet.* **7**, 22–28.

Walter, M. R. (2004). Structural analysis of IL-10 and Type I interferon family members and their complexes with receptor. *Adv. Protein Chem.* **68**, 171–223.

Walter, M. R., and Nagabhushan, T. L. (1995). Crystal structure of interleukin 10 reveals an interferon gamma-like fold. *Biochemistry* **34**, 12118–12125.

Walter, M. R., Windsor, W. T., Nagabhushan, T. L., Lundell, D. J., Lunn, C. A., Zauodny, P. J., and Narula, S. K. (1995). Crystal structure of a complex between interferon-gamma and its soluble high-affinity receptor. *Nature* **376**, 230–235.

Wei, C. C., Ho, T. W., Liang, W. G., Chen, G. Y., and Chang, M. S. (2003). Cloning and characterization of mouse IL-22 binding protein. *Genes Immun.* **4**, 204–211.

Weiss, B., Wolk, K., Grunberg, B. H., Volk, H. D., Sterry, W., Asadullah, K., and Sabat, R. (2004). Cloning of murine IL-22 receptor alpha 2 and comparison with its human counterpart. *Genes Immun.* **5**, 330–336.

Whittington, H. A., Armstrong, L., Uppington, K. M., and Millar, A. B. (2004). Interleukin-22: A potential immunomodulatory molecule in the lung. *Am. J. Respir. Cell. Mol. Biol.* **31**, 220–226.

Wolk, K., Kunz, S., Witte, E., Friedrich, M., Asadullah, K., and Sabat, R. (2004). IL-22 increases the innate immunity of tissues. *Immunity* **21**, 241–254.

Wolk, K., Witte, E., Reineke, U., Witte, K., Friedrich, M., Sterry, W., Asadullah, K., Volk, H. D., and Sabat, R. (2005). Is there an interaction between interleukin-10 and interleukin-22? *Genes Immun.* **6**, 8–18.

Xie, M. H., Aggarwal, S., Ho, W. H., Foster, J., Zhang, Z., Stinson, J., Wood, W. I., Goddard, A. D., and Gurney, A. L. (2000). Interleukin (IL)-22, a novel human cytokine that signals through the interferon receptor-related proteins CRF2-4 and IL-22R. *J. Biol. Chem.* **275**, 31335–31339.

Xu, T., Logsdon, N. J., and Walter, M. R. (2004). Crystallization and X-ray diffraction analysis of insect-cell-derived IL-22. *Acta Crystallogr. D Biol. Crystallogr.* **60**, 1295–1298.

Xu, T., Logsdon, N. J., and Walter, M. R. (2005). Structure of insect-cell-derived IL-22. *Acta Crystallogr. D Biol. Crystallogr.* **61**, 942–950.

Xu, W., Presnell, S. R., Parrish-Novak, J., Kindsvogel, W., Jaspers, S., Chen, Z., Dillon, S. R., Gao, Z., Gilbert, T., Madden, K., Schlutsmeyer, S., Yao, S., et al. (2001). A soluble class II cytokine receptor, IL-22RA2, is a naturally occurring IL-22 antagonist. *Proc. Natl. Acad. Sci. USA* **98**, 9511–9516.

Zasloff, M. (2002). Antimicrobial peptides of multicellular organisms. *Nature* **415**, 389–395.

Zdanov, A. (2004). Structural features of the interleukin-10 family of cytokines. *Curr. Pharm. Des.* **10**, 3873–3884.

Zdanov, A., Schalk-Hihi, C., Gustchina, A., Tsang, M., Weatherbee, J., and Wlodawer, A. (1995). Crystal structure of interleukin-10 reveals the functional dimer with an unexpected topological similarity to interferon gamma. *Structure* **3**, 591–601.

Zdanov, A., Schalk-Hihi, C., and Wlodawer, A. (1996). Crystal structure of human interleukin-10 at 1.6 A resolution and a model of a complex with its soluble receptor. *Protein Sci.* **5**, 1955–1962.

5

CONTROL OF INTERLEUKIN-2 GENE TRANSCRIPTION: A PARADIGM FOR INDUCIBLE, TISSUE-SPECIFIC GENE EXPRESSION

KAREN BUNTING, JUN WANG, AND M. FRANCES SHANNON

Division of Molecular Bioscience, John Curtin School of Medical Research
Australian National University, Canberra, ACT, Australia

Vitamins and Hormones, Volume 74
0083-6729/06 $35.00
DOI: 10.1016/S0083-6729(06)74005-5

Interleukin-2 (IL-2) is a key cytokine that controls immune cell function, in particular the adaptive arm of the immune system, through its ability to control the clonal expansion and homeostasis of peripheral T cells. IL-2 is produced almost exclusively by T cells in response to antigenic stimulation and thus provides an excellent example of a cell-specific inducible gene. The mechanisms that control *IL-2* gene transcription have been studied in detail for the past 20 years and our current understanding of the nature of the inducible and tissue-specific controls will be discussed. © 2006 Elsevier Inc.

I. INTERLEUKIN-2: DIVERSE ROLES IN IMMUNITY AND PATHOGENESIS

Interleukin-2 (IL-2) is a cytokine belonging to a family of short-chain, four-helix bundle cytokines, including IL-4, IL-7, IL-9, and IL-15, that all share a common receptor chain for signal transduction and have overlapping and complex roles in immunity (Kelso, 1998). IL-2 was first identified as a growth-promoting factor for bone marrow–derived T lymphocytes and has since been shown to be a critical mediator in the development and function of a variety of immune cell types (summarized in Fig. 1B; Gaffen and Liu, 2004). Produced exclusively by T cells, IL-2 principally serves as an initiator of T cell clonal expansion, as a regulator of T cell homeostasis, and in T cell tolerance. The autocrine and paracrine functions of IL-2 on CD4+ and CD8+ T lymphocytes drive T cell proliferation through the ability of IL-2 to promote progression from G_1 to S phase of the cell cycle (Crabtree, 1989; Gesbert *et al.*, 2005). In addition to inducing CD4+ and CD8+ T cell clonal expansion and concomitant cytokine production, IL-2 has been implicated in the

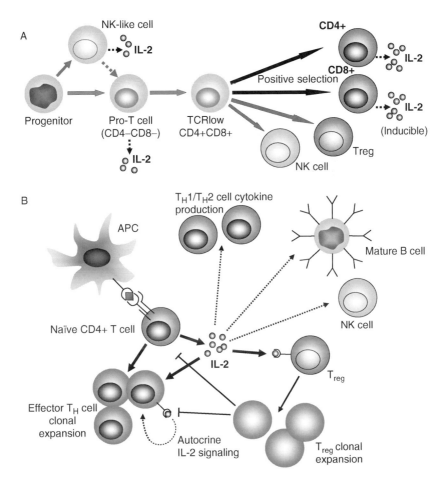

FIGURE 1. IL-2 expression during T cell development and actions on immune cells. (A) IL-2 is expressed at low levels during early T cell development by pro-T cells and by NK-like precursors, then inducibly at high levels in mature peripheral CD4+ and CD8+ T cells that have undergone prior activation. (B) Naïve CD4+ T cells encounter antigen in the context of antigen presenting cells (APC) which drives the production of large quantities of IL-2, leading to T_H effector cell clonal expansion and activation of T cells via autocrine signaling and upregulation of surface IL-2Rα. IL-2 can also trigger a negative feedback loop by stimulating T regulatory cell (T_{reg}) proliferation which suppress CD4+ effector cells. IL-2 also regulates cytokine production by mature T_H1/T_H2 effector cells and the proliferation of B cells and NK cells.

development and maintenance of CD4+CD25+ T regulatory (Treg) cells and is required for activation-induced cell death (AICD) in T cells (Malek, 2003; Maloy and Powrie, 2005; Schimpl *et al.*, 2002). IL-2 also promotes the proliferation of natural killer (NK) cells and B cells, as well as enhancing the production of antibody during humoral immune responses (Gaffen and Liu, 2004). In addition, IL-2 has also been shown to exert an effect on T cell development in the thymus (Bayer *et al.*, 2005; Wang *et al.*, 1998; Yang-Snyder and Rothenberg, 1993). Like other growth factors, IL-2 often acts in synergy with other cytokines to promote effector cell responses (Ben Aribia *et al.*, 1987; Bream *et al.*, 2003; Parada *et al.*, 1998; Rodriguez-Galan *et al.*, 2005).

The potent nature of IL-2 and the central role it plays in the development, differentiation, and regulation of T cells makes it an important contributing factor in a variety of acute and chronic pathological conditions, including leukemia, inflammatory disease, autoimmunity, and viral pathogenesis, where IL-2 expression is dysregulated. *IL-2*-deficient mice develop normal immune systems and do not display any evidence of immunodeficiency. Rather, these mice exhibit lymphoid hyperplasia and produce excessive amounts of autoantibodies, which leads to conditions such as hemolytic anemia, chronic inflammatory bowel disease, and severe autoimmunity in ageing mice (Reya *et al.*, 1998; Sadlack *et al.*, 1993, 1995; Schorle *et al.*, 1991). Similar autoimmune defects are observed in *IL-2 receptor-alpha* (*IL-2Rα*)- and *IL-2Rβ*-knockout mice (Suzuki *et al.*, 1995; Willerford *et al.*, 1995). *IL-2* deficiency has been associated with the absence of CD4+CD25+ Treg cells and defective AICD, which are likely to contribute to increased numbers of autoreactive lymphocytes and to uncontrolled T cell accumulation in the periphery (Kneitz *et al.*, 1995; Schimpl *et al.*, 2002). The nonredundant role of IL-2, therefore, appears to be in the maintenance of T cell homeostasis and promotion of peripheral tolerance.

IL-2 dysregulation is also thought to play a key role in the promotion of inflammatory responses and immune cell dysfunction in a number of disorders, including experimental autoimmune encephalomyelitis (EAE) in mice, Crohn's disease, rheumatoid arthritis, type I diabetes, and systemic lupus erythematosus (SLE) (Crispin and Alcocer-Varela, 1998; Eerligh *et al.*, 2004; Pawlik *et al.*, 2005; Petitto *et al.*, 2000; Radford-Smith and Jewell, 1996), although the underlying mechanisms for these conditions have not been fully characterized. Inappropriate expression of IL-2 has also been implicated in certain forms of leukemia—the best example of this is adult T cell leukemia which is associated with human T cell leukemia virus type 1 (HTLV-1) infection and the constitutive upregulation of IL-2-producing and IL-2-responsive T cells (Niinuma *et al.*, 2005; Tsuda *et al.*, 1993).

Single nucleotide polymorphism (SNP) mapping techniques have also suggested that dysregulated cytokine expression could be associated with mutations in control regions of loci encoding cytokine genes and, thus, may increase the susceptibility of individuals to diseases such as autoimmunity or diabetes or infection with virus. A well-studied example of this in the *IL-2* gene is an SNP at position −330 within the *IL-2* gene promoter which has been linked to acute renal and bone marrow transplant rejection and susceptibility to multiple sclerosis, rheumatoid arthritis, and gastric atrophy induced by Helicobacter pylori infection (MacMillan *et al.*, 2003; Matesanz *et al.*, 2004;

Morgun *et al.*, 2003; Pawlik *et al.*, 2005; Togawa *et al.*, 2005). There remains some debate, however, as to which genotypes (and subsequent clinical manifestations) can be attributed to higher or lower IL-2 production, owing to inconsistencies between experiments performed with stimulated cell lines and lymphocytes from patients. A study has even suggested that *IL-2* may be a candidate gene in schizophrenia (Schwarz *et al.*, 2005). In mice, it is well known that the *IL-2* gene resides within Idd3, a susceptibility locus for insulin-dependent diabetes in the nonobese diabetic (NOD) mouse.

In response to infection with some viruses, such as human immunodeficiency virus (HIV), HTLV-1, and mosquito-borne flaviviruses, virus-infected cells produce abnormal patterns and quantities of cytokines—often in response to the actions of particular viral proteins expressed inside the infected cell. For example, the Tax-1 gene product in HTLV-1 infection induces the upregulation of IL-2 and IL-2Rα in T cells (McGuire *et al.*, 1993; Niinuma *et al.*, 2005; Okayama *et al.*, 1997). In HIV, suppression of IL-2 contributes to the pathogenesis of disease by impairing cell-mediated (T_H1) immunity (clearance of virus) and inducing higher levels of virus infection and replication (Clerici *et al.*, 2000; Gaffen and Liu, 2004). In light of this finding, IL-2 is being evaluated as an adjunctive therapy to antiretroviral therapy in HIV patients (Kedzierska and Crowe, 2001).

Clearly, control over the cell-specific, inducible nature of IL-2 expression, either during an active immune response or during immune cell development, is a critical and ongoing process. The fine balance between the proinflammatory, antiviral and immunosuppressive functions of IL-2 that determine whether an infection is cleared or is augmented by various immunopathological states associated with IL-2 dysregulation, highlights the importance of understanding the various control mechanisms which serve to regulate the expression of the *IL-2* gene.

II. *IL-2*: AN EXAMPLE OF A T CELL–RESTRICTED INDUCIBLE GENE

There are two major characteristics of the expression pattern of the *IL-2* gene that has seen it subjected to intense investigation. First, IL-2 expression is almost exclusively restricted to the T cell lineage although there have been a few reports of IL-2 expression in other cells types (Jain *et al.*, 1995; Serfling *et al.*, 1995). For example, IL-2 expression has been reported in dendritic cells and has been postulated to have a role in linking the innate and adaptive immune systems (Granucci *et al.*, 2003). Second, IL-2 cannot be expressed in resting T cells and requires the activation of these cells through the T cell receptor (TCR) or other activation signals (Granucci *et al.*, 2003; Serfling *et al.*, 1995). These characteristics imply that the *IL-2* gene is subjected to developmental control during T cell differentiation in the thymus to generate a permissive state exclusive to T cells, thus allowing the gene to respond to activation signals.

During T cell development, the ability to express IL-2 is acquired very early following the migration of hematopoietic precursors to the thymus. Pre-T cells that are CD4–CD8– and have not yet rearranged their TCR genes already have the capacity to express IL-2 and in addition to signals that mimic TCR activation, IL-1 treatment is required for IL-2 expression (Chen and Rothenberg, 1993; Lugo et al., 1986). These populations of cells are thought to represent pluripotent precursors and NK-like cells (Fig. 1A; Chen and Rothenberg, 1993; Lugo et al., 1986). Conversely, during specific stages of development when the thymocytes are undergoing negative and positive selection and are classified as CD4+CD8+TCRlow, IL-2 expression cannot be induced even by pharmacological stimuli (Chen and Rothenberg, 1993; Rothenberg et al., 1990). Subsequent to these events, however, mature peripheral T cells of both the CD4+ and CD8+ lineages regain the potential to express IL-2 and activation of these cells leads to IL-2 gene expression and the production of large amounts of IL-2 protein (Fig. 1A; Chen and Rothenberg, 1993; Rothenberg and Ward, 1996).

While mature naïve T cells emerge from the thymus with the capacity to express IL-2, this expression requires a complex series of signaling events. The key activation signals occur through ligation of the TCR which, together with the activation of costimulators such as CD28 on CD4+ T cells, leads to high-level transcriptional activation of the gene (Favero and Lafont, 1998). Other forms of costimulation such as cytokine treatment and activation of adhesion molecules have also been shown to generate increased IL-2 expression (Chirathaworn et al., 2002; Novak et al., 1990). The expression of the gene is transient and mRNA levels decline within 10–16 h of activation. The composition and amplitude of the activation signals are critical for IL-2 gene transcription. A partial activation signal or a low level of signal can lead to T cell anergy and the inability to express IL-2 (Powell et al., 1998). The IL-2 gene, like other cytokine genes, has been shown to exhibit monoallelic expression (Hollander et al., 1998) but the molecular basis of this restriction is still to be determined and leads to a discussion on the stochastic nature of cytokine gene transcription which is outside the scope of this chapter (Hollander, 1999).

III. GENOMIC REGIONS THAT CONTROL IL-2 GENE TRANSCRIPTION

The genes encoding mouse and human IL-2 were first isolated in the mid-1980s (Devos et al., 1983; Fujita et al., 1983; Holbrook et al., 1984; Taniguchi et al., 1983) and shortly after this, the potential control regions of the genes were defined by DNaseI hypersensitive (DH) site mapping (Siebenlist et al., 1986). Many detailed studies since then have mapped

DNaseI hypersensitivity regions in both resting and activated T cells as far upstream of the transcription start site (TSS) as –10 kilobases (kb) (summarized in Fig. 2A). Of particular interest was the increased hypersensitivity that occurred in response to T cell activation in the first 300 base pairs (bp) upstream from the TSS and the constitutive hypersensitivity from –300 to –600bp that was initially proposed to be involved in tissue specificity (Ward et al., 1998). Fine mapping studies with DNaseI, MNase, or restriction enzymes (REs) and dimethyl sulphate (DMS) footprinting across these regions identified more specific areas of promoter occupation, but results from different cell types do not always correlate (Brunvand et al., 1993; Ward et al., 1998). Sequence comparison across species has also helped to identify potential control regions in the IL-2 locus and in some cases there is a clear correspondence between the DH sites and the cross-species conserved regions (Fig. 2A). Promoter mapping studies using reporter assays complimented these DNaseI studies and defined a 300bp region, corresponding to the DH sites immediately upstream from the TSS, as the functional inducible promoter region (Fig. 2B; Durand et al., 1987; Fujita et al., 1986). The transcription factors that operate here and the chromatin structure across this region have been the subject of intensive study and this promoter has served as a model to elucidate the complex nature of inducible gene transcription.

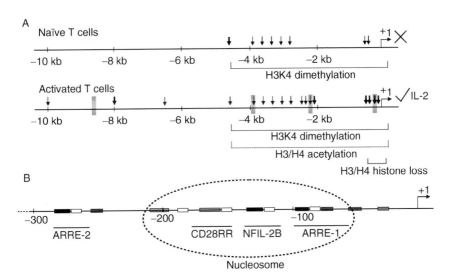

FIGURE 2.   Schematic representation of histone modifications and positioned nucleosome on the murine IL-2 locus. (A) IL-2 promoter regions with DNase hypersensitive sites (arrows), H3K4 dimethylation, H3/H4 acetylation and H3/H4 histone loss before and after T cell activation. Regions of high homology with the human IL-2 gene are shaded. Note that H3/H4 histone loss occurs only at the distal/proximal region of the IL-2 promoter (−500 to +100bp). (B) IL-2 proximal promoter with transcription factor regulatory elements showing the location of a highly positioned nucleosome (dashed ellipse) from −210 to −60 bp.

The detailed operations of this promoter region are discussed later but there are a few salient features that will be noted here. The promoter is highly cell specific and has no activity outside the T cell lineage. Thus, at least in transient transfection assays, it mimics the major expression features of the endogenous *IL-2* gene, that is, cell-specific and inducible expression. This promoter region, like the endogenous *IL-2* gene, requires a combination of signals for activity. If a single signal or transcription factor is removed or a transcription factor binding site is mutated, the promoter suffers a dramatic loss in activity and conversely, it cannot be activated by expression of a single transcription factor (Avots *et al.*, 1995; Rothenberg and Ward, 1996). These features imply a cooperative nature of promoter activity that will be discussed in more detail later.

A region between –300 and –600bp shows some interesting features that distinguish it from the proximal 300bp promoter region. This region is accessible to digestion with DNaseI in resting T cells implying a possible role in maintaining the gene in a permissive or "available" transcription state (Briegel *et al.*, 1991; Serfling *et al.*, 1995; Ward *et al.*, 1998). This region binds high-mobility group (HMG) box factors, octamer (Oct) factors, and the Ets factor, GA binding protein alpha (GABPα) (Avots *et al.*, 1997; Ward *et al.*, 1998). The role of this region and the binding of these factors have not been investigated in great detail but given the conservation of these binding sites across species it is likely that they play an important role in *IL-2* gene regulation.

However, when the proximal 300bp promoter region or a fragment up to 600bp was used to generate transgenic mice, *IL-2* transcription was variable across different founder lines implying an integration site effect (Martensson and Leanderson, 1989). These studies indicated that while the proximal promoter region could mimic the expression pattern of the endogenous gene in transient transfections, other regions were required to give consistent expression in a transgenic context, implying a role for chromatin in this process. Attention then turned to the far upstream regions where DH sites had previously been mapped as there was no evidence for DH sites or areas of cross-species conservation in the intronic regions or downstream of the *IL-2* gene (Yui *et al.*, 2001). It was found that an 8kb region was required for consistent T cell–specific inducible expression in all founder lines (Yui *et al.*, 2001). Thus, it is likely that this 8kb fragment contains all of the control regions required for correct IL-2 expression since this transgene also mimicked IL-2 expression patterns in developing thymocytes (Yui *et al.*, 2001). The only discrepancy noted between the transgene expression and the endogenous gene was that there was lower expression of the transgene in CD8+ cells compared with CD4+ cells, in contrast to the endogenous gene which usually has similar levels of expression in these two cell types. Both constitutive and inducible DH sites have been mapped upstream of the proximal promoter within this 8kb region and represent possible functional regions responsible for correct developmental expression but their exact role requires further investigation. Of particular note is the region of hypersensitivity between –3 and –4kb from the TSS as well as inducible DH sites between –3 and –2kb whose functions have yet to be determined (Yui et al., 2001).

While the proximal promoter plays a critical role in inducible expression of the *IL-2* gene, there are many other upstream regions that appear to be important for correct developmental and T cell–specific expression.

IV. T CELL LINEAGE SPECIFICITY OF *IL-2* GENE EXPRESSION

It had been envisaged that a T cell–specific factor(s) might account for the restricted and specific expression of IL-2 from T cell lineages; however, none of the factors identified to date, which are essential for activation of the *IL-2* proximal promoter or that bind to the distal region, have been demonstrated to be T cell specific. Evidence of the nature of T cell restriction of IL-2 expression has come from studies of the populations of thymocytes that can or cannot express IL-2 (Chen and Rothenberg, 1993; Wang et al., 1998; Yui et al., 2004). All of the regulatory proteins critical for initiation of *IL-2* transcription (Oct, NF-κB, NFAT, and AP-1) are present in immature thymocytes early during T cell development and IL-2 can be induced in these cells. However, as the cells mature in the thymus to double positive (DP) CD4+CD8+ thymocytes, they lose the ability to induce nuclear factor of activated T cells (NFAT) and activating protein-1 (AP-1) activity which prevents expression of IL-2 prior to positive selection (Fig. 1A; Rincon and Flavell, 1996). Similarly, in the periphery, a block in the transcriptional activity of AP-1 at a specific region of the IL-2 promoter has been identified both in mature CD8+ lymphocytes, which have lost the ability to express IL-2 in response to antigen stimulation, and in anergized CD4+ lymphocytes (Finch et al., 2001; Heisel and Keown, 2001). The simplest explanation for the failure of these cells to activate the correct cohort of inducible factors leading to *IL-2* transcription is altered signaling responses, especially by costimulatory molecules such as CD28, which may be intrinsic to the T cell subset or directed by specific developmental signals in the intrathymic milieu.

Studies of T cells or cell lines using inhibitors of specific transcription factors known to block one transcription factor or the use of T cells from mice with deletions in specific transcription factors have also shown that the *IL-2* promoter is nonfunctional in the absence of any one factor (Garrity et al., 1994; Randak et al., 1990; Rao et al., 2003; Rothenberg and Ward, 1996; Smith et al., 2003; Wang et al., 1997). The requirement for all activated factors to be present for IL-2 expression during T cell development or in mature activated T cells supports a model whereby the precise combination of nuclear factors, forming an enhanceosome at the minimal promoter in response to

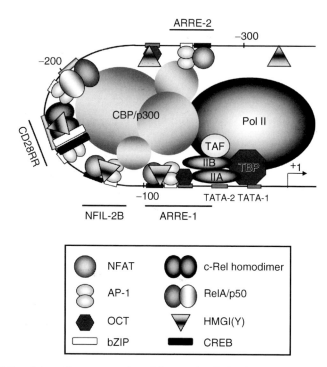

FIGURE 3. Schematic representation of the putative IL-2 enhanceosome assembled at the proximal promoter following T cell activation. Shows positions of activator regulatory sites and composite elements with bound transcription factors, architectural proteins, coactivator proteins and the RNA Pol II transcription machinery. For simplicity, the NF-κB proteins are depicted as a c-Rel homodimer and the canonical RelA/p50 heterodimer, however, many other dimer combinations are possible.

specific activating signals, governs expression of the *IL-2* gene (Fig. 3). This view is complicated, however, by several studies which show that there is in fact a diverse array of factors able to bind to the *IL-2* promoter and enhancer regions under a variety of signal-specific and cell type–specific conditions (Hughes and Pober, 1993; Mouzaki *et al.*, 1995; Pan *et al.*, 2004; Rooney *et al.*, 1995; Thompson *et al.*, 1992; Ward *et al.*, 1998) and that it may not be so much the precise combination of factors as the occupation of the correct set of binding sites that governs cell specificity and induction.

While negative regulators have been shown to silence IL-2 expression, *in vivo* footprinting studies have shown that nuclear factors fail to occupy the *IL-2* minimal promoter region in unstimulated T cells (Garrity *et al.*, 1994). This suggests that while competing activators and repressors might act as an on/off switch for *IL-2* transcription, repressor proteins do not play a role in maintaining the gene in an inactive but permissive state. Rather, this suggests that additional, epigenetic mechanisms exist that are specific for the T cell and for its state of activation. This additional layer of control is determined by T cell–specific changes in chromatin, which modify the structure of the *IL-2* locus into a permissive (resting T cell) or nonpermissive (non-T cell) state and an activated state (activated T cell), depending on the appropriate stimulating or developmental conditions. There are now a growing number of studies which have documented these *IL-2* gene-specific chromatin changes *in vivo* (Adachi and Rothenberg, 2005; Rao *et al.*, 2003; Thomas *et al.*, 2005; Wang *et al.*, 2005; Ward *et al.*, 1998).

Thus, T cell–restricted expression of IL-2 is governed not only by the correct arrangement of transcription factors binding to the *IL-2* promoter but is also critically regulated by T cell–lineage specific *IL-2* gene architecture, which can be further modified on T cell activation.

V. THE ROLE OF CHROMATIN IN CONTROLLING *IL-2* GENE TRANSCRIPTION

In a resting naïve T cell, the *IL-2* locus is in a permissive but inactive chromatin configuration and as discussed earlier, there are specific regions of the gene locus that are DH (Fig. 2). These include the region between –300 and –600bp, a large region stretching from approximately –3 to –4kb and a discreet region at –4.5kb (Ward *et al.*, 1998; Yui *et al.*, 2001). There is no detailed functional data suggesting how these regions may be involved in the regulation of the *IL-2* gene nor is there any evidence as to the point at which these DH sites appear prior to or during T cell development. Following T cell activation, other regions of the gene become hypersensitive to digestion with DNaseI, MNase, or REs and DMS modification (Ward *et al.*, 1998; Yui *et al.*, 2001). There are two major regions of change: one represents the proximal functional promoter and has been well characterized by a number of groups; the second is a region between –2.0 and –3.0kb whose function has not been determined (Siebenlist *et al.*, 1986; Ward *et al.*, 1998; Yui *et al.*, 2001). In addition, discreet regions of DNaseI hypersensitivity occur upstream between –6.0 and –10kb (Yui *et al.*, 2001). It is likely that some of these regions may play a role in controlling the availability of the gene only in the T cell lineage and maintaining the locus in a permissive state but this requires further investigation.

The proximal promoter region has been studied in detail in regard to chromatin structure and the mechanisms by which changes in chromatin structure may occur in response to activation. In a resting T cell this region is inaccessible to DNaseI, MNase, and RE digestion but becomes highly accessible following activation (Brunvand *et al.*, 1993; Rao *et al.*, 2001, 2003; Siebenlist *et al.*, 1986; Ward *et al.*, 1998). In attempting to understand the mechanisms that control this increase in accessibility, many studies have shown that it is the presence of the correct cohort of transcription factors that is essential for chromatin remodeling (Rao *et al.*, 2003; Rothenberg and

Ward, 1996). First, non-T cells or T cells incapable of expressing IL-2 do not show this increase in accessibility implying that it is closely linked with transcription from the gene. For example, CD4+CD25+ Treg cells that cannot express IL-2 do not remodel the *IL-2* proximal promoter following activation (Su *et al.*, 2004). Cells stimulated through the TCR alone also show no change in chromatin structure at the *IL-2* promoter but require CD28 signals for these changes (Thomas *et al.*, 2005). This mimics the need for CD28 to generate high-level transcription from the *IL-2* gene and prevent anergy. Second, inhibiting the activation of specific transcription factors, for example, treatment with cyclosporine to inhibit NFAT or increases in cyclic adenosine monophosphate (cAMP), leads to a loss of accessibility (Rothenberg and Ward, 1996). While these drug treatments are never entirely specific [e.g., cyclosporin A (CsA) can inhibit NF-κB at high doses], other experiments have shown that in T cells where the *c-Rel* gene has been deleted, MNase accessibility is blocked across the entire promoter although RE access shows a more complex pattern (Rao *et al.*, 2003). In many instances, these cells contain the majority of the transcription factors needed to drive transcription but it appears that in the absence of even one of these factors, chromatin cannot be remodeled on the *IL-2* proxiclose relationship between recruitment of the correct transcription complexes on the promoter and the detection of chromatin remodeling, and supports the idea that the formation of an enhanceosome is required for correct gene activation and changes to chromatin structure.

It was speculated that histone modification might play a role in chromatin remodeling at the *IL-2* promoter since a number of coactivators of transcription with histone acetylase activity can interact with the transcription factors that drive *IL-2* transcription. Two studies examining histone modification across the *IL-2* gene have made some interesting observations (summarized in Fig. 2A). First, it was shown that in resting T cells permissive for IL-2 expression, a region spreading from the TSS upstream to –4.6kb had a relatively high level of dimethylation of histone H3 on lysine 4 (diMeH3K4) (Adachi and Rothenberg, 2005). This modification was not observed in cells incapable of expressing IL-2, whether of the T cell lineage or not, and the level of this dimethylation did not change in response to activation (Adachi and Rothenberg, 2005). diMeH3K4 is a marker of a permissive gene and it has previously been shown that this modification is associated with active genes (Peters and Schubeler, 2005). The –4.6kb region, which marks the boundary of the diMeH3K4 region, is marked by a constitutive DH site that remains intact, but is less intense, following activation. This DS may represent a boundary element and may also explain the requirement for this region in order to generate high-frequency expression in transgenic mouse lines (Adachi and Rothenberg, 2005).

The resting state of chromatin appears to be critical for correct gene activation with the specific placement of nucleosomes across promoter or enhancer regions playing a critical role in addition to the histone modification status discussed earlier. It appears that inducible genes often have highly positioned nucleosomes placed across critical control regions. This is well illustrated by studies of the *interferon* (*IFN*)-β gene (Lomvardas and Thanos, 2002) and the *PHO5* gene in yeast (Martinez-Campa *et al.*, 2004). We have shown that the *IL-2* promoter can assemble a highly positioned nucleosome at least in *in vitro* studies and have provided some evidence that a similar nucleosome exists in resting T cells (Attema *et al.*, 2002). This is not a common property of all inducible T cell promoters since the *granulocyte-macrophage colony-stimulating factor* (*GM-CSF*) gene promoter cannot assemble positioned nucleosomes *in vitro* (Attema *et al.*, 2002). The positioned nucleosome on the *IL-2* promoter covers a region from –210 to –60bp, spanning several important transcription factor binding sites (Fig. 2B). It is assumed that this nucleosome plays an important role in maintaining the correct chromatin structure in resting T cells to maintain a permissive but inactive gene.

On activation of *IL-2* transcription, the region marked by diMeH3K4 modification becomes acetylated on histones H3 and H4 and this occurs both in T cell lines and in primary T cells isolated from spleens (Fig. 2A; Adachi and Rothenberg, 2005). These findings are consistent with many studies showing an association between histone acetylation and active gene transcription and the idea that histone acetyltransferases (HATs) may be recruited to the gene on activation (Eberharter and Becker, 2002; Liang *et al.*, 2004; Roh *et al.*, 2005). Results from our own laboratory suggest that this increase in acetylation (at least as measured at –2kb) is transient in nature and decreases in intensity by 6–8 h following activation; the same time frame in which mRNA levels peak and start to decline (Chen *et al.*, 2005). The transient nature of this increase in acetylation may reflect the replacement of activator proteins recruiting HATs with repressors which can recruit histone deacetylases, although it has not yet been shown whether this can occur on the *IL-2* promoter. An exception to the general increase in acetylation across the region to –4.6kb was noted at the proximal promoter where no increase or even slight decreases in acetylation were observed (Adachi and Rothenberg, 2005). Our own studies, where strong decreases in acetylation and phosphorylation of H3 and H4 were observed following activation, have shed light on this unexpected result (Chen *et al.*, 2005). We have shown that these apparent decreases in histone modification were in fact the result of histone loss at the proximal promoter region (Chen *et al.*, 2005). This loss of histones was shown to occur in the same time frame and in response to the same signals as the increase in MNase accessibility and suggests that the increase in MNase accessibility is a measure of histone loss (Chen *et al.*, 2005; Rao *et al.*, 2003). The histone loss was limited to a region of 300–400bp upstream from the TSS, equates with the functional proximal promoter region, and includes the region encompassed by the positioned nucleosome discussed earlier. There is no evidence of significant histone loss further upstream or downstream (Chen *et al.*, 2005).

This loss of histones appears to be transient and by 20 h following activation, histones reappear on the proximal promoter. In addition, if the stimulus is removed at 4 h following activation, histones reappear within a few hours (Chen *et al.*, 2005). A similar phenomenon has been observed on a highly inducible gene, the *PHO5* gene, in yeast following phosphate starvation (Boeger *et al.*, 2003; Reinke and Horz, 2003) and many of the characteristics of activation of this gene and the accompanying histone loss appear very reminiscent of the *IL-2* gene. The mechanism of this histone loss has not yet been elucidated but will be of interest to understand the general mechanisms of proximal promoter function for inducible genes.

DNA methylation has been associated with gene repression and removal of cytosine methylation is associated with gene activation (Hendrich and Tweedie, 2003; Robertson, 2002). The *IL-2* gene has been shown to be methylated on CpG residues in resting T cells (Bruniquel and Schwartz, 2003). Demethylation was shown to accompany gene activation but this demethylation occurred with fast kinetics being observed for some sites within 20 min of cell activation (Bruniquel and Schwartz, 2003). It is unclear as to how such demethylation might occur since a cytosine demethylase has not been isolated. Because of its fast kinetics it appears to be a prelude to histone loss, histone modification, and gene transcription, but any relationship here remains to be determined. The loss of methylation, unlike the other events described earlier, appears to be permanent and may form the basis of the molecular memory of IL-2 expression and T cell activation.

In the future, it will be important to determine the molecular mechanism of chromatin remodeling events at the *IL-2* gene promoter and to understand the role of the upstream regions in maintaining a permissive but inducible chromatin state in T cells.

VI. MULTIPLE SIGNALS ARE REQUIRED FOR ACTIVATION OF *IL-2* GENE TRANSCRIPTION

The transient and exclusive nature of IL-2 expression in T cells during thymocyte development and in mature peripheral immune responses suggests that a highly organized and complex set of signals is required to initiate gene transcription. The way in which this combination of signals is integrated and coordinated—at the level of both T cell activation and the assembly of transcription factor complexes on the *IL-2* promoter—will be the focus of this section.

A. T CELL ACTIVATION AND SIGNALING
PATHWAYS TO *IL-2*

The primary trigger for *de novo* IL-2 expression, both in developing thymocytes and from naïve CD4+ and CD8+ T cells, is a direct and specific interaction of the TCR/CD3 complex with antigen in the context of an antigen-presenting cell (APC) and its associated major histocompatibility complex (MHC) (Santana and Rosenstein, 2003). A secondary stimulus is provided by costimulatory signals—the canonical pathway involves engagement of the B7.1/B7.2 ligands on the APC with the CD28 costimulatory molecule on the surface of the T lymphocyte. This second signal is essential for the induction of IL-2: in the absence of costimulation, TCR engagement fails to induce a productive T cell response leading to a state of unresponsiveness known as clonal anergy (Powell *et al.*, 1998). At least one aspect of this state of anergy is failure to produce IL-2. The intensity and duration of the TCR interaction is also important. Studies have shown that there is a lower requirement for costimulation when the TCR signal is maximized (Murtaza *et al.*, 1999). Conversely, strong costimulation can convert a weak or partial TCR agonist into a full agonist, which is concomitant with enhanced IL-2 production (Murtaza *et al.*, 1999).

Early investigations into the kinetics of T cell activation and gene expression showed that in addition to antigen-specific signals via the TCR/CD28 pathway, pharmacological agents and mitogens, such as phorbol esters (PMA, PHA), calcium ionophores (ionomycin), and lectins (ConA), could induce expression of *IL-2* (and other genes) independently of the TCR (Isakov and Altman, 1985; Lugo *et al.*, 1986; Mohr *et al.*, 1986). Moreover, T cell activation could be mimicked by stimulation with antibodies against the TCR, CD3 (TCR signaling component), or CD28 surface molecules (Bjorndahl *et al.*, 1989; Verweij *et al.*, 1991). All of these modes of activation are commonly used in studies of *IL-2* gene transcription and it is important to note here that while the profiles and expression patterns of genes in response to these different stimuli are virtually identical, the magnitude of their induction has been shown to differ (Diehn *et al.*, 2002).

CD28 costimulation plays an important amplifying role during T cell activation and has been shown to enhance and sustain signaling to a number of genes including *IL-2* (Diehn *et al.*, 2002; Fraser and Weiss, 1992; Michel *et al.*, 2001; Murtaza *et al.*, 1999). At the level of transcription, the CD28 cosignal is thought to act by sustaining the nuclear accumulation of a number of transcription factors involved in the maintenance of *IL-2* transcription and by prolonging the half-life of the *IL-2* mRNA (Coyle and Gutierrez-Ramos, 2001; Powell *et al.*, 1998). Moreover, there is considerable evidence that the CD28 costimulatory signal functions by converging on specific CD28-responsive *cis* elements in the *IL-2* gene promoter to drive transcription (discussed in greater detail in a later section). While it is generally accepted that CD28 acts to augment TCR signals, there are also reports that CD28 can deliver a unique signal to the cell, independently of the TCR (Marinari *et al.*, 2004; Siefken *et al.*, 1997).

In addition to CD28, many other T cell surface molecules provide costimulatory signals to T cells, including CD4, ICAM-1, CD2, CD43, CD69, IL-1, CD5, and CD9 (Coyle and Gutierrez-Ramos, 2001; D'Ambrosio *et al.*, 1993; Dubey *et al.*, 1995; Novak *et al.*, 1990; Zhou *et al.*, 2002). Stimulation of human T lymphocytes with a combination of CD2 and CD28 induces long-term nuclear expression of NF-κB, driving sustained IL-2 and IL-2Rα production (Costello *et al.*, 1993). Likewise, intercellular adhesion molecule 1 (ICAM-1) molecules residing on the T cell surface deliver a costimulatory signal via enhanced cell-to-cell contact which promotes T cell proliferation and increased IL-2 expression (Chirathaworn *et al.*, 2002; Dubey *et al.*, 1995). Conversely, the integrin lymphocyte function-associated antigen 1 (LFA-1), which is also expressed on T cells and is a ligand for ICAM-1 expressed on APCs, can upregulate *IL-2* gene expression independently of mRNA stabilization (Abraham and Miller, 2001). The macrophage-derived cytokine IL-1 has also been shown to be a potent "second signal," eliciting the production of IL-2 from T helper cells (Novak *et al.*, 1990). A new member of the costimulatory molecule family was identified—the glucocorticoid-induced TNF-related gene receptor (GITR)—which is expressed on resting Treg cells and activated CD4+ T cells and, in combination with CD28, is thought to play a role in T cell proliferation and effector function by modulating IL-2 expression (Kohm *et al.*, 2005). In contrast, the cytotoxic T lymphocyte antigen 4 (CTLA-4) and suppressor of cytokine signaling 3 (SOCS3) signaling molecules contribute to downregulation of the IL-2 response (Egen and Allison, 2002; Matsumoto *et al.*, 2003). Activation of IL-2 by alternate signals, such as the HTLV-1 gene product Tax, the human cytomegalovirus immediate early gene (IE2), and the viral proteins Nef and Tat produced during HIV-1 infection, have also been demonstrated in human CD4+ T cells and lead to hyperresponsiveness of the *IL-2* promoter (Curtiss *et al.*, 1996; Fortin *et al.*, 2004; Geist *et al.*, 1991).

Subsequent to the engagement of the TCR complex and adjacent costimulatory molecules on the T cell surface, IL-2-activating signals are relayed via intracellular signaling cascades, which culminate at the T cell nucleus. Briefly, membrane-associated protein tyrosine kinases (ZAP-70, SYK, SRC, and TEC family kinases) are recruited to the transmembrane receptor molecules (CD3, CD4, and CD28), followed by the phosphorylation of adaptor proteins (LAT, SLP-76, and Grb2), GTP/GDP exchange factors (Vav, Sos), and PLCγ1 (Iwashima, 2003). Interactions between transmembrane receptors and cytosolic signaling molecules have been shown to be mediated by rearrangements in the T cell cytoskeleton and aided by glycolipid microdomains or "lipid rafts" which aggregate at the T cell-APC interface to enhance the magnitude of the transmitted signal (Koretzky and Myung, 2001). Downstream of these events, intermediate signaling molecules, including the small GTPases, Ras and Rac, and the secondary messengers, diacylglycerol (DAG) and inositol triphosphate (IP3), activate the major protein kinases: MEKK1, PKC, IKK, and PKA which, in turn, activate pathways leading to transcription factor induction. The mitogen activated protein kinase (MAPK)- or MAP kinase-ERK kinase kinase (MEKK)-induced extracellular regulated MAP kinase (ERK) and Jun kinase (JNK) pathways lead to activation of an Ets family member, Elk-1, and to induction of AP-1 complexes containing c-Jun and c-Fos. Increases in intracellular calcium (Ca^{2+}) activate calcineurin and PKC, which feed into pathways that activate the NFAT family of transcription factors or, via PKC-θ, induce IKK activation, targeting IκB complexes for degradation, and releasing active NF-κB dimers (Gaffen and Liu, 2004; Iwashima, 2003; Sedwick and Altman, 2004). The three major classes of transcription factors activated by these TCR/CD28-mediated intracellular signaling pathways—AP-1, NFAT, and NF-κB—translocate to the T cell nucleus, where they play a primary role in inducing IL-2 expression by binding to specific elements within the IL-2 proximal promoter and enhancer regions (Garrity et al., 1994).

B. THE *IL-2* PROMOTER BINDS A COMPLEX SET OF TRANSCRIPTION FACTORS

Soon after the initial characterization of the 300bp control region immediately upstream of the TSS of the *IL-2* gene, several reports emerged with the first evidence of nuclear factors that could bind specifically to mitogen-responsive elements in the *IL-2* promoter (Brunvand et al., 1988; Granelli-Piperno and Nolan, 1991; Shibuya and Taniguchi, 1989). The identities of these nuclear proteins were delineated in subsequent investigations, which found that inducible NFAT, AP-1, and NF-κB transcription factor complexes and the constitutively expressed factor Oct-1 could bind specifically to individual promoter elements to activate *IL-2* transcription (Fig. 4; Jain et al., 1995; Serfling et al., 1995). Together, these early investigations also showed that these three classes of inducible transcription factors could directly link signals initiated at the TCR to transcription of *IL-2*.

NFAT, originally—but no longer—believed to be the T cell–specific factor driving *IL-2* transcription, plays a key role in transduction of the Ca^{2+} signal following TCR engagement and is specifically blocked by a number of potent immunosuppressant drugs (including CsA and FK506) which inhibit calcineurin phosphatase activity (Emmel et al., 1989; Granelli-Piperno and Nolan, 1991; Serfling et al., 1995; Shaw et al., 1988). The *IL-2* proximal promoter contains three well-characterized NFAT binding sites (regions are denoted ARRE-1, NFIL-2B, and ARRE-2), which are bound by NFAT1 and NFAT2 in stimulated T cells (Fig. 4) (Garrity et al., 1994). Additional NFAT sites have also been identified by footprinting and reporter analysis

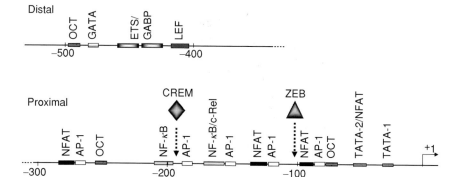

FIGURE 4. Transcription factor binding to the murine *IL-2* minimal promoter region. The distal and proximal *IL-2* promoter regions show locations of well defined activator binding sites, the CD28-responsive region (CD28RR), antigen receptor-responsive elements (ARRE-1 and ARRE-2) and the NFIL-2B composite element. Sites for the binding of repressor proteins (CREM and ZEB) to the proximal region are also indicated.

(Rooney *et al.*, 1995). While the targeted disruption of NFAT1 and NFAT2 genes individually in mice does not cause a decrease in IL-2 production, a dominant-negative NFAT mutant was shown to selectively inhibit NFAT-mediated IL-2 expression implying redundant use of the family members (Chow *et al.*, 1999). A characteristic feature of NFAT proteins is that they bind cooperatively with AP-1 proteins (Yaseen *et al.*, 1994) and this is clearly illustrated at the composite NFIL-2B site and at the two antigen receptor-responsive elements, ARRE-1 and ARRE-2, within the *IL-2* promoter (Fig. 4; Durand *et al.*, 1988).

   The Oct factors also regulate *IL-2* transcription by binding to two Oct binding sites within the proximal and distal regions of the *IL-2* promoter (Kamps *et al.*, 1990). Mutation of either of these Oct sites reduces *IL-2* promoter activity, but mutation of both abolishes expression. Oct factors have also been demonstrated to bind upstream of the minimal *IL-2* promoter in the distal –600 to –300bp region, although less is understood about these interactions here (Fig. 4; Ward *et al.*, 1998). While Oct-1 is expressed constitutively, Oct-2 requires cell stimulation; however, the role of Oct-2 is not so clear since mice deficient in Oct-2 do not show any defects in their peripheral T cell responses (Corcoran and Karvelas, 1994). Like the NFAT sites, the proximal Oct site forms a composite element with AP-1 (ARRE-1) and these factors, in addition to NFAT, can bind cooperatively (de Grazia *et al.*, 1994; Pfeuffer *et al.*, 1994).

   The NF-κB/Rel family of transcription factors which includes five members: NF-κB1 (p50), RelB, NF-κB2 (p52), RelA (p65), and c-Rel, function as homo- and heterodimers and bind to two canonical sites in the *IL-2* promoter (Fig. 4).

One of these sites—the CD28-responsive element, or CD28RE—forms a composite element with an AP-1 site (the CD28RR) which has been extensively characterized and is critical for integration of the CD28 cosignal (Ghosh et al., 1993; McGuire and Iacobelli, 1997; Shapiro et al., 1997). The actual proteins that bind to this AP-1 element are controversial and other related factors such as the CREB family of bZIP proteins also play a role here (Curtiss et al., 1996). In response to a variety of extracellular stimuli, RelA/p50 dimers are released from inhibitory IκB complexes into the nucleus, where they bind to the IL-2 promoter and help to drive transcription. The available evidence suggests that RelA/p50 activity on the IL-2 promoter occurs immediately following T cell stimulation, while complexes containing c-Rel proteins are induced later and could contribute to the maintenance of IL-2 promoter activity (Bryan et al., 1994). Antisense experiments have also shown that c-Rel activity is critical for CD28-mediated activation of IL-2 and preferentially binds to and activates the IL-2 CD28RE site (Himes et al., 1996). While RelA knockout is embryonic lethal in mice, mice lacking the c-Rel gene have distinct defects in mature T cell responses and have reduced expression of IL-2 and other cytokines (Gerondakis et al., 1996; Grossmann et al., 1999). Specifically, c-Rel has been shown to play a role in chromatin remodeling events across the CD28RR region of the IL-2 promoter in CD4+ T cells and can cooperate with other transcription factors to drive transcription from reporters containing multimerized IL-2 CD28RR sites (Butscher et al., 1998; Harant and Lindley, 2004; Rao et al., 2003).

As seen earlier, AP-1 cooperates with all of the other major factors that control IL-2 transcription and thus plays a critical role in IL-2 transcription. It is therefore considered the primary integrator and coordinator of information from extracellular signals and is even thought to respond to various developmental stages of the T cell (Chen and Rothenberg, 1993; Rincon and Flavell, 1994, 1996). A combination of signaling via the PKC and Ca^{2+} pathways is required for maximal induction and DNA binding of AP-1 factors to the IL-2 promoter (Jain et al., 1992b; Rincon and Flavell, 1994). In addition, AP-1 transcriptional activity requires costimulation, either through CD28 or other surface molecules (described earlier), which can also modulate the composition of subunits that constitute the AP-1 dimer. AP-1 binding sites, which bind dimers of c-Fos and c-Jun family members, predominantly function as composite elements within the Oct/NFAT (ARRE-1), NFAT (ARRE-2), and CD28RE (CD28RR) sites (Fig. 4; Jain et al., 1992a; Serfling et al., 1995).

In addition to the four classes of IL-2 regulatory factors described previously, roles for a variety of other factors—some novel—have been described in IL-2 promoter function. These include Sp1, Egr1, ETS family transcription factors, Elf1 and GABP, the HMG box protein LEF-1, NF-45/ILF2, and NF-90/ILF3, Schnurri-3, myocyte enhancer factor 2 (MEF2), and Kruppel-like factor 2 (KLF2) (Avots et al., 1997; Oukka et al., 2004; Pan et al., 2004; Skerka et al., 1995; Thompson et al., 1992; Ward et al., 1998;

Wu and Lingrel, 2005; Zhao *et al.*, 2005) but their precise functions are still to be determined.

C. COMBINATORIAL CONTROL OF THE PROXIMAL
IL-2 PROMOTER

It is evident from these investigations that induced transcription of the *IL-2* gene in activated T cells relies on the binding of multiple, distinct transcription factors to many adjacent and overlapping elements within the *IL-2* proximal and distal promoter regions. In resting T cells, footprinting analysis across the promoter has shown that all the binding sites for these factors are unoccupied. In contrast, in activated, IL-2-expressing cells there appears to be an "all or nothing" occupation of the promoter sites. However, when any one regulatory element is blocked in activated cells, IL-2 expression is completely abrogated, indicating nonredundancy among these distinct groups of activating factors and the requirement for coordinated occupancy of all of the sites (Briegel *et al.*, 1991). This can be explained by the fact that, individually, the *IL-2* regulatory proteins bind relatively weakly to their cognate sites and do not appear to interact stably with the DNA unless all factors are present (Garrity *et al.*, 1994; Hentsch *et al.*, 1992). This is evident in experiments where the entire *IL-2* footprint is lost using inhibitors which specifically block a distinct signaling pathway or the DNA binding of only a subset of factors (Garrity *et al.*, 1994). In addition, if the weak binding sites are changed to canonical sites, the correct regulation of the promoter is disrupted, suggesting that multiple weak interactions are important for correct transcriptional activation of the gene (Hentsch *et al.*, 1992).

Another notable feature of *IL-2* transcription is its regulation by several composite promoter elements and the cooperative binding of transcription factors as described earlier. This combinatorial control enables the integration of many different, cell-specific signals which dictate the specific expression of IL-2 in T cells. Cooperative binding of factors to gene promoter elements that are nonconsensus sites or "weak binders," as is the case for *IL-2*, could represent a control mechanism to prevent inappropriate expression of the gene. This is particularly pertinent for synthesis of IL-2 considering its role as a potent inducer of T cell immunity.

AP-1 is the best example of this coordinate binding, forming composite complexes right across the *IL-2* proximal and distal promoter regions, it works in close association with the Oct, NFAT, and NF-κB regulatory factors to drive transcription (Serfling *et al.*, 1995). Studies by Shapiro and colleagues (Shapiro *et al.*, 1997) have elegantly demonstrated the requirement for coordinated binding of AP-1 and NF-κB/Rel proteins to the composite CD28RE/AP-1 (CD28RR or RE/AP) element in the proximal region of the *IL-2* promoter. c-Rel associates specifically with the CD28RE site in response to CD28 signaling but alone, cannot account for full activation of the *IL-2* gene, requiring cooperation with AP-1 binding to the adjacent AP-1 element (Shapiro *et al.*, 1997). In addition, when c-Rel was overexpressed in T cells, AP-1 activity was significantly enhanced, thus providing an example of a feed-forward loop where one factor controls the level of a second factor and, together, they regulate the expression of a downstream gene (Shapiro *et al.*, 1996, 1998).

NFAT binds cooperatively with the AP-1 components, c-Fos and c-Jun, to the distal NFAT/AP-1 site (ARRE-2). Specifically, the family members Fra-1 and JunB form a heterodimer, which has been identified in the NFAT1 DNA binding complex (Boise *et al.*, 1993). Cooperation between NFAT and AP-1 on the *IL-2* promoter is thought to be directed by a leucine zipper in the AP-1 dimer which orientates the two proteins for interaction (Erlanson *et al.*, 1996). Modification of the variant AP-1 element within this composite site has been shown to eliminate *IL-2* transcription, despite the presence of an intact NFAT site further downstream (Zhang and Nabel, 1994). This is supported by studies which show that a dominant-negative form of c-Jun can inhibit NFAT-mediated *IL-2* transcription, while overexpression of AP-1 family members significantly augments this action (Jain *et al.*, 1992c; Petrak *et al.*, 1994; Yaseen *et al.*, 1994). Likewise, Oct-1 functionally cooperates with AP-1 proteins at the proximal AP-1/Oct site (ARRE-1). Mutation of this element also abolishes *IL-2* transcription, and this also cannot be overcome by binding to an Oct-1 site further upstream (de Grazia, 1994).

It was demonstrated that the early growth response proteins, Egr1 and Egr4, synergistically interact with NFAT factors to activate *IL-2* transcription. In addition to requiring both adjacent sites (NFAT and bZIP sequences) to be intact, Egr and NFAT can form stable heterodimers to regulate expression of both the *IL-2* and *tumour necrosis factor-α* (*TNF-α*) genes (Decker *et al.*, 1998). It has also been shown that Egr can directly associate with RelA and p50 to either transactivate or inhibit *IL-2* promoter activity (Wieland *et al.*, 2005).

Thus, the cooperativity of transcription factor complexes on the *IL-2* promoter can help to overcome the absence of canonical, independent binding sequences and forms the basis of a precise means of controlling transcriptional activation of the *IL-2* gene in T cells.

D. COACTIVATOR RECRUITMENT TO THE *IL-2* PROMOTER

The cooperative effects of transcription factors on the *IL-2* gene promoter do not necessarily arise from direct contact between the factors themselves at adjacent sites but may be mediated by coactivator complexes which help to bridge groups of factors bound to a promoter. These coactivators form large multiprotein/DNA complexes or "enhanceosomes" which generally assist in the recruitment of the basal transcription machinery, the modification of the DNA or histones to alter chromatin structure, or help to stabilize all of the components of the transcriptionally active complex at the promoter.

The HMGI(Y) family of small nuclear proteins is known to play an important role in chromatin architecture and in inducible gene expression. HMGI(Y) has been implicated in the transcriptional control of a number of inducible immune genes, such as *IFN-β, E-selectin, IL-4, IL-2, IL-2Rα* and *GM-CSF*, functioning either as a positive or negative regulator of gene expression (Shannon *et al.*, 1998, 2001). With respect to *IL-2* transcription, studies from our own lab have shown that HMGI(Y) binds to the CD28RE of the *IL-2* promoter and is critical for the specific recruitment and binding of c-Rel—but not RelA—to this region (Himes *et al.*, 1996). Moreover, CD28-driven IL-2 activation is blocked by HMGI(Y) antisense RNA, both in the context of a reporter plasmid and at the level of the endogenous *IL-2* gene, implying an important role for this nuclear protein in *IL-2* promoter activity (Himes *et al.*, 1996). Subsequent investigations have identified A: T-rich binding sites for this protein at many sites across the *IL-2* promoter and distal –600 to –300bp region and these overlap many of the elements bound by transcription factor complexes (Fig. 3). It was found that HMGI (Y) could also modulate the binding of NFAT and AP-1; however, DNA binding of HMGI(Y) is not essential for binding of c-Rel and AP-1 proteins to the *IL-2* promoter (Himes *et al.*, 1996). Furthermore, a non-DNA-binding mutant of HMGI(Y) can still interact with transcription factor complexes, suggesting a role for HMGI(Y) in promoting transcription factor binding by protein–protein interactions (Himes *et al.*, 1996). This idea is supported by experiments performed on the *IL-2Rα* promoter, which show that HMGI(Y) and Elf-1 act together in a complex to drive transcription (John *et al.*, 1995). Likewise, HMGI(Y) is essential for the formation of an enhanceosome on the *IFN-β* promoter (Yie *et al.*, 1999). It is clearly evident from these studies that HMGI(Y) serves an important regulatory function in *IL-2* activation; by facilitating or modulating the binding of the NF-κB, NFAT, and AP-1 transcription factors to their relatively weak-affinity sites within the *IL-2* promoter, it can help to establish the cooperative assembly of promoter-specific factors which drive expression of IL-2.

The CD28RR enhancer element within the *IL-2* proximal promoter is also targeted by the CREB-binding protein (CBP)/p300 coactivator complex in association with c-Rel and cAMP-responsive element (CRE)-binding protein (CREB) factors (Fig. 3) (Butscher *et al.*, 1998, 2001; Smith *et al.*, 2003). The intrinsic HAT activity of p300 appears to be dispensable for *IL-2* promoter activity; rather, p300 may play a role in the assembly of an enhanceosome-like complex in combination with many other DNA-binding and non-DNA-binding factors and can integrate signals from mitogenic and oncogenic stimuli (Butscher *et al.*, 2001). Chromatin immunoprecipitation (ChIP) experiments have shown that p300 is recruited to the *IL-2* promoter within 30 min of activation by mitogenic stimuli (PMA and ionophore) (Smith *et al.*, 2004).

Detailed analysis of the temporal and signal-dependent recruitment of these complexes and transcription factors to the endogenous *IL-2* gene by ChIP will certainly be an important step toward understanding the sequence of events which occurs on activation of the *IL-2* promoter, both at the level of gene transcription and in the context of chromatin remodeling.

VII. MECHANISMS TO REPRESS THE *IL-2* GENE IN T CELLS

Concomitant with the requirement for tight regulation and restriction of *IL-2* gene activation in T cells is the need for repressors or "silencers" of *IL-2* transcription. A number of transcription factors, steroids, and other molecules have been identified as negative regulators of *IL-2* gene expression. These have been proposed to contribute to *IL-2* gene regulation by restricting or silencing *IL-2* transcription in tissues that are nonpermissive for IL-2 expression and in T cell lineages or subsets which do not express IL-2 or have undergone clonal anergy. In addition, repressors may play a role in maintaining a permissive but inactive gene in T cell lineages, although there is still some debate about transcription factor occupancy of the promoter in resting T cells. While a cell-specific repressor of *IL-2* transcription has not been identified, it is clear that in cells where the *IL-2* gene is not expressed, the components of the *IL-2* transcriptional complexes are altered to favor a repressed chromatin state. These repressive mechanisms have already been utilized to inhibit IL-2 expression in specific disease situations and may also be perturbed in situations of aberrant IL-2 expression.

A. STEROID-MEDIATED *IL-2* REPRESSION

Glucocorticoids (GCs) have played a major role in the treatment of allograft rejection and in autoimmune, allergic, and malignant diseases. The extensive use of GCs is based on their dramatic effects on inflammatory and immune responses. GCs affect the growth, differentiation, and function of monocytes and lymphocytes as well as the production of cytokines (Boumpas *et al.*, 1991). Dexamethasone (Dex), a synthetic GC hormone, inhibits the transcription of the *IL-2* gene in primary human T cells (Paliogianni *et al.*, 1993). However, in the *IL-2* promoter region there are no GC response elements (GREs) which could bind the GC receptor (GR) and negatively regulate transcription. Studies toward understanding the molecular mechanisms of GC-mediated inhibition of the *IL-2* gene in T cells suggest that the inhibitory effect is mainly mediated by interference with AP-1 and NFAT since T cells treated with GCs exhibited significantly reduced binding of AP-1 and NFAT to their respective sites on the *IL-2* promoter. Maximum inhibition of *IL-2* promoter transcription involves interaction with both transcription factors, but AP-1 is thought to be the primary target of GCs since inhibition of AP-1 site function does not require the presence of other motifs from the *IL-2* promoter (Paliogianni *et al.*, 1993). Mutation of NFAT and the proximal AP-1-like motifs impairs the ability of the promoter to be inhibited by GCs. Direct protein–protein interactions between AP-1 and GR have been shown to repress several genes (Jonat *et al.*, 1990; Schule *et al.*, 1990) and it is assumed that the same occurs for the *IL-2* gene, although this remains to be directly shown. Whether the *IL-2* gene is controlled in T cells by the balance between GCs and the activating transcription complexes remains to be determined but the use of synthetic steroids to inhibit the expression of IL-2 and other similarly controlled cytokines has clearly been of clinical significance already.

B. CAMP-MEDIATED SUPPRESSION OF THE *IL-2* GENE

Cyclic AMP-triggered expression of numerous genes is largely mediated by CREB which belongs to a large superfamily of immediate early transcription factors with bZIP motifs (Gonzalez and Montminy, 1989). The response begins with the cAMP-mediated dissociation of the inactive tetrameric protein kinase A (PKA) complex into active catalytic and regulatory subunits (Stopka *et al.*, 2005). Catalytic subunits then migrate into the nucleus, where they phosphorylate and activate transcriptional activators, including CREB, which then interacts as a dimer with CREs in the promoters of cAMP-responsive genes and activates their transcription (Sassone-Corsi, 1998). cAMP is able to either downregulate or upregulate expression of a number of cytokine genes, generally having upregulatory effects on the production of T_H2 cytokines, such as IL-10 and IL-6, whereas it downregulates T_H1 type cytokines, including IL-2 and IFN-γ (Novak and Rothenberg, 1990). This correlates with the observation that significantly higher amounts of cAMP are present in T_H2 compared to T_H1 cell lines. CD4+ T cells, which preferentially make IL-2, have particularly low levels of cAMP per cell and a low capacity to elevate cAMP in response to forskolin (Novak and Rothenberg, 1990).

The mechanism by which increased cAMP levels repress IL-2 has been investigated by several groups (Tenbrock and Tsokos, 2004). Paradoxically, as described earlier, CREB has been shown to have an activating function on the *IL-2* promoter (Solomou *et al.*, 2001) and other related bZIP proteins have been implicated as repressors of *IL-2* promoter activity (Bodor *et al.*, 2001). CREB, cAMP response element modulator (CREM) and inducible cAMP early repressor (ICER) are members of the cAMP-responsive family of the basic leucine zipper transcription factors, all of which bind to CREs (Foulkes *et al.*, 1991; Hoeffler *et al.*, 1989). CREM has various isoforms regulated by four different promoters and alternative splicing (Daniel and Habener, 1998).

These isoforms can function as either transcriptional repressors or activators depending on the presence or the absence of specific transactivating domains (Foulkes *et al.*, 1991). One of the four promoters regulates the expression of ICER, which lacks the upstream transactivation domain of CREM (Bodor *et al.*, 1996, 2000). Both CREM and ICER are expressed in the immune system and act as repressors of T cell proliferation via inhibition of IL-2 expression (Bodor *et al.*, 1996). In the *IL-2* proximal promoter region, the AP-1-like element of the CD28RR (at −150bp) has been shown to bind CREB and other family members including CREM and ICER (Bodor and Habener, 1998). As ICER does not have a transactivation domain required for the recruitment of CBP/p300, binding of ICER to the *IL-2* promoter may fail to target the CBP/p300 complex to the promoter. Therefore, transcription cannot be initiated due to the lack of CBP/p300 which is needed as a scaffold protein for the *IL-2* enhanceosome and could also be involved in histone acetylation (Fig. 3) (Garcia-Rodriguez and Rao, 1998). Transgenic mice overexpressing ICER showed a significant reduction of IL-2 and a severe defect in T cell proliferation (Bodor *et al.*, 2001). Mice expressing a dominant-negative mutant of CREB exhibited the same phenotype (Barton *et al.*, 1996). In fact, CBP-deficient mice also show a general proliferation defect (Yao *et al.*, 1998), supporting the concept that the dominant-negative mutant of CREB or overexpression of ICER may compete with endogenous CREB and interfere with recruitment of CBP/p300.

Other studies have provided further evidence that CREM is a repressor of IL-2 (Tenbrock *et al.*, 2002, 2003). In normal T cells, CREM is induced on T cell activation and binds to the −180bp position of *IL-2* promoter to repress its transcriptional activity (Fig. 4). It has been shown that blocking CREM production can enhance and extend IL-2 production (Juang *et al.*, 2005). It has also been shown using ChIP assays that CREB binds to the −180bp region in resting T cells and that it is phosphorylated *in situ* on activation. This phosphorylated CREB is later replaced by CREM (Solomou *et al.*, 2001). Following the binding of CREM to the *IL-2* promoter, there is an elevated association of histones to the proximal promoter and increased inaccessibility of the promoter region to endonucleases implying that the chromatin structure reverts to a repressive configuration (Tenbrock, 2003). Although CREM can recruit CBP/p300 to the *IL-2* promoter through its kinase inducible domain, it is unable to stimulate its HAT activity because CREM lacks the transactivating domain Q2 (De Cesare *et al.*, 1999). Other studies have shown, however, that the HAT activity of CBP/p300 is not necessary for the induction of *IL-2* transcription (Butscher *et al.*, 2001) so this discrepancy remains to be resolved. Furthermore, CREM does not activate transcription factor IID (TFIID) which is an essential step in transcription (Ferreri *et al.*, 1994). These results imply that the balance between CREB and CREM/ICER may modulate the level of IL-2 expression.

A study revealed that T cells from patients with SLE produce less IL-2 and this appears to be due to the altered balance between activators and repressors in these SLE T cells. In fact, SLE T cells are thought to have an anergic phenotype (Tenbrock and Tsokos, 2004). CREM is highly expressed in unstimulated T cells from SLE patients whereas other transcription factors such as NF-κB, AP-1, and CREB are downregulated compared with normal T cells (Kyttaris *et al.*, 2004; Wong *et al.*, 1999). Increased binding of CREM to the –180bp site (an AP-1 site in Fig. 4) of the *IL-2* promoter correlates with accumulation of nuclear CREM whereas CREB binding appears to be underrepresented in these cells. This may reflect, in part, disproportional elevation in nuclear CREM in SLE T cells (Juang *et al.*, 2005). Ca^{2+}/calmodulin-dependent kinase IV (CaMKIV) was shown to play an important role in regulating CREM expression associated with suppression of IL-2 in SLE T cells (Juang *et al.*, 2005). CaMKIV is located in the cytoplasm in normal T cells but resides primarily in the nucleus in SLE T cells. Therefore, abnormally regulated CaMKIV in SLE T cells may relate to the dysregulation of *IL-2* gene expression. CaMKIV significantly upregulates expression of CREM and enhances its binding to the –180bp site of the *IL-2* promoter in SLE T cells to suppress *IL-2* transcription (Juang *et al.*, 2005). In SLE T cells, only anti-TCR/CD3 antibodies which can activate CaMKIV are responsible for the increased expression of CREM and the suppression of *IL-2* transcription. This increased nuclear CREM could function to repress transcription in several ways. It is possible that increased amounts of CREM sequester the CBP/p300 coactivators, making them unavailable to CREB or other transcription factors. It is also possible that CREM has a higher binding affinity than CREB to –180bp site, thereby preferentially occupying the –180bp site in SLE T cells and subsequently repressing *IL-2* transcription using the same mechanism described earlier in normal T cells.

It is appears that reduction of IL-2 expression in SLE T cells is a combinatorial effect of decreased activators (such as NF-κB and AP-1) and excessive expression of repressors (CREM) and is a good model to study the balancing act that is needed to generate appropriate levels of *IL-2* gene expression.

C. REPRESSIVE ACTIVITY OF ZEB ON THE *IL-2* GENE

ZEB is a zinc finger/homeodomain transcription factor which contains two C2H2 zinc finger clusters located close to N- and C-termini and a homeodomain in between. It is also called δ-EF-1 in mouse, ZFH-1 in *Drosophila*, AREB6 and Nil-2-a in human, and BZP in hamster. ZEB was originally identified as a transcriptional repressor which binds to the negative regulatory element (NRE) of the *IL-2* promoter to reduce the transcriptional activity of the *IL-2* gene (Williams *et al.*, 1991). Furthermore,

ZEB was shown to repress other genes such as *immunoglobulin μ heavy chain, CD4, GATA-3, integrin-α4,* and *p73* (Postigo and Dean, 2000). In both T_H1 and T_H2 type cells, the transcription factors—AP-1, NFAT, and NF-κB—required for activation of the *IL-2* gene are present in the nucleus of activated cells but IL-2 is generally not expressed in T_H2 cells. Activated T_H2 cells treated with cycloheximide (CHX) give rise to transcription of the *IL-2* gene (Munoz *et al.*, 1989), and further, treatment of both a mouse T cell line (EL-4) and T_H1 cells with CHX results in a superinduction of IL-2 production (Zubiaga *et al.*, 1991), indicating that a transcriptional repressor that requires ongoing synthesis is controlling *IL-2* gene expression. The binding of nuclear ZEB to the NRE of the *IL-2* promoter in polarized T_H cells shows that following activation, T_H1 cells have reduced binding activity to the NRE, while in T_H2 cells NRE binding activity remains high, perhaps explaining the lack of IL-2 expression in T_H2 cells. Mutation of the NRE ZEB binding site in the context of the *IL-2* promoter results in significantly enhanced *IL-2* reporter gene activity in T_H2, suggesting that binding of ZEB to the NRE can repress *IL-2* transcriptional activity in a cell type which normally does not produce IL-2 on activation. Cells transfected with anti-sense ZEB show a dramatic increase in *IL-2* reporter gene activity, whereas the activity of the *IL-2* NRE mutant promoter was much less affected (Yasui *et al.*, 1998). All of these studies suggest that ZEB is an inducible, CHX-sensitive repressor of *IL-2* transcription in T_H2 cells, and to a lesser extent in T_H1 cells.

It appears that ZEB binding to the *IL-2* promoter disrupts the formation of a stable transcription complex, thereby inhibiting IL-2 expression. It has been shown that ZEB strongly interacts with CtBP, a corepressor, to suppress various genes (Postigo and Dean, 1999). Our own studies have shown that ZEB cooperates with CtBP to significantly repress *IL-2* promoter activity in EL-4 cells (unpublished data). A recently identified CtBP complex which contains ZEB, histone deacetylase, histone methytransferase, and demethylase play an important role in converting an open, active chromatin state to a compacted repressive chromatin state, thereby silencing gene expression (Shi *et al.*, 2003). It will be of interest to determine the role of ZEB in many aspects of *IL-2* gene regulation, including maintenance of a permissive but inactive gene, the repression of the gene immediately following activation, and in repressing IL-2 in other cell populations such as Tregs.

There are a number of other transcription factors which have been shown to negatively regulate *IL-2* transcription, including Ets1 (Romano-Spica *et al.*, 1995), T-bet (Hwang *et al.*, 2005), and p21[SNFT] (Iacobelli *et al.*, 2000) but much less is known about their function. 5-Aminoimidazole-4-carboxamide ribonucleoside (AICAR), an intermediate of purine biosynthesis, is also known to suppress IL-2 expression and *IL-2* promoter activity by inhibiting GSK-3 phosphorylation and NFAT activation (Jhun *et al.*, 2005).

Experiments have shown that the transcriptional repressor DREAM (down-stream regulatory element antagonist modulator) can directly bind to the *IL-2* promoter to repress IL-2 production in TCR-transgenic T lymphocytes (Savignac *et al.*, 2005). Binding of DREAM to specific DRE sequences within the promoter is thought to be regulated by interactions with other nucleoproteins such as CREM and CREB (Ledo *et al.*, 2000, 2002). Similarly, there is evidence implicating SATB1, a T cell–specific global gene regulator, in repression of the *IL-2* and *IL-2Rα* genes, where recruitment of HDAC1 by SATB1 to the human *IL-2* promoter leads to downregulation of IL-2 expression (Kumar *et al.*, 2005). These repressive effects can be overcome by the competitive displacement of HDAC1 by the HIV Tat transactivator, suggesting that there is also a dynamic interplay between repressor and activator complexes.

D. *IL-2* REPRESSION AND T CELL ANERGY

Repression of IL-2 synthesis is most commonly seen in activated T cells which have undergone clonal anergy. While the mechanisms responsible for the induction of T cell anergy are not well understood, it is generally thought to be caused by the engagement of the TCR in the absence of costimulation signals such as CD28/B7 (Schwartz, 2003). The resulting hallmark features of T cell anergy are attenuated proliferation and the failure of T cells to produce IL-2. Engagement of the CD28 costimulatory molecules, however, is unable to directly protect T cells from anergy; rather effects downstream of costimulation are thought to prevent anergy. These downstream events are initiated by the upregulation of IL-2 which drives proliferation of the T cell and a consequential "dilution" of TCR activation-induced anergic factors (Powell *et al.*, 1998). This was demonstrated in early experiments by Schwartz and colleagues, who found that the anergic state could be induced by incubating purified T cells with anti-CD3 or anti-TCR antibodies and could subsequently be reversed by the addition of exogenous IL-2 (Beverly *et al.*, 1992). Thus, in addition to being repressed in anergic T cells, IL-2 itself plays a key role in T cell anergy. Anergy has also been shown to be induced in effector T cells by Hepatitis C virus core protein and drugs such as rapamycin (Powell *et al.*, 1998; Sundstrom *et al.*, 2005), and is a notable feature of Treg cells which are hyporesponsive to stimulation and do not produce IL-2 (Li *et al.*, 2005). Treg cells can in turn act to induce suppression or anergy in effector T cells by way of a negative feedback loop in response to IL-2/IL-2Rα signaling.

The molecular basis for T cell anergy has not been extensively characterized; however, there is some evidence to suggest that a number of negative regulatory factors described earlier, such as ZEB, CREM, and ICER, are involved in direct repression of *IL-2* transcription in anergized T cells (Bodor *et al.*, 2000; Powell *et al.*, 1998, 1999; Yasui *et al.*, 1998). Overexpression experiments have also shown that sustained Egr-2 and Egr-3 expression leads to inhibition of IL-2 expression and inhibits T cell function (Harris *et al.*, 2004; Safford *et al.*, 2005). There is significant evidence showing that anergy is accompanied by a reduction in AP-1 binding to the –180bp CD28RR composite element of the *IL-2* proximal promoter and that this region is in fact a target for transcriptional repression in anergic T cells (Heisel and Keown, 2001; Powell *et al.*, 1999). It is possible that proteins, such as ICER or CREM, may replace AP-1/CREB at the CD28RR in anergic T cells and lead to an inactive promoter by blocking chromatin remodeling.

Control of *IL-2* gene expression during an immune response is mediated not only by the coordinated binding of transcription factor complexes to the *IL-2* promoter to initiate transcription but also by the signal-dependent binding of negative regulators which function to suppress IL-2 in a tissue-specific manner. The balance between activators and repressors needs to be critically maintained in order to achieve correct temporal and cell-specific expression of IL-2.

VIII. CONCLUSIONS

The overall mechanism of activation and expression of the *IL-2* gene, which is highly specific to T cells that are responsive to an immune signal, is clearly contingent on a distinct hierarchy and interplay of events. In the T cell, this begins with information from extracellular stimuli which is translated through TCR-mediated signaling cascades and integrated at the level of transcription factor binding to individual elements within the *IL-2* promoter region. CD28-mediated signaling noticeably plays a central role in full and enhanced activation of the *IL-2* gene. Perhaps the most striking feature of *IL-2* transcription activation is that it absolutely requires all of the DNA elements and factors binding to the DNA to be intact, and it is the precise, cooperative actions of multiple proteins and other higher-order complexes which can ultimately initiate *IL-2* transcription. Likewise, there is increasing evidence that the chromatin architecture of the *IL-2* locus plays a critical role in controlling activation-dependent induction of IL-2 and that the necessary basal chromatin architecture is likely to be established during T cell development. Thus, IL-2 synthesis is tightly and explicitly regulated in T cells such that the rapid expression of this cytokine is limited to immune responses generated only by an appropriate activating signal.

REFERENCES

Abraham, C., and Miller, J. (2001). Molecular mechanisms of IL-2 gene regulation following costimulation through LFA-1. *J. Immunol.* **167**, 5193–5201.

Adachi, S., and Rothenberg, E. V. (2005). Cell-type-specific epigenetic marking of the IL2 gene at a distal cis-regulatory region in competent, nontranscribing T-cells. *Nucleic Acids Res.* **33**, 3200–3210.

Attema, J. L., Reeves, R., Murray, V., Levichkin, I., Temple, M. D., Tremethick, D. J., and Shannon, M. F. (2002). The human IL-2 gene promoter can assemble a positioned nucleosome that becomes remodeled upon T cell activation. *J. Immunol.* **169**, 2466–2476.

Avots, A., Escher, C., Muller-Deubert, S., Neumann, M., and Serfling, E. (1995). The interplay between lymphoid-specific and ubiquitous transcription factors controls the expression of interleukin 2 gene in T lymphocytes. *Immunobiology* **193**, 254–258.

Avots, A., Hoffmeyer, A., Flory, E., Cimanis, A., Rapp, U. R., and Serfling, E. (1997). GABP factors bind to a distal interleukin 2 (IL-2) enhancer and contribute to c-Raf-mediated increase in IL-2 induction. *Mol. Cell. Biol.* **17**, 4381–4389.

Barton, K., Muthusamy, N., Chanyangam, M., Fischer, C., Clendenin, C., and Leiden, J. M. (1996). Defective thymocyte proliferation and IL-2 production in transgenic mice expressing a dominant-negative form of CREB. *Nature* **379**, 81–85.

Bayer, A. L., Yu, A., Adeegbe, D., and Malek, T. R. (2005). Essential role for interleukin-2 for CD4(+)CD25(+) T regulatory cell development during the neonatal period. *J. Exp. Med.* **201**, 769–777.

Ben Aribia, M. H., Leroy, E., Lantz, O., Metivier, D., Autran, B., Charpentier, B., Hercend, T., and Senik, A. (1987). rIL 2-induced proliferation of human circulating NK cells and T lymphocytes: Synergistic effects of IL 1 and IL 2. *J. Immunol.* **139**, 443–451.

Beverly, B., Kang, S. M., Lenardo, M. J., and Schwartz, R. H. (1992). Reversal of *in vitro* T cell clonal anergy by IL-2 stimulation. *Int. Immunol.* **4**, 661–671.

Bjorndahl, J. M., Sung, S. S., Hansen, J. A., and Fu, S. M. (1989). Human T cell activation: Differential response to anti-CD28 as compared to anti-CD3 monoclonal antibodies. *Eur. J. Immunol.* **19**, 881–887.

Bodor, J., and Habener, J. F. (1998). Role of transcriptional repressor ICER in cyclic AMP-mediated attenuation of cytokine gene expression in human thymocytes. *J. Biol. Chem.* **273**, 9544–9551.

Bodor, J., Spetz, A. L., Strominger, J. L., and Habener, J. F. (1996). cAMP inducibility of transcriptional repressor ICER in developing and mature human T lymphocytes. *Proc. Natl. Acad. Sci. USA* **93**, 3536–3541.

Bodor, J., Bodorova, J., and Gress, R. E. (2000). Suppression of T cell function: A potential role for transcriptional repressor ICER. *J. Leukoc. Biol.* **67**, 774–779.

Bodor, J., Feigenbaum, L., Bodorova, J., Bare, C., Reitz, M. S., Jr., and Gress, R. E. (2001). Suppression of T-cell responsiveness by inducible cAMP early repressor (ICER). *J. Leukoc. Biol.* **69**, 1053–1059.

Boeger, H., Griesenbeck, J., Strattan, J. S., and Kornberg, R. D. (2003). Nucleosomes unfold completely at a transcriptionally active promoter. *Mol. Cell* **11**, 1587–1598.

Boise, L. H., Petryniak, B., Mao, X., June, C. H., Wang, C. Y., Lindsten, T., Bravo, R., Kovary, K., Leiden, J. M., and Thompson, C. B. (1993). The NFAT-1 DNA binding complex in activated T cells contains Fra-1 and JunB. *Mol. Cell. Biol.* **13**, 1911–1919.

Boumpas, D. T., Anastassiou, E. D., Older, S. A., Tsokos, G. C., Nelson, D. L., and Balow, J. E. (1991). Dexamethasone inhibits human interleukin 2 but not interleukin 2 receptor gene expression *in vitro* at the level of nuclear transcription. *J. Clin. Invest.* **87**, 1739–1747.

Bream, J. H., Curiel, R. E., Yu, C. R., Egwuagu, C. E., Grusby, M. J., Aune, T. M., and Young, H. A. (2003). IL-4 synergistically enhances both IL-2- and IL-12-induced IFN-gamma expression in murine NK cells. *Blood* **102**, 207–214.

Briegel, K., Hentsch, B., Pfeuffer, I., and Serfling, E. (1991). One base pair change abolishes the T cell-restricted activity of a kB-like proto-enhancer element from the interleukin 2 promoter. *Nucleic Acids Res.* **19,** 5929–5936.

Bruniquel, D., and Schwartz, R. H. (2003). Selective, stable demethylation of the interleukin-2 gene enhances transcription by an active process. *Nat. Immunol.* **4,** 235–240.

Brunvand, M. W., Schmidt, A., and Siebenlist, U. (1988). Nuclear factors interacting with the mitogen-responsive regulatory region of the interleukin-2 gene. *J. Biol. Chem.* **263,** 18904–18910.

Brunvand, M. W., Krumm, A., and Groudine, M. (1993). *In vivo* footprinting of the human IL-2 gene reveals a nuclear factor bound to the transcription start site in T cells. *Nucleic Acids Res.* **21,** 4824–4829.

Bryan, R. G., Li, Y., Lai, J. H., Van, M., Rice, N. R., Rich, R. R., and Tan, T. H. (1994). Effect of CD28 signal transduction on c-Rel in human peripheral blood T cells. *Mol. Cell. Biol.* **14,** 7933–7942.

Butscher, W. G., Powers, C., Olive, M., Vinson, C., and Gardner, K. (1998). Coordinate transactivation of the interleukin-2 CD28 response element by c-Rel and ATF-1/CREB2. *J. Biol. Chem.* **273,** 552–560.

Butscher, W. G., Haggerty, C. M., Chaudhry, S., and Gardner, K. (2001). Targeting of p300 to the interleukin-2 promoter via CREB-Rel cross-talk during mitogen and oncogenic molecular signaling in activated T-cells. *J. Biol. Chem.* **276,** 27647–27656.

Chen, D., and Rothenberg, E. V. (1993). Molecular basis for developmental changes in interleukin-2 gene inducibility. *Mol. Cell. Biol.* **13,** 228–237.

Chen, X., Wang, J., Woltring, D., Gerondakis, S., and Shannon, M. F. (2005). Histone dynamics on the interleukin-2 gene in response to T-cell activation. *Mol. Cell. Biol.* **25,** 3209–3219.

Chirathaworn, C., Kohlmeier, J. E., Tibbetts, S. A., Rumsey, L. M., Chan, M. A., and Benedict, S. H. (2002). Stimulation through intercellular adhesion molecule-1 provides a second signal for T cell activation. *J. Immunol.* **168,** 5530–5537.

Chow, C. W., Rincon, M., and Davis, R. J. (1999). Requirement for transcription factor NFAT in interleukin-2 expression. *Mol. Cell. Biol.* **19,** 2300–2307.

Clerici, M., Galli, M., Bosis, S., Gervasoni, C., Moroni, M., and Norbiato, G. (2000). Immunoendocrinologic abnormalities in human immunodeficiency virus infection. *Ann. N. Y. Acad. Sci.* **917,** 956–961.

Corcoran, L. M., and Karvelas, M. (1994). Oct-2 is required early in T cell-independent B cell activation for G1 progression and for proliferation. *Immunity* **1,** 635–645.

Costello, R., Lipcey, C., Algarte, M., Cerdan, C., Baeuerle, P. A., Olive, D., and Imbert, J. (1993). Activation of primary human T-lymphocytes through CD2 plus CD28 adhesion molecules induces long-term nuclear expression of NF-kappa B. *Cell Growth Differ.* **4,** 329–339.

Coyle, A. J., and Gutierrez-Ramos, J. C. (2001). The expanding B7 superfamily: Increasing complexity in costimulatory signals regulating T cell function. *Nat. Immunol.* **2,** 203–209.

Crabtree, G. R. (1989). Contingent genetic regulatory events in T lymphocyte activation. *Science* **243,** 355–361.

Crispin, J. C., and Alcocer-Varela, J. (1998). Interleukin-2 and systemic lupus erythematosus–fifteen years later. *Lupus* **7,** 214–222.

Curtiss, V. E., Smilde, R., and McGuire, K. L. (1996). Requirements for interleukin 2 promoter transactivation by the Tax protein of human T-cell leukemia virus type 1. *Mol. Cell. Biol.* **16,** 3567–3575.

D'Ambrosio, D., Trotta, R., Vacca, A., Frati, L., Santoni, A., Gulino, A., and Testi, R. (1993). Transcriptional regulation of interleukin-2 gene expression by CD69-generated signals. *Eur. J. Immunol.* **23,** 2993–2997.

De Cesare, D., Fimia, G. M., and Sassone-Corsi, P. (1999). Signaling routes to CREM and CREB: Plasticity in transcriptional activation. *Trends Biochem. Sci.* **24,** 281–285.

de Grazia, U., Felli, M. P., Vacca, A., Farina, A. R., Maroder, M., Cappabianca, L., Meco, D., Farina, M., Screpanti, I., Frati, L., and Gulino, A. (1994). Positive and negative regulation of the composite octamer motif of the interleukin 2 enhancer by AP-1, Oct-2, and retinoic acid receptor. *J. Exp. Med.* **180**, 1485–1497.

Daniel, P. B., and Habener, J. F. (1998). Cyclical alternative exon splicing of transcription factor cyclic adenosine monophosphate response element-binding protein (CREB) messenger ribonucleic acid during rat spermatogenesis. *Endocrinology* **139**, 3721–3729.

Decker, E. L., Skerka, C., and Zipfel, P. F. (1998). The early growth response protein (EGR-1) regulates interleukin-2 transcription by synergistic interaction with the nuclear factor of activated T cells. *J. Biol. Chem.* **273**, 26923–26930.

Devos, R., Plaetinck, G., Cheroutre, H., Simons, G., Degrave, W., Tavernier, J., Remaut, E., and Fiers, W. (1983). Molecular cloning of human interleukin 2 cDNA and its expression in *E. coli. Nucleic Acids Res.* **11**, 4307–4323.

Diehn, M., Alizadeh, A. A., Rando, O. J., Liu, C. L., Stankunas, K., Botstein, D., Crabtree, G. R., and Brown, P. O. (2002). Genomic expression programs and the integration of the CD28 costimulatory signal in T cell activation. *Proc. Natl. Acad. Sci. USA* **99**, 11796–11801.

Dubey, C., Croft, M., and Swain, S. L. (1995). Costimulatory requirements of naive CD4+ T cells. ICAM-1 or B7-1 can costimulate naive CD4 T cell activation but both are required for optimum response. *J. Immunol.* **155**, 45–57.

Durand, D. B., Bush, M. R., Morgan, J. G., Weiss, A., and Crabtree, G. R. (1987). A 275 basepair fragment at the 5' end of the interleukin 2 gene enhances expression from a heterologous promoter in response to signals from the T cell antigen receptor. *J. Exp. Med.* **165**, 395–407.

Durand, D. B., Shaw, J. P., Bush, M. R., Replogle, R. E., Belagaje, R., and Crabtree, G. R. (1988). Characterization of antigen receptor response elements within the interleukin-2 enhancer. *Mol. Cell. Biol.* **8**, 1715–1724.

Eberharter, A., and Becker, P. B. (2002). Histone acetylation: A switch between repressive and permissive chromatin. Second in review series on chromatin dynamics. *EMBO Rep.* **3**, 224–229.

Eerligh, P., Koeleman, B. P., Dudbridge, F., Jan Bruining, G., Roep, B. O., and Giphart, M. J. (2004). Functional genetic polymorphisms in cytokines and metabolic genes as additional genetic markers for susceptibility to develop type 1 diabetes. *Genes Immun.* **5**, 36–40.

Egen, J. G., and Allison, J. P. (2002). Cytotoxic T lymphocyte antigen-4 accumulation in the immunological synapse is regulated by TCR signal strength. *Immunity* **16**, 23–35.

Emmel, E. A., Verweij, C. L., Durand, D. B., Higgins, K. M., Lacy, E., and Crabtree, G. R. (1989). Cyclosporin A specifically inhibits function of nuclear proteins involved in T cell activation. *Science* **246**, 1617–1620.

Erlanson, D. A., Chytil, M., and Verdine, G. L. (1996). The leucine zipper domain controls the orientation of AP-1 in the NFAT.AP-1.DNA complex. *Chem. Biol.* **3**, 981–991.

Favero, J., and Lafont, V. (1998). Effector pathways regulating T cell activation. *Biochem. Pharmacol.* **56**, 1539–1547.

Ferreri, K., Gill, G., and Montminy, M. (1994). The cAMP-regulated transcription factor CREB interacts with a component of the TFIID complex. *Proc. Natl. Acad. Sci. USA* **91**, 1210–1213.

Finch, R. J., Fields, P. E., and Greenberg, P. D. (2001). A transcriptional block in the IL-2 promoter at the –150 AP-1 site in effector CD8+ T cells. *J. Immunol.* **166**, 6530–6536.

Fortin, J. F., Barat, C., Beausejour, Y., Barbeau, B., and Tremblay, M. J. (2004). Hyper-responsiveness to stimulation of human immunodeficiency virus-infected CD4+ T cells requires Nef and Tat virus gene products and results from higher NFAT, NF-kappaB, and AP-1 induction. *J. Biol. Chem.* **279**, 39520–39531.

Foulkes, N. S., Laoide, B. M., Schlotter, F., and Sassone-Corsi, P. (1991). Transcriptional antagonist cAMP-responsive element modulator (CREM) down-regulates c-fos cAMP-induced expression. *Proc. Natl. Acad. Sci. USA* **88**, 5448–5452.

Fraser, J. D., and Weiss, A. (1992). Regulation of T-cell lymphokine gene transcription by the accessory molecule CD28. *Mol. Cell. Biol.* **12**, 4357–4363.

137

Fujita, T., Takaoka, C., Matsui, H., and Taniguchi, T. (1983). Structure of the human interleukin 2 gene. *Proc. Natl. Acad. Sci. USA* **80**, 7437–7441.

Fujita, T., Shibuya, H., Ohashi, T., Yamanishi, K., and Taniguchi, T. (1986). Regulation of human interleukin-2 gene: Functional DNA sequences in the 5′ flanking region for the gene expression in activated T lymphocytes. *Cell* **46**, 401–405.

Gaffen, S. L., and Liu, K. D. (2004). Overview of interleukin-2 function, production and clinical applications. *Cytokine* **28**, 109–123.

Garcia-Rodriguez, C., and Rao, A. (1998). Nuclear factor of activated T cells (NFAT)-dependent transactivation regulated by the coactivators p300/CREB-binding protein (CBP). *J. Exp. Med.* **187**, 2031–2036.

Garrity, P. A., Chen, D., Rothenberg, E. V., and Wold, B. J. (1994). Interleukin-2 transcription is regulated *in vivo* at the level of coordinated binding of both constitutive and regulated factors. *Mol. Cell. Biol.* **14**, 2159–2169.

Geist, L. J., Monick, M. M., Stinski, M. F., and Hunninghake, G. W. (1991). The immediate early genes of human cytomegalovirus upregulate expression of the interleukin-2 and interleukin-2 receptor genes. *Am. J. Respir. Cell. Mol. Biol.* **5**, 292–296.

Gerondakis, S., Strasser, A., Metcalf, D., Grigoriadis, G., Scheerlinck, J. Y., and Grumont, R. J. (1996). Rel-deficient T cells exhibit defects in production of interleukin 3 and granulocyte-macrophage colony-stimulating factor. *Proc. Natl. Acad. Sci. USA* **93**, 3405–3409.

Gesbert, F., Moreau, J. L., and Theze, J. (2005). IL-2 responsiveness of CD4 and CD8 lymphocytes: Further investigations with human IL-2Rbeta transgenic mice. *Int. Immunol.* **17**, 1093–1102.

Ghosh, P., Tan, T. H., Rice, N. R., Sica, A., and Young, H. A. (1993). The interleukin 2 CD28-responsive complex contains at least three members of the NF kappa B family: c-Rel, p50, and p65. *Proc. Natl. Acad. Sci. USA* **90**, 1696–1700.

Gonzalez, G. A., and Montminy, M. R. (1989). Cyclic AMP stimulates somatostatin gene transcription by phosphorylation of CREB at serine 133. *Cell* **59**, 675–680.

Granelli-Piperno, A., and Nolan, P. (1991). Nuclear transcription factors that bind to elements of the IL-2 promoter. Induction requirements in primary human T cells. *J. Immunol.* **147**, 2734–2739.

Granucci, F., Zanoni, I., Feau, S., and Ricciardi-Castagnoli, P. (2003). Dendritic cell regulation of immune responses: A new role for interleukin 2 at the intersection of innate and adaptive immunity. *EMBO J.* **22**, 2546–2551.

Grossmann, M., Metcalf, D., Merryfull, J., Beg, A., Baltimore, D., and Gerondakis, S. (1999). The combined absence of the transcription factors Rel and RelA leads to multiple hemopoietic cell defects. *Proc. Natl. Acad. Sci. USA* **96**, 11848–11853.

Harant, H., and Lindley, I. J. (2004). Negative cross-talk between the human orphan nuclear receptor Nur77/NAK-1/TR3 and nuclear factor-kappaB. *Nucleic Acids Res.* **32**, 5280–5290.

Harris, J. E., Bishop, K. D., Phillips, N. E., Mordes, J. P., Greiner, D. L., Rossini, A. A., and Czech, M. P. (2004). Early growth response gene-2, a zinc-finger transcription factor, is required for full induction of clonal anergy in CD4+ T cells. *J. Immunol.* **173**, 7331–7338.

Heisel, O., and Keown, P. (2001). Alterations in transcription factor binding at the IL-2 promoter region in anergized human CD4+ T lymphocytes. *Transplantation* **72**, 1416–1422.

Hendrich, B., and Tweedie, S. (2003). The methyl-CpG binding domain and the evolving role of DNA methylation in animals. *Trends Genet.* **19**, 269–277.

Hentsch, B., Mouzaki, A., Pfeuffer, I., Rungger, D., and Serfling, E. (1992). The weak, fine-tuned binding of ubiquitous transcription factors to the Il-2 enhancer contributes to its T cell-restricted activity. *Nucleic Acids Res.* **20**, 2657–2665.

Himes, S. R., Coles, L. S., Reeves, R., and Shannon, M. F. (1996). High mobility group protein I(Y) is required for function and for c-Rel binding to CD28 response elements within the GM-CSF and IL-2 promoters. *Immunity* **5**, 479–489.

Hoeffler, J. P., Deutsch, P. J., Lin, J., and Habener, J. F. (1989). Distinct adenosine 3′, 5′-monophosphate and phorbol ester-responsive signal transduction pathways converge at the level of transcriptional activation by the interactions of DNA-binding proteins. *Mol. Endocrinol.* **3,** 868–880.

Holbrook, N. J., Smith, K. A., Fornace, A. J., Jr., Comeau, C. M., Wiskocil, R. L., and Crabtree, G. R. (1984). T-cell growth factor: Complete nucleotide sequence and organization of the gene in normal and malignant cells. *Proc. Natl. Acad. Sci. USA* **81,** 1634–1638.

Hollander, G. A. (1999). On the stochastic regulation of interleukin-2 transcription. *Semin. Immunol.* **11,** 357–367.

Hollander, G. A., Zuklys, S., Morel, C., Mizoguchi, E., Mobisson, K., Simpson, S., Terhorst, C., Wishart, W., Golan, D. E., Bhan, A. K., and Burakoff, S. J. (1998). Monoallelic expression of the interleukin-2 locus. *Science* **279,** 2118–2121.

Hughes, C. C., and Pober, J. S. (1993). Costimulation of peripheral blood T cell activation by human endothelial cells. Enhanced IL-2 transcription correlates with increased c-fos synthesis and increased Fos content of AP-1. *J. Immunol.* **150,** 3148–3160.

Hwang, E. S., Hong, J. H., and Glimcher, L. H. (2005). IL-2 production in developing Th1 cells is regulated by heterodimerization of RelA and T-bet and requires T-bet serine residue 508. *J. Exp. Med.* **202,** 1289–1300.

Iacobelli, M., Wachsman, W., and McGuire, K. L. (2000). Repression of IL-2 promoter activity by the novel basic leucine zipper p21SNFT protein. *J. Immunol.* **165,** 860–868.

Isakov, N., and Altman, A. (1985). Tumor promoters in conjunction with calcium ionophores mimic antigenic stimulation by reactivation of alloantigen-primed murine T lymphocytes. *J. Immunol.* **135,** 3674–3680.

Iwashima, M. (2003). Kinetic perspectives of T cell antigen receptor signaling. A two-tier model for T cell full activation. *Immunol. Rev.* **191,** 196–210.

Jain, J., Loh, C., and Rao, A. (1995). Transcriptional regulation of the IL-2 gene. *Curr. Opin. Immunol.* **7,** 333–342.

Jain, J., Valge-Archer, V. E., and Rao, A. (1992a). Analysis of the AP-1 sites in the IL-2 promoter. *J. Immunol.* **148,** 1240–1250.

Jain, J., Valge-Archer, V. E., Sinskey, A. J., and Rao, A. (1992b). The AP-1 site at −150 bp, but not the NF-kappa B site, is likely to represent the major target of protein kinase C in the interleukin 2 promoter. *J. Exp. Med.* **175,** 853–862.

Jain, J., McCaffrey, P. G., Valge-Archer, V. E., and Rao, A. (1992c). Nuclear factor of activated T cells contains Fos and Jun. *Nature* **356,** 801–804.

Jhun, B. S., Oh, Y. T., Lee, J. Y., Kong, Y., Yoon, K. S., Kim, S. S., Baik, H. H., Ha, J., and Kang, I. (2005). AICAR suppresses IL-2 expression through inhibition of GSK-3 phosphorylation and NF-AT activation in Jurkat T cells. *Biochem. Biophys. Res. Commun.* **332,** 339–346.

John, S., Reeves, R. B., Lin, J. X., Child, R., Leiden, J. M., Thompson, C. B., and Leonard, W. J. (1995). Regulation of cell-type-specific interleukin-2 receptor alpha-chain gene expression: Potential role of physical interactions between Elf-1, HMG-I(Y), and NF-kappa B family proteins. *Mol. Cell. Biol.* **15,** 1786–1796.

Jonat, C., Rahmsdorf, H. J., Park, K. K., Cato, A. C., Gebel, S., Ponta, H., and Herrlich, P. (1990). Antitumor promotion and antiinflammation: Down-modulation of AP-1 (Fos/Jun) activity by glucocorticoid hormone. *Cell* **62,** 1189–1204.

Juang, Y. T., Wang, Y., Solomou, E. E., Li, Y., Mawrin, C., Tenbrock, K., Kyttaris, V. C., and Tsokos, G. C. (2005). Systemic lupus erythematosus serum IgG increases CREM binding to the IL-2 promoter and suppresses IL-2 production through CaMKIV. *J. Clin. Invest.* **115,** 996–1005.

Kamps, M. P., Corcoran, L., LeBowitz, J. H., and Baltimore, D. (1990). The promoter of the human interleukin-2 gene contains two octamer-binding sites and is partially activated by the expression of Oct-2. *Mol. Cell. Biol.* **10,** 5464–5472.

Kedzierska, K., and Crowe, S. M. (2001). Cytokines and HIV-1: Interactions and clinical implications. *Antivir. Chem. Chemother.* **12**, 133–150.

Kelso, A. (1998). Cytokines: Principles and prospects. *Immunol. Cell. Biol.* **76**, 300–317.

Kneitz, B., Herrmann, T., Yonehara, S., and Schimpl, A. (1995). Normal clonal expansion but impaired Fas-mediated cell death and anergy induction in interleukin-2-deficient mice. *Eur. J. Immunol.* **25**, 2572–2577.

Kohm, A. P., Podojil, J. R., Williams, J. S., McMahon, J. S., and Miller, S. D. (2005). CD28 regulates glucocorticoid-induced TNF receptor family-related gene expression on CD4+ T cells via IL-2-dependent mechanisms. *Cell. Immunol.* **235**, 56–64.

Koretzky, G. A., and Myung, P. S. (2001). Positive and negative regulation of T-cell activation by adaptor proteins. *Nat. Rev. Immunol.* **1**, 95–107.

Kumar, P. P., Purbey, P. K., Ravi, D. S., Mitra, D., and Galande, S. (2005). Displacement of SATB1-bound histone deacetylase 1 corepressor by the human immunodeficiency virus type 1 transactivator induces expression of interleukin-2 and its receptor in T cells. *Mol. Cell. Biol.* **25**, 1620–1633.

Kyttaris, V. C., Juang, Y. T., Tenbrock, K., Weinstein, A., and Tsokos, G. C. (2004). Cyclic adenosine 5′-monophosphate response element modulator is responsible for the decreased expression of c-fos and activator protein-1 binding in T cells from patients with systemic lupus erythematosus. *J. Immunol.* **173**, 3557–3563.

Ledo, F., Carrion, A. M., Link, W. A., Mellstrom, B., and Naranjo, J. R. (2000). DREAM-alphaCREM interaction via leucine-charged domains derepresses downstream regulatory element-dependent transcription. *Mol. Cell. Biol.* **20**, 9120–9126.

Ledo, F., Kremer, L., Mellstrom, B., and Naranjo, J. R. (2002). Ca^{2+}-dependent block of CREB-CBP transcription by repressor DREAM. *EMBO J.* **21**, 4583–4592.

Li, L., Godfrey, W. R., Porter, S. B., Ge, Y., June, C. H., Blazar, B. R., and Boussiotis, V. A. (2005). CD4+CD25+ regulatory T-cell lines from human cord blood have functional and molecular properties of T-cell anergy. *Blood* **106**, 3068–3073.

Liang, G., Lin, J. C., Wei, V., Yoo, C., Cheng, J. C., Nguyen, C. T., Weisenberger, D. J., Egger, G., Takai, D., Gonzales, F. A., and Jones, P. A. (2004). Distinct localization of histone H3 acetylation and H3-K4 methylation to the transcription start sites in the human genome. *Proc. Natl. Acad. Sci. USA* **101**, 7357–7362.

Lomvardas, S., and Thanos, D. (2002). Modifying gene expression programs by altering core promoter chromatin architecture. *Cell* **110**, 261–271.

Lugo, J. P., Krishnan, S. N., Sailor, R. D., and Rothenberg, E. V. (1986). Early precursor thymocytes can produce interleukin 2 upon stimulation with calcium ionophore and phorbol ester. *Proc. Natl. Acad. Sci. USA* **83**, 1862–1866.

MacMillan, M. L., Radloff, G. A., Kiffmeyer, W. R., DeFor, T. E., Weisdorf, D. J., and Davies, S. M. (2003). High-producer interleukin-2 genotype increases risk for acute graft-versus-host disease after unrelated donor bone marrow transplantation. *Transplantation* **76**, 1758–1762.

Malek, T. R. (2003). The main function of IL-2 is to promote the development of T regulatory cells. *J. Leukoc. Biol.* **74**, 961–965.

Maloy, K. J., and Powrie, F. (2005). Fueling regulation: IL-2 keeps CD4+ Treg cells fit. *Nat. Immunol.* **6**, 1071–1072.

Marinari, B., Costanzo, A., Marzano, V., Piccolella, E., and Tuosto, L. (2004). CD28 delivers a unique signal leading to the selective recruitment of RelA and p52 NF-kappaB subunits on IL-8 and Bcl-xL gene promoters. *Proc. Natl. Acad. Sci. USA* **101**, 6098–6103.

Martensson, I. L., and Leanderson, T. (1989). Regulation of interleukin 2 gene expression: Discrepancy between enhancer activity and endogenous gene expression. *Eur. J. Immunol.* **19**, 145–149.

Martinez-Campa, C., Politis, P., Moreau, J. L., Kent, N., Goodall, J., Mellor, J., and Goding, C. R. (2004). Precise nucleosome positioning and the TATA box dictate requirements for the histone H4 tail and the bromodomain factor Bdf1. *Mol. Cell* **15**, 69–81.

Matesanz, F., Fedetz, M., Leyva, L., Delgado, C., Fernandez, O., and Alcina, A. (2004). Effects of the multiple sclerosis associated −330 promoter polymorphism in IL2 allelic expression. *J. Neuroimmunol.* **148**, 212–217.

Matsumoto, A., Seki, Y., Watanabe, R., Hayashi, K., Johnston, J. A., Harada, Y., Abe, R., Yoshimura, A., and Kubo, M. (2003). A role of suppressor of cytokine signaling 3 (SOCS3/CIS3/SSI3) in CD28-mediated interleukin 2 production. *J. Exp. Med.* **197**, 425–436.

McGuire, K. L., and Iacobelli, M. (1997). Involvement of Rel, Fos, and Jun proteins in binding activity to the IL-2 promoter CD28 response element/AP-1 sequence in human T cells. *J. Immunol.* **159**, 1319–1327.

McGuire, K. L., Curtiss, V. E., Larson, E. L., and Haseltine, W. A. (1993). Influence of human T-cell leukemia virus type I tax and rex on interleukin-2 gene expression. *J. Virol.* **67**, 1590–1599.

Michel, F., Attal-Bonnefoy, G., Mangino, G., Mise-Omata, S., and Acuto, O. (2001). CD28 as a molecular amplifier extending TCR ligation and signaling capabilities. *Immunity* **15**, 935–945.

Mohr, H., Monner, D., and Plessing, A. (1986). Calcium ionophore A 23 187 in the presence of phorbol ester PMA: A potent inducer of interleukin 2 and interferon-gamma synthesis by human blood cells. *Immunobiology* **171**, 195–204.

Morgun, A., Shulzhenko, N., Rampim, G. F., Medina, J. O., Machado, P. G., Diniz, R. V., Almeida, D. R., and Gerbase-DeLima, M. (2003). Interleukin-2 gene polymorphism is associated with renal but not cardiac transplant outcome. *Transplant. Proc.* **35**, 1344–1345.

Mouzaki, A., Serfling, E., and Zubler, R. H. (1995). Interleukin-2 promoter activity in Epstein-Barr virus-transformed B lymphocytes is controlled by nuclear factor-chi B. *Eur. J. Immunol.* **25**, 2177–2182.

Munoz, E., Zubiaga, A., Olson, D., and Huber, B. T. (1989). Control of lymphokine expression in T helper 2 cells. *Proc. Natl. Acad. Sci. USA* **86**, 9461–9464.

Murtaza, A., Kuchroo, V. K., and Freeman, G. J. (1999). Changes in the strength of co-stimulation through the B7/CD28 pathway alter functional T cell responses to altered peptide ligands. *Int. Immunol.* **11**, 407–416.

Niinuma, A., Higuchi, M., Takahashi, M., Oie, M., Tanaka, Y., Gejyo, F., Tanaka, N., Sugamura, K., Xie, L., Green, P. L., and Fujii, M. (2005). Aberrant activation of the interleukin-2 autocrine loop through the nuclear factor of activated T cells by nonleukemogenic human T-cell leukemia virus type 2 but not by leukemogenic type 1 virus. *J. Virol.* **79**, 11925–11934.

Novak, T. J., and Rothenberg, E. V. (1990). cAMP inhibits induction of interleukin 2 but not of interleukin 4 in T cells. *Proc. Natl. Acad. Sci. USA* **87**, 9353–9357.

Novak, T. J., Chen, D., and Rothenberg, E. V. (1990). Interleukin-1 synergy with phosphoinositide pathway agonists for induction of interleukin-2 gene expression: Molecular basis of costimulation. *Mol. Cell. Biol.* **10**, 6325–6334.

Okayama, A., Tachibana, N., Ishihara, S., Nagatomo, Y., Murai, K., Okamoto, M., Shima, T., Sagawa, K., Tsubouchi, H., Stuver, S., and Mueller, N. (1997). Increased expression of interleukin-2 receptor alpha on peripheral blood mononuclear cells in HTLV-I tax/rex mRNA-positive asymptomatic carriers. *J. Acquir. Immune. Defic. Syndr. Hum. Retrovirol.* **15**, 70–75.

Oukka, M., Wein, M. N., and Glimcher, L. H. (2004). Schnurri-3 (KRC) interacts with c-Jun to regulate the IL-2 gene in T cells. *J. Exp. Med.* **199**, 15–24.

Paliogianni, F., Raptis, A., Ahuja, S. S., Najjar, S. M., and Boumpas, D. T. (1993). Negative transcriptional regulation of human interleukin 2 (IL-2) gene by glucocorticoids through interference with nuclear transcription factors AP-1 and NF-AT. *J. Clin. Invest.* **91,** 1481–1489.

Pan, F., Ye, Z., Cheng, L., and Liu, J. O. (2004). Myocyte enhancer factor 2 mediates calcium-dependent transcription of the interleukin-2 gene in T lymphocytes: A calcium signaling module that is distinct from but collaborates with the nuclear factor of activated T cells (NFAT). *J. Biol. Chem.* **279,** 14477–14480.

Parada, N. A., Center, D. M., Kornfeld, H., Rodriguez, W. L., Cook, J., Vallen, M., and Cruikshank, W. W. (1998). Synergistic activation of CD4+ T cells by IL-16 and IL-2. *J. Immunol.* **160,** 2115–2120.

Pawlik, A., Kurzawski, M., Florczak, M., Gawronska Szklarz, B., and Herczynska, M. (2005). IL1beta+3953 exon 5 and IL-2 –330 promoter polymorphisms in patients with rheumatoid arthritis. *Clin. Exp. Rheumatol.* **23,** 159–164.

Peters, A. H., and Schubeler, D. (2005). Methylation of histones: Playing memory with DNA. *Curr. Opin. Cell. Biol.* **17,** 230–238.

Petitto, J. M., Streit, W. J., Huang, Z., Butfiloski, E., and Schiffenbauer, J. (2000). Interleukin-2 gene deletion produces a robust reduction in susceptibility to experimental autoimmune encephalomyelitis in C57BL/6 mice. *Neurosci. Lett.* **285,** 66–70.

Petrak, D., Memon, S. A., Birrer, M. J., Ashwell, J. D., and Zacharchuk, C. M. (1994). Dominant negative mutant of c-Jun inhibits NF-AT transcriptional activity and prevents IL-2 gene transcription. *J. Immunol.* **153,** 2046–2051.

Pfeuffer, I., Klein-Hessling, S., Heinfling, A., Chuvpilo, S., Escher, C., Brabletz, T., Hentsch, B., Schwarzenbach, H., Matthias, P., and Serfling, E. (1994). Octamer factors exert a dual effect on the IL-2 and IL-4 promoters. *J. Immunol.* **153,** 5572–5585.

Postigo, A. A., and Dean, D. C. (1999). ZEB represses transcription through interaction with the corepressor CtBP. *Proc. Natl. Acad. Sci. USA* **96,** 6683–6688.

Postigo, A. A., and Dean, D. C. (2000). Differential expression and function of members of the zfh-1 family of zinc finger/homeodomain repressors. *Proc. Natl. Acad. Sci. USA* **97,** 6391–6396.

Powell, J. D., Ragheb, J. A., Kitagawa-Sakakida, S., and Schwartz, R. H. (1998). Molecular regulation of interleukin-2 expression by CD28 co-stimulation and anergy. *Immunol. Rev.* **165,** 287–300.

Powell, J. D., Lerner, C. G., Ewoldt, G. R., and Schwartz, R. H. (1999). The –180 site of the IL-2 promoter is the target of CREB/CREM binding in T cell anergy. *J. Immunol.* **163,** 6631–6639.

Radford-Smith, G., and Jewell, D. P. (1996). Cytokines and inflammatory bowel disease. *Baillieres Clin. Gastroenterol.* **10,** 151–164.

Rao, S., Procko, E., and Shannon, M. F. (2001). Chromatin remodeling, measured by a novel real-time polymerase chain reaction assay, across the proximal promoter region of the IL-2 gene. *J. Immunol.* **167,** 4494–4503.

Rao, S., Gerondakis, S., Woltring, D., and Shannon, M. F. (2003). c-Rel is required for chromatin remodeling across the IL-2 gene promoter. *J. Immunol.* **170,** 3724–3731.

Randak, C., Brabletz, T., Hergenrother, M., Sobotta, I., and Serfling, E. (1990). Cyclosporin A suppresses the expression of the interleukin 2 gene by inhibiting the binding of lymphocyte-specific factors to the IL-2 enhancer. *EMBO J.* **9,** 2529–2536.

Reinke, H., and Horz, W. (2003). Histones are first hyperacetylated and then lose contact with the activated PHO5 promoter. *Mol. Cell* **11,** 1599–1607.

Reya, T., Bassiri, H., Biancaniello, R., and Carding, S. R. (1998). Thymic stromal-cell abnormalities and dysregulated T-cell development in IL-2-deficient mice. *Dev. Immunol.* **5,** 287–302.

Rincon, M., and Flavell, R. A. (1994). AP-1 transcriptional activity requires both T-cell receptor-mediated and co-stimulatory signals in primary T lymphocytes. *EMBO J.* **13,** 4370–4381.

Rincon, M., and Flavell, R. A. (1996). Regulation of AP-1 and NFAT transcription factors during thymic selection of T cells. *Mol. Cell. Biol.* **16,** 1074–1084.

Robertson, K. D. (2002). DNA methylation and chromatin—unraveling the tangled web. *Oncogene* **21,** 5361–5379.

Rodriguez-Galan, M. C., Bream, J. H., Farr, A., and Young, H. A. (2005). Synergistic effect of IL-2, IL-12, and IL-18 on thymocyte apoptosis and Th1/Th2 cytokine expression. *J. Immunol.* **174,** 2796–2804.

Roh, T. Y., Cuddapah, S., and Zhao, K. (2005). Active chromatin domains are defined by acetylation islands revealed by genome-wide mapping. *Genes Dev.* **19,** 542–552.

Romano-Spica, V., Georgiou, P., Suzuki, H., Papas, T. S., and Bhat, N. K. (1995). Role of ETS1 in IL-2 gene expression. *J. Immunol.* **154,** 2724–2732.

Rooney, J. W., Sun, Y. L., Glimcher, L. H., and Hoey, T. (1995). Novel NFAT sites that mediate activation of the interleukin-2 promoter in response to T-cell receptor stimulation. *Mol. Cell. Biol.* **15,** 6299–6310.

Rothenberg, E. V., and Ward, S. B. (1996). A dynamic assembly of diverse transcription factors integrates activation and cell-type information for interleukin 2 gene regulation. *Proc. Natl. Acad. Sci. USA* **93,** 9358–9365.

Rothenberg, E. V., Diamond, R. A., Pepper, K. A., and Yang, J. A. (1990). IL-2 gene inducibility in T cells before T cell receptor expression. Changes in signaling pathways and gene expression requirements during intrathymic maturation. *J. Immunol.* **144,** 1614–1624.

Sadlack, B., Merz, H., Schorle, H., Schimpl, A., Feller, A. C., and Horak, I. (1993). Ulcerative colitis-like disease in mice with a disrupted interleukin-2 gene. *Cell* **75,** 253–261.

Sadlack, B., Lohler, J., Schorle, H., Klebb, G., Haber, H., Sickel, E., Noelle, R. J., and Horak, I. (1995). Generalized autoimmune disease in interleukin-2-deficient mice is triggered by an uncontrolled activation and proliferation of CD4+ T cells. *Eur. J. Immunol.* **25,** 3053–3059.

Safford, M., Collins, S., Lutz, M. A., Allen, A., Huang, C. T., Kowalski, J., Blackford, A., Horton, M. R., Drake, C., Schwartz, R. H., and Powell, J. D. (2005). Egr-2 and Egr-3 are negative regulators of T cell activation. *Nat. Immunol.* **6,** 472–480.

Santana, M. A., and Rosenstein, Y. (2003). What it takes to become an effector T cell: The process, the cells involved, and the mechanisms. *J. Cell. Physiol.* **195,** 392–401.

Sassone-Corsi, P. (1998). Coupling gene expression to cAMP signalling: Role of CREB and CREM. *Int. J. Biochem. Cell Biol.* **30,** 27–38.

Savignac, M., Pintado, B., Gutierrez-Adan, A., Palczewska, M., Mellstrom, B., and Naranjo, J. R. (2005). Transcriptional repressor DREAM regulates T-lymphocyte proliferation and cytokine gene expression. *EMBO J.* **24,** 3555–3564.

Schimpl, A., Berberich, I., Kneitz, B., Kramer, S., Santner-Nanan, B., Wagner, S., Wolf, M., and Hunig, T. (2002). IL-2 and autoimmune disease. *Cytokine Growth Factor Rev.* **13,** 369–378.

Schorle, H., Holtschke, T., Hunig, T., Schimpl, A., and Horak, I. (1991). Development and function of T cells in mice rendered interleukin-2 deficient by gene targeting. *Nature* **352,** 621–624.

Schule, R., Rangarajan, P., Kliewer, S., Ransone, L. J., Bolado, J., Yang, N., Verma, I. M., and Evans, R. M. (1990). Functional antagonism between oncoprotein c-Jun and the glucocorticoid receptor. *Cell* **62,** 1217–1226.

Schwartz, R. H. (2003). T cell anergy. *Annu. Rev. Immunol.* **21,** 305–334.

Schwarz, M. J., Kronig, H., Riedel, M., Dehning, S., Douhet, A., Spellmann, I., Ackenheil, M., Moller, H. J., and Muller, N. (2006). IL-2 and IL-4 polymorphisms as candidate genes in schizophrenia. *Eur. Arch. Psychiatry Clin. Neurosci.* **256,** 72–76.

Sedwick, C. E., and Altman, A. (2004). Perspectives on PKCtheta in T cell activation. *Mol. Immunol.* **41,** 675–686.

Serfling, E., Avots, A., and Neumann, M. (1995). The architecture of the interleukin-2 promoter: A reflection of T lymphocyte activation. *Biochim. Biophys. Acta* **1263**, 181–200.

Shannon, M. F., Himes, S. R., and Attema, J. (1998). A role for the architectural transcription factors HMGI(Y) in cytokine gene transcription in T cells. *Immunol. Cell Biol.* **76**, 461–466.

Shannon, M. F., Coles, L. S., Attema, J., and Diamond, P. (2001). The role of architectural transcription factors in cytokine gene transcription. *J. Leukoc. Biol.* **69**, 21–32.

Shapiro, V. S., Mollenauer, M. N., Greene, W. C., and Weiss, A. (1996). c-rel regulation of IL-2 gene expression may be mediated through activation of AP-1. *J. Exp. Med.* **184**, 1663–1669.

Shapiro, V. S., Truitt, K. E., Imboden, J. B., and Weiss, A. (1997). CD28 mediates transcriptional upregulation of the interleukin-2 (IL-2) promoter through a composite element containing the CD28RE and NF-IL-2B AP-1 sites. *Mol. Cell. Biol.* **17**, 4051–4058.

Shapiro, V. S., Mollenauer, M. N., and Weiss, A. (1998). Nuclear factor of activated T cells and AP-1 are insufficient for IL-2 promoter activation: Requirement for CD28 up-regulation of RE/AP. *J. Immunol.* **161**, 6455–6458.

Shaw, J. P., Utz, P. J., Durand, D. B., Toole, J. J., Emmel, E. A., and Crabtree, G. R. (1988). Identification of a putative regulator of early T cell activation genes. *Science* **241**, 202–205.

Shi, Y., Sawada, J., Sui, G., Affar el, B., Whetstine, J. R., Lan, F., Ogawa, H., Luke, M. P., and Nakatani, Y. (2003). Coordinated histone modifications mediated by a CtBP co-repressor complex. *Nature* **422**, 735–738.

Shibuya, H., and Taniguchi, T. (1989). Identification of multiple cis-elements and trans-acting factors involved in the induced expression of human IL-2 gene. *Nucleic Acids Res.* **17**, 9173–9184.

Siebenlist, U., Durand, D. B., Bressler, P., Holbrook, N. J., Norris, C. A., Kamoun, M., Kant, J. A., and Crabtree, G. R. (1986). Promoter region of interleukin-2 gene undergoes chromatin structure changes and confers inducibility on chloramphenicol acetyltransferase gene during activation of T cells. *Mol. Cell. Biol.* **6**, 3042–3049.

Siefken, R., Kurrle, R., and Schwinzer, R. (1997). CD28-mediated activation of resting human T cells without costimulation of the CD3/TCR complex. *Cell. Immunol.* **176**, 59–65.

Skerka, C., Decker, E. L., and Zipfel, P. F. (1995). A regulatory element in the human interleukin 2 gene promoter is a binding site for the zinc finger proteins Sp1 and EGR-1. *J. Biol. Chem.* **270**, 22500–22506.

Smith, J. L., Collins, I., Chandramouli, G. V., Butscher, W. G., Zaitseva, E., Freebern, W. J., Haggerty, C. M., Doseeva, V., and Gardner, K. (2003). Targeting combinatorial transcriptional complex assembly at specific modules within the interleukin-2 promoter by the immunosuppressant SB203580. *J. Biol. Chem.* **278**, 41034–41046.

Smith, J. L., Freebern, W. J., Collins, I., De Siervi, A., Montano, I., Haggerty, C. M., McNutt, M. C., Butscher, W. G., Dzekunova, I., Petersen, D. W., Kawasaki, E., Merchant, J. L., et al. (2004). Kinetic profiles of p300 occupancy in vivo predict common features of promoter structure and coactivator recruitment. *Proc. Natl. Acad. Sci. USA* **101**, 11554–11559.

Solomou, E. E., Juang, Y. T., and Tsokos, G. C. (2001). Protein kinase C-theta participates in the activation of cyclic AMP-responsive element-binding protein and its subsequent binding to the −180 site of the IL-2 promoter in normal human T lymphocytes. *J. Immunol.* **166**, 5665–5674.

Stopka, T., Amanatullah, D. F., Papetti, M., and Skoultchi, A. I. (2005). PU.1 inhibits the erythroid program by binding to GATA-1 on DNA and creating a repressive chromatin structure. *EMBO J.* **24**, 3712–3723.

Su, L., Creusot, R. J., Gallo, E. M., Chan, S. M., Utz, P. J., Fathman, C. G., and Ermann, J. (2004). Murine CD4+CD25+ regulatory T cells fail to undergo chromatin remodeling across the proximal promoter region of the IL-2 gene. *J. Immunol.* **173**, 4994–5001.

Sundstrom, S., Ota, S., Dimberg, L. Y., Masucci, M. G., and Bergqvist, A. (2005). Hepatitis C virus core protein induces an anergic state characterized by decreased interleukin-2 production and perturbation of mitogen-activated protein kinase responses. *J. Virol.* **79,** 2230–2239.

Suzuki, H., Kundig, T. M., Furlonger, C., Wakeham, A., Timms, E., Matsuyama, T., Schmits, R., Simard, J. J., Ohashi, P. S., Griesser, H., Taniguchi, T., Paige, C. J., *et al.* (1995). Deregulated T cell activation and autoimmunity in mice lacking interleukin-2 receptor beta. *Science* **268,** 1472–1476.

Taniguchi, T., Matsui, H., Fujita, T., Takaoka, C., Kashima, N., Yoshimoto, R., and Hamuro, J. (1983). Structure and expression of a cloned cDNA for human interleukin-2. *Nature* **302,** 305–310.

Tenbrock, K., and Tsokos, G. C. (2004). Transcriptional regulation of interleukin 2 in SLE T cells. *Int. Rev. Immunol.* **23,** 333–345.

Tenbrock, K., Juang, Y. T., Gourley, M. F., Nambiar, M. P., and Tsokos, G. C. (2002). Antisense cyclic adenosine 5′-monophosphate response element modulator up-regulates IL-2 in T cells from patients with systemic lupus erythematosus. *J. Immunol.* **169,** 4147–4152.

Tenbrock, K., Juang, Y. T., Tolnay, M., and Tsokos, G. C. (2003). The cyclic adenosine 5′-monophosphate response element modulator suppresses IL-2 production in stimulated T cells by a chromatin-dependent mechanism. *J. Immunol.* **170,** 2971–2976.

Thomas, R. M., Gao, L., and Wells, A. D. (2005). Signals from CD28 induce stable epigenetic modification of the IL-2 promoter. *J. Immunol.* **174,** 4639–4646.

Thompson, C. B., Wang, C. Y., Ho, I. C., Bohjanen, P. R., Petryniak, B., June, C. H., Miesfeldt, S., Zhang, L., Nabel, G. J., Karpinski, B., and Leiden, J. M. (1992). cis-acting sequences required for inducible interleukin-2 enhancer function bind a novel Ets-related protein, Elf-1. *Mol. Cell. Biol.* **12,** 1043–1053.

Togawa, S., Joh, T., Itoh, M., Katsuda, N., Ito, H., Matsuo, K., Tajima, K., and Hamajima, N. (2005). Interleukin-2 gene polymorphisms associated with increased risk of gastric atrophy from Helicobacter pylori infection. *Helicobacter.* **10,** 172–178.

Tsuda, H., Huang, R. W., and Takatsuki, K. (1993). Interleukin-2 prevents programmed cell death in adult T-cell leukemia cells. *Jpn. J. Cancer Res.* **84,** 431–437.

Verweij, C. L., Geerts, M., and Aarden, L. A. (1991). Activation of interleukin-2 gene transcription via the T-cell surface molecule CD28 is mediated through an NF-kB-like response element. *J. Biol. Chem.* **266,** 14179–14182.

Wang, H., Diamond, R. A., Yang-Snyder, J. A., and Rothenberg, E. V. (1998). Precocious expression of T cell functional response genes *in vivo* in primitive thymocytes before T lineage commitment. *Int. Immunol.* **10,** 1623–1635.

Wang, L., Kametani, Y., Katano, I., and Habu, S. (2005). T-cell specific enhancement of histone H3 acetylation in 5′ flanking region of the IL-2 gene. *Biochem. Biophys. Res. Commun.* **331,** 589–594.

Wang, W., Tam, W. F., Hughes, C. C., Rath, S., and Sen, R. (1997). c-Rel is a target of pentoxifylline-mediated inhibition of T lymphocyte activation. *Immunity* **6,** 165–174.

Ward, S. B., Hernandez-Hoyos, G., Chen, F., Waterman, M., Reeves, R., and Rothenberg, E. V. (1998). Chromatin remodeling of the interleukin-2 gene: Distinct alterations in the proximal versus distal enhancer regions. *Nucleic Acids Res.* **26,** 2923–2934.

Wieland, G. D., Nehmann, N., Muller, D., Eibel, H., Siebenlist, U., Suhnel, J., Zipfel, P. F., and Skerka, C. (2005). Early growth response proteins EGR-4 and EGR-3 interact with immune inflammatory mediators NF-kappaB p50 and p65. *J. Cell. Sci.* **118,** 3203–3212.

Willerford, D. M., Chen, J., Ferry, J. A., Davidson, L., Ma, A., and Alt, F. W. (1995). Interleukin-2 receptor alpha chain regulates the size and content of the peripheral lymphoid compartment. *Immunity* **3,** 521–530.

Williams, T. M., Moolten, D., Burlein, J., Romano, J., Bhaerman, R., Godillot, A., Mellon, M., Rauscher, F. J., III, and Kant, J. A. (1991). Identification of a zinc finger protein that inhibits IL-2 gene expression. *Science* **254,** 1791–1794.

Wong, H. K., Kammer, G. M., Dennis, G., and Tsokos, G. C. (1999). Abnormal NF-kappa B activity in T lymphocytes from patients with systemic lupus erythematosus is associated with decreased p65-RelA protein expression. *J. Immunol.* **163,** 1682–1689.

Wu, J., and Lingrel, J. B. (2005). Kruppel-like factor 2, a novel immediate-early transcriptional factor, regulates IL-2 expression in T lymphocyte activation. *J. Immunol.* **175,** 3060–3066.

Yang-Snyder, J. A., and Rothenberg, E. V. (1993). Developmental and anatomical patterns of IL-2 gene expression *in vivo* in the murine thymus. *Dev. Immunol.* **3,** 85–102.

Yao, T. P., Oh, S. P., Fuchs, M., Zhou, N. D., Ch'ng, L. E., Newsome, D., Bronson, R. T., Li, E., Livingston, D. M., and Eckner, R. (1998). Gene dosage-dependent embryonic development and proliferation defects in mice lacking the transcriptional integrator p300. *Cell* **93,** 361–372.

Yaseen, N. R., Park, J., Kerppola, T., Curran, T., and Sharma, S. (1994). A central role for Fos in human B- and T-cell NFAT (nuclear factor of activated T cells): An acidic region is required for *in vitro* assembly. *Mol. Cell. Biol.* **14,** 6886–6895.

Yasui, D. H., Genetta, T., Kadesch, T., Williams, T. M., Swain, S. L., Tsui, L. V., and Huber, B. T. (1998). Transcriptional repression of the IL-2 gene in Th cells by ZEB. *J. Immunol.* **160,** 4433–4440.

Yie, J., Merika, M., Munshi, N., Chen, G., and Thanos, D. (1999). The role of HMG I(Y) in the assembly and function of the IFN-beta enhanceosome. *EMBO J.* **18,** 3074–3089.

Yui, M. A., Hernandez-Hoyos, G., and Rothenberg, E. V. (2001). A new regulatory region of the IL-2 locus that confers position-independent transgene expression. *J. Immunol.* **166,** 1730–1739.

Yui, M. A., Sharp, L. L., Havran, W. L., and Rothenberg, E. V. (2004). Preferential activation of an IL-2 regulatory sequence transgene in TCR gamma delta and NKT cells: Subset-specific differences in IL-2 regulation. *J. Immunol.* **172,** 4691–4699.

Zhang, L., and Nabel, G. J. (1994). Positive and negative regulation of IL-2 gene expression: Role of multiple regulatory sites. *Cytokine* **6,** 221–228.

Zhao, G., Shi, L., Qiu, D., Hu, H., and Kao, P. N. (2005). NF45/ILF2 tissue expression, promoter analysis, and interleukin-2 transactivating function. *Exp. Cell. Res.* **305,** 312–323.

Zhou, X. Y., Yashiro-Ohtani, Y., Nakahira, M., Park, W. R., Abe, R., Hamaoka, T., Naramura, M., Gu, H., and Fujiwara, H. (2002). Molecular mechanisms underlying differential contribution of CD28 versus non-CD28 costimulatory molecules to IL-2 promoter activation. *J. Immunol.* **168,** 3847–3854.

Zubiaga, A. M., Munoz, E., and Huber, B. T. (1991). Superinduction of IL-2 gene transcription in the presence of cycloheximide. *J. Immunol.* **146,** 3857–3863.

6

Transcription Factors Mediating Interleukin-3 Survival Signals

Jeffrey Jong-Young Yen* and Hsin-Fang Yang-Yen[†]

*Institute of Biomedical Sciences, Academia Sinica, Taipei 11529, Taiwan
[†]Institute of Molecular Biology, Academia Sinica, Taipei 11529, Taiwan

Interleukin-3 (IL-3) is one of the major hematopoietic cytokines that regulate the survival of hematopoietic cells of various lineages. Although the mechanism underlying the survival effect of IL-3 has been investigated intensively for more than a decade, our knowledge of the survival-signaling network remains incomplete. Binding of IL-3 to its cognate receptors initiates rapid tyrosine phosphorylation of Janus

0083-6729/06 $35.00
DOI: 10.1016/S0083-6729(06)74006-7

kinases (JAKs) and of signal transducer and activator of transcription (STAT) proteins, as well as activation of the phosphatidylinositol-3 kinase (PI-3K)/Akt and Ras/Raf/MAPK kinase (MEK)/mitogen-activated protein kinase (MAPK) pathways. These signals culminate in induction of a constellation of antiapoptotic genes and prevent cell death from occurring. Thus IL-3 signaling has substantial effects on kinase activation and gene transcription. Previous articles have summarized the roles of these kinase pathways in cell proliferation and survival. In this chapter, we will focus on the role of several newly characterized transcriptional factors, which are targets of these initial kinase cascades and bridge the gap between kinases and survival effector genes, in transducing the IL-3 survival signal. The biological significance of the existence of these multiple survival-specific transcription pathways will also be discussed. © 2006 Elsevier Inc.

I. INTRODUCTION

Interleukin-3 (IL-3) is a pleiotropic cytokine that can stimulate proliferation, differentiation, secretion, and survival of multiple target cell types, including immunological and hematopoietic cells. Binding of IL-3 to its cognate high-affinity cell surface receptors causes specific phosphorylation of the receptor's common β chain as well as many other signaling intermediate molecules, such as JAK, STAT proteins, src kinase, phosphatidylinositol-3 kinase (PI-3K), Akt, and MAPK. Studies have revealed that the proliferation and survival signals of IL-3 are distinct and dissociable. In IL-3-dependent pro-B or pro-myeloid cells, genistein treatment specifically blocks induction of DNA synthesis, without altering the survival activity of IL-3 (Kinoshita *et al.*, 1995). On the other hand, IL-5 was able to stimulate DNA synthesis in a human erythroleukemic TF-1 cell line, but was not able to suppress apoptosis (Yen *et al.*, 1995), wherein Bcl-2 overexpression renders TF-1 cells dependent on IL-5 for growth (Huang *et al.*, 1999). Furthermore, the distinction between survival and mitogenesis pathways has been well documented in studies examining the phenotypes of deletion mutants of receptor common β chain (Kinoshita *et al.*, 1995; Sato *et al.*, 1993). Removal of the membrane distal domain of the common β chain results in receptors which retain the ability to promote DNA synthesis upon granulocyte-macrophage colony-stimulating factor (GM-CSF) stimulation, but fail to mediate activation of the Ras and Raf/MAP kinase pathway, and fail to suppress apoptosis. Meanwhile receptors lacking the membrane proximal domain are unable to bind JAK2 kinase, and unable to mediate induction of DNA synthesis.

The importance of Ras and Raf-1/MAP kinase pathways in mediating the survival response to IL-3 binding has been further demonstrated in experiments expressing a constitutively active form of Ras (Kinoshita *et al.*, 1997; Nicola *et al.*, 1996; Terada *et al.*, 1995). The survival defect observed in cells expressing the β chain mutant protein that lacks the membrane distal domain could be restored by coexpression of the activated Ras mutant, presumably through the activating effects of Ras mutant on Raf-1. Consistent with this interpretation, overexpression of constitutively active Raf-1 has also been shown to suppress apoptosis in IL-3-dependent cells (Cleveland *et al.*, 1994; Kinoshita *et al.*, 1997). The existence of a Raf-1-independent survival pathway is also evident, since expression of an activated Ras mutant, which is unable to activate Raf-1, can still suppress apoptosis (Kinoshita *et al.*, 1997). Apoptosis suppression via the Raf-1-independent pathway is sensitive to the PI-3K inhibitor, wortmannin, suggesting that the PI-3K/Akt pathway may be involved in mediating the IL-3 survival signal. Therefore, the survival signal initiated from an activated receptor common β chain in IL-3/GM-CSF/IL-5 receptor complexes is perhaps transmitted by at least two distinct pathways: a PI-3K/Akt pathway and a Raf/MEK/MAPK pathway.

The identification of the above-mentioned two pathways as mediators of IL-3 signaling however does not fully define the downstream processes involved as many intracellular signals converge at both the PI-3K/Akt and Raf/MEK/MAPK pathway nodes, including cell cycle, proliferation, differentiation, migration, inflammation, and programmed cell death. Intracellular signals that are integrated at PI-3K and Akt regulate the phosphorylation of several downstream effectors, such as NF-κB, mTOR, Forkhead, Bad, GSK-3, and MDM-2, that in turn mediate the effects of Akt on cell growth, proliferation, protection from proapoptotic stimuli, and stimulation of neoangiogenesis (Coffer *et al.*, 1998; Datta *et al.*, 1999). Likewise, MAPK pathways can be activated by a multitude of effectors including neurotransmitters, cytokines, growth factors, and chemical and mechanical stresses, and in turn phosphorylate at least four distinct mitogen kinase cascades and numerous downstream kinase substrates, including transcription factors, kinases, phosphatases and phospholipases, as well as cytoskeletal proteins. Activation or inhibition of these pathways can affect proliferation, morphological changes, survival, death, and cell cycle arrest (Wada and Penninger, 2004). Numerous studies have also indicated that the mitochondrion can be a direct target of these major kinase-signaling pathways, including protein kinase A (PKA), Akt/PKB, PKC, MAPK/ERK, c-Jun N-terminal kinase (JNK), and p38 MAPK (Horbinski and Chu, 2005). Therefore, the effector genes downstream of the PI-3K/Akt and/or Raf/MEK/MAPK pathways that are involved in IL-3 survival signaling are much more complicated than initially perceived.

As summarized herein, transcription factors have been implicated in mediating the survival effects of IL-3 by two approaches: (1) identifying mammalian orthologs of *Caenorhabditis elegans* Ces2/Ces1 in IL-3-dependent hematopoietic cells, and (2) characterizing the promoter element-binding proteins responsible for IL-3 induction of the *mcl-1* gene. Examination of these studies reveals that several specific protein kinases and transcription factors show an unexpected connection between IL-3 receptors and survival genes when mapped. We will also discuss the biological significance of the existence of multiple survival-specific transcription pathways in terms of tissue-specific regulation, differential subcellular localization, and specific interaction between antiapoptotic proteins and BH3-only Bcl-2 family members on the mitochondrial membrane.

II. MAMMALIAN ORTHOLOGS OF *C. ELEGANS* CES2/CES1 PROTEINS

In early embryo development of *C. elegans*, the fate of two sister neurose-cretory motor neurons is determined by the expression of two cell death specification genes, *ces-1* and *ces-2* (Ellis and Horvitz, 1991). Genetic evidence suggests that *ces-2* induces cell death by negatively regulating the cell-specific survival activity of *ces-1* (Ellis and Horvitz, 1991). The *ces-2* gene encodes a basic leucine-zipper (bZIP) transcription factor (Metzstein *et al.*, 1996), and *ces-1* encodes a snail family zinc finger protein (Metzstein and Horvitz, 1999). The Ces-1 protein was shown to suppress the expression of the BH3-only cell death activator gene *egl-1* by directly binding to an *egl-1* enhancer element (Thellmann *et al.*, 2003). However, *ces-1* is itself repressed by the ces-2 bZIP transcription factor. The fact that this transcription regulator pathway identified in *C. elegans* is highly evolutionarily conserved across species underscores the importance of this pathway. Like many genes whose muta-tion affects programmed cell death in *C. elegans*, Ces-2 and Ces-1 also have their counterparts in mammals. Slug, a snail family zinc finger transcription factor, was identified as the mammalian ortholog of *C. elegans* Ces-1 (Inukai *et al.*, 1999). There are several putative mammalian bZIP transcription factor orthologs of Ces-2, such as E4BP4 (Ikushima *et al.*, 1997; Kuribara *et al.*, 1999), cyclic adenosine monophosphate response element (CRE)-binding protein (CREB) (Chen *et al.*, 2001), and TEF (Inukai *et al.*, 2005). As discussed in later sections, many of these mammalian orthologs have been demonstrated to be involved in apoptosis prevention in IL-3-dependent cells (Fig. 1).

A. CREB

The Ces-2/E2A-HLF-binding element (CBE) in *C. elegans* can be recog-nized by the human acute lymphocytic leukemia oncoprotein E2A-HLF as well as the protein product of the *C. elegans* death specification gene *ces-2*. We and others have searched for cellular transcription factors which can bind specifically to this CBE site and potentially mediate IL-3 survival

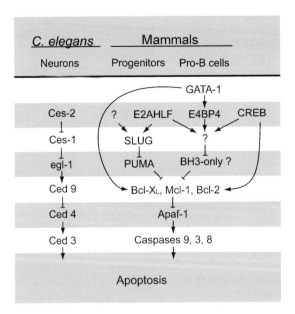

FIGURE 1. Conservation of the apoptosis pathway from *C. elegans* to mammals. Genes at the same level are orthologs. Positive effects are indicated by arrows and negative effects are indicated by blocks. The unidentified factors are indicated as "?". In mammals, the signaling pathway in hematopoietic progenitor cells differs from that in pro-B cells. SLUG only plays a critical role in regulation of DNA damage-induced apoptosis.

responses. We found in experiments using an electrophoretic mobility shift assay that there were many molecules in mammalian cells with CBE-binding activity. Several CBE-binding protein factors were subsequently identified by screening cDNA libraries with labeled CBE probes, such as E4BP4, C/EBPβ, PAR domain factors (TEF and HLF), and CREB family proteins (CREB and ATF2) (Chen *et al.*, 2001).

We first focused on CREB since it was known to be a major CBE-binding transcription factor in IL-3-dependent pro-B cells, and has been suggested to mediate neurotransmitter-dependent neuron protection (Finkbeiner *et al.*, 1997). Our data indicated that IL-3 stimulation can activate CBE-driven luciferase reporter gene expression via a PKA-dependent pathway and that activation or overexpression of the active form of PKA can prevent cell death. Coexpression of a dominant negative CREB mutant with PKA revealed that the survival effects of IL-3 and PKA are partly mediated through actions of the CREB protein (Chen *et al.*, 2001). Intriguingly, we identified a putative CBE site in the promoter of the *bcl-2* gene, which can be bound by CREB and be activated by both PKA and IL-3. The role of CREB in protecting cells from apoptosis induced by various stimuli has been reported in widely diverse cell types, including cardiac myocytes

(Maldonado *et al.*, 2005), macrophages (Park *et al.*, 2005), primary hippo-campal neurons (Glover *et al.*, 2004), and colon cancer cells (Nishihara *et al.*, 2004). It would be interesting to explore the role of CBE-containing genes in these CREB-dependent survival effects.

B. E4BP4

E4BP4 was initially identified as a transcription repressor by virtue of its ability to bind to the CRE/ATF site located in the adenovirus E4 gene promoter and to repress transcription in a DNA-binding site-dependent manner (Cowell *et al.*, 1992). Its peptide sequence is identical to the tran-scriptional activator NF-IL3A, which binds specifically to a region of the IL-3 promoter and transactivates expression of an IL-3 reporter gene in response to T cell stimulation (Zhang *et al.*, 1995). This E4BP4-binding site is identical to the consensus CBE sequence recognized by Ces-2 and E2A-HLF transcription factors (Chen *et al.*, 2001; Inaba *et al.*, 1996; Metzstein *et al.*, 1996). Although E4BP4 is better known as a circadian cycle regulatory gene (Cowell, 2002; Mitsui *et al.*, 2001), subsequent studies in a pro-B cell line have indicated that E4BP4/NFIL3 expression is highly inducible by IL-3 and mediates IL-3-dependent viability (Ikushima *et al.*, 1997). Forced expression of wild-type E4BP4 substantially prolonged cell viability in the absence of IL-3, without affecting Bcl-XL expression. In contrast, expression of a dominant negative form of E4BP4 reduced the growth response to IL-3. Furthermore, the expression of E4BP4 was found to be regulated by onco-genic Ras mutants through both the Raf/MAPK and PI-3K/Akt pathways, suggesting that both pathways are involved in IL-3-induction (Kuribara *et al.*, 1999). E4BP4 expression was shown to correlate with survival ability in rat and chicken motor neurons, and overexpression of E4BP4 in purified cultured motor neurons protected the cells against cell death in the absence of neurotrophic factors (Junghans *et al.*, 2004). Apparently, in some cell contexts, E4BP4 is still capable of initiating a survival signal and suppressing programmed cell death.

C. GATA-1

It is quite intriguing to find that the master gene of erythrocyte differ-entiation, GATA-1, functions as a survival gene via regulation of E4BP4 expression. As mentioned earlier, the expression of the mammalian Ces-2 ortholog E4BP4 is tightly regulated by IL-3 stimulation. The IL-3 responsive element in the e4bp4 promoter was identified to be a GATA transcription factor-binding site, and GATA-1 was found to be the major cellular factor binding to the e4bp4 promoter (Yu *et al.*, 2002). Overexpression of GATA-1 in IL-3-dependent pro-B cells suppresses apoptosis and upregulates e4bp4 mRNA levels (Yu *et al.*, 2002). The transactivation activity of GATA-1 in turn is stimulated by IL-3 via MAPK-dependent phosphorylation of a serine residue within the transactivation domain of the N-terminus of GATA-1 (Yu *et al.*, 2005). Surprisingly, while this MAPK-mediated phosphorylation is essential for GATA-1 transactivation of the *e4bp4* gene (Yu *et al.*, 2005), it is not required for induction of the expression of several red blood cell–specific genes, nor for induction of red blood cell differentiation of a murine erythroid leukemia cell line (our unpublished data). Finally, activation of the GATA-1-estrogen receptor fusion protein by β-estradiol revealed that phosphorylation of GATA-1 at serine-26 is essential for the survival effect of the GATA-1 protein; this survival effect strongly correlated with the induction of the antiapoptotic protein Bcl-XL (Yu *et al.*, 2005).

This scenario is reminiscent of a previous study on the antiapoptotic mechanism of GATA-1 in a GATA-1-deficient erythroid cell line (Gregory *et al.*, 1999). In that study, a special GATA-1-deficient erythroid cell line G1E was used. The G1E cells were derived from *in vitro* differentiated GATA-1$^{-/-}$ embryonic stem cells and represent primary erythroblasts (Weiss *et al.*, 1997). While G1E cells normally proliferate continuously in culture in the presence of erythropoietin, expression of functional GATA-1 proteins causes terminal erythroid maturation in G1E cells. G1E cells that stably express GATA-1-estrogen receptor fusion protein can undergo erythroid differentiation in the presence of estradiol. However in the absence of erythropoietin, Bcl-XL expression and survival of the differentiated erythroid cells are severely compromised (Gregory *et al.*, 1999). The observed cooperation between GATA-1 and erythropoietin suggest that erythropoietin stimulation induces phosphorylation of GATA-1, possibly at serine 26, and that this phosphorylation event manifests the antiapoptotic ability of GATA-1 and concomitantly confers Bcl-XL transactivation. This hypothesis remains to be investigated further.

D. SLUG

The E2A-HLF oncoprotein not only promotes the growth of murine fibroblasts in soft agar (Yoshihara *et al.*, 1995) but also suppresses apoptosis in lymphoid and myeloid cells (Inaba *et al.*, 1996). Research with the aim of elucidating the molecular mechanism mediating the antiapoptotic effects of the E2A-HLF oncoprotein identified the *slug* gene as the downstream target of E2A-HLF and the mediator of E2A-HLF associated survival activity (Inukai *et al.*, 1999). The Slug protein is a member of the highly evolutionarily conserved snail family of zinc finger transcription factors. The predicted protein sequences in five zinc fingers of Slug are remarkably homologous to Ces-1 of *C. elegans*, suggesting conservation in biological function.

Snail family members have been implicated in many developmental processes including mesoderm differentiation, neural crest formation, cell motility, tumor progression, and cell survival (Nieto, 2002). Slug in particular

has been shown to play an important role in protecting hematopoietic progenitor cells from apoptotic insult by γ-irradiation (Inoue *et al.*, 2002). These
protective effects of Slug are mediated by an inhibition of the apoptotic effect
of *p53-u*pregulated *m*odulator of *A*poptosis (PUMA) induced by irradiation-
dependent p53 activation (Wu *et al.*, 2005). The lack of Slug expression in
normal pro-B cells however argues that the antiapoptotic signals activated by
the E2A-HLF oncoprotein are not a normal pathway in B lymphocytes but
rather an aberrant Slug-dependent pathway normally used by primitive
hematopoietic progenitors (Inoue *et al.*, 2002). It remains to be investigated
whether Slug is under cytokine regulation in the early progenitor cells.

III. REGULATORY MACHINERY OF THE *MCL-1* GENE

Mcl-1 is a prosurvival Bcl-2 family member initially identified during a
myeloid cell differentiation (Kozopas *et al.*, 1993). Mcl-1 expression can be
readily induced in response to stimulation by many survival factors including GM-CSF (Derouet *et al.*, 2004), vascular endothelial cell growth factor
(Le Gouill *et al.*, 2004), stem cell factor (Huang *et al.*, 2000), IL-5
(Huang *et al.*, 2000), IL-3 (Wang *et al.*, 1999), and hypoxia-inducible
factor-1 (Piret *et al.*, 2005). Furthermore, the Mcl-1 protein is very labile
in both the presence and absence of cytokines, possibly due to the existence
of PEST [P (proline), E (glutamic acid), S (serine), T (threonine)] sequences
(Chao *et al.*, 1998; Yang *et al.*, 1995).

The ease by which Mcl-1 expression is induced enables it to function in
many systems as an early responder to apoptosis induced by environmental
insults and stresses. As an early responder, Mcl-1 serves as a critical survival
factor which can determine the fate of cells in various physiological and
pathological conditions. Studies examining transcriptional regulation of the
mcl-1 gene have revealed the involvement of known transcription factors in
mediating the intracellular signal transduction from IL-3 binding to the
expression of the antiapoptotic Mcl-1 protein (Fig. 2). Analysis of the entire
mcl-1 promoter region reveals that there are two promoter elements, SIE at
nt -87 and CRE-2 at nt -70, which contribute to IL-3 induced *mcl-1* gene
expression (Wang *et al.*, 1999). In the following sections, there will be
discussion on the regulation of these two elements.

A. CRE-2-BINDING FACTORS

In the IL-3-dependent pro-B cell line Ba/F3, induction of *mcl-1* is dependent on the activation of the PI-3K/Akt pathway. There is a CRE-2 site,
which is bound by a transcription factor complex containing CREB, within
the IL-3 responsive promoter region (Wang *et al.*, 1999). CRE-2-binding
activity is low in the absence of IL-3 but increases dramatically within 1 h of

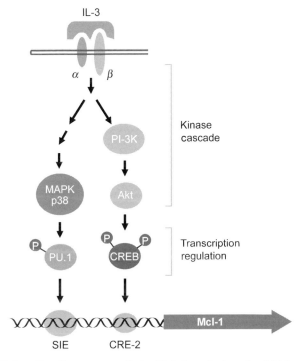

FIGURE 2.   Signaling events mediating IL-3-dependent murine Mcl-1 expression.

cytokine stimulation via a PI-3K/Akt-dependent mechanism (Wang *et al.*, 1999). IL-3 activation of CRE-2 reporter gene expression is mediated via the PI-3K/Akt pathway and is suppressed by a dominant negative CREB mutant, suggesting that CREB also plays an important role in *mcl-1* regulation (Wang *et al.*, 1999). Of special note, CREB proteins only present in a small portion of the total CRE-2-binding activity whereas the whole complexes are highly induced in response to IL-3 treatment. Furthermore, a reporter gene driven by multiple copies of the consensus CRE site does not respond to cytokine stimulation, although it responds to the adenylate cyclin stimulator forskolin and db-cAMP very well (our unpublished data). Therefore, the *mcl-1* CRE-2-binding complexes may contain additional factors, which are required to coordinate with CREB and achieve IL-3 responsiveness.

B. PU.1 TRANSACTIVATION OF *MCL-1* VIA THE *C-SIS*-INDUCIBLE ELEMENT (SIE) SITE

While the binding activity of CRE-2-binding complexes is dramatically induced upon IL-3 treatment, the binding activity of SIE-binding complexes remains constant throughout the course of cytokine stimulation. However, reporter gene analyses indicate that the transcription activity of the SIE promoter significantly increases when p38 MAPK is activated (Wang *et al.*, 2003). Screening of an expression cDNA library with an SIE promoter sequence revealed that PU.1 specifically bound to the *mcl-1* SIE site and transactivated SIE-driven reporter activity (Wang *et al.*, 2003). PU.1 belongs to the family of Est transcription factors and is expressed selectively in cells of the hematopoietic lineage, including B cells, macrophages, mast cells, neutrophils, and early erythroblasts (Oikawa *et al.*, 1999). The *PU.1* gene is identical to the oncogene, *Spi-1*, uncovered in the common proviral insertion site in murine erythroleukemic (MEL) cell by spleen focus-forming virus (Moreau-Gachelin *et al.*, 1988; Paul *et al.*, 1989), which suggests that it may contribute to leukemogenesis. PU.1 was previously shown to be involved in apoptosis regulation in macrophages (Hu *et al.*, 2001) and in mature B cells (Sevilla *et al.*, 2001). Wang *et al.* (2003) have since demonstrated that PU.1 plays an essential role in transactivating the *mcl-1* gene in response to the IL-3 survival signal. PU.1 is activated by p38 MAPK-dependent Ser142 phosphorylation, which increases the transcription activity, rather than DNA-binding activity, of PU.1 (Wang *et al.*, 2003).

IV. DISCUSSIONS

IL-3 can activate multiple survival signaling pathways, which result in the induction of several Bcl-2 family member proteins, including Bcl-2, Mcl-1, Bcl-XL, and A1 (Fig. 3). Since many IL-3-responsive cell lines are derived from different cell lineages, it is conceivable some pathways may be cell type specific rather than being common to all IL-3 responsive cells. For instance, Bcl-XL is highly inducible by IL-3 in the pro-B cell line Ba/F3, whereas in the erythroleukemic cell line TF-1, its expression remains unchanged regardless the challenges encountered (Huang *et al.*, 2000). This discrepancy could be explained by the presence of GATA-1 pathway in Ba/F3 cells, but not in TF-1 cells. Thus, studies examining the upstream transcription regulatory mechanisms of Bcl-2 family genes may greatly help us to interpret the phenotypic outcomes. Furthermore, establishing the relationship between specific transcription pathways and hematopoietic cell lineages may ultimately help predict disease prognosis and therapeutic efficacy.

The recognition of GATA-1 as a potent anti-apoptotic effector in our research has great significance. It underscores a fact that a powerful differentiation master gene in a multicellular organism should have the capability to simultaneously promote differentiation and maintain cellular homeostasis. For example, the GATA-1 knockout mouse has an embryonic lethal phenotype due to the absence of mature red blood cells (Pevny *et al.*, 1991). Subsequent *in vitro* experiments demonstrated that GATA-1$^{-/-}$ embryonic stem (ES) cells gave rise to proerythroblast colonies with normal lineage markers of red blood cells which underwent developmental arrest and

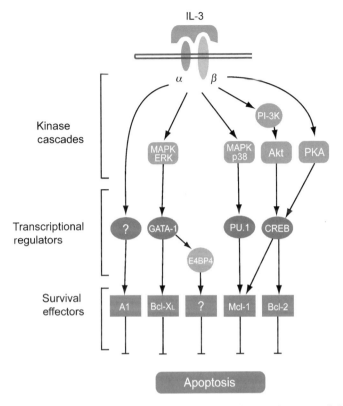

FIGURE 3. Multiple antiapoptotic effector genes are simultaneously expressed via distinct transcriptional factors. Unidentified factors are indicated as "?".

apoptosis (Weiss and Orkin, 1995; Weiss *et al.*, 1994). On the other hand, our data suggest that in *C. elegans* the genetic step upstream of the death specification gene *ces-2* may well be a developmental master gene that supports both neuronal differentiation and cell viability.

Usually multiple Bcl-2 family proteins are induced by IL-3 in an IL-3-dependent cell line. For example, in Ba/F3 cells, Bcl-2, Mcl-1, Bcl-XL, and A1 are all induced by signals derived from IL-3 receptor complexes. It seems highly redundant to have at least four similar proteins in mammalian cells to do the same job as a single protein (Ced-9) in *C. elegans* cells. This apparent redundancy in mammals may be due to gene or pathway multiplication that was selected for or conserved as the cells of higher organisms with supplementary survival signaling pathways may have been more likely to survive the insults of various genotoxic agents. However, differences in both their subcellular localization and the way they interact with the BH3-only proapoptotic proteins suggest that these prosurvival Bcl-2 family proteins are not functionally equivalent. For example, Bcl-2 stably associates with the outer membrane of mitochondria and other extramitochondrial membranes (Kaufmann *et al.*, 2003; Krajewski *et al.*, 1993; Lithgow *et al.*, 1994; Nguyen *et al.*, 1993); meanwhile Bcl-XL is present in both the cytosol and the mitochondrial membrane (Hausmann *et al.*, 2000; Hsu *et al.*, 1997), and cytosolic Bcl-XL translocates to mitochondria in response to apoptotic stimulation (Hsu *et al.*, 1997; Nijhawan *et al.*, 2003). Mcl-1 is present in multiple membrane compartments, including mitochondria and cell nuclei (Yang *et al.*, 1995). In contrast to the apoptotic insult-driven relocation of Bcl-XL, Mcl-1 localization within different subcellular compartments seems to be dependent on cell cycle stage (Liu *et al.*, 2005). It has been shown that Bcl-2 molecularly engineered to be targeted exclusively to the endoplasmic reticulum or the mitochondria showed differential resistance to various apoptotic challenges (Lee *et al.*, 1999; Zhu *et al.*, 1996). Therefore, it is conceivable that the differential subcellular destinations of various Bcl-2 family members reflect their nonidentical antiapoptotic spectrum.

Furthermore, interaction among the Bcl-2 proteins is not homogenous. While Bax, one of two major proapoptotic Bcl-2 proteins, can interact with all prosurvival family members (Wang *et al.*, 1998), Bak, a major proapoptotic Bcl-2 relative, can associate with Mcl-1 and Bcl-XL, but not with Bcl-2, Bcl-W, or A1 (Willis *et al.*, 2005). In healthy cells, Bak is mostly sequestered on the mitochondrial membrane via association with Mcl-1 and Bcl-XL. Loss of Mcl-1 activity by siRNA or Noxa overexpression only leads to apoptosis when Bcl-XL is also deficient (Willis *et al.*, 2005). On the other hand, the BH3-only proteins, in responding to external stimuli, can regulate the availability of Mcl-1 or Bcl-XL and thereby unleash Bak by altering its association with Mcl-1 and Bcl-XL (Adams, 2003). The functional nonequivalency of Bcl-2 members is also clearly documented by *in vivo* gene-targeting studies which have shown that embryonic lethality arises in mice that lack either Mcl-1 or Bcl-XL, while those that lack Bcl-2, Bcl-W, or A1 only exhibit tissue specific effects (Ranger *et al.*, 2001).

In conclusion, it is clear that the functions of Bcl-2 members are determined by several factors, including the differing affinities among the Bcl-2 family members, the cell types in which they are expressed, the subcellular compartments where they reside, and the particular developmental stage during which they are present. Studying the transcriptional regulation of each family member and possible cross-talk between pathways involved in each gene's regulation would greatly help elucidate the complex cell death regulatory networks.

ACKNOWLEDGMENTS

This work was supported in part by an intramural fund from the Academia Sinica and by grants NSC 94-2320-B-001-013 and NSC 94-2320-B-001-007 from the National Science Council of Taiwan to J. J. Y. Y., and by grants NHRI-EX93-9119BN and NSC 92-3112-B-001-016 from the National Health Research Institutes and the National Science Council of Taiwan to H. F. Y. Y., respectively.

REFERENCES

Adams, J. M. (2003). Ways of dying: Multiple pathways to apoptosis. *Genes Dev.* **17**, 2481–2495.

Chao, J. R., Wang, J. M., Lee, S. F., Peng, H. W., Lin, Y. H., Chou, C. H., Li, J. C., Huang, H. M., Chou, C. K., Kuo, M. L., Yen, J. J. Y., and Yang-Yen, H. F. (1998). mcl-1 is an immediate-early gene activated by the granulocyte-macrophage colony-stimulating factor (GM-CSF) signaling pathway and is one component of the GM-CSF viability response. *Mol. Cell. Biol.* **18**, 4883–4898.

Chen, W., Yu, Y. L., Lee, S. F., Chiang, Y. J., Chao, J. R., Huang, J. H., Chiong, J. H., Huang, C. J., Lai, M. Z., Yang-Yen, H. F., and Yen, J. J. (2001). CREB is one component of the binding complex of the Ces-2/E2A-HLF-binding element and is an integral part of the interleukin-3 survival signal. *Mol. Cell. Biol.* **21**, 4636–4646.

Cleveland, J. L., Troppmair, J., Packham, G., Askew, D. S., Lloyd, P., Gonzalez-Garcia, M., Nunez, G., Ihle, J. N., and Rapp, U. R. (1994). v-raf suppresses apoptosis and promotes growth of interleukin-3-dependent myeloid cells. *Oncogene* **9**, 2217–2226.

Coffer, P. J., Jin, J., and Woodgett, J. R. (1998). Protein kinase B (c-Akt): A multifunctional mediator of phosphatidylinositol 3-kinase activation. *Biochem. J.* **335**(Pt. 1), 1–13.

Cowell, I. G. (2002). E4BP4/NFIL3, a PAR-related bZIP factor with many roles. *Bioessays* **24**, 1023–1029.

Cowell, I. G., Skinner, A., and Hurst, H. C. (1992). Transcriptional repression by a novel member of the bZIP family of transcription factors. *Mol. Cell. Biol.* **12**, 3070–3077.

Datta, S. R., Brunet, A., and Greenberg, M. E. (1999). Cellular survival: A play in three Akts. *Genes Dev.* **13**, 2905–2927.

Derouet, M., Thomas, L., Cross, A., Moots, R. J., and Edwards, S. W. (2004). Granulocyte-macrophage colony-stimulating factor signaling and proteasome inhibition delay neutrophil apoptosis by increasing the stability of Mcl-1. *J. Biol. Chem.* **279**, 26915–26921.

Ellis, R. E., and Horvitz, H. R. (1991). Two *C. elegans* genes control the programmed deaths of specific cells in the pharynx. *Development* **112**, 591–603.

Finkbeiner, S., Tavazoie, S. F., Maloratsky, A., Jacobs, K. M., Harris, K. M., and Greenberg, M. E. (1997). CREB: A major mediator of neuronal neurotrophin responses. *Neuron* **19**, 1031–1047.

Glover, C. P., Heywood, D. J., Bienemann, A. S., Deuschle, U., Kew, J. N., and Uney, J. B. (2004). Adenoviral expression of CREB protects neurons from apoptotic and excitotoxic stress. *Neuroreport* **15**, 1171–1175.

Gregory, T., Yu, C., Ma, A., Orkin, S. H., Blobel, G. A., and Weiss, M. J. (1999). GATA-1 and erythropoietin cooperate to promote erythroid cell survival by regulating bcl-xL expression. *Blood* **94**, 87–96.

Hausmann, G., O'Reilly, L. A., van Driel, R., Beaumont, J. G., Strasser, A., Adams, J. M., and Huang, D. C. (2000). Pro-apoptotic apoptosis protease-activating factor 1 (Apaf-1) has a cytoplasmic localization distinct from Bcl-2 or Bcl-x(L). *J. Cell Biol.* **149**, 623–634.

Horbinski, C., and Chu, C. T. (2005). Kinase signaling cascades in the mitochondrion: A matter of life or death. *Free Radic. Biol. Med.* **38**, 2–11.

Hsu, Y. T., Wolter, K. G., and Youle, R. J. (1997). Cytosol-to-membrane redistribution of Bax and Bcl-X(L) during apoptosis. *Proc. Natl. Acad. Sci. USA* **94**, 3668–3672.

Hu, C. J., Rao, S., Ramirez-Bergeron, D. L., Garrett-Sinha, L. A., Gerondakis, S., Clark, M. R., and Simon, M. C. (2001). PU.1/Spi-B regulation of c-rel is essential for mature B cell survival. *Immunity* **15**, 545–555.

Huang, H. M., Li, J. C., Hsieh, Y. C., Yang-Yen, H. F., and Yen, J. J. (1999). Optimal proliferation of a hematopoietic progenitor cell line requires either costimulation with stem cell factor or increase of receptor expression that can be replaced by overexpression of Bcl-2. *Blood* **93,** 2569–2577.

Huang, H. M., Huang, C. J., and Yen, J. J. (2000). Mcl-1 is a common target of stem cell factor and interleukin-5 for apoptosis prevention activity via MEK/MAPK and PI-3K/Akt pathways. *Blood* **96,** 1764–1771.

Ikushima, S., Inukai, T., Inaba, T., Nimer, S. D., Cleveland, J. L., and Look, A. T. (1997). Pivotal role for the NFIL3/E4BP4 transcription factor in interleukin 3-mediated survival of pro-B lymphocytes. *Proc. Natl. Acad. Sci. USA* **94,** 2609–2614.

Inaba, T., Inukai, T., Yoshihara, T., Seyschab, H., Ashmun, R. A., Canman, C. E., Laken, S. J., Kastan, M. B., and Look, A. T. (1996). Reversal of apoptosis by the leukaemia-associated E2A-HLF chimaeric transcription factor. *Nature* **382,** 541–544.

Inoue, A., Seidel, M. G., Wu, W., Kamizono, S., Ferrando, A. A., Bronson, R. T., Iwasaki, H., Akashi, K., Morimoto, A., Hitzler, J. K., Pestina, T. I., Jackson, C. W., *et al.* (2002). Slug, a highly conserved zinc finger transcriptional repressor, protects hematopoietic progenitor cells from radiation-induced apoptosis *in vivo. Cancer Cell* **2,** 279–288.

Inukai, T., Inoue, A., Kurosawa, H., Goi, K., Shinjyo, T., Ozawa, K., Mao, M., Inaba, T., and Look, A. T. (1999). SLUG, a ces-1-related zinc finger transcription factor gene with antiapoptotic activity, is a downstream target of the E2A-HLF oncoprotein. *Mol. Cell* **4,** 343–352.

Inukai, T., Inaba, T., Dang, J., Kuribara, R., Ozawa, K., Miyajima, A., Wu, W., Look, A. T., Arinobu, Y., Iwasaki, H., Akashi, K., Kagami, K., *et al.* (2005). TEF, an antiapoptotic bZIP transcription factor related to the oncogenic E2A-HLF chimera, inhibits cell growth by down-regulating expression of the common beta chain of cytokine receptors. *Blood* **105,** 4437–4444.

Junghans, D., Chauvet, S., Buhler, E., Dudley, K., Sykes, T., and Henderson, C. E. (2004). The CES-2-related transcription factor E4BP4 is an intrinsic regulator of motoneuron growth and survival. *Development* **131,** 4425–4434.

Kaufmann, T., Schlipf, S., Sanz, J., Neubert, K., Stein, R., and Borner, C. (2003). Characterization of the signal that directs Bcl-x(L), but not Bcl-2, to the mitochondrial outer membrane. *J. Cell Biol.* **160,** 53–64.

Kinoshita, T., Yokota, T., Arai, K., and Miyajima, A. (1995). Suppression of apoptotic death in hematopoietic cells by signalling through the IL-3/GM-CSF receptors. *EMBO J.* **14,** 266–275.

Kinoshita, T., Shirouzu, M., Kamiya, A., Hashimoto, K., Yokoyama, S., and Miyajima, A. (1997). Raf/MAPK and rapamycin-sensitive pathways mediate the anti-apoptotic function of p21Ras in IL-3-dependent hematopoietic cells. *Oncogene* **15,** 619–627.

Kozopas, K. M., Yang, T., Buchan, H. L., Zhou, P., and Craig, R. W. (1993). MCL1, a gene expressed in programmed myeloid cell differentiation, has sequence similarity to BCL2. *Proc. Natl. Acad. Sci. USA* **90,** 3516–3520.

Krajewski, S., Tanaka, S., Takayama, S., Schibler, M. J., Fenton, W., and Reed, J. C. (1993). Investigation of the subcellular distribution of the bcl-2 oncoprotein: Residence in the nuclear envelope, endoplasmic reticulum, and outer mitochondrial membranes. *Cancer Res.* **53,** 4701–4714.

Kuribara, R., Kinoshita, T., Miyajima, A., Shinjyo, T., Yoshihara, T., Inukai, T., Ozawa, K., Look, A. T., and Inaba, T. (1999). Two distinct interleukin-3-mediated signal pathways, Ras-NFIL3 (E4BP4) and Bcl-xL, regulate the survival of murine pro-B lymphocytes. *Mol. Cell. Biol.* **19,** 2754–2762.

Le Gouill, S., Podar, K., Amiot, M., Hideshima, T., Chauhan, D., Ishitsuka, K., Kumar, S., Raje, N., Richardson, P. G., Harousseau, J. L., and Anderson, K. C. (2004). VEGF induces

Mcl-1 up-regulation and protects multiple myeloma cells against apoptosis. *Blood* **104,** 2886–2892.

Lee, S. T., Hoeflich, K. P., Wasfy, G. W., Woodgett, J. R., Leber, B., Andrews, D. W., Hedley, D. W., and Penn, L. Z. (1999). Bcl-2 targeted to the endoplasmic reticulum can inhibit apoptosis induced by Myc but not etoposide in Rat-1 fibroblasts. *Oncogene* **18,** 3520–3528.

Lithgow, T., van Driel, R., Bertram, J. F., and Strasser, A. (1994). The protein product of the oncogene bcl-2 is a component of the nuclear envelope, the endoplasmic reticulum, and the outer mitochondrial membrane. *Cell Growth Differ.* **5,** 411–417.

Liu, H., Peng, H. W., Cheng, Y. S., Yuan, H. S., and Yang-Yen, H. F. (2005). Stabilization and enhancement of the antiapoptotic activity of mcl-1 by TCTP. *Mol. Cell. Biol.* **25,** 3117–3126.

Maldonado, C., Cea, P., Adasme, T., Collao, A., Diaz-Araya, G., Chiong, M., and Lavandero, S. (2005). IGF-1 protects cardiac myocytes from hyperosmotic stress-induced apoptosis via CREB. *Biochem. Biophys. Res. Commun.* **336,** 1112–1118.

Metzstein, M. M., and Horvitz, H. R. (1999). The *C. elegans* cell death specification gene ces-1 encodes a snail family zinc finger protein. *Mol. Cell* **4,** 309–319.

Metzstein, M. M., Hengartner, M. O., Tsung, N., Ellis, R. E., and Horvitz, H. R. (1996). Transcriptional regulator of programmed cell death encoded by *Caenorhabditis elegans* gene ces-2. *Nature* **382,** 545–547.

Mitsui, S., Yamaguchi, S., Matsuo, T., Ishida, Y., and Okamura, H. (2001). Antagonistic role of E4BP4 and PAR proteins in the circadian oscillatory mechanism. *Genes Dev.* **15,** 995–1006.

Moreau-Gachelin, F., Tavitian, A., and Tambourin, P. (1988). Spi-1 is a putative oncogene in virally induced murine erythroleukaemias. *Nature* **331,** 277–280.

Nguyen, M., Millar, D. G., Yong, V. W., Korsmeyer, S. J., and Shore, G. C. (1993). Targeting of Bcl-2 to the mitochondrial outer membrane by a COOH-terminal signal anchor sequence. *J. Biol. Chem.* **268,** 25265–25268.

Nicola, N. A., Robb, L., Metcalf, D., Cary, D., Drinkwater, C. C., and Begley, C. G. (1996). Functional inactivation in mice of the gene for the interleukin-3 (IL-3)-specific receptor beta-chain: Implications for IL-3 function and the mechanism of receptor transmodulation in hematopoietic cells. *Blood* **87,** 2665–2674.

Nieto, M. A. (2002). The snail superfamily of zinc-finger transcription factors. *Nat. Rev. Mol. Cell. Biol.* **3,** 155–166.

Nijhawan, D., Fang, M., Traer, E., Zhong, Q., Gao, W., Du, F., and Wang, X. (2003). Elimination of Mcl-1 is required for the initiation of apoptosis following ultraviolet irradiation. *Genes Dev.* **17,** 1475–1486.

Nishihara, H., Hwang, M., Kizaka-Kondoh, S., Eckmann, L., and Insel, P. A. (2004). Cyclic AMP promotes cAMP-responsive element-binding protein-dependent induction of cellular inhibitor of apoptosis protein-2 and suppresses apoptosis of colon cancer cells through ERK1/2 and p38 MAPK. *J. Biol. Chem.* **279,** 26176–26183.

Oikawa, T., Yamada, T., Kihara-Negishi, F., Yamamoto, H., Kondoh, N., Hitomi, Y., and Hashimoto, Y. (1999). The role of Ets family transcription factor PU.1 in hematopoietic cell differentiation, proliferation and apoptosis. *Cell Death Differ.* **6,** 599–608.

Park, J. M., Greten, F. R., Wong, A., Westrick, R. J., Arthur, J. S., Otsu, K., Hoffmann, A., Montminy, M., and Karin, M. (2005). Signaling pathways and genes that inhibit pathogen-induced macrophage apoptosis—CREB and NF-kappaB as key regulators. *Immunity* **23,** 319–329.

Paul, R., Schuetze, S., Kozak, S. L., and Kabat, D. (1989). A common site for immortalizing proviral integrations in Friend erythroleukemia: Molecular cloning and characterization. *J. Virol.* **63,** 4958–4961.

Pevny, L., Simon, M. C., Robertson, E., Klein, W. H., Tsai, S. F., D'Agati, V., Orkin, S. H., and Costantini, F. (1991). Erythroid differentiation in chimaeric mice blocked by a targeted mutation in the gene for transcription factor GATA-1. *Nature* **349,** 257–260.

Piret, J. P., Minet, E., Cosse, J. P., Ninane, N., Debacq, C., Raes, M., and Michiels, C. (2005). Hypoxia-inducible factor-1-dependent overexpression of myeloid cell factor-1 protects hypoxic cells against tert-butyl hydroperoxide-induced apoptosis. *J. Biol. Chem.* **280**, 9336–9344.

Ranger, A. M., Malynn, B. A., and Korsmeyer, S. J. (2001). Mouse models of cell death. *Nat. Genet.* **28**, 113–118.

Sato, N., Sakamaki, K., Terada, N., Arai, K., and Miyajima, A. (1993). Signal transduction by the high-affinity GM-CSF receptor: Two distinct cytoplasmic regions of the common beta subunit responsible for different signaling. *EMBO J.* **12**, 4181–4189.

Sevilla, L., Zaldumbide, A., Carlotti, F., Dayem, M. A., Pognonec, P., and Boulukos, K. E. (2001). Bcl-XL expression correlates with primary macrophage differentiation, activation of functional competence, and survival and results from synergistic transcriptional activation by Ets2 and PU.1. *J. Biol. Chem.* **276**, 17800–17807.

Terada, K., Kaziro, Y., and Satoh, T. (1995). Ras is not required for the interleukin 3-induced proliferation of a mouse pro-B cell line, BaF3. *J. Biol. Chem.* **270**, 27880–27886.

Thellmann, M., Hatzold, J., and Conradt, B. (2003). The Snail-like CES-1 protein of *C. elegans* can block the expression of the BH3-only cell-death activator gene *egl-1* by antagonizing the function of bHLH proteins. *Development* **130**, 4057–4071.

Wada, T., and Penninger, J. M. (2004). Mitogen-activated protein kinases in apoptosis regulation. *Oncogene* **23**, 2838–2849.

Wang, J. M., Chao, J. R., Chen, W., Kuo, M. L., Yen, J. J., and Yang-Yen, H. F. (1999). The antiapoptotic gene mcl-1 is up-regulated by the phosphatidylinositol 3-kinase/Akt signaling pathway through a transcription factor complex containing CREB. *Mol. Cell. Biol.* **19**, 6195–6206.

Wang, J. M., Lai, M. Z., and Yang-Yen, H. F. (2003). Interleukin-3 stimulation of mcl-1 gene transcription involves activation of the PU.1 transcription factor through a p38 mitogen-activated protein kinase-dependent pathway. *Mol. Cell. Biol.* **23**, 1896–1909.

Wang, K., Gross, A., Waksman, G., and Korsmeyer, S. J. (1998). Mutagenesis of the BH3 domain of BAX identifies residues critical for dimerization and killing. *Mol. Cell. Biol.* **18**, 6083–6089.

Weiss, M. J., and Orkin, S. H. (1995). Transcription factor GATA-1 permits survival and maturation of erythroid precursors by preventing apoptosis. *Proc. Natl. Acad. Sci. USA* **92**, 9623–9627.

Weiss, M. J., Keller, G., and Orkin, S. H. (1994). Novel insights into erythroid development revealed through *in vitro* differentiation of GATA-1 embryonic stem cells. *Genes Dev.* **8**, 1184–1197.

Weiss, M. J., Yu, C., and Orkin, S. H. (1997). Erythroid-cell-specific properties of transcription factor GATA-1 revealed by phenotypic rescue of a gene-targeted cell line. *Mol. Cell. Biol.* **17**, 1642–1651.

Willis, S. N., Chen, L., Dewson, G., Wei, A., Naik, E., Fletcher, J. I., Adams, J. M., and Huang, D. C. (2005). Proapoptotic Bak is sequestered by Mcl-1 and Bcl-xL, but not Bcl-2, until displaced by BH3-only proteins. *Genes Dev.* **19**, 1294–1305.

Wu, W. S., Heinrichs, S., Xu, D., Garrison, S. P., Zambetti, G. P., Adams, J. M., and Look, A. T. (2005). Slug antagonizes p53-mediated apoptosis of hematopoietic progenitors by repressing puma. *Cell* **123**, 641–653.

Yang, T., Kozopas, K. M., and Craig, R. W. (1995). The intracellular distribution and pattern of expression of Mcl-1 overlap with, but are not identical to, those of Bcl-2. *J. Cell Biol.* **128**, 1173–1184.

Yen, J. J., Hsieh, Y. C., Yen, C. L., Chang, C. C., Lin, S., and Yang-Yen, H. F. (1995). Restoring the apoptosis suppression response to IL-5 confers on erythroleukemic cells a phenotype of IL-5-dependent growth. *J. Immunol.* **154**, 2144–2152.

Yoshihara, T., Inaba, T., Shapiro, L. H., Kato, J. Y., and Look, A. T. (1995). E2A-HLF-mediated cell transformation requires both the *trans*-activation domains of E2A and the leucine zipper dimerization domain of HLF. *Mol. Cell. Biol.* **15,** 3247–3255.

Yu, Y. L., Chiang, Y. J., and Yen, J. J. (2002). GATA factors are essential for transcription of the survival gene E4bp4 and the viability response of interleukin-3 in Ba/F3 hematopoietic cells. *J. Biol. Chem.* **277,** 27144–27153.

Yu, Y. L., Chiang, Y. J., Chen, Y. C., Papetti, M., Juo, C. G., Skoultchi, A. I., and Yen, J. J. (2005). MAPK-mediated phosphorylation of GATA-1 promotes Bcl-XL expression and cell survival. *J. Biol. Chem.* **280,** 29533–29542.

Zhang, W., Zhang, J., Kornuc, M., Kwan, K., Frank, R., and Nimer, S. D. (1995). Molecular cloning and characterization of NF-IL3A, a transcriptional activator of the human interleukin-3 promoter. *Mol. Cell. Biol.* **15,** 6055–6063.

Zhu, W., Cowie, A., Wasfy, G. W., Penn, L. Z., Leber, B., and Andrews, D. W. (1996). Bcl-2 mutants with restricted subcellular location reveal spatially distinct pathways for apoptosis in different cell types. *EMBO J.* **15,** 4130–4141.

7

INTERLEUKINS AND STAT SIGNALING

S. JAHARUL HAQUE[*,†,‡] AND PANKAJ SHARMA[*,†]

*Department of Cancer Biology, Lerner Research Institute
Cleveland Clinic Foundation, Cleveland, Ohio 44195
†Department of Pulmonary, Allergy, and Critical Care Medicine
Cleveland Clinic Foundation, Cleveland, Ohio 44195
‡Brain Tumor Institute, Cleveland Clinic Foundation, Cleveland, Ohio 44195

Metazoan cells secrete small proteins termed cytokines that execute a variety of biological functions essential for the survival of organisms. Binding of cytokines that belong to the hematopoietin- or interferon-family, to their cognate receptors on the surface of target cells, induces receptor aggregation, which in turn sequentially triggers tyrosine-phosphorylation-dependent activation of receptor-associated Janus-family tyrosine kinases (JAKs), receptors, and signal transducers and activators of transcription (STATs). Phosphorylated STATs form dimers that migrate to the nucleus, bind to cognate enhancer elements and activate transcription of target genes. Each cytokine activates a specific set of genes to execute its biological functions with a certain degree of redundancy. Cytokine signals are, in general, transient in nature. Therefore, under normal physiological conditions, initiation and attenuation of cytokine signals are tightly controlled via multiple cellular and molecular mechanisms. Aberrant activation of cytokine signaling pathways is, however, found under a variety of patho-physiological conditions including cancer and immune diseases. © 2006 Elsevier Inc.

I. INTERLEUKINS: STRUCTURE, CLASSIFICATION, AND MODE OF ACTION

The term "interleukin (IL)" was originally coined to refer to a family of structurally related proteins, which are secreted by certain leukocytes (producer cells) and act on other leukocytes (target cells) (Abbas and Litchman, 2003; Boulay et al., 2003; Rozwarski et al., 1994). Subsequent studies have shown that many interleukins as well as interleukin-related proteins are produced by and act on cells other than leukocytes. Therefore, the generic term "cytokine" represents a family of proteins that include interleukins (1 through 31), interferons (IFNs, both type I and type II), erythropoietin (EPO), thrombopoietin (TPO), prolactin (PRL), growth hormone (GH), granulocyte colony stimulating factor (G-CSF), granulocyte macrophage colony stimulating factor (GM-CSF), leptin, leukemia inhibitory factor (LIF), oncostatin M (OSM), ciliary neurotropic factor (CNTF), cardiotrophin-1 (CT-1), cardiotrophin-like cytokine (CLC), and tumor necrosis factor (TNF) (Boulay *et al.*, 2003; Goldsby *et al.*, 2003; Ozaki and Leonard, 2002; O'Shea *et al.*, 2005b).

Based on their protein structures, cytokines are classified into four families: hematopoietin, IFN, chemokine, and TNF (Goldsby *et al.*, 2003). Here, we will discuss about hematopoietins and IFN-family of cytokines that have helix-loop-helix bundle structures (Bazan, 1990a; Mitsui and Senda, 1997; Rozwarski *et al.*, 1994; Uze *et al.*, 1995). The hematopietin family of cytokines contains four α helices labeled A through D, which are connected by two long loops (AB and CD) and a short loop (BC) with up-up–down-down topology (Fig. 1A) (Mitsui and Senda, 1997; Uze *et al.*, 1995). IFN-family of cytokines also contain four α helices termed A, C, D, and F that form a bundle structure, in which helix-pairs AC and DF are linked by two long overhand connections (B and E), which pack against each other on one edge of the bundle (Fig. 1B) (Pestka *et al.*, 2004). Of note, the conformation of the helix F is straight in type I IFNs (IFNα/β), whereas it is bent at ∼50° in IFN-γ and IL-10 (Pestka *et al.*, 2004).

A cytokine may act on its producer cells in an autocrine fashion and/or it may act on neighboring target cells in a paracrine fashion (Abbas and Litchman, 2003; Goldsby *et al.*, 2003). Depending on lineages of target cells,

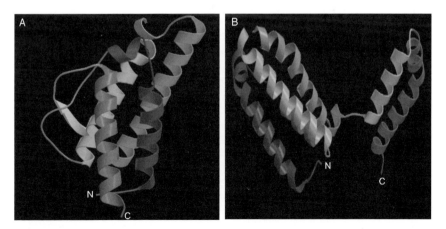

FIGURE 1. Ribbon structures of human IL-4 (A) and IL-10 (B). Both illustrations are "rainbow" colored, with the N-terminus colored violet, running through to the C-terminus colored red. The figures were prepared automatically from the 3-D coordinates of the proteins using NAOMI to drive Molscript/Raster3D. It is to be noted that human IL-10 is biologically functional as a dimer. (See Color Insert.)

a single cytokine may produce multiple biological outcomes by a pleiotropic mechanism. For example, IL-4 induces the differentiation of naïve T helper cells to type 2 (Th2) phenotype, whereas in B cells it induces immunoglobulin class-switching (Coffman *et al.*, 1986; Gascan *et al.*, 1991; Vitetta *et al.*, 1985). In addition, IL-4 attenuates activation of macrophages (Abbas and Litchman, 2003; Crawford *et al.*, 1987; Nelms *et al.*, 1999; Zlotnik *et al.*, 1987). More than one cytokine may produce the same biological outcome in a given target cell. An example of such redundant cytokine action is the induction of B cell proliferation by IL-2, IL-4, and IL-5 (Abbas and Litchman, 2003). Moreover, more than one cytokine may simultaneously act on a given single cell. In this case, one cytokine may augment the action of the other in a synergistic way; for example, both TNF-α and IFN-γ increase the expression of class I MHC in a variety of cells (Abbas and Litchman, 2003). Further, one cytokine may also inhibit the action of others by acting as an antagonist. For example, IL-10 inhibits IFN-γ-mediated activation of macrophages (Abbas and Litchman, 2003; Tebo *et al.*, 1998).

II. CYTOKINE RECEPTORS: STRUCTURE AND CLASSIFICATION

Receptors for hematopoietins and IFN-family cytokines are classified as class I and class II receptors, respectively. Cytokines that belong to the hematopoietin family include IL-2, IL-3, IL-4, IL-5, IL-6, IL-7, IL-9, IL-11, IL-12, IL-13, IL-15, IL-23, IL-27, IL-31, CLC, CNTF, CT-1, EPO, G-CSF, GH, GM-CSF, leptin, LIF, OSM, PRL, and TPO (O'Shea *et al.*, 2005b). Many interleukins including IL-10, IL-19, IL-20, IL-21, IL-22, IL-24, IL-26, IL-28A (IFN-λ2), IL-28B (IFN-λ3), IL-29 (IFN-λ1), and limitin use class II receptors for cell signaling (Kotenko *et al.*, 2003; O'Shea *et al.*, 2005b; Sheppard *et al.*, 2003; Vilcek, 2003). Some interleukins like IL-1, IL-8, IL-17, IL-18, and IL-25 use receptors that do not belong to either class I or class II cytokine receptors. Both class I and class II receptors are transmembrane glycoproteins with a single membrane spanning region of 20–25 amino acids (Bazan, 1990b; Haque and Williams, 1998; Heldin, 1995; Kishimoto *et al.*, 1994). These receptors contain one or two characteristic external domain structure(s) termed D200 that consists of two homologous subdomains (SD100) of approximately 100 amino acids. Each SD100 adopts an immunoglobulin-like fold with seven β strands (s1–s7) organized into two β sheets (Bazan, 1990a). The D200 module of class I receptors contains a set of four cysteine residues and a WSXWS (W = tryptophan, S = serine, and X = any amino acid) motif, whereas class II receptors share one cysteine-pair with the class I receptors and contain an additional conserved cysteine-pair

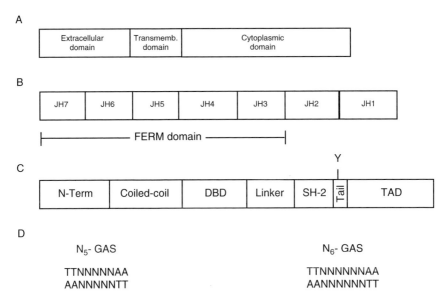

FIGURE 2.   Schematic representation of the components of the JAK–STAT pathway. (A) Type I and Type II cytokine receptors. The cytokine receptor comprises an extracellular domain, a short transmembrane domain, and a C-terminal cytoplasmic domain that contains docking sites for all signaling components. (B) Janus kinases (JAKs) have JH1–JH7 domains of which the N-terminal JH3–JH7 domains constitute the FERM domain. (C) Signal transducers and activators of transcription (STATs). The STAT proteins are composed of N-terminal oligomerization domain followed by a coiled-coil domain that is likely involved in the nuclear translocation of STATs. This is followed by a DNA-binding domain that is important for binding to cognate sequences on the DNA, an SH2 domain responsible for binding to the tyrosine-phosphorylated receptors followed by the tail segment that includes the conserved tyrosine residue, and is followed by the C-terminal transactivation domain responsible for the activation of STAT-responsive genes. (D) DNA sequences recognized by STATs. The conserved N5-GAS and N6-GAS sequences present in the promoter regions of cognate genes that are recognized by STAT dimers for binding through their DNA-binding domains.

and several conserved proline and tryptophan residues, but lack the WSXWS motif (Bazan, 1990a).

   The human genome encodes a total of 34 class I receptor proteins, whereas the mouse genome encodes 35. Twenty-five human receptors exhibit perfect consensus of class I receptors (Boulay et al., 2003). Class II receptor genes identified in humans include type I IFN receptors (IFNAR1 and IFNAR2), type II IFN receptors (IFNGR1 and IFNGR2), IL-10 receptors (IL-10Rα and IL-10Rβ), IL-19 receptors (IL-20Rα and IL-20Rβ), IL-20 receptors (IL-20Rα/IL-22Rα and IL-20Rβ), IL-22 receptors (IL-22Rα and IL-10Rβ), IL-24 receptors (IL-20Rα/IL-22Rα and IL-20Rβ), and IL-28 receptors (IL-28Rα and IL-10Rβ) (Gadina et al., 2001; Kotenko *et al.*, 2003; Ozaki and Leonard, 2002; Sheppard *et al.*, 2003; Vilcek, 2003). Extracellular domains of both classes of receptors confer specificity for ligand binding (Fig. 2A).

The three-dimensional structure of cytoplasmic domains of cytokine receptors is not available. Most information on the structure–function relationship has been derived from receptor mutagenesis studies. Although structurally more diverse, cytoplasmic domains of these receptors, in general, contain short α helices designated as box I and box II motifs that are located proximally to transmembrane regions (Fig. 2A) (Bazan, 1990c; Ihle, 1995; Kishimoto *et al.*, 1994; Leonard and O'Shea, 1998). These motifs are responsible for stable association of Janus-family tyrosine kinases (JAKs) to cytokine receptor subunits (Ihle, 1995). Cytoplasmic regions of these receptors also contain a number of tyrosine residues that become phosphorylated upon cytokine stimulation of cells, which in turn serve as docking sites for cognate downstream signaling proteins (Domanski and Colamonici, 1996; Haque and Williams, 1998; Stark *et al.*, 1998).

III. FUNCTIONAL CYTOKINE-RECEPTOR COMPLEXES

Based on subunit-compositions of functional receptor complexes formed upon cytokine binding, cytokines and their cognate receptors can be categorized as follows.

A. CATEGORY I

Binding of a cytokine of this category consisting of IL-4, IL-7, IL-9, IL-13, and IFN-α/β, to its cognate receptor that is constitutively associated with a JAK, recruits a secondary receptor chain that is also constitutively associated with another JAK, in order to form a functional receptor complex.

B. CATEGORY II

Binding of a cytokine of the second category (IL-2, IL-6, IL-11, and CNTF) to its cognate receptor that does not bind to JAK, recruits two secondary receptor subunits that are bound to JAKs, to form a functional receptor complex of three receptor subunits. Two secondary receptors are identical for IL-6, IL-11, and CNTF, whereas they are different for IL-2.

C. CATEGORY III

Binding of EPO, PRL, or GH to its cognate receptor that is associated with JAK2, forms a homodimer in order to constitute a functional receptor complex.

D. CATEGORY IV

In order to form a signaling receptor complex, IFN-γ-dimer binds to two molecules of JAK1-bound IFNGR1, which then recruit two molecules of JAK2-associated IFNGR2. It is possible that other cytokines like IL-5 that may exist as dimers, also allow the formation of a tetrameric receptor complex for cell signaling (Geijsen et al., 2001).

Thus, it is apparent that at least two receptor subunits (identical or different) both of which are physically associated with cognate JAKs, are required for the formation of a functional receptor complex, and the possible reason for this requirement is discussed later.

IV. SHARING OF RECEPTOR-SUBUNITS BY CYTOKINES

Although each cytokine has its own specific receptor, sharing of receptor subunits for cell signaling is a unique feature of both hematopoietins and IFN-family of cytokines, as discussed later.

(1) IL-4 shares its primary receptor IL-4Rα, with IL-13. IL-4 forms two types of receptor complexes, type I and type II, for cell signaling. The type I IL-4 receptor complex that is composed of IL-4Rα and the gamma common (γc) chain, is not shared by IL-13, because neither of these receptor subunits binds to IL-13 (Nelms et al., 1999). IL-13 binds to IL-13Rα1 that recruits IL-4Rα or IL-4 binds to IL-4Rα that recruits IL-13Rα1 in order to form the type II IL-4 receptor complex (Nelms et al., 1999). In both types of IL-4 receptor complexes, IL-4Rα is the key signaling receptor subunit, whereas either γc-associated JAK3 or IL-13Rα1-associated JAK2 (or TYK2) is likely involved in catalyzing phosphorylation of IL-4Rα-associated JAK1 (mechanisms discussed in a later section). Thus, IL-4 and IL-13 exhibit many overlapping biological outcomes in cells expressing all components of type II IL-4 receptor complex. However, nonhematopoietic cells that do not express γc and JAK3, fail to form type I IL-4 receptor complex; on the other hand, murine B and T cells and human T cells, which lack IL-13Rα1 expression, cannot respond to IL-13 (Jiang et al., 2000; Nelms et al., 1999).

(2) IL-2, IL-4, IL-7, IL-9, IL-15, and possibly IL-21 share γc for cell signaling. Therefore, deficiency of γc expression severely impairs biological functions of these cytokines in relevant cells (O'Shea et al.,

2005b). JAK3 specifically binds to γc; therefore, deficiency of JAK3 mirrors that of γc (Yamaoka *et al.*, 2004). In addition, loss-of-function mutations in γc results in X-linked severe combined immunodeficiency (X-SCID) in humans and mice (DiSanto *et al.*, 1995; Leonard and O'Shea, 1998; Nakajima *et al.*, 1997; Nosaka *et al.*, 1995; O'Shea *et al.*, 2005b; Park *et al.*, 1995; Thomis *et al.*, 1995).

(3) IL-6 family of cytokines including IL-6 itself, IL-11, OSM, LIF, CNTF, CT-1, and CLC share gp130 for signaling their target cells. IL-6 and IL-11 bind to their cognate receptors IL-6Rα and IL-11Rα respectively, which do not bind to JAK. These ligand–receptor complexes recruit two bipartite molecules of JAK-associated gp130, in order to form functional receptors (Heinrich *et al.*, 2003). Similarly, binding of CNTF or CLC with CNTFR that does not bind to JAK, recruits one molecule of JAK-associated gp130 and one molecule of JAK-associated LIFR to constitute their respective functional receptor complexes (Heinrich *et al.*, 2003). In contrast, LIF or OSM shares a heterodimer of LIFR and gp130 for signal transduction. OSM may also form a functional receptor by engaging a heterodimer of OSMR and gp130 (Heinrich *et al.*, 2003). All three signaling receptors gp130, LIFR, and OSMR can bind to JAK1, JAK2, or TYK2; however, JAK1 is found to play an essential role in gp130-mediated signal transduction and consequent gene expression (Heinrich *et al.*, 2003). Due to sharing of gp130, the IL-6 subfamily of cytokines show many overlapping biological outcomes in their target cells (Heinrich *et al.*, 2003).

(4) IL-3, IL-5, and GM-CSF bind to their specific receptors IL-3Rα, IL-5Rα, and GM-CSFRα, respectively (Geijsen *et al.*, 2001). This allows them to recruit a common β chain termed βc that has constitutive, physical association with JAK2 (Quelle *et al.*, 1994). Of note, the mouse genome encodes an additional IL-3-specific β chain termed $βc_{IL-3}$ (van Dijk *et al.*, 1998). It is presumed that two heterodimers of α and β-common chains constitute a functional receptor complex allowing two JAK2 molecules to trans-phosphorylate each other (Muto *et al.*, 1995). Moreover, IL-5Rα binds to JAK2 by virtue of having a box I-like proline-rich motif in its cytoplasmic domain (Adachi and Alam, 1998; Geijsen *et al.*, 2001).

(5) Sharing of receptor subunits among class II cytokines including IL-10, IL-19, IL-20, IL-22, IL-24, IL-28, and IL-29, results in a wide range of redundancy in their biological outcomes. For example, IL-10Rβ that remains physically associated with TYK2, dimerizes with: (i) JAK1-bound IL-10Rα to form a functional IL-10 receptor complex, and (ii) JAK1-bound IL-22Rα to form a functional IL-22 receptor (Kotenko *et al.*, 2001). Similarly, IL-20Rβ that is bound to JAK2 or TYK2 heterodimerizes with: (i) JAK1-associated IL-20Rα to form functional receptors for IL-19, IL-20 and IL-24, and (ii) JAK1-bound IL-22Rα to form functional receptors for

IL-20 and IL-24 (Ozaki and Leonard, 2002). Ligation of IL-28 and IL-29 with IL-28Rα that is bound to JAK1, recruits TYK2-bound IL-10Rβ in order to form functional receptor complexes for these cytokines (Kotenko et al., 2003; Sheppard et al., 2003).

(6) Like IL-6 that binds to its cognate receptor (soluble or membrane-bound IL-6Rα), IL-12 (p35) binds to p40 that structurally resembles a soluble form of cytokine receptor. A p35/p40 heterodimer forms a functional receptor by recruiting IL-12Rβ1 and IL-12Rβ2, which are physically associated with JAK2 and TYK2, respectively (Ozaki and Leonard, 2002). IL-23 (p19) also forms a heterodimer with p40, which recruits IL-23R and IL-12Rβ1 to form a functional receptor (Gately et al., 1998). Both IL-12 and IL-23 promote the differentiation of naïve T helper cells to Th1 phenotype (Oppmann et al., 2000; Parham et al., 2002).

V. JAKS: CYTOKINE RECEPTOR-ASSOCIATED PROTEIN TYROSINE KINASES

The mammalian genome encodes four members of the Janus family: TYK2, JAK1, JAK2, and JAK3 (Ihle, 2001; Leonard and O'Shea, 1998; O'Shea et al., 2002). Tyrosine kinase 2 (TYK2), the first member of the family was originally identified by screening a human T cell–derived cDNA library using human c-fms kinase domain as a probe (Velazquez et al., 1992). Others were subsequently identified by PCR screening of cDNA libraries using primers derived from conserved motifs located in the catalytic domain of protein-tyrosine kinase (Harpur et al., 1992; Kawamura et al., 1994; Rane and Reddy, 1994; Takahashi and Shirasawa, 1994; Wilks et al., 1991; Witthuhn et al., 1994). Molecular weights of these intracellular protein tyrosine kinases range from 120 to 140 kD (Leonard and O'Shea, 1998). JAK3 is primarily expressed in hematopoietic cells, whereas others are expressed in most cell types (Ihle, 2001). In humans, JAK1 is located on chromosome 1, JAK2 on chromosome 9, JAK3 on chromosome 19, and TYK2 on chromosome 19. In mice, JAK1 is mapped to chromosome 4, JAK2 to chromosome 19, JAK3 to chromosome 8, and TYK2 to chromosome 9 (Table IA) (Leonard and O'Shea, 1998). Importantly, TYK2 was identified as a component of IFN-α/β signaling pathway by using somatic cell genetics approaches, and subsequent studies revealed roles for JAK1 and JAK2 in the activation of many class I and class II cytokine receptors (Muller et al., 1993; Velazquez et al., 1992; Watling et al., 1993). JAK3 specifically binds to γc and is involved in IL-2-, IL-4-, IL-7-, IL-9-, IL-15-, and possibly IL-21-mediated cell signaling (Leonard and O'Shea, 1998). The primary importance of different JAKs has been elucidated by the phenotypes of

TABLE I.   Chromosomal Location of JAKs and STATs

	Human	Mouse	References
A: JAKs			
JAK1	1p31.3	4C6	(Gough et al., 1995; Parganas et al., 1998)
JAK2	9p24	19C1	(Gough et al., 1995; Parganas et al., 1998)
JAK3	19p13.1	8B3.3	(Kono et al., 1996; Kumar et al., 1996; Riedy et al., 1996)
TYK2	19p13.2	9A3	(Firmbach-Kraft et al., 1990)
B: STATs			
STAT1	2q32.2	1C1.1	(Copeland et al., 1995; Yamamoto et al., 1997)
STAT2	12q13.3	10D3	(Copeland et al., 1995)
STAT3	17q21.31	8B3.3	(Akira et al., 1994; Copeland et al., 1995)
STAT4	2q32.2-q32.3	1C1.1	(Copeland et al., 1995; Yamamoto et al., 1997)
STAT5A	17q11.2	11D	(Copeland et al., 1995; Lin et al., 1996)
STAT5B	17q11.2	11D	(Copeland et al., 1995; Lin et al., 1996)
STAT6	12q13	10D3	(Copeland et al., 1995; Leek et al., 1997)

knockout mice that are listed in Table II. Protein tyrosine phosphorylation is essential for cytokine signal transduction, which is catalyzed by receptor-associated JAKs (Velazquez et al., 1992; Watling et al., 1993). Unlike growth factor receptors including EGFR and PDGF, receptors for class I and class II cytokines do not possess any tyrosine-kinase activity. Each signal transducing receptor subunit constitutively associates with its cognate JAK partner in order to constitute a bipartite receptor tyrosine kinase molecule, which is functionally equivalent to a receptor tyrosine kinase like EGFR or PDGFR.

Based on amino acid sequence similarities in JAK-family members, seven JAK homology regions (JH1 through JH7) are defined (Haque and Williams, 1998; Ihle, 1995) (Fig. 2B). A functional protein kinase domain (JH1) is located at the C-terminus of each JAK (Haque and Williams, 1998; Leonard and O'Shea, 1998). JH1 domain comprises 279–302 amino acids, which contains all structural signatures of a classical tyrosine kinase domain (Hanks et al., 1988). Like all other protein tyrosine kinases, JAKs require the phosphorylation of conserved tyrosine residue(s) located in their activation segments, for the activation of their catalytic activity. In the absence of this phosphorylation, JAKs possess a basal kinase activity, which is, however, not sufficient for activation of cytokine receptors in vivo. This is in part, due to association of protein tyrosine phosphatase(s) (PTPs) with cytokine receptor complexes (Haque et al., 1997). A single JAK molecule cannot catalyze the

TABLE II. Phenotypes of JAK-Deficient Mice

JAK kinase	Phenotype	Cytokines affected	References
JAK1	Die perinatally; 40% smaller; fail to nurse; primary defect in thymocyte production; profound defect in lymphoid development	IL-2, IL-4, IL-6, IL-7, IL-9, IL-15, IL-6, LIF, CNTF, OSM, CT-1, IFN-γ	(Rodig *et al.*, 1998)
JAK2	Embryonic lethal at E12.5 p.c; no erythropoeisis; delay in heart development	IFN-γ, EPO, TPO, IL-3, IL-5, GM-CSF	(Neubauer *et al.*, 1998; Parganas *et al.*, 1998)
JAK3	Viable, fertile; SCID due to marked reduction in both B-cell and T-cell populations	IL-2, IL-4, IL-7, IL-9, IL-15	(Nosaka *et al.*, 1995; Park *et al.*, 1995; Thomis *et al.*, 1995)
TYK2	Viable, fertile; defective Th1 differentiation; defective IL-12/IL-18-induced IFN-γ production by T and NK cells	Partial response to IFN-α, IL-12, IL-18	(Shimoda *et al.*, 2000, 2002)

phosphorylation of cognate tyrosine residue (underlined in Fig. 3) located in its own activation segment, because the binding of ATP (phosphate donor substrate) and accessibility of the tyrosine residue to be phosphorylated (phosphate acceptor substrate) are believed to be mutually exclusive (Hubbard *et al.*, 1994), which is a unique characteristic of all RD kinases (Fig. 3) (Hanks *et al.*, 1988). An RD kinase is defined by the presence of an arginine (R) adjacent to the catalytic aspartic acid (D) present in all tyrosine kinases and in many serine/threonine kinases like c-AMP-dependent protein kinase (Johnson *et al.*, 1996). Therefore, at least two JAK molecules are required for their mutual trans-phosphorylation *in vivo* and hence, at least two bipartite receptor chains are required for cell signaling by a given cytokine receptor complex, as discussed in an earlier section. Adjacent to JH1, there is a pseudokinase (kinase-related) domain JH2 that has a number of protein kinase signature motifs characteristic of a functional catalytic domain but is missing some conserved amino acids including the catalytic aspartic acid residue (Haque and Williams, 1998). Studies have shown that JH2 plays a regulatory role in JAK function (O'Shea *et al.*, 2005b).

The N-terminal half of JAK comprising of five regions (JH3–JH7) shares amino acid sequence homology among the family members, which predicts a FERM (Band-4.1, ezrin, radixin, moesin) domain (Fig. 2B) (Girault *et al.*, 1998). An SH2-like domain is also found in this region, whose function

IR	RD	(X)19 DFG	(X)8	D<u>Y</u>Y	(X)10	RWM	APE
FGFR1	RD	(X)19 DFG	(X)8	D<u>Y</u>Y	(X)10	KWM	APE
PDGFRβ	RD	(X)19 DFG	(X)9	N<u>YI</u>	(X)9	KWM	APE
CSF1R	RD	(X)19 DFG	(X)9	N<u>YI</u>	(X)9	KWM	APE
TYK2	RD	(X)19 DFG	(X)9	E<u>YY</u>	(X)10	FWY	APE
JAK1	RD	(X)19 DFG	(X)9	E<u>YY</u>	(X)10	FWY	APE
JAK2	RD	(X)19 DFG	(X)9	E<u>YY</u>	(X)10	FWY	APE
JAK3	RD	(X)19 DFG	(X)9	E<u>YY</u>	(X)10	FWY	APE
cAPK	RD	(X)19 DFG	(X)9	W<u>TL</u>	(X)4	EYL	APE

FIGURE 3. Activation segments of three classes of RD (arginine aspartic acid) protein kinases. Insulin receptor kinase (IRK), fibroblast growth factor receptor 1 (FGFR1), platelet-derived growth factor receptor-(PDGFR), and colony-stimulating factor 1 receptor (CSF1R) represent the receptor tyrosine kinases. Janus kinases (JAKs) and cyclic-AMP-dependent protein kinase (cAPK) represent nonreceptor tyrosine kinases and serine/threonine kinase respectively. These kinases are activated by autophosphorylation of conserved tyrosine/threonine residues (underlined). The activation segment (boxed) is located between the highly conserved triplets DFG of kinase subdomain VII and APE of kinase subdomain VIII. RD is located 19 amino acids upstream of DFG. The activation segment of IRK, which causes autoinhibition has five extra amino acids and adopts a different conformation of the segment in cAPK.

is not clear. The FERM domain is responsible for the stable physical association of JAK to its cognate receptors (Haan *et al.*, 2001; Hilkens *et al.*, 2001). Like class I and class II cytokine receptors, a number of growth factor receptors including EGFR, also form complexes with JAKs (Leaman *et al.*, 1996). Specificity of JAK recognition by cytokine receptors is shown in Table III.

VI. SIGNAL TRANSDUCERS AND ACTIVATORS OF TRANSCRIPTION

An IFNα/β-inducible DNA-binding activity, known as IFN-stimulated gene factor 3 (ISGF3) was shown to contain four proteins of molecular weights 48, 84, 91, and 113 kD (Levy *et al.*, 1989). Subsequently, molecular cloning revealed that p91 and p84 components of ISGF3 are derived from spliced variants of a single transcript and are named STAT1α and STAT1β, respectively, and p113 is named STAT2 (Fu *et al.*, 1992). The smallest ISGF3-subunit p48 (IRF-9) is a member of IFN regulatory factor (IRF)-family proteins (Levy *et al.*, 1986). STAT1 and STAT2 play dual roles in IFN

TABLE III. Utililization of JAKs and STATs and Receptors by Cytokines

Cytokine	JAKs	STATs	References
Hematopoeitin family			
IL-3, IL-5, GM-CSF	JAK2	STAT5	(Miyajima et al., 1993)
IL-4	JAK1, JAK2/TYK2/JAK3	STAT6	(Leonard, 2001;
			Nelms et al., 1999)
IL-6, IL-11, LIF, CT-1, CNTF, OsM, CLCG	JAK1/JAK2/TYK2	STAT1, STAT3	(Heinrich et al., 2003)
IL-7, IL-9, IL-15, IL-21	JAK1, JAK3	STAT5	(Leonard, 2001)
IL-12	JAK2, TYK2	STAT4	(Gately et al., 1998)
IL-13	JAK1, JAK2/TYK2	STAT6	(Nelms et al., 1999)
IL-23	JAK1, JAK2	STAT1, STAT3	(Oppmann et al., 2000)
IL-31	JAK1, JAK2	STAT1, STAT3, STAT5	(Dillon et al., 2004;
			Dreuw et al., 2004)
EPO, GH, PRL, TPO	JAK2	STAT5	(Leonard and O'Shea, 1998)
Leptin	JAK2	STAT1, STAT3, STAT5	(Bendinelli et al., 2000)
Interferon family			
Type I IFNs (IFN-α, -β, -δ, -ε, -κ, -τ, -ω)	JAK1, TYK2	STAT1, STAT2, STAT3	(Kotenko and Pestka, 2000)
Type II IFN (IFN-γ)	JAK1, JAK2	STAT1	(Kotenko and Pestka, 2000)
IL-10	JAK1, TYK2	STAT1, STAT3, STAT5	(Kotenko and Pestka, 2000)
IL-19	JAK1, JAK2/TYK2	STAT1, STAT3	(Dumoutier et al., 2001)
IL-20	JAK1, JAK2/TYK2	STAT1, STAT3	(Blumberg et al., 2001;
			Dumoutier et al., 2001)

(Continues)

TABLE III. (*Continued*)

Cytokine	JAKs	STATs	References
IL-22	JAK1, JAK2/TYK2	STAT1, STAT3, STAT5	(Kotenko et al., 2001; Xie et al., 2000)
IL-24	JAK1, JAK2/TYK2	STAT1, STAT3	(Parrish-Novak et al., 2002)
IL-26	Not known	Unknown	(Sheikh et al., 2004)
Limitin	JAK1, TYK2	STAT1, STAT2, STAT3	(Aoki et al., 2003; Oritani et al., 2000)
IL-28A	JAK1, TYK2	STAT1, STAT2, STAT3, STAT5	(Dumoutier et al., 2003; Kotenko et al., 2003; Sheppard et al., 2003)
IL-28B	JAK1, TYK2	STAT1, STAT2, STAT3, STAT5	(Dumoutier et al., 2003; Kotenko et al., 2003; Sheppard et al., 2003)
IL-29	JAK1, TYK2	STAT1, STAT2, STAT3, STAT5	(Dumoutier et al., 2003; Kotenko et al., 2003; Sheppard et al., 2003)

signaling: they transduce signals from IFN receptor to the nucleus and bind to IFN-inducible enhancer element and activate transcription; hence they are termed *signal transducers and activator of transcription* (STATs). Subsequent studies identified five other STATs: STAT3, -4, -5a, -5b, and -6, each one encoded by an individual gene (Darnell, 1997). Chromosomal location of human and murine STAT genes are described in Table IB.

STATs share a striking amino acid sequence homology throughout the molecule except the C-terminal regions (Fig. 2C) (Darnell, 1997; Shuai, 1999). Each STAT contains an N-terminal domain ($\sim$130 amino acids) that is responsible for the oligomerization of STATs that binds to the tandem recognition sites located in promoters of many STAT-responsive genes. This domain is flanked by a coiled-coil domain, which is shown to have a role in the nuclear translocation of STATs (Liu *et al.*, 2005b), followed by a DNA-binding domain. Next to the DNA-binding domain is a linker region of unknown functions. Adjacent to the linker, is located an SH2 domain ($\sim$100 amino acids), which is flanked by a short tail ($\sim$10 amino acids) containing a conserved tyrosine residue that becomes phosphorylated in response to cytokine stimulation of cells (discussed later). The SH2 domain is responsible for the dimerization of tyrosine-phosphorylated STAT molecules, which is mediated by intermolecular interaction between SH2 domain and a phosphotyrosine residue located in the tail (Darnell, 1997).

Three-dimensional structures of DNA-bound STAT1 and STAT3 have been solved (Becker *et al.*, 1998; Chen *et al.*, 1998). Like STAT3-dimer, STAT1-dimer forms a contiguous C-shaped clamp around the cognate DNA, which is stabilized by the reciprocal interaction between the SH2 domain of one monomer and the C-terminal segment of the second monomer that is phosphorylated at Tyr701 (Chen *et al.*, 1998). This structure has been determined in a STAT1 protein that lacks the C-terminal transactivation domain (TAD) (Fig. 4).

The C-terminal TADs of STATs have the most diverse primary structures with variable sizes (Fig. 2C). The TADs of STAT1, STAT3, STAT4, STAT5a, and STAT5b contain a consensus serine phosphorylation motif, which could be phosphorylated by proline-directed kinases (Decker and Kovarik, 2000; Park *et al.*, 2001; Yamashita *et al.*, 1998). Phosphorylation of Ser727 residues in the TAD of STAT1 and STAT3 enhances their transcriptional activities (Decker and Kovarik, 2000). STAT proteins may also be phosphorylated at Ser residues distinct from those present in the conserved Pro-Met-Ser-Pro motif (Chung *et al.*, 1997b); however, the biological outcome of this phosphorylation is not known (Decker and Kovarik, 2000). Recent studies have shown that phosphorylation of multiple Ser residues located in the STAT3-TAD (other than Ser727) and STAT6-TAD inhibits their DNA-binding activity (Ghosh *et al.*, 2005; Maiti *et al.*, 2005; Woetmann *et al.*, 1999, 2003).

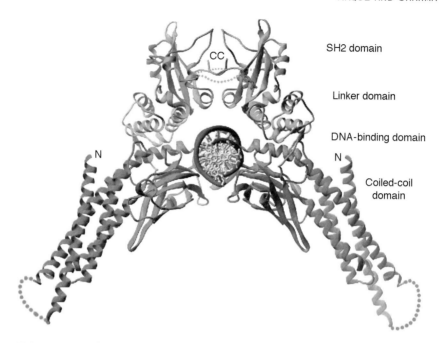

SH2 domain

Linker domain

DNA-binding domain

Coiled-coil
domain

FIGURE 4.   Ribbon structure of the STAT1 core dimer on DNA. The component domains are colored green (coiled-coil domain), red (DNA-binding domain), orange (linker domain), and cyan (SH2 domain). The tail segments are shown in magenta and yellow. Disordered loops (one in the coiled-coil domain, and one connecting the SH2 domain to the tail segment) are shown in dotted lines. The phosphotyrosine residue is shown in a stick representation. The N- and C-termini of STAT1 core are indicated by "N" and "C." The DNA backbone is shown in gray. (Reprinted from Chang *et al.* (1998). *Cell* **93**, 827–839, copyright (1998) with permission from Elsevier.) (See Color Insert.)

VII. MECHANISM OF JAK-STAT SIGNAL TRANSDUCTION

Binding of a given cytokine to its cognate receptor induces an aggregation of at least two receptor chains, each of which is constitutively bound to a cognate JAK molecule (Fig. 5). Receptor aggregation is believed to induce a conformational change that allows the receptor complex to bring two JAK molecules to an approximate proximity, which allows them to trans-phosphorylate each other on conserved tyrosine residues located in their activation segments (underlined residue in Fig. 3). This results in an increment of basal catalytic activities of these two kinase molecules. Like all other protein tyrosine kinases, as mentioned earlier, JAKs belong to the RD kinase family (Fig. 3), in which the catalytic aspartic acid (D) is preceded by an arginine (R), whose positive charge needs to be neutralized by the

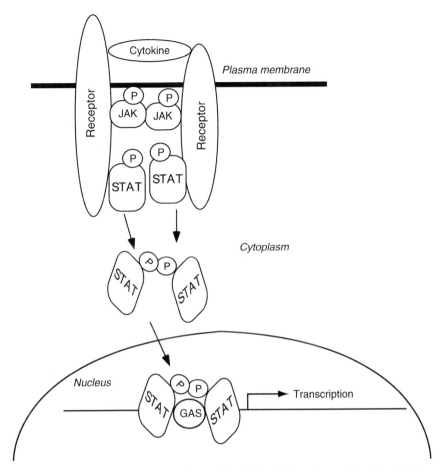

FIGURE 5. Schematic representation of the JAK–STAT pathway. Cytokines bind to homodimeric or heterodimeric receptors to which the Janus kinases (JAKs) are constitutively associated. After receptor dimerization, JAKs transphosphorylate each other. This, in turn, leads to phosphorylation of cognate tyrosines on the receptors, allowing STATs to bind via SH2-phosphotyrosine interactions. As a result, STAT proteins become phosphorylated at conserved tyrosine residues allowing them to dimerize and translocate to the nucleus where they bind to cognate GAS sites on the DNA and regulate gene expression.

negatively charged phosphate moiety that is covalently linked to the tyrosine (Y) in the activation segment (Haque *et al.*, 1997). However, a single kinase molecule does not have the structural freedom to access both its substrates—an ATP (phosphate donor substrate) and the tyrosine (phosphate acceptor substrate) located in its own activation segment (Johnson *et al.*, 1996). It is believed that due to this structural restraint, at least two RD kinase molecules are required for the phosphorylation of each other on the target tyrosine residues (Hubbard *et al.*, 1994). Due to the presence of a functional kinase domain (JH1) in JAKs, one can assume that a JAK molecule should have some basal catalytic activity in the absence of tyrosine phosphorylation of the activation segment. In fact, it has been shown in the case of IL-4 receptor activation, receptor-associated PTPs are responsible for the attenuation of cytokine (ligand)-independent receptor activation catalyzed by the basal kinase activity of IL-4Rα-associated JAK1 (Haque *et al.*, 1997). Once the JAKs' catalytic activities are augmented, they can phosphorylate multiple tyrosine residues that are located in the cytoplasmic domain of the cognate receptor chains. The phoshorylated tyrosine residues then serve as docking sites for downstream signaling proteins that include STATs, and various adapter proteins like IRS, Shc, and Grb2. Adapter proteins couple the activated receptor to multiple signaling pathways that include Ras-MAPK, PI3K-AKT, and PKC (Nelms *et al.*, 1999). Receptor-associated JAKs phosphorylate the conserved tyrosine residues of STATs (Fig. 4). An activated receptor complex may phosphorylate more than one STAT protein. Phosphorylated STAT proteins are then released from the receptor by an unknown mechanism and form dimers (homodimers and/or heterodimers), which migrate to the nucleus and bind to cognate DNA element, known as γ IFN *a*ctivation *s*ite (GAS), which was originally identified as IFN-γ-responsive enhancer element (Shuai *et al.*, 1992). GAS is a palindromic enhancer with a consensus sequence TTNNNNNAA (N5-GAS), that is present in promoters of many cytokine-responsive genes (Fig. 2D) (Darnell *et al.*, 1994; Schindler *et al.*, 1995). All activated STAT-dimers except STAT6-homodimer can bind to N5-GAS, whereas STAT6-homodimer but not other STAT-dimers binds only to TTNNNNNNAA (N6-GAS), which contains an extra nucleotide between AA and TT. In the literature, N5-GAS is also referred to as N3-GAS that has TTCNNNGAA consensus sequence (Fig. 2D). Likewise, N6-GAS is also designated as N4-GAS with TTCNNNNGAA consensus sequence (Mikita *et al.*, 1996). Stimulation of cells with type I IFNs induces the transcription of genes, whose promoters contain another enhancer element designated as IFN-stimulated response element (ISRE) (Levy *et al.*, 1989). An ISRE contains a direct repeat of GAAA flanked by either one or two nucleotides (GAAAN$_{1-2}$GAAA) (Darnell *et al.*, 1994; Levy *et al.*, 1986; Schindler and Darnell, 1995). As mentioned in an earlier section, the protein complex that binds to an ISRE in IFN−α/β-stimulated cells is known as IFN-stimulated gene factor 3 (ISGF3) that is composed of a complex of activated STAT1 (α and/or β), STAT2 and IRF-9 (originally identified as ISGF-3γ, a 48-kD protein (p48), whose expression is increased by IFN-γ treatment of cells) (Darnell *et al.*, 1994). Of note, upon activation many growth factor receptors including EGFR and PDGFR can recruit and activate STAT1 and STAT3 proteins as efficiently as an activated cytokine receptor (Lang *et al.*, 2003; Vignais *et al.*, 1996; Zhong *et al.*, 1994). The promoter of c-fos proto-oncogene contains a *sis* (PDGFβ)-inducible enhancer (SIE) that binds to homodimers and heterodimers of STAT1 and STAT3, which are collectively known as *sis*-inducible factors (SIF) (Wagner *et al.*, 1990).

Like other transcription factors, STATs must pass through nuclear pore complexes (NPC) to enter the nucleus (Rout *et al.*, 2003). Proteins larger than 40–50 kDa require specific signaling motifs to traverse the NPC, which are recognized by karyopherin superfamily of proteins also known as importins/exportins (Rout *et al.*, 2003). STAT proteins associate with importins that recognize nuclear localization signals (NLS) usually rich in basic residues (McBride *et al.*, 2000, 2002; Sekimoto *et al.*, 1997). The binding site for importin $\alpha 5$ recognizes a dimer-specific NLS within the DNA-binding domain of STAT1 (McBride *et al.*, 2002). In addition, the N-terminal oligomerization (Strehlow and Schindler, 1998) and coiled-coil domains (Ma *et al.*, 2003) of STAT are also implicated in nuclear import. It has been demonstrated that STAT dephosphorylation is blocked when it is bound to DNA (Meyer *et al.*, 2003; Shuai and Liu, 2003), and this may be responsible for the nuclear accumulation of tyrosine-phosphorylated STATs after cytokine stimulation. Exportins, such as CRM1, may recognize leucine-rich export signals identified in STATs that have fallen off the DNA and are subsequently dephosphorylated (Begitt *et al.*, 2000; Bhattacharya and Schindler, 2003; Liu *et al.*, 2005b; McBride *et al.*, 2000, 2002) and facilitate their exit through the NPC. Surprisingly, unphosphorylated STAT proteins are found to shuttle continuously between the cytosol and the nucleus (Chatterjee-Kishore *et al.*, 2000; Meyer *et al.*, 2002).

VIII. SPECIFICITY OF CYTOKINE SIGNALING

More than 50 cytokines can activate the canonical JAK–STAT pathway and more than one cytokine can activate a single STAT. Yet, each cytokine or a group of functionally related cytokines is able to activate a fairly unique set of genes, although some overlaps occur. How does a cell maintain the specificity of JAK–STAT-mediated gene expression? It is believed that signal specificity is maintained at multiple levels through a number of specific macromolecular interactions. Specificity may be provided by the selective recruitment of STAT protein(s) to the activated receptor subunits via specific interactions between phosphotyrosine and SH2 domain (Haque and Williams, 1998). For example, IFNAR1 molecule contains STAT2-specific docking site and IL-4Rα contains docking sites that are specific for STAT6 (Krishnan *et al.*, 1998; Nelms *et al.*, 1999). Physical association of other proteins to a given STAT-dimer may confer the specificity of DNA–protein interactions. Sequence heterogeneity found in the GAS and ISRE also renders specificity for STAT-specific gene expression. For example, the GAS sequence present in the promoter of β casein gene preferably binds to STAT5 (Hannigan and Williams, 1992). Recent studies indicate that novel posttranslational modifications of STATs like acetylation, sumoylation, and methylation, may regulate the specificity of STAT function at the chromatin level (O'Shea *et al.*, 2005a).

IX. HOMEOSTATIC CONTROL OF CYTOKINE PRODUCTION AND CYTOKINE SIGNALING

As mentioned in the beginning, cytokine producer cells synthesize and secrete cytokines for communication with neighboring cells in order to fulfill the specific requirements for the development and survival of the organism. Specific requirements that include induction of mitosis, induction or inhibition of cell death, and induction of cell differentiation along a particular lineage of target cells, are determined by a complex mechanism that controls the physiological homoeostasis. Once a secreted cytokine engages its receptor on the surface of a target cell, its actions are controlled by a variety of intracellular mechanisms. In the following section we will discuss general mechanisms by which cytokine synthesis and cytokine action are controlled at cellular and molecular levels.

X. REGULATION OF CYTOKINE SYNTHESIS

More than 50 cytokines belong to the hematopoietin- and IFN-family, which are produced by a variety of cells in response to multiple internal and/or external signals. It is beyond our scope to discuss how the production of each cytokine is controlled. Here, we use the paradigm of helper T cell differentiation to illustrate the regulation of cytokine production. CD4-expressing T helper cells are classified into two functionally distinct subtypes, Th1 and Th2. This concept was originally proposed in 1986 by Mosmann and Coffman (Mosmann *et al.*, 1986). It is now a dominant paradigm that provides a framework for a better understanding of the differentiation of helper T cells and the molecular and cellular bases of cytokine production. According to this paradigm, Th1 and Th2 cells derive from a common precursor cell (ThP) depending upon the cytokine signals it receives at the time of first antigen exposure. Th1 cells emerge typically in the presence of IL-12, whereas Th2 cells expand in an IL-4-dominated microenvironment. Upon reexposure to an antigen Th1 and Th2 cells secrete two distinct sets of cytokines that orchestrate different immune responses. Th1-derived cytokines (IL-2, IFN-γ, and TNF) promote defense against intracellular pathogens. On the other hand, Th2-derived cytokines that include IL-4, IL-5, IL-6, IL-9, and IL-13, provide protection against extracellular organisms (O'Shea *et al.*, 2004, 2005b). Importantly, a majority, if not all, Th2-specific cytokines have been implicated in the pathogenesis of atopic disorders. Interestingly, many Th2-specific cytokine genes such as IL-3, IL-4, IL-5, IL-9, and IL-13 are located in the long arm of human chromosome 5 (Kelleher *et al.*, 1991). When stimulated with antigen, naïve T cells support very low levels of nonselective transcription of both Th1- and Th2-specific cytokine genes that encode IFN-γ, IL-4, IL-5, and IL-13, indicating that chromatin architectures of these genes are poised for responding to signals that induce the differentiation (Ansel *et al.*, 2003). Upon differentiation Th1 cells epigenetically silence the Th2-specific genes and express the Th1-specific genes at more than 100-fold greater level than naïve T cells, and Th2 cells show a converse pattern of gene expression (Ansel *et al.*, 2003).

XI. NEGATIVE REGULATION OF CYTOKINE SIGNALING

Cytokine signal is, in general, limited in both duration and magnitude. Thus, the regulation of cytokine signaling requires a delicate balance between biochemical events that activate and amplify the signal initiated by the activation of cytokine receptor and the mechanisms that attenuate or terminate the signal. Here, we will discuss how a cytokine-activated JAK–STAT pathway is negatively controlled at molecular levels. In principle, the JAK–STAT signaling can be controlled at multiple levels by a number of molecules that act through distinct mechanisms (Starr and Hilton, 1999). For instance, a receptor antagonist may compete with the cytokine for receptor occupation or a decoy receptor may compete with the functional receptor for cytokine binding, and blocks the initiation of cytokine signaling. Many key components of the JAK–STAT pathway are activated by protein tyrosine phosphorylation. Therefore, dephosphorylation of phosphotyrosine residues of signaling proteins by PTP activity is a major means of negatively regulating the pathway. Two families of proteins, the *s*uppressor *o*f *c*ytokine *s*ignaling (SOCS) and the *p*rotein *i*nhibitor of *a*ctivated *S*TATs (PIAS) can downregulate the pathway through distinct mechanisms. SOCS-family proteins do so by inhibiting the JAK activity and/or blocking the recruitment of the downstream signaling proteins to activated cytokine receptors, whereas PIAS-family proteins inhibit JAK–STAT mediated gene expression by blocking the DNA-binding activity of the activated STAT proteins (Starr and Hilton, 1999; Wormald and Hilton, 2004). Proteolytic degradation of signaling proteins also causes attenuation or termination of cytokine signals.

A. DECOY RECEPTORS

Decoy receptors are soluble or transmembrane proteins that bind to cytokines with high affinity and high specificity but are incapable of generating and transducing cytokine signals. Thus, they limit cytokine binding to the cognate-signaling receptors by sequestering cytokines with high affinity, and thereby act as negative regulators of cytokine signaling (Heaney and Golde, 1996; Levine, 2004; Mantovani et al., 2001; Rahaman et al., 2002b). Soluble cytokine receptors can be generated by proteolytic cleavage of extracellular regions of functional receptors, alternate splicing of receptor mRNA or expression of distinct genes (Heaney and Golde, 1996; Levine, 2004; Mantovani et al., 2001; Rahaman et al., 2002b). Alternate splicing of mRNA generates receptor transcripts that encode extracellular domains containing leader signals but not transmembrane domains, and are secreted by producer cells. Soluble IL-4Rα detected in biological fluids is produced by an alternate splicing of mRNA (Chilton and Fernandez-Botran, 1993; Heaney and Golde, 1996; Levine, 2004). Additional examples of alternate splicing-mediated expression of soluble receptors include GM-CSFRα, G-CSFRα, EPOR, LIFR, IL-5Rα, IL-7Rα, IL-9Rα (Heaney and Golde, 1996). IL-13Rα2, a distinct gene product is a nonsignaling transmembrane protein that binds to IL-13 with high affinity, thus it competes with IL-13Rα1 (a low-affinity receptor for IL-13) for ligand binding and inhibits IL-13 signaling (Rahaman et al., 2002b; Zhang et al., 1997). We have shown that IL-13Rα2 can also inhibit IL-4 signaling through the type II receptor complex comprising of IL-4Rα and IL-13Rα1 (Rahaman et al., 2002b).

B. PROTEIN TYROSINE PHOSPHATASES

A number of studies have shown that PTP activity is a major, primary negative regulator of the JAK–STAT pathway. It has been noted that a continuous presence of the cytokine IL-4 is required for sustained signaling through the JAK–STAT pathway (Haque and Sharma, unpublished data). Based on biochemical studies on the negative regulation of IFN-γ-activated JAK–STAT signaling, it was postulated that more than one protein-tyrosine phosphatase activity is required for the negative regulation of cytokine signaling: an upstream phosphatase activity, termed PTP-x, is responsible for the dephosphorylation of activated JAKs and associated cytokine receptor subunits, whereas PTP-y dephosphorylates activated STAT proteins in the nucleus (Haque et al., 1995). PTP-x and PTP-y may represent two families of PTPs rather than two individual enzymes. Subsequent studies have shown that an SH2 domain containing PTP, Shp-1, is a potent negative regulator of JAK–STAT pathway activated by a number of cytokines (Haque et al., 1995, 1998). Shp-1 physically associates with many cytokine receptor complexes via direct interaction with receptor subunits and/or with receptor-associated JAKs. The Shp-1 gene in mouse chromosome 6 encodes a 68-kD protein that has two tandem SH2 domains and a catalytic domain (Yi et al., 1992a). Spontaneous mutations are found in the Shp-1 gene in C57BL/6J mice, which are associated with the motheaten and the viable motheaten phenotypes that develop severe combined immunodeficiency and systemic autoimmunity

(Shultz *et al.*, 1993). The motheaten phenotype is caused by a point mutation in the N-terminal SH2 domain resulting in the absence of Shp-1 protein expression, whereas, the viable motheaten phenotype is caused by point mutations in the phosphatase domain, which result in the generation of two mutant Shp-1 proteins, one with a 5 amino acid deletion (with molecular weight of 67 kD) and another with a 23 amino acid insertion (with molecular weight of 71 kD), with little or no catalytic activity (Shultz *et al.*, 1993). Shp-1 is primarily expressed in cells of hematopoietic lineages (Yi *et al.*, 1992b). CD45 that dephosphorylates JAK and attenuate STAT activation is also expressed only in hematopoietic cells (Irie-Sasaki *et al.*, 2001; Hermiston *et al.*, 2003). Then question arises, which PTP acts as a negative regulator of cytokine signaling in nonhematopoietic cells. To this end, Shp-2 a ubiquitously expressed, SH2-domain containing PTP, has been implicated in the negative regulation of a number of cytokine signaling pathways (Lehmann *et al.*, 2003; Ohtani *et al.*, 2000; Schaper *et al.*, 1998; Wu *et al.*, 2002). Shp-2 has also been found to act as an adapter in PDGFR-mediated cell signaling (Qu, 2000). Shp2 does not downregulate IL-4/IL-13-mediated activation of JAK–STAT pathway (Haque and Sharma, unpublished data). We have recently found that PTP1B, a ubiquitously expressed PTP is involved in the negative regulation of IL-4/IL-13-mediated JAK–STAT signaling (Sharma and Haque, unpublished data). We have also found that PTP1B associates with IL-4Rα (Sharma *et al.*, unpublished data). Interestingly, TCPTP, which is closely related to PTP1B, is found to dephosphorylate STAT1, STAT3, and STAT5 but not STAT6 (Bourdeau *et al.*, 2005; ten Hoeve *et al.*, 2002).

C. SUPPRESSOR OF CYTOKINE SIGNALING

Suppressor of cytokine signaling family proteins were originally identified as cytokine-inducible inhibitors of cytokine signaling (Endo *et al.*, 1997; Naka *et al.*, 1997; Starr *et al.*, 1997). Eight members have been identified in the SOCS-family: SOCS-1 through SOCS-7 and cytokine inducible SH2 containing protein (CIS). These proteins are characterized by the presence of three structural domains (Alexander and Hilton, 2004). The N-terminal domain that varies in length and primary structure seems to regulate the JAK kinase activity (Haque *et al.*, 2000). The central SH2 domain binds to cognate phosphotyrosine residues of target proteins (Alexander and Hilton, 2004; Ozaki and Leonard, 2002). The C-terminal homology domain is known as SOCS-BOX (Kile *et al.*, 2002). It is apparent from a number of studies that all three domains of SOCS play roles in the attenuation of cytokine signaling. For example, N-terminal Pre-SH2 domains of SOCS-1 and SOCS-3 are implicated in the inhibition of IL-4 and IL-6 signaling (Haque *et al.*, 2000; Narazaki *et al.*, 1998; Nicholson *et al.*, 1999). SH2 domains of SOCS-2, SOCS-3, and CIS bind to phosphotyrosine residues in cytokine receptors and that of SOCS-1 and SOCS-3 bind to JAKs and inhibit cytokine signaling

(Endo *et al.*, 1997; Haque *et al.*, 2000; Naka *et al.*, 1997; Starr *et al.*, 1997; Wormald and Hilton, 2004). SOCS-BOX mediates interactions with elongins B and C, which in turn target SOCS and SOCS-associated proteins to proteasomal degradation (Kamura *et al.*, 1998; Zhang *et al.*, 1999). SOCS-1 targets TEL-JAK2 fusion protein to ubiquitination and proteasomal degradation in a SOCS-BOX–dependent manner (Frantsve *et al.*, 2001; Kamizono *et al.*, 2001; Ungureanu *et al.*, 2002). SOCS-1-deficient mice exhibit enhanced response to IFN-γ, and die within 3 weeks of age, whereas mice that are deficient in both SOCS-1 and IFN-γ survive (Alexander *et al.*, 1999; Marine *et al.*, 1999b). SOCS-2-deficient mice exhibit enhanced signaling through GH and IGF-1 and grow significantly bigger than control animals (Metcalf *et al.*, 2000). Deletion of SOCS-3 gene results in embryonic lethality at 12–16 days associated with marked erythrocytosis (Marine *et al.*, 1999a). Generation of mice lacking SOCS-3 in specific tissues has allowed to demonstrate that SOCS-3 is involved in the attenuation of IL-6-mediated signal transduction (Croker *et al.*, 2003; Lang *et al.*, 2003; Yasukawa *et al.*, 2003). We have found that SOCS-1 and SOCS-3 but not SOCS-2 or CIS inhibit IL-4-dependent activation of STAT6, when overexpressed in 293T cells (Haque *et al.*, 2000). It has been shown that IL-4 signaling is suppressed by SOCS-5 expression during Th1 differentiation (Alexander and Hilton, 2004; Seki *et al.*, 2002).

D. PROTEIN INHIBITOR OF ACTIVATED STATS

The PIAS-family consisting of four members (PIAS1, PIAS3, PIASx/PIAS2, and PIASy/PIAS4) was originally identified as negative regulator of STAT signaling (Chung *et al.*, 1997a; Liu *et al.*, 1998; O'Shea and Watford, 2004; Shuai and Liu, 2005). Subsequent studies have shown that PIAS proteins also interact with a variety of cellular proteins, most of which are transcription factors including STATs, and regulate transcription via multiple mechanisms (Reviewed in Shuai and Liu, 2005). PIAS1 can inhibit the DNA-binding activity of STAT1; accordingly, STAT1-binding to cognate DNA is increased in PIAS-deficient cells, as examined by chromatin immunoprecipitation (Liu *et al.*, 2004, 2005a). IL-12-dependent activation of STAT4 is inhibited by PIASx, which could be restored by treating cells with trichostatin A, an inhibitor of histone deacetylase 3 (HDAC3) (Arora *et al.*, 2003). HDAC enzymes play important roles in chromatin modification and gene regulation by removing acetyl groups from lysine residues in histone and nonhistone proteins (Tussie-Luna *et al.*, 2002). PIASx-b is found to interact with HDAC3 (Tussie-Luna *et al.*, 2002). PIAS proteins repress gene expression by inducing the sumoylation of transcription factors including STAT1 (Shuai and Liu, 2005). PIAS1 interacts with the N-terminal region of STAT1 that has an arginine residue, which is methylated and negatively controls PIAS interaction with STAT1 (Mowen *et al.*, 2001). PIAS3 blocks the DNA-binding activity of STAT3 homodimer and

STAT1–STAT3 heterodimer but not STAT1 homodimer (Chung *et al.*, 1997b; Schindler, 1999).

E. PROTEOLYSIS OF STATS

The ubiquitin-proteasome pathway has been shown to negatively control the stability of activated STAT1 and increase the amount of DNA-bound STAT1 in MG132-treated HeLa cells (Kim and Maniatis, 1996). Studies have also demonstrated that activated forms of STAT4, STAT5, and STAT6 are stabilized in cells that are exposed to MG132 (Maiti *et al.*, 2005; Wang *et al.*, 2000; Woctmann *et al.*, 1999, 2003). It has been reported that STAT3-, STAT5-, and STAT6-specific nuclear proteases exist, which cleave cognate STATs at the C-termini to generate dominant negative STAT molecules that inhibit STAT functions (Chakraborty and Tweardy, 1998; Lee *et al.*, 1999; Nakajima *et al.*, 2003; Sherman *et al.*, 2002; Suzuki *et al.*, 2002).

XII. STATS IN HUMAN DISEASES

Persistent activation of STAT1, STAT3, and STAT5 has been documented in a number of malignancies (reviewed in Yu and Jove, 2004). STAT1 has been shown to have antiproliferative activity (Ramana *et al.*, 2002). However, a study has demonstrated that activated STAT1 confers resistance to radiation-induced cell death (Khodarev *et al.*, 2004). STAT3 remains persistently activated in cancer cells via aberrant activation of cytokine and growth factor signaling pathways, and by oncogenic activation of Src in many cancer cell types, which in turn promotes the expression of bcl-2 family of prosurvival genes including bcl-2, bcl-x, and mcl-1, and cell cycle regulatory genes like cyclin D1 and c-myc (reviewed in Yu and Jove, 2004), (Ghosh *et al.*, 2005; Rahaman *et al.*, 2002a). STAT3 also induces the expression of *VEGF*, thus promotes angiogenesis in experimental pancreatic cancer model (Niu *et al.*, 2002; Wei *et al.*, 2003). Constitutive activation of STAT5 in chronic myelogenous leukemia is catalyzed by either TEL-JAK2 or by BCR-ABL fusion kinase (Huang *et al.*, 2002; Schwaller *et al.*, 2000). STAT1 and STAT2 play key roles in the establishment of antiviral state (Stark *et al.*, 1998).

STAT6 that is activated by IL-4 and IL-13, plays a key role in the production of IgE that initiates immediate hypersensitivity reaction, a powerful trigger for allergic diseases including asthma, eczema, hay fever, and food allergy (Pernis and Rothman, 2002). Airways of atopic (allergic) asthma patients contain more STAT6-expressing cells than those of nonatopic asthmatics (Christodoulopoulos *et al.*, 2001). STAT6-deficient mice fail to develop airway hyperresponsiveness, IgE production, and mucus secretion in response to antigen provocation (Akimoto *et al.*, 1998; Kuperman *et al.*,

TABLE IV. Phenotypes of STAT-Deficient Mice

STAT protein	Phenotype	References
STAT1	Viable, fertile; defects in responses to IFN-α/β and IFN-γ; increased susceptibility to bacterial and viral infections; increased susceptibility to tumor formation	(Durbin et al., 1996; Kaplan et al., 1998; Meraz et al., 1996)
STAT2	Viable, fertile; defects in responses to IFN-α/β; increased susceptibility to bacterial and viral infections	(Park et al., 2000)
STAT3	Embryonic lethal at E6.5–7.5; defective IL-6-induced T cell proliferation due to defective apoptosis (thymoctye-specific deletion); impaired IL-2-induced proliferation of thymocytes and splenic T cells (thymoctye-specific deletion) Impaired skin remodeling (keratinocyte-specific deletion); enhanced Th1 activity; suppression of mammary epithelial apoptosis; delayed mammary gland involution (breast-specific deletion) Impaired acute phase immune response; lack of mature thymocytes (interferon-induced deletion) Overly pseudoactivated innate immune response; significantly increased proliferation of cells of myeloid lineage; Crohn's disease-like pathogenesis (bone marrow-specific deletion during hematopoeisis)	(Akaishi et al., 1998; Alonzi et al., 2001; Chapman et al., 1999; Sano et al., 1999, 2001, Takeda et al., 1997, 1998, 1999; Welte et al., 2003)

STAT4	Impaired Th1 differentiation; impaired IL-12-induced response of thymocytes	(Kaplan et al., 1996b; Thierfelder et al., 1996)
STAT5A	Impaired mammary gland development due to loss of PRL signaling; defective lactation; defective GM-CSF-induced proliferation and gene expression	(Feldman et al., 1997; Liu et al., 1997)
STAT5B	Loss of sexually dimorphic growth due to defective GH signaling	(Udy et al., 1997)
STAT5A/STAT5B	Female infertility; defective mammary gland development; reduced body mass; no NK cells; defective IL-2-induced T cell proliferation; fetal anemia and enhanced apoptosis of erythroid progenitors; reduced responsiveness to IL-7; lymphopenia, neutrophelia, modest anemia, thrombocytopenia, reduced numbers of B-cell precursors and mature B cells	(Bunting et al., 2002; Cui et al., 2004; Miyoshi et al., 2001; Moriggl et al., 1999; Sexl et al., 2000; Snow et al., 2002; Socolovsky et al., 1999; Teglund et al., 1998)
STAT6	Defective Th2 development; impaired IL-4/IL-13 signaling leading to defective Th2 development, surface expression of CD23 and MHC class II in resting B cells, and lack of immunoglobulin class-switching to IgE; abrogation of bronchial eosinophilic inflammation and airway hyperreactivity	(Akimoto et al., 1998; Kaplan et al., 1996a; Shimoda et al., 1996; Takeda et al., 1996)

1998; Miyata *et al.*, 1999). However, injection of STAT6-deficient mice with IL-5 restored eosinophil infiltration to airways and AHR in response to antigen challenge, indicating that STAT6 plays a key role in Th2 differentiation and IL-5 production (Tomkinson *et al.*, 1999). As expected, STAT4 deficiency in mice are resistant to autoimmune disorders that results from Th1 response, which may implicate that STAT4 may be involved in autoimmune diseases (Table IV).

XIII. PERSPECTIVE

Cytokine secretion and cytokine action are intimately coupled in the whole organism. However, our understanding of cytokine production and signaling is based on studies that were performed in isolated systems. In order to better understand the biology of cytokine network we need to study cytokine functions in model systems where secretion and action of cytokines are coupled. A single cell may simultaneously be targeted by more than one cytokine, which may result in cross-talk among many intracellular signaling pathways. Moreover, aberrant cytokine production and aberrant cytokine signaling occur in many pathological conditions including cancer and immune diseases. Therefore, it is important to identify molecular and cellular mechanisms that control cytokine production, cytokine signaling, and cytokine cross-talk under physiological conditions. STAT proteins are major mediators of cytokine action, which migrate from cytoplasm to nucleus, upon activation by tyrosine phosphorylation in response to cytokine stimulation of cells. By contrast, studies find that nuclear translocation of STATs may also occur in the absence of tyrosine phosphorylation. Therefore, it is important to understand molecular bases of subcellular distribution of STATs in health and disease. STAT proteins are also phosphorylated on serine residues; however, its biological outcomes remain mostly unclear. Gene regulation requires coordinated interaction of chromatin-modulating proteins and specific transcription factors. To this end, little information is available on the role of chromatin modulating enzymes and structural proteins in STAT-mediated expression of cytokine-responsive genes.

ACKNOWLEDGMENTS

We would like to acknowledge Drs. Serpil Erzurum, Fred Hsieh, Atreyi Dasgupta, Baisakhi Raychaudhuri, and Ms. Phyllis Harbor for critical reading of the article. This work is supported by NIH grants GM060533 and CA095006 to SJH. We regret for being unable to cite many important references due to lack of space.

REFERENCES

Abbas, A. K., and Litchman, A. H. (2003). "Cellular and Molecular Immunolgy." Elsevier Science, Philadelphia, PA.

Adachi, T., and Alam, R. (1998). The mechanism of IL-5 signal transduction. *Am. J. Physiol.* **275**, C623–C633.

Akaishi, H., Takeda, K., Kaisho, T., Shineha, R., Satomi, S., Takeda, J., and Akira, S. (1998). Defective IL-2-mediated IL-2 receptor alpha chain expression in Stat3-deficient T lymphocytes. *Int. Immunol.* **10**, 1747–1751.

Akimoto, T., Numata, F., Tamura, M., Takata, Y., Higashida, N., Takashi, T., Takeda, K., and Akira, S. (1998). Abrogation of bronchial eosinophilic inflammation and airway hyperreactivity in signal transducers and activators of transcription (STAT)6-deficient mice. *J. Exp. Med.* **187**, 1537–1542.

Akira, S., Nishio, Y., Inoue, M., Wang, X. J., Wei, S., Matsusaka, T., Yoshida, K., Sudo, T., Naruto, M., and Kishimoto, T. (1994). Molecular cloning of APRF, a novel IFN-stimulated gene factor 3 p91-related transcription factor involved in the gp130-mediated signaling pathway. *Cell* **77**, 63–71.

Alexander, W. S., and Hilton, D. J. (2004). The role of suppressors of cytokine signaling (SOCS) proteins in regulation of the immune response. *Annu. Rev. Immunol.* **22**, 503–529.

Alexander, W. S., Starr, R., Fenner, J. E., Scott, C. L., Handman, E., Sprigg, N. S., Corbin, J. E., Cornish, A. L., Darwiche, R., Owczarek, C. M., Kay, T. W., Nicola, N. A., *et al.* (1999). SOCS1 is a critical inhibitor of interferon gamma signaling and prevents the potentially fatal neonatal actions of this cytokine. *Cell* **98**, 597–608.

Alonzi, T., Maritano, D., Gorgoni, B., Rizzuto, G., Libert, C., and Poli, V. (2001). Essential role of STAT3 in the control of the acute-phase response as revealed by inducible gene inactivation [correction of activation] in the liver. *Mol. Cell. Biol.* **21**, 1621–1632.

Ansel, K. M., Lee, D. U., and Rao, A. (2003). An epigenetic view of helper T cell differentiation. *Nat. Immunol.* **4**, 616–623.

Aoki, K., Shimoda, K., Oritani, K., Matsuda, T., Kamezaki, K., Muromoto, R., Numata, A., Tamiya, S., Haro, T., Ishikawa, F., Takase, K., Yamamoto, T., *et al.* (2003). Limitin, an interferon-like cytokine, transduces inhibitory signals on B-cell growth through activation of Tyk2, but not Stat1, followed by induction and nuclear translocation of Daxx. *Exp. Hematol.* **31**, 1317–1322.

Arora, T., Liu, B., He, H., Kim, J., Murphy, T. L., Murphy, K. M., Modlin, R. L., and Shuai, K. (2003). PIASx is a transcriptional co-repressor of signal transducer and activator of transcription 4. *J. Biol. Chem.* **278**, 21327–21330.

Bazan, J. F. (1990a). Haemopoietic receptors and helical cytokines. *Immunol. Today* **11**, 350–354.

Bazan, J. F. (1990b). Shared architecture of hormone binding domains in type I and II interferon receptors. *Cell* **61**, 753–754.

Bazan, J. F. (1990c). Structural design and molecular evolution of a cytokine receptor superfamily. *Proc. Natl. Acad. Sci. USA* **87**, 6934–6938.

Becker, S., Groner, B., and Muller, C. W. (1998). Three-dimensional structure of the Stat3beta homodimer bound to DNA. *Nature* **394**, 145–151.

Begitt, A., Meyer, T., van Rossum, M., and Vinkemeier, U. (2000). Nucleocytoplasmic translocation of Stat1 is regulated by a leucine-rich export signal in the coiled-coil domain. *Proc. Natl. Acad. Sci. USA* **97**, 10418–10423.

Bendinelli, P., Maroni, P., Pecori Giraldi, F., and Piccoletti, R. (2000). Leptin activates Stat3, Stat1 and AP-1 in mouse adipose tissue. *Mol. Cell. Endocrinol.* **168**, 11–20.

Bhattacharya, S., and Schindler, C. (2003). Regulation of Stat3 nuclear export. *J. Clin. Invest.* **111**, 553–559.

Blumberg, H., Conklin, D., Xu, W. F., Grossmann, A., Brender, T., Carollo, S., Eagan, M., Foster, D., Haldeman, B. A., Hammond, A., Haugen, H., Jelinek, L., *et al.* (2001). Interleukin 20: Discovery, receptor identification, and role in epidermal function. *Cell* **104**, 9–19.

Boulay, J. L., O'Shea, J. J., and Paul, W. E. (2003). Molecular phylogeny within type I cytokines and their cognate receptors. *Immunity* **19**, 159–163.

Bourdeau, A., Dube, N., and Tremblay, M. L. (2005). Cytoplasmic protein tyrosine phosphatases, regulation and function: The roles of PTP1B and TC-PTP. *Curr. Opin. Cell. Biol.* **17**, 203–209.

Bunting, K. D., Bradley, H. L., Hawley, T. S., Moriggl, R., Sorrentino, B. P., and Ihle, J. N. (2002). Reduced lymphomyeloid repopulating activity from adult bone marrow and fetal liver of mice lacking expression of STAT5. *Blood* **99**, 479–487.

Chakraborty, A., and Tweardy, D. J. (1998). Granulocyte colony-stimulating factor activates a 72-kDa isoform of STAT3 in human neutrophils. *J. Leukoc. Biol.* **64**, 675–680.

Chapman, R. S., Lourenco, P. C., Tonner, E., Flint, D. J., Selbert, S., Takeda, K., Akira, S., Clarke, A. R., and Watson, C. J. (1999). Suppression of epithelial apoptosis and delayed mammary gland involution in mice with a conditional knockout of Stat3. *Genes Dev.* **13**, 2604–2616.

Chatterjee-Kishore, M., Wright, K. L., Ting, J. P., and Stark, G. R. (2000). How Stat1 mediates constitutive gene expression: A complex of unphosphorylated Stat1 and IRF1 supports transcription of the LMP2 gene. *EMBO J.* **19**, 4111–4122.

Chen, X., Vinkemeier, U., Zhao, Y., Jeruzalmi, D., Darnell, J. E., Jr., and Kuriyan, J. (1998). Crystal structure of a tyrosine phosphorylated STAT-1 dimer bound to DNA. *Cell* **93**, 827–839.

Chilton, P. M., and Fernandez-Botran, R. (1993). Production of soluble IL-4 receptors by murine spleen cells is regulated by T cell activation and IL-4. *J. Immunol.* **151**, 5907–5917.

Christodoulopoulos, P., Cameron, L., Nakamura, Y., Lemiere, C., Muro, S., Dugas, M., Boulet, L. P., Laviolette, M., Olivenstein, R., and Hamid, Q. (2001). TH2 cytokine-associated transcription factors in atopic and nonatopic asthma: Evidence for differential signal transducer and activator of transcription 6 expression. *J. Allergy Clin. Immunol.* **107**, 586–591.

Chung, C. D., Liao, J., Liu, B., Rao, X., Jay, P., Berta, P., and Shuai, K. (1997a). Specific inhibition of Stat3 signal transduction by PIAS3. *Science* **278**, 1803–1805.

Chung, J., Uchida, E., Grammer, T. C., and Blenis, J. (1997b). STAT3 serine phosphorylation by ERK-dependent and -independent pathways negatively modulates its tyrosine phosphorylation. *Mol. Cell. Biol.* **17**, 6508–6516.

Coffman, R. L., Ohara, J., Bond, M. W., Carty, J., Zlotnik, A., and Paul, W. E. (1986). B cell stimulatory factor-1 enhances the IgE response of lipopolysaccharide-activated B cells. *J. Immunol.* **136**, 4538–4541.

Copeland, N. G., Gilbert, D. J., Schindler, C., Zhong, Z., Wen, Z., Darnell, J. E., Jr., Mui, A. L., Miyajima, A., Quelle, F. W., Ihle, J. N., and Jenkins, N. A. (1995). Distribution of the mammalian Stat gene family in mouse chromosomes. *Genomics* **29**, 225–228.

Crawford, R. M., Finbloom, D. S., Ohara, J., Paul, W. E., and Meltzer, M. S. (1987). B cell stimulatory factor-1 (interleukin 4) activates macrophages for increased tumoricidal activity and expression of Ia antigens. *J. Immunol.* **139**, 135–141.

Croker, B. A., Krebs, D. L., Zhang, J. G., Wormald, S., Willson, T. A., Stanley, E. G., Robb, L., Greenhalgh, C. J., Forster, I., Clausen, B. E., Nicola, N. A., Metcalf, D., *et al.* (2003). SOCS3 negatively regulates IL-6 signaling *in vivo*. *Nat. Immunol.* **4**, 540–545.

Cui, Y., Riedlinger, G., Miyoshi, K., Tang, W., Li, C., Deng, C. X., Robinson, G. W., and Hennighausen, L. (2004). Inactivation of Stat5 in mouse mammary epithelium during pregnancy reveals distinct functions in cell proliferation, survival, and differentiation. *Mol. Cell Biol.* **24**, 8037–8047.

Darnell, J. E., Jr. (1997). STATs and gene regulation. *Science* **277**, 1630–1635.

Darnell, J. E., Jr., Kerr, I. M., and Stark, G. R. (1994). Jak-STAT pathways and transcriptional activation in response to IFNs and other extracellular signaling proteins. *Science* **264**, 1415–1421.

Decker, T., and Kovarik, P. (2000). Serine phosphorylation of STATs. *Oncogene* **19**, 2628–2637.

Dillon, S. R., Sprecher, C., Hammond, A., Bilsborough, J., Rosenfeld-Franklin, M., Presnell, S. R., Haugen, H. S., Maurer, M., Harder, B., Johnston, J., Bort, S., Mudri, S., et al. (2004). Interleukin 31, a cytokine produced by activated T cells, induces dermatitis in mice. *Nat. Immunol.* **5**, 752–760.

DiSanto, J. P., Muller, W., Guy-Grand, D., Fischer, A., and Rajewsky, K. (1995). Lymphoid development in mice with a targeted deletion of the interleukin 2 receptor gamma chain. *Proc. Natl. Acad. Sci. USA* **92**, 377–381.

Domanski, P., and Colamonici, O. R. (1996). The type-I interferon receptor. The long and short of it. *Cytokine Growth Factor Rev.* **7**, 143–151.

Dreuw, A., Radtke, S., Pflanz, S., Lippok, B. E., Heinrich, P. C., and Hermanns, H. M. (2004). Characterization of the signaling capacities of the novel gp130-like cytokine receptor. *J. Biol. Chem.* **279**, 36112–36120.

Dumoutier, L., Leemans, C., Lejeune, D., Kotenko, S. V., and Renauld, J. C. (2001). Cutting edge: STAT activation by IL-19, IL-20 and mda-7 through IL-20 receptor complexes of two types. *J. Immunol.* **167**, 3545–3549.

Dumoutier, L., Lejeune, D., Hor, S., Fickenscher, H., and Renauld, J. C. (2003). Cloning of a new type II cytokine receptor activating signal transducer and activator of transcription (STAT)1, STAT2 and STAT3. *Biochem. J.* **370**, 391–396.

Durbin, J. E., Hackenmiller, R., Simon, M. C., and Levy, D. E. (1996). Targeted disruption of the mouse Stat1 gene results in compromised innate immunity to viral disease. *Cell* **84**, 443–450.

Endo, T. A., Masuhara, M., Yokouchi, M., Suzuki, R., Sakamoto, H., Mitsui, K., Matsumoto, A., Tanimura, S., Ohtsubo, M., Misawa, H., Miyazaki, T., Leonor, N., et al. (1997). A new protein containing an SH2 domain that inhibits JAK kinases. *Nature* **387**, 921–924.

Feldman, G. M., Rosenthal, L. A., Liu, X., Hayes, M. P., Wynshaw-Boris, A., Leonard, W. J., Hennighausen, L., and Finbloom, D. S. (1997). STAT5A-deficient mice demonstrate a defect in granulocyte-macrophage colony-stimulating factor-induced proliferation and gene expression. *Blood* **90**, 1768–1776.

Firmbach-Kraft, I., Byers, M., Shows, T., Dalla-Favera, R., and Krolewski, J. J. (1990). tyk2, prototype of a novel class of non-receptor tyrosine kinase genes. *Oncogene* **5**, 1329–1336.

Frantsve, J., Schwaller, J., Sternberg, D. W., Kutok, J., and Gilliland, D. G. (2001). Socs-1 inhibits TEL-JAK2-mediated transformation of hematopoietic cells through inhibition of JAK2 kinase activity and induction of proteasome-mediated degradation. *Mol. Cell. Biol.* **21**, 3547–3557.

Fu, X. Y., Schindler, C., Improta, T., Aebersold, R., and Darnell, J. E., Jr. (1992). The proteins of ISGF-3, the interferon alpha-induced transcriptional activator, define a gene family involved in signal transduction. *Proc. Natl. Acad. Sci. USA* **89**, 7840–7843.

Gadina, M., Hilton, D., Johnston, J. A., Morinobu, A., Lighvani, A., Zhou, Y. J., Visconti, R., and O'Shea, J. J. (2001). Signaling by type I and II cytokine receptors: Ten years after. *Curr. Opin. Immunol.* **13**, 363–373.

Gascan, H., Gauchat, J. F., Roncarolo, M. G., Yssel, H., Spits, H., and de Vries, J. E. (1991). Human B cell clones can be induced to proliferate and to switch to IgE and IgG4 synthesis by interleukin 4 and a signal provided by activated CD4 + T cell clones. *J. Exp. Med.* **173**, 747–750.

Gately, M. K., Renzetti, L. M., Magram, J., Stern, A. S., Adorini, L., Gubler, U., and Presky, D. H. (1998). The interleukin-12/interleukin-12-receptor system: Role in normal and pathologic immune responses. *Annu. Rev. Immunol.* **16**, 495–521.

Geijsen, N., Koenderman, L., and Coffer, P. J. (2001). Specificity in cytokine signal transduction: Lessons learned from the IL-3/IL-5/GM-CSF receptor family. *Cytokine Growth Factor Rev.* **12,** 19–25.

Ghosh, M. K., Sharma, P., Harbor, P. C., Rahaman, S. O., and Haque, S. J. (2005). PI3K-AKT pathway negatively controls EGFR-dependent DNA-binding activity of Stat3 in glioblastoma multiforme cells. *Oncogene* **24,** 7290–7300.

Girault, J. A., Labesse, G., Mornon, J. P., and Callebaut, I. (1998). Janus kinases and focal adhesion kinases play in the 4.1 band: A superfamily of band 4.1 domains important for cell structure and signal transduction. *Mol. Med.* **4,** 751–769.

Goldsby, R. A., Kindt, T. A., Osborne, B. A., and Kuby, J. (2003). "Immunology." W. H. Freeman and Company, New York, NY.

Gough, N. M., Rakar, S., Harpur, A., and Wilks, A. F. (1995). Localization of genes for two members of the JAK family of protein tyrosine kinases to murine chromosomes 4 and 19. *Mamm. Genome* **6,** 247–248.

Haan, C., Is'harc, H., Hermanns, H. M., Schmitz-Van De Leur, H., Kerr, I. M., Heinrich, P. C., Grotzinger, J., and Behrmann, I. (2001). Mapping of a region within the N terminus of Jak1 involved in cytokine receptor interaction. *J. Biol. Chem.* **276,** 37451–37458.

Hanks, S. K., Quinn, A. M., and Hunter, T. (1988). The protein kinase family: Conserved features and deduced phylogeny of the catalytic domains. *Science* **241,** 42–52.

Hannigan, G. E., and Williams, B. R. (1992). Interferon-alpha activates binding of nuclear factors to a sequence element in the c-fos proto-oncogene 5'-flanking region. *J. Interferon Res.* **12,** 355–361.

Haque, S. J., and Williams, B. R. (1998). Signal transduction in the interferon system. *Semin. Oncol.* **25,** 14–22.

Haque, S. J., Flati, V., Deb, A., and Williams, B. R. (1995). Roles of protein-tyrosine phosphatases in Stat1 alpha-mediated cell signaling. *J. Biol. Chem.* **270,** 25709–25714.

Haque, S. J., Wu, Q., Kammer, W., Friedrich, K., Smith, J. M., Kerr, I. M., Stark, G. R., and Williams, B. R. (1997). Receptor-associated constitutive protein tyrosine phosphatase activity controls the kinase function of JAK1. *Proc. Natl. Acad. Sci. USA* **94,** 8563–8568.

Haque, S. J., Harbor, P., Tabrizi, M., Yi, T., and Williams, B. R. (1998). Protein-tyrosine phosphatase Shp-1 is a negative regulator of IL-4- and IL-13-dependent signal transduction. *J. Biol. Chem.* **273,** 33893–33896.

Haque, S. J., Harbor, P. C., and Williams, B. R. (2000). Identification of critical residues required for suppressor of cytokine signaling-specific regulation of interleukin-4 signaling. *J. Biol. Chem.* **275,** 26500–26506.

Harpur, A. G., Andres, A. C., Ziemiecki, A., Aston, R. R., and Wilks, A. F. (1992). JAK2, a third member of the JAK family of protein tyrosine kinases. *Oncogene* **7,** 1347–1353.

Heaney, M. L., and Golde, D. W. (1996). Soluble cytokine receptors. *Blood* **87,** 847–857.

Heinrich, P. C., Behrmann, I., Haan, S., Hermanns, H. M., Muller-Newen, G., and Schaper, F. (2003). Principles of interleukin (IL)-6-type cytokine signalling and its regulation. *Biochem. J.* **374,** 1–20.

Heldin, C. H. (1995). Dimerization of cell surface receptors in signal transduction. *Cell* **80,** 213–223.

Hermiston, M. L., Xu, Z., and Weiss, A. (2003). CD45: A critical regulator of signaling thresholds in immune cells. *Annu. Rev. Immunol.* **21,** 107–137.

Hilkens, C. M., Is'harc, H., Lillemeier, B. F., Strobl, B., Bates, P. A., Behrmann, I., and Kerr, I. M. (2001). A region encompassing the FERM domain of Jak1 is necessary for binding to the cytokine receptor gp130. *FEBS Lett.* **505,** 87–91.

Huang, M., Dorsey, J. F., Epling-Burnette, P. K., Nimmanapalli, R., Landowski, T. H., Mora, L. B., Niu, G., Sinibaldi, D., Bai, F., Kraker, A., Yu, H., Moscinski, L., *et al.* (2002). Inhibition of Bcr-Abl kinase activity by PD180970 blocks constitutive activation of Stat5 and growth of CML cells. *Oncogene* **21,** 8804–8816.

Hubbard, S. R., Wei, L., Ellis, L., and Hendrickson, W. A. (1994). Crystal structure of the tyrosine kinase domain of the human insulin receptor. *Nature* **372**, 746–754.

Ihle, J. N. (1995). Cytokine receptor signalling. *Nature* **377**, 591–594.

Ihle, J. N. (2001). The Stat family in cytokine signaling. *Curr. Opin. Cell Biol.* **13**, 211–217.

Irie-Sasaki, J., Sasaki, T., Matsumoto, W., Opavsky, A., Cheng, M., Welstead, G., Griffiths, E., Krawczyk, C., Richardson, C. D., Aitken, K., Iscove, N., Koretzky, G., et al. (2001). CD45 is a JAK phosphatase and negatively regulates cytokine receptor signalling. *Nature* **409**, 349–354.

Jiang, H., Harris, M. B., and Rothman, P. (2000). IL-4/IL-13 signaling beyond JAK/STAT. *J. Allergy Clin. Immunol.* **105**, 1063–1070.

Johnson, L. N., Noble, M. E., and Owen, D. J. (1996). Active and inactive protein kinases: Structural basis for regulation. *Cell* **85**, 149–158.

Kamizono, S., Hanada, T., Yasukawa, H., Minoguchi, S., Kato, R., Minoguchi, M., Hattori, K., Hatakeyama, S., Yada, M., Morita, S., Kitamura, T., and Kato, H. (2001). The SOCS box of SOCS-1 accelerates ubiquitin-dependent proteolysis of TEL-JAK2. *J. Biol. Chem.* **276**, 12530–12538.

Kamura, T., Sato, S., Haque, D., Liu, L., Kaelin, W. G., Jr., Conaway, R. C., and Conaway, J. W. (1998). The Elongin BC complex interacts with the conserved SOCS-box motif present in members of the SOCS, ras, WD-40 repeat, and ankyrin repeat families. *Genes Dev.* **12**, 3872–3881.

Kaplan, D. H., Shankaran, V., Dighe, A. S., Stockert, E., Aguet, M., Old, L. J., and Schreiber, R. D. (1998). Demonstration of an interferon gamma-dependent tumor surveillance system in immunocompetent mice. *Proc. Natl. Acad. Sci. USA* **95**, 7556–7561.

Kaplan, M. H., Schindler, U., Smiley, S. T., and Grusby, M. J. (1996a). Stat6 is required for mediating responses to IL-4 and for development of Th2 cells. *Immunity* **4**, 313–319.

Kaplan, M. H., Sun, Y. L., Hoey, T., and Grusby, M. J. (1996b). Impaired IL-12 responses and enhanced development of Th2 cells in Stat4-deficient mice. *Nature* **382**, 174–177.

Kawamura, M., McVicar, D. W., Johnston, J. A., Blake, T. B., Chen, Y. Q., Lal, B. K., Lloyd, A. R., Kelvin, D. J., Staples, J. E., Ortaldo, J. R., and O'Shea, J. J. (1994). Molecular cloning of L-JAK, a Janus family protein-tyrosine kinase expressed in natural killer cells and activated leukocytes. *Proc. Natl. Acad. Sci. USA* **91**, 6374–6378.

Kelleher, K., Bean, K., Clark, S. C., Leung, W. Y., Yang-Feng, T. L., Chen, J. W., Lin, P. F., Luo, W., and Yang, Y. C. (1991). Human interleukin-9: Genomic sequence, chromosomal location, and sequences essential for its expression in human T-cell leukemia virus (HTLV)-I-transformed human T cells. *Blood* **77**, 1436–1441.

Khodarev, N. N., Beckett, M., Labay, E., Darga, T., Roizman, B., and Weichselbaum, R. R. (2004). STAT1 is overexpressed in tumors selected for radioresistance and confers protection from radiation in transduced sensitive cells. *Proc. Natl. Acad. Sci. USA* **101**, 1714–1719.

Kile, B. T., Schulman, B. A., Alexander, W. S., Nicola, N. A., Martin, H. M., and Hilton, D. J. (2002). The SOCS box: A tale of destruction and degradation. *Trends Biochem. Sci.* **27**, 235–241.

Kim, T. K., and Maniatis, T. (1996). Regulation of interferon-gamma-activated STAT1 by the ubiquitin-proteasome pathway. *Science* **273**, 1717–1719.

Kishimoto, T., Taga, T., and Akira, S. (1994). Cytokine signal transduction. *Cell* **76**, 253–262.

Kono, D. H., Owens, D. G., and Wechsler, A. R. (1996). Jak3 maps to chromosome 8. *Mamm. Genome* **7**, 476–477.

Kotenko, S. V., and Pestka, S. (2000). Jak-Stat signal transduction pathway through the eyes of cytokine class II receptor complexes. *Oncogene* **19**, 2557–2565.

Kotenko, S. V., Izotova, L. S., Mirochnitchenko, O. V., Esterova, E., Dickensheets, H., Donnelly, R. P., and Pestka, S. (2001). Identification of the functional interleukin-22 (IL-22) receptor complex: The IL-10R2 chain (IL-10Rbeta) is a common chain of both the IL-10 and IL-22 (IL-10-related T cell-derived inducible factor, IL-TIF) receptor complexes. *J. Biol. Chem.* **276**, 2725–2732.

Kotenko, S. V., Gallagher, G., Baurin, V. V., Lewis-Antes, A., Shen, M., Shah, N. K., Langer, J. A., Sheikh, F., Dickensheets, H., and Donnelly, R. P. (2003). IFN-lambdas mediate antiviral protection through a distinct class II cytokine receptor complex. *Nat. Immunol.* **4**, 69–77.

Krishnan, K., Singh, B., and Krolewski, J. J. (1998). Identification of amino acid residues critical for the Src-homology 2 domain-dependent docking of Stat2 to the interferon alpha receptor. *J. Biol. Chem.* **273**, 19495–19501.

Kumar, A., Toscani, A., Rane, S., and Reddy, E. P. (1996). Structural organization and chromosomal mapping of JAK3 locus. *Oncogene* **13**, 2009–2014.

Kuperman, D., Schofield, B., Wills-Karp, M., and Grusby, M. J. (1998). Signal transducer and activator of transcription factor 6 (Stat6)-deficient mice are protected from antigen-induced airway hyperresponsiveness and mucus production. *J. Exp. Med.* **187**, 939–948.

Lang, R., Pauleau, A. L., Parganas, E., Takahashi, Y., Mages, J., Ihle, J. N., Rutschman, R., and Murray, P. J. (2003). SOCS3 regulates the plasticity of gp130 signaling. *Nat. Immunol.* **4**, 546–550.

Leaman, D. W., Pisharody, S., Flickinger, T. W., Commane, M. A., Schlessinger, J., Kerr, I. M., Levy, D. E., and Stark, G. R. (1996). Roles of JAKs in activation of STATs and stimulation of c-fos gene expression by epidermal growth factor. *Mol. Cell. Biol.* **16**, 369–375.

Lee, C., Piazza, F., Brutsaert, S., Valens, J., Strehlow, I., Jarosinski, M., Saris, C., and Schindler, C. (1999). Characterization of the Stat5 protease. *J. Biol. Chem.* **274**, 26767–26775.

Leek, J. P., Hamlin, P. J., Bell, S. M., and Lench, N. J. (1997). Assignment of the STAT6 gene (STAT6) to human chromosome band 12q13 by *in situ* hybridization. *Cytogenet. Cell Genet.* **79**, 208–209.

Lehmann, U., Schmitz, J., Weissenbach, M., Sobota, R. M., Hortner, M., Friederichs, K., Behrmann, I., Tsiaris, W., Sasaki, A., Schneider-Mergener, J., Yoshimura, A., Neel, B. G., et al. (2003). SHP2 and SOCS3 contribute to Tyr-759-dependent attenuation of interleukin-6 signaling through gp130. *J. Biol. Chem.* **278**, 661–671.

Leonard, W. J. (2001). Cytokines and immunodeficiency diseases. *Nat. Rev. Immunol.* **1**, 200–208.

Leonard, W. J., and O'Shea, J. J. (1998). Jaks and STATs: Biological implications. *Annu. Rev. Immunol.* **16**, 293–322.

Levine, S. J. (2004). Mechanisms of soluble cytokine receptor generation. *J. Immunol.* **173**, 5343–5348.

Levy, D., Larner, A., Chaudhuri, A., Babiss, L. E., and Darnell, J. E., Jr. (1986). Interferon-stimulated transcription: Isolation of an inducible gene and identification of its regulatory region. *Proc. Natl. Acad. Sci. USA* **83**, 8929–8933.

Levy, D. E., Kessler, D. S., Pine, R., and Darnell, J. E., Jr. (1989). Cytoplasmic activation of ISGF3, the positive regulator of interferon-alpha-stimulated transcription, reconstituted *in vitro*. *Genes Dev.* **3**, 1362–1371.

Lin, J. X., Mietz, J., Modi, W. S., John, S., and Leonard, W. J. (1996). Cloning of human Stat5B. Reconstitution of interleukin-2-induced Stat5A and Stat5B DNA binding activity in COS-7 cells. *J. Biol. Chem.* **271**, 10738–10744.

Liu, B., Liao, J., Rao, X., Kushner, S. A., Chung, C. D., Chang, D. D., and Shuai, K. (1998). Inhibition of Stat1-mediated gene activation by PIAS1. *Proc. Natl. Acad. Sci. USA* **95**, 10626–10631.

Liu, B., Mink, S., Wong, K. A., Stein, N., Getman, C., Dempsey, P. W., Wu, H., and Shuai, K. (2004). PIAS1 selectively inhibits interferon-inducible genes and is important in innate immunity. *Nat. Immunol.* **5**, 891–898.

Liu, B., Yang, R., Wong, K. A., Getman, C., Stein, N., Teitell, M. A., Cheng, G., Wu, H., and Shuai, K. (2005a). Negative regulation of NF-kappaB signaling by PIAS1. *Mol. Cell. Biol.* **25**, 1113–1123.

Liu, L., McBride, K. M., and Reich, N. C. (2005b). STAT3 nuclear import is independent of tyrosine phosphorylation and mediated by importin-alpha3. *Proc. Natl. Acad. Sci. USA* **102**, 8150–8155.

Liu, X., Robinson, G. W., Wagner, K. U., Garrett, L., Wynshaw-Boris, A., and Hennighausen, L. (1997). Stat5a is mandatory for adult mammary gland development and lactogenesis. *Genes Dev.* **11**, 179–186.

Ma, J., Zhang, T., Novotny-Diermayr, V., Tan, A. L., and Cao, X. (2003). A novel sequence in the coiled-coil domain of Stat3 essential for its nuclear translocation. *J. Biol. Chem.* **278**, 29252–29260.

Maiti, N. R., Sharma, P., Harbor, P. C., and Haque, S. J. (2005). Serine phosphorylation of Stat6 negatively controls its DNA-binding function. *J. Interferon. Cytokine. Res.* **25**, 553–563.

Mantovani, A., Locati, M., Vecchi, A., Sozzani, S., and Allavena, P. (2001). Decoy receptors: A strategy to regulate inflammatory cytokines and chemokines. *Trends Immunol.* **22**, 328–336.

Marine, J. C., McKay, C., Wang, D., Topham, D. J., Parganas, E., Nakajima, H., Pendeville, H., Yasukawa, H., Sasaki, A., Yoshimura, A., and Ihle, J. N. (1999a). SOCS3 is essential in the regulation of fetal liver erythropoiesis. *Cell* **98**, 617–627.

Marine, J. C., Topham, D. J., McKay, C., Wang, D., Parganas, E., Stravopodis, D., Yoshimura, A., and Ihle, J. N. (1999b). SOCS1 deficiency causes a lymphocyte-dependent perinatal lethality. *Cell* **98**, 609–616.

McBride, K. M., McDonald, C., and Reich, N. C. (2000). Nuclear export signal located within the DNA-binding domain of the STAT1transcription factor. *EMBO J.* **19**, 6196–6206.

McBride, K. M., Banninger, G., McDonald, C., and Reich, N. C. (2002). Regulated nuclear import of the STAT1 transcription factor by direct binding of importin-alpha. *EMBO J.* **21**, 1754–1763.

Meraz, M. A., White, J. M., Sheehan, K. C., Bach, E. A., Rodig, S. J., Dighe, A. S., Kaplan, D. H., Riley, J. K., Greenlund, A. C., Campbell, D., Carver-Moore, K., DuBois, R. N., *et al.* (1996). Targeted disruption of the Stat1 gene in mice reveals unexpected physiologic specificity in the JAK-STAT signaling pathway. *Cell* **84**, 431–442.

Metcalf, D., Greenhalgh, C. J., Viney, E., Willson, T. A., Starr, R., Nicola, N. A., Hilton, D. J., and Alexander, W. S. (2000). Gigantism in mice lacking suppressor of cytokine signalling-2. *Nature* **405**, 1069–1073.

Meyer, T., Gavenis, K., and Vinkemeier, U. (2002). Cell type-specific and tyrosine phosphorylation-independent nuclear presence of STAT1 and STAT3. *Exp. Cell. Res.* **272**, 45–55.

Meyer, T., Marg, A., Lemke, P., Wiesner, B., and Vinkemeier, U. (2003). DNA binding controls inactivation and nuclear accumulation of the transcription factor Stat1. *Genes Dev.* **17**, 1992–2005.

Mikita, T., Campbell, D., Wu, P., Williamson, K., and Schindler, U. (1996). Requirements for interleukin-4-induced gene expression and functional characterization of Stat6. *Mol. Cell. Biol.* **16**, 5811–5820.

Mitsui, Y., and Senda, T. (1997). Elucidation of the basic three-dimensional structure of type I interferons and its functional and evolutionary implications. *J. Interferon Cytokine Res.* **17**, 319–326.

Miyajima, A., Mui, A. L., Ogorochi, T., and Sakamaki, K. (1993). Receptors for granulocyte-macrophage colony-stimulating factor, interleukin-3, and interleukin-5. *Blood* **82**, 1960–1974.

Miyata, S., Matsuyama, T., Kodama, T., Nishioka, Y., Kuribayashi, K., Takeda, K., Akira, S., and Sugita, M. (1999). STAT6 deficiency in a mouse model of allergen-induced airways inflammation abolishes eosinophilia but induces infiltration of CD8+ T cells. *Clin. Exp. Allergy* **29**, 114–123.

Miyoshi, K., Shillingford, J. M., Smith, G. H., Grimm, S. L., Wagner, K. U., Oka, T., Rosen, J. M., Robinson, G. W., and Hennighausen, L. (2001). Signal transducer and activator of transcription (Stat) 5 controls the proliferation and differentiation of mammary alveolar epithelium. *J. Cell. Biol.* **155**, 531–542.

Moriggl, R., Topham, D. J., Teglund, S., Sexl, V., McKay, C., Wang, D., Hoffmeyer, A., van Deursen, J., Sangster, M. Y., Bunting, K. D., Grosveld, G. C., and Ihle, J. N. (1999). Stat5 is required for IL-2-induced cell cycle progression of peripheral T cells. *Immunity* **10**, 249–259.

Mosmann, T. R., Cherwinski, H., Bond, M. W., Giedlin, M. A., and Coffman, R. L. (1986). Two types of murine helper T cell clone. I. Definition according to profiles of lymphokine activities and secreted proteins. *J. Immunol.* **136**, 2348–2357.

Mowen, K. A., Tang, J., Zhu, W., Schurter, B. T., Shuai, K., Herschman, H. R., and David, M. (2001). Arginine methylation of STAT1 modulates IFNalpha/beta-induced transcription. *Cell* **104**, 731–741.

Muller, M., Briscoe, J., Laxton, C., Guschin, D., Ziemiecki, A., Silvennoinen, O., Harpur, A. G., Barbieri, G., Witthuhn, B. A., Schindler, C., Pellegrini, S., Wilks, A. F., *et al.* (1993). The protein tyrosine kinase JAK1 complements defects in interferon-alpha/beta and -gamma signal transduction. *Nature* **366**, 129–135.

Muto, A., Watanabe, S., Itoh, T., Miyajima, A., Yokota, T., and Arai, K. (1995). Roles of the cytoplasmic domains of the alpha and beta subunits of human granulocyte-macrophage colony-stimulating factor receptor. *J. Allergy Clin. Immunol.* **96**, 1100–1114.

Naka, T., Narazaki, M., Hirata, M., Matsumoto, T., Minamoto, S., Aono, A., Nishimoto, N., Kajita, T., Taga, T., Yoshizaki, K., Akira, S., and Kishimoto, T. (1997). Structure and function of a new STAT-induced STAT inhibitor. *Nature* **387**, 924–929.

Nakajima, H., Shores, E. W., Noguchi, M., and Leonard, W. J. (1997). The common cytokine receptor gamma chain plays an essential role in regulating lymphoid homeostasis. *J. Exp. Med.* **185**, 189–195.

Nakajima, H., Suzuki, K., and Iwamoto, I. (2003). Lineage-specific negative regulation of STAT-mediated signaling by proteolytic processing. *Cytokine Growth Factor Rev.* **14**, 375–380.

Narazaki, M., Fujimoto, M., Matsumoto, T., Morita, Y., Saito, H., Kajita, T., Yoshizaki, K., Naka, T., and Kishimoto, T. (1998). Three distinct domains of SSI-1/SOCS-1/JAB protein are required for its suppression of interleukin 6 signaling. *Proc. Natl. Acad. Sci. USA* **95**, 13130–13134.

Nelms, K., Keegan, A. D., Zamorano, J., Ryan, J. J., and Paul, W. E. (1999). The IL-4 receptor: Signaling mechanisms and biologic functions. *Annu. Rev. Immunol.* **17**, 701–738.

Neubauer, H., Cumano, A., Muller, M., Wu, H., Huffstadt, U., and Pfeffer, K. (1998). Jak2 deficiency defines an essential developmental checkpoint in definitive hematopoiesis. *Cell* **93**, 397–409.

Nicholson, S. E., Willson, T. A., Farley, A., Starr, R., Zhang, J. G., Baca, M., Alexander, W. S., Metcalf, D., Hilton, D. J., and Nicola, N. A. (1999). Mutational analyses of the SOCS proteins suggest a dual domain requirement but distinct mechanisms for inhibition of LIF and IL-6 signal transduction. *EMBO J.* **18**, 375–385.

Niu, G., Wright, K. L., Huang, M., Song, L., Haura, E., Turkson, J., Zhang, S., Wang, T., Sinibaldi, D., Coppola, D., Heller, R., Ellis, L. M., *et al.* (2002). Constitutive Stat3 activity up-regulates VEGF expression and tumor angiogenesis. *Oncogene* **21**, 2000–2008.

Nosaka, T., van Deursen, J. M., Tripp, R. A., Thierfelder, W. E., Witthuhn, B. A., McMickle, A. P., Doherty, P. C., Grosveld, G. C., and Ihle, J. N. (1995). Defective lymphoid development in mice lacking Jak3. *Science* **270**, 800–802.

O'Shea, J. J., and Watford, W. (2004). A peek at PIAS. *Nat. Immunol.* **5**, 875–876.

O'Shea, J. J., Gadina, M., and Schreiber, R. D. (2002). Cytokine signaling in 2002: New surprises in the Jak/Stat pathway. *Cell* **109**(Suppl.), S121–S131.

O'Shea, J. J., Pesu, M., Borie, D. C., and Changelian, P. S. (2004). A new modality for immunosuppression: Targeting the JAK/STAT pathway. *Nat. Rev. Drug Discov.* **3**, 555–564.

O'Shea, J. J., Kanno, Y., Chen, X., and Levy, D. E. (2005a). Cell signaling. Stat acetylation: A key facet of cytokine signaling? *Science* **307**, 217–218.

O'Shea, J. J., Park, H., Pesu, M., Borie, D., and Changelian, P. (2005b). New strategies for immunosuppression: Interfering with cytokines by targeting the Jak/Stat pathway. *Curr. Opin. Rheumatol.* **17**, 305–311.

Ohtani, T., Ishihara, K., Atsumi, T., Nishida, K., Kaneko, Y., Miyata, T., Itoh, S., Narimatsu, M., Maeda, H., Fukada, T., Itoh, M., Okano, H., *et al.* (2000). Dissection of signaling cascades through gp130 *in vivo*: Reciprocal roles for STAT3- and SHP2-mediated signals in immune responses. *Immunity* **12**, 95–105.

Oppmann, B., Lesley, R., Blom, B., Timans, J. C., Xu, Y., Hunte, B., Vega, F., Yu, N., Wang, J., Singh, K., Zonin, F., Vaisberg, E., *et al.* (2000). Novel p19 protein engages IL-12p40 to form a cytokine, IL-23, with biological activities similar as well as distinct from IL-12. *Immunity* **13**, 715–725.

Oritani, K., Medina, K. L., Tomiyama, Y., Ishikawa, J., Okajima, Y., Ogawa, M., Yokota, T., Aoyama, K., Takahashi, I., Kincade, P. W., and Matsuzawa, Y. (2000). Limitin: An interferon-like cytokine that preferentially influences B-lymphocyte precursors. *Nat. Med.* **6**, 659–666.

Ozaki, K., and Leonard, W. J. (2002). Cytokine and cytokine receptor pleiotropy and redundancy. *J. Biol. Chem.* **277**, 29355–29358.

Parganas, E., Wang, D., Stravopodis, D., Topham, D. J., Marine, J. C., Teglund, S., Vanin, E. F., Bodner, S., Colamonici, O. R., van Deursen, J. M., Grosveld, G., and Ihle, J. N. (1998). Jak2 is essential for signaling through a variety of cytokine receptors. *Cell* **93**, 385–395.

Parham, C., Chirica, M., Timans, J., Vaisberg, E., Travis, M., Cheung, J., Pflanz, S., Zhang, R., Singh, K. P., Vega, F., To, W., Wagner, J., *et al.* (2002). A receptor for the heterodimeric cytokine IL-23 is composed of IL-12Rbeta1 and a novel cytokine receptor subunit, IL-23R. *J. Immunol.* **168**, 5699–5708.

Park, C., Li, S., Cha, E., and Schindler, C. (2000). Immune response in Stat2 knockout mice. *Immunity* **13**, 795–804.

Park, S. H., Yamashita, H., Rui, H., and Waxman, D. J. (2001). Serine phosphorylation of GH-activated signal transducer and activator of transcription 5a (STAT5a) and STAT5b: Impact on STAT5 transcriptional activity. *Mol. Endocrinol.* **15**, 2157–2171.

Park, S. Y., Saijo, K., Takahashi, T., Osawa, M., Arase, H., Hirayama, N., Miyake, K., Nakauchi, H., Shirasawa, T., and Saito, T. (1995). Developmental defects of lymphoid cells in Jak3 kinase-deficient mice. *Immunity* **3**, 771–782.

Parrish-Novak, J., Xu, W., Brender, T., Yao, L., Jones, C., West, J., Brandt, C., Jelinek, L., Madden, K., McKernan, P. A., Foster, D. C., Jaspers, S., *et al.* (2002). Interleukins 19, 20, and 24 signal through two distinct receptor complexes. Differences in receptor-ligand interactions mediate unique biological functions. *J. Biol. Chem.* **277**, 47517–47523.

Pernis, A. B., and Rothman, P. B. (2002). JAK-STAT signaling in asthma. *J. Clin. Invest.* **109**, 1279–1283.

Pestka, S., Krause, C. D., Sarkar, D., Walter, M. R., Shi, Y., and Fisher, P. B. (2004). Interleukin-10 and related cytokines and receptors. *Annu. Rev. Immunol.* **22**, 929–979.

Qu, C. K. (2000). The SHP-2 tyrosine phosphatase: Signaling mechanisms and biological functions. *Cell Res.* **10**, 279–288.

Quelle, F. W., Sato, N., Witthuhn, B. A., Inhorn, R. C., Eder, M., Miyajima, A., Griffin, J. D., and Ihle, J. N. (1994). JAK2 associates with the beta c chain of the receptor for granulocyte-macrophage colony-stimulating factor, and its activation requires the membrane-proximal region. *Mol. Cell. Biol.* **14**, 4335–4341.

Rahaman, S. O., Harbor, P. C., Chernova, O., Barnett, G. H., Vogelbaum, M. A., and Haque, S. J. (2002a). Inhibition of constitutively active Stat3 suppresses proliferation and induces apoptosis in glioblastoma multiforme cells. *Oncogene* **21,** 8404–8413.

Rahaman, S. O., Sharma, P., Harbor, P. C., Aman, M. J., Vogelbaum, M. A., and Haque, S. J. (2002b). IL-13R(alpha)2, a decoy receptor for IL-13 acts as an inhibitor of IL-4-dependent signal transduction in glioblastoma cells. *Cancer Res.* **62,** 1103–1109.

Ramana, C. V., Gil, M. P., Schreiber, R. D., and Stark, G. R. (2002). Stat1-dependent and -independent pathways in IFN-gamma-dependent signaling. *Trends Immunol.* **23,** 96–101.

Rane, S. G., and Reddy, E. P. (1994). JAK3: A novel JAK kinase associated with terminal differentiation of hematopoietic cells. *Oncogene* **9,** 2415–2423.

Riedy, M. C., Dutra, A. S., Blake, T. B., Modi, W., Lal, B. K., Davis, J., Bosse, A., O'Shea, J. J., and Johnston, J. A. (1996). Genomic sequence, organization, and chromosomal localization of human JAK3. *Genomics* **37,** 57–61.

Rodig, S. J., Meraz, M. A., White, J. M., Lampe, P. A., Riley, J. K., Arthur, C. D., King, K. L., Sheehan, K. C., Yin, L., Pennica, D., Johnson, E. M., Jr., and Schreiber, R. D. (1998). Disruption of the Jak1 gene demonstrates obligatory and nonredundant roles of the Jaks in cytokine-induced biologic responses. *Cell* **93,** 373–383.

Rout, M. P., Aitchison, J. D., Magnasco, M. O., and Chait, B. T. (2003). Virtual gating and nuclear transport: The hole picture. *Trends Cell Biol.* **13,** 622–628.

Rozwarski, D. A., Gronenborn, A. M., Clore, G. M., Bazan, J. F., Bohm, A., Wlodawer, A., Hatada, M., and Karplus, P. A. (1994). Structural comparisons among the short-chain helical cytokines. *Structure* **2,** 159–173.

Sano, S., Itami, S., Takeda, K., Tarutani, M., Yamaguchi, Y., Miura, H., Yoshikawa, K., Akira, S., and Takeda, J. (1999). Keratinocyte-specific ablation of Stat3 exhibits impaired skin remodeling, but does not affect skin morphogenesis. *EMBO J.* **18,** 4657–4668.

Sano, S., Takahama, Y., Sugawara, T., Kosaka, H., Itami, S., Yoshikawa, K., Miyazaki, J., van Ewijk, W., and Takeda, J. (2001). Stat3 in thymic epithelial cells is essential for postnatal maintenance of thymic architecture and thymocyte survival. *Immunity* **15,** 261–273.

Schaper, F., Gendo, C., Eck, M., Schmitz, J., Grimm, C., Anhuf, D., Kerr, I. M., and Heinrich, P. C. (1998). Activation of the protein tyrosine phosphatase SHP2 via the interleukin-6 signal transducing receptor protein gp130 requires tyrosine kinase Jak1 and limits acute-phase protein expression. *Biochem. J.* **335**(Part 3), 557–565.

Schindler, C. (1999). Cytokines and JAK-STAT signaling. *Exp. Cell Res.* **253,** 7–14.

Schindler, C., and Darnell, J. E., Jr. (1995). Transcriptional responses to polypeptide ligands: The JAK-STAT pathway. *Annu. Rev. Biochem.* **64,** 621–651.

Schindler, U., Wu, P., Rothe, M., Brasseur, M., and McKnight, S. L. (1995). Components of a Stat recognition code: Evidence for two layers of molecular selectivity. *Immunity* **2,** 689–697.

Schwaller, J., Parganas, E., Wang, D., Cain, D., Aster, J. C., Williams, I. R., Lee, C. K., Gerthner, R., Kitamura, T., Frantsve, J., Anastasiadou, E., Loh, M. L., *et al.* (2000). Stat5 is essential for the myelo- and lymphoproliferative disease induced by TEL/JAK2. *Mol. Cell* **6,** 693–704.

Seki, Y., Hayashi, K., Matsumoto, A., Seki, N., Tsukada, J., Ransom, J., Naka, T., Kishimoto, T., Yoshimura, A., and Kubo, M. (2002). Expression of the suppressor of cytokine signaling-5 (SOCS5) negatively regulates IL-4-dependent STAT6 activation and Th2 differentiation. *Proc. Natl. Acad. Sci. USA* **99,** 13003–13008.

Sekimoto, T., Imamoto, N., Nakajima, K., Hirano, T., and Yoneda, Y. (1997). Extracellular signal-dependent nuclear import of Stat1 is mediated by nuclear pore-targeting complex formation with NPI-1, but not Rch1. *EMBO J.* **16,** 7067–7077.

Sexl, V., Piekorz, R., Moriggl, R., Rohrer, J., Brown, M. P., Bunting, K. D., Rothammer, K., Roussel, M. F., and Ihle, J. N. (2000). Stat5a/b contribute to interleukin 7-induced B-cell precursor expansion, but abl- and bcr/abl-induced transformation are independent of stat5. *Blood* **96,** 2277–2283.

Sheikh, F., Baurin, V. V., Lewis-Antes, A., Shah, N. K., Smirnov, S. V., Anantha, S., Dickensheets, H., Dumoutier, L., Renauld, J. C., Zdanov, A., Donnelly, R. P., and Kotenko, S. V. (2004). Cutting edge: IL-26 signals through a novel receptor complex composed of IL-20 receptor 1 and IL-10 receptor 2. *J. Immunol.* **172**, 2006–2010.

Sheppard, P., Kindsvogel, W., Xu, W., Henderson, K., Schlutsmeyer, S., Whitmore, T. E., Kuestner, R., Garrigues, U., Birks, C., Roraback, J., Ostrander, C., Dong, D., *et al.* (2003). IL-28, IL-29 and their class II cytokine receptor IL-28R. *Nat. Immunol.* **4**, 63–68.

Sherman, M. A., Powell, D. R., and Brown, M. A. (2002). IL-4 induces the proteolytic processing of mast cell STAT6. *J. Immunol.* **169**, 3811–3818.

Shimoda, K., van Deursen, J., Sangster, M. Y., Sarawar, S. R., Carson, R. T., Tripp, R. A., Chu, C., Quelle, F. W., Nosaka, T., Vignali, D. A., Doherty, P. C., Grosveld, G., *et al.* (1996). Lack of IL-4-induced Th2 response and IgE class switching in mice with disrupted Stat6 gene. *Nature* **380**, 630–633.

Shimoda, K., Kato, K., Aoki, K., Matsuda, T., Miyamoto, A., Shibamori, M., Yamashita, M., Numata, A., Takase, K., Kobayashi, S., Shibata, S., Asano, Y., *et al.* (2000). Tyk2 plays a restricted role in IFN alpha signaling, although it is required for IL-12-mediated T cell function. *Immunity* **13**, 561–571.

Shimoda, K., Tsutsui, H., Aoki, K., Kato, K., Matsuda, T., Numata, A., Takase, K., Yamamoto, T., Nukina, H., Hoshino, T., Asano, Y., Gondo, H., *et al.* (2002). Partial impairment of interleukin-12 (IL-12) and IL-18 signaling in Tyk2-deficient mice. *Blood* **99**, 2094–2099.

Shuai, K. (1999). The STAT family of proteins in cytokine signaling. *Prog. Biophys. Mol. Biol.* **71**, 405–422.

Shuai, K., and Liu, B. (2003). Regulation of JAK-STAT signalling in the immune system. *Nat. Rev. Immunol.* **3**, 900–911.

Shuai, K., and Liu, B. (2005). Regulation of gene-activation pathways by PIAS proteins in the immune system. *Nat. Rev. Immunol.* **5**, 593–605.

Shuai, K., Schindler, C., Prezioso, V. R., and Darnell, J. E., Jr. (1992). Activation of transcription by IFN-gamma: Tyrosine phosphorylation of a 91-kD DNA binding protein. *Science* **258**, 1808–1812.

Shultz, L. D., Schweitzer, P. A., Rajan, T. V., Yi, T., Ihle, J. N., Matthews, R. J., Thomas, M. L., and Beier, D. R. (1993). Mutations at the murine motheaten locus are within the hematopoietic cell protein-tyrosine phosphatase (Hcph) gene. *Cell* **73**, 1445–1454.

Snow, J. W., Abraham, N., Ma, M. C., Abbey, N. W., Herndier, B., and Goldsmith, M. A. (2002). STAT5 promotes multilineage hematolymphoid development *in vivo* through effects on early hematopoietic progenitor cells. *Blood* **99**, 95–101.

Socolovsky, M., Fallon, A. E., Wang, S., Brugnara, C., and Lodish, H. F. (1999). Fetal anemia and apoptosis of red cell progenitors in Stat5a-/-5b-/- mice: A direct role for Stat5 in Bcl-X (L) induction. *Cell* **98**, 181–191.

Stark, G. R., Kerr, I. M., Williams, B. R., Silverman, R. H., and Schreiber, R. D. (1998). How cells respond to interferons. *Annu. Rev. Biochem.* **67**, 227–264.

Starr, R., and Hilton, D. J. (1999). Negative regulation of the JAK/STAT pathway. *Bioessays* **21**, 47–52.

Starr, R., Willson, T. A., Viney, E. M., Murray, L. J., Rayner, J. R., Jenkins, B. J., Gonda, T. J., Alexander, W. S., Metcalf, D., Nicola, N. A., and Hilton, D. J. (1997). A family of cytokine-inducible inhibitors of signalling. *Nature* **387**, 917–921.

Strehlow, I., and Schindler, C. (1998). Amino-terminal signal transducer and activator of transcription (STAT) domains regulate nuclear translocation and STAT deactivation. *J. Biol. Chem.* **273**, 28049–28056.

Suzuki, K., Nakajima, H., Kagami, S., Suto, A., Ikeda, K., Hirose, K., Hiwasa, T., Takeda, K., Saito, Y., Akira, S., and Iwamoto, I. (2002). Proteolytic processing of Stat6 signaling in mast cells as a negative regulatory mechanism. *J. Exp. Med.* **196**, 27–38.

Takahashi, T., and Shirasawa, T. (1994). Molecular cloning of rat JAK3, a novel member of the JAK family of protein tyrosine kinases. *FEBS Lett.* **342**, 124–128.

Takeda, K., Tanaka, T., Shi, W., Matsumoto, M., Minami, M., Kashiwamura, S., Nakanishi, K., Yoshida, N., Kishimoto, T., and Akira, S. (1996). Essential role of Stat6 in IL-4 signalling. *Nature* **380**, 627–630.

Takeda, K., Noguchi, K., Shi, W., Tanaka, T., Matsumoto, M., Yoshida, N., Kishimoto, T., and Akira, S. (1997). Targeted disruption of the mouse Stat3 gene leads to early embryonic lethality. *Proc. Natl. Acad. Sci. USA* **94**, 3801–3804.

Takeda, K., Kaisho, T., Yoshida, N., Takeda, J., Kishimoto, T., and Akira, S. (1998). Stat3 activation is responsible for IL-6-dependent T cell proliferation through preventing apoptosis: Generation and characterization of T cell-specific Stat3-deficient mice. *J. Immunol.* **161**, 4652–4660.

Takeda, K., Clausen, B. E., Kaisho, T., Tsujimura, T., Terada, N., Forster, I., and Akira, S. (1999). Enhanced Th1 activity and development of chronic enterocolitis in mice devoid of Stat3 in macrophages and neutrophils. *Immunity* **10**, 39–49.

Tebo, J. M., Kim, H. S., Gao, J., Armstrong, D. A., and Hamilton, T. A. (1998). Interleukin-10 suppresses IP-10 gene transcription by inhibiting the production of class I interferon. *Blood* **92**, 4742–4749.

Teglund, S., McKay, C., Schuetz, E., van Deursen, J. M., Stravopodis, D., Wang, D., Brown, M., Bodner, S., Grosveld, G., and Ihle, J. N. (1998). Stat5a and Stat5b proteins have essential and nonessential, or redundant, roles in cytokine responses. *Cell* **93**, 841–850.

ten Hoeve, J., de Jesus Ibarra-Sanchez, M., Fu, Y., Zhu, W., Tremblay, M., David, M., and Shuai, K. (2002). Identification of a nuclear Stat1 protein tyrosine phosphatase. *Mol. Cell. Biol.* **2B**, 5662–5668.

Thierfelder, W. E., van Deursen, J. M., Yamamoto, K., Tripp, R. A., Sarawar, S. R., Carson, R. T., Sangster, M. Y., Vignali, D. A., Doherty, P. C., Grosveld, G. C., and Ihle, J. N. (1996). Requirement for Stat4 in interleukin-12-mediated responses of natural killer and T cells. *Nature* **382**, 171–174.

Thomis, D. C., Gurniak, C. B., Tivol, E., Sharpe, A. H., and Berg, L. J. (1995). Defects in B lymphocyte maturation and T lymphocyte activation in mice lacking Jak3. *Science* **270**, 794–797.

Tomkinson, A., Kanehiro, A., Rabinovitch, N., Joetham, A., Cieslewicz, G., and Gelfand, E. W. (1999). The failure of STAT6-deficient mice to develop airway eosinophilia and airway hyperresponsiveness is overcome by interleukin-5. *Am. J. Respir. Crit. Care Med.* **160**, 1283–1291.

Tussie-Luna, M. I., Bayarsaihan, D., Seto, E., Ruddle, F. H., and Roy, A. L. (2002). Physical and functional interactions of histone deacetylase 3 with TFII-I family proteins and PIASxbeta. *Proc. Natl. Acad. Sci. USA* **99**, 12807–12812.

Udy, G. B., Towers, R. P., Snell, R. G., Wilkins, R. J., Park, S. H., Ram, P. A., Waxman, D. J., and Davey, H. W. (1997). Requirement of STAT5b for sexual dimorphism of body growth rates and liver gene expression. *Proc. Natl. Acad. Sci. USA* **94**, 7239–7244.

Ungureanu, D., Saharinen, P., Junttila, I., Hilton, D. J., and Silvennoinen, O. (2002). Regulation of Jak2 through the ubiquitin-proteasome pathway involves phosphorylation of Jak2 on Y1007 and interaction with SOCS-1. *Mol. Cell. Biol.* **22**, 3316–3326.

Uze, G., Lutfalla, G., and Mogensen, K. E. (1995). Alpha and beta interferons and their receptor and their friends and relations. *J. Interferon Cytokine Res.* **15**, 3–26.

van Dijk, T. B., Baltus, B., Caldenhoven, E., Handa, H., Raaijmakers, J. A., Lammers, J. W., Koenderman, L., and de Groot, R. P. (1998). Cloning and characterization of the human interleukin-3 (IL-3)/IL-5/granulocyte-macrophage colony-stimulating factor receptor betac gene: Regulation by Ets family members. *Blood* **92**, 3636–3646.

Velazquez, L., Fellous, M., Stark, G. R., and Pellegrini, S. (1992). A protein tyrosine kinase in the interferon alpha/beta signaling pathway. *Cell* **70**, 313–322.

Vignais, M. L., Sadowski, H. B., Watling, D., Rogers, N. C., and Gilman, M. (1996). Platelet-derived growth factor induces phosphorylation of multiple JAK family kinases and STAT proteins. *Mol. Cell. Biol.* **16**, 1759–1769.

Vilcek, J. (2003). Novel interferons. *Nat. Immunol.* **4**, 8–9.

Vitetta, E. S., Ohara, J., Myers, C. D., Layton, J. E., Krammer, P. H., and Paul, W. E. (1985). Serological, biochemical, and functional identity of B cell-stimulatory factor 1 and B cell differentiation factor for IgG1. *J. Exp. Med.* **162**, 1726–1731.

Wagner, B. J., Hayes, T. E., Hoban, C. J., and Cochran, B. H. (1990). The SIF binding element confers sis/PDGF inducibility onto the c-fos promoter. *EMBO J.* **9**, 4477–4484.

Wang, D., Moriggl, R., Stravopodis, D., Carpino, N., Marine, J. C., Teglund, S., Feng, J., and Ihle, J. N. (2000). A small amphipathic alpha-helical region is required for transcriptional activities and proteasome-dependent turnover of the tyrosine-phosphorylated Stat5. *EMBO J.* **19**, 392–399.

Watling, D., Guschin, D., Muller, M., Silvennoinen, O., Witthuhn, B. A., Quelle, F. W., Rogers, N. C., Schindler, C., Stark, G. R., Ihle, J. N., and Kerr, L. M. (1993). Complementation by the protein tyrosine kinase JAK2 of a mutant cell line defective in the interferon-gamma signal transduction pathway. *Nature* **366**, 166–170.

Wei, D., Le, X., Zheng, L., Wang, L., Frey, J. A., Gao, A. C., Peng, Z., Huang, S., Xiong, H. Q., Abbruzzese, J. L., and Xie, K. (2003). Stat3 activation regulates the expression of vascular endothelial growth factor and human pancreatic cancer angiogenesis and metastasis. *Oncogene* **22**, 319–329.

Welte, T., Zhang, S. S., Wang, T., Zhang, Z., Hesslein, D. G., Yin, Z., Kano, A., Iwamoto, Y., Li, E., Craft, J. E., Bothwell, A. L., Fikrig, E., *et al.* (2003). STAT3 deletion during hematopoiesis causes Crohn's disease-like pathogenesis and lethality: A critical role of STAT3 in innate immunity. *Proc. Natl. Acad. Sci. USA* **100**, 1879–1884.

Wilks, A. F., Harpur, A. G., Kurban, R. R., Ralph, S. J., Zurcher, G., and Ziemiecki, A. (1991). Two novel protein-tyrosine kinases, each with a second phosphotransferase-related catalytic domain, define a new class of protein kinase. *Mol. Cell. Biol.* **11**, 2057–2065.

Witthuhn, B. A., Silvennoinen, O., Miura, O., Lai, K. S., Cwik, C., Liu, E. T., and Ihle, J. N. (1994). Involvement of the Jak-3 Janus kinase in signalling by interleukins 2 and 4 in lymphoid and myeloid cells. *Nature* **370**, 153–157.

Woetmann, A., Nielsen, M., Christensen, S. T., Brockdorff, J., Kaltoft, K., Engel, A. M., Skov, S., Brender, C., Geisler, C., Svejgaard, A., Rygaard, J., Leick, V., *et al.* (1999). Inhibition of protein phosphatase 2A induces serine/threonine phosphorylation, subcellular redistribution, and functional inhibition of STAT3. *Proc. Natl. Acad. Sci. USA* **96**, 10620–10625.

Woetmann, A., Brockdorff, J., Lovato, P., Nielsen, M., Leick, V., Rieneck, K., Svejgaard, A., Geisler, C., and Odum, N. (2003). Protein phosphatase 2A (PP2A) regulates interleukin-4-mediated STAT6 signaling. *J. Biol. Chem.* **278**, 2787–2791.

Wormald, S., and Hilton, D. J. (2004). Inhibitors of cytokine signal transduction. *J. Biol. Chem.* **279**, 821–824.

Wu, T. R., Hong, Y. K., Wang, X. D., Ling, M. Y., Dragoi, A. M., Chung, A. S., Campbell, A. G., Han, Z. Y., Feng, G. S., and Chin, Y. E. (2002). SHP-2 is a dual-specificity phosphatase involved in Stat1 dephosphorylation at both tyrosine and serine residues in nuclei. *J. Biol. Chem.* **277**, 47572–47580.

Xie, M. H., Aggarwal, S., Ho, W. H., Foster, J., Zhang, Z., Stinson, J., Wood, W. I., Goddard, A. D., and Gurney, A. L. (2000). Interleukin (IL)-22, a novel human cytokine that signals through the interferon receptor-related proteins CRF2–4 and IL-22R. *J. Biol. Chem.* **275**, 31335–31339.

Yamamoto, K., Kobayashi, H., Arai, A., Miura, O., Hirosawa, S., and Miyasaka, N. (1997). cDNA cloning, expression and chromosome mapping of the human STAT4 gene: Both

STAT4 and STAT1 genes are mapped to 2q32.2–>q32.3. *Cytogenet. Cell Genet.* **77,** 207–210.

Yamaoka, K., Saharinen, P., Pesu, M., Holt, V. E., 3rd, Silvennoinen, O., and O'Shea, J. J. (2004). The Janus kinases (Jaks). *Genome Biol.* **5,** 253.

Yamashita, H., Xu, J., Erwin, R. A., Farrar, W. L., Kirken, R. A., and Rui, H. (1998). Differential control of the phosphorylation state of proline-juxtaposed serine residues Ser725 of Stat5a and Ser730 of Stat5b in prolactin-sensitive cells. *J. Biol. Chem.* **273,** 30218–30224.

Yasukawa, H., Ohishi, M., Mori, H., Murakami, M., Chinen, T., Aki, D., Hanada, T., Takeda, K., Akira, S., Hoshijima, M., Hirano, T., Chien, K. R., *et al.* (2003). IL-6 induces an anti-inflammatory response in the absence of SOCS3 in macrophages. *Nat. Immunol.* **4,** 551–556.

Yi, T., Gilbert, D. J., Jenkins, N. A., Copeland, N. G., and Ihle, J. N. (1992a). Assignment of a novel protein tyrosine phosphatase gene (Hcph) to mouse chromosome 6. *Genomics* **14,** 793–795.

Yi, T. L., Cleveland, J. L., and Ihle, J. N. (1992b). Protein tyrosine phosphatase containing SH2 domains: Characterization, preferential expression in hematopoietic cells, and localization to human chromosome 12p12-p13. *Mol. Cell. Biol.* **12,** 836–846.

Yu, H., and Jove, R. (2004). The STATs of cancer: New molecular targets come of age. *Nat. Rev. Cancer* **4,** 97–105.

Zhang, J. G., Hilton, D. J., Willson, T. A., McFarlane, C., Roberts, B. A., Moritz, R. L., Simpson, R. J., Alexander, W. S., Metcalf, D., and Nicola, N. A. (1997). Identification, purification, and characterization of a soluble interleukin (IL)-13-binding protein. Evidence that it is distinct from the cloned Il-13 receptor and Il-4 receptor alpha-chains. *J. Biol. Chem.* **272,** 9474–9480.

Zhang, J. G., Farley, A., Nicholson, S. E., Willson, T. A., Zugaro, L. M., Simpson, R. J., Moritz, R. L., Cary, D., Richardson, R., Hausmann, G., Kile, B. J., Kent, S. B., *et al.* (1999). The conserved SOCS box motif in suppressors of cytokine signaling binds to elongins B and C and may couple bound proteins to proteasomal degradation. *Proc. Natl. Acad. Sci. USA* **96,** 2071–2076.

Zhong, Z., Wen, Z., and Darnell, J. E., Jr. (1994). Stat3: A STAT family member activated by tyrosine phosphorylation in response to epidermal growth factor and interleukin-6. *Science* **264,** 95–98.

Zlotnik, A., Fischer, M., Roehm, N., and Zipori, D. (1987). Evidence for effects of interleukin 4 (B cell stimulatory factor 1) on macrophages: Enhancement of antigen presenting ability of bone marrow-derived macrophages. *J. Immunol.* **138,** 4275–4279.

8

THE NEWEST INTERLEUKINS: RECENT ADDITIONS TO THE EVER-GROWING CYTOKINE FAMILY

QIAN CHEN, HELEN P. CARROLL,
AND MASSIMO GADINA

Division of Infection and Immunity
Centre for Cancer Research and Cell Biology
Queen's University Belfast, Belfast, United Kingdom

Cytokines play a critical role in the control of the innate and adaptive immune responses. The most recent additions to the ever-growing family of cytokines include interleukin (IL)-27, IL-28A, IL-28B, IL-29, IL-31, IL-32, and IL-33. Many of the newly identified cytokines and/or their specific receptors have been identified using bioinformatics. The coming of age of this discipline has coincided with completion of the sequencing of the human genome thus enabling the identification of new

0083-6729/06 $35.00
DOI: 10.1016/S0083-6729(06)74008-0

uncharacterized proteins. The latest additions to the interleukin family have shed new light on the intricacies of immune system regulation. These novel cytokines have pleiotrophic actions ranging from antiviral immunity to the regulation of Th2 immune responses. For example, the discovery of IL-27 has greatly improved our understanding of the factors regulating the polarization of the T helper cell responses and IL-31 appears to be an important regulator of Th2 responses. On the other hand, IL-28 and IL-29 are considered to be critical for mounting an efficient antiviral response and IL-32 and IL-33, which are yet to be fully characterized, are emerging as important components of the inflammatory response in allergy and autoimmunity. These new cytokine/receptor combinations may therefore serve as novel targets for the treatment and control of allergy, autoimmune diseases, and some cancers.

I. THE NEW INTERLEUKINS

Cytokines are secreted molecules which allow communication between cells without direct contact. These molecules have been shown to have a pivotal role in the functionality of the immune system. They are utilized by leukocytes for their communication and are often referred to as interleukins. These molecules also allow immune cells to deliver and/or receive messages from other types of cells including endothelial cells. The completion of the human genome sequence and the subsequent dramatic development of the bioinformatics field have allowed the discovery of several new cytokines and cytokine receptors. Through database searches for predicted proteins encoding putative receptor sequences several new cytokine receptors have been identified and characterized. Moreover, analysis of similar intron-exon structures as well as analysis of the structural information of the typical four-helix bundle structure of cytokines has allowed the recognition as cytokines of previously uncharacterized molecules.

In this chapter, we will cover the very latest addition to the interleukin family. Molecules such as IL-27 and interferon (IFN)-λs are examples of these new cytokines which have been shown to have an important role in the functionality of our immune system.

The discovery and characterization of new cytokines, and of new receptors, and the characterization of their signaling cascades is providing us not only with a better understanding of how the immune cells develop, differentiate, and function but also are providing us with new targets for the treatment of several immune-related disorders.

A. INTERLEUKIN-27

IL-27 is the most recent addition to the IL-12 family of cytokines. Like the other two members of the family, IL-12 and IL-23, IL-27 is also a hetero-dimeric cytokine (Pflanz et al., 2004). It comprises two subunits designated Epstein-Barr induced molecule 3 (EBI3) and a novel protein p28, now officially designated IL-30.

The EBI3 subunit of IL-27 is homologous to IL-12p40 (Devergne et al., 1996, 1997). It was first identified in B cells infected with Epstein-Barr virus but, like IL-12, it was later demonstrated to be expressed in macrophages and monocytes on activation with mitogenic stimuli. EBI3 has also been reported to be expressed in fetal cells and trophoblasts but the significance of this expression is still unclear.

The discovery of p28 was the result of a bioinformatics approach search-ing for molecules with homology to IL-12p35 and IL-6. The p28 subunit of IL-27 is secreted as a helical protein which is related to IL-12p35. However, its secretion is dependent upon the coexpression of EBI3, a feature similar to the secretion of heterodimeric IL-12.

IL-27 is produced by antigen-presenting cells with the highest levels of p28 and EBI3 occurring in lipopolysaccharide (LPS)-activated monocytes and monocyte-derived dendritic cells (DCs) or on exposure to gram-positive bacteria. IL-27 expression is also induced by several inflammatory stimuli and by interferons (IFNs).

1. Interleukin-27 Receptor and Signaling

IL-27 binds WSX-1/T cell cytokine receptor (TCCR), previously an orphan receptor, which is a type I cytokine receptor with homology to the gp130 family (Fig. 1). WSX-1 is mainly expressed in hematopoietic cells especially cells of the lymphoid lineage such as T cells and natural killer (NK) cells. Although it was initially reported that WSX-1 was preferentially expressed in naïve T cells, reports have shown that in fact, the highest levels are found on effector and memory T cells (Villarino et al., 2005).

The second chain of the IL-27 receptor is gp130, a receptor chain which is utilized by many other cytokines including IL-6, making IL-27 a member of two families of cytokines (Pflanz et al., 2004). Given that gp130 is a broadly expressed molecule, the expression of the IL-27 receptor is therefore con-trolled by WSX-1 expression. Contrary to what has been observed for other gp130-utilizing cytokines, soluble gp130 cannot inhibit IL-27 signaling rais-ing the question of relative importance of the two chains of the receptor (Scheller et al., 2005).

The signaling pathways activated by IL-12 and IL-27 largely overlap. Activation of Janus kinase (JAK)1, signal transducer and activator of tran-scription 1(STAT)1, STAT3, and STAT5 has been reported (Fig. 2), and activation of different sets of STATs and other transcription factors has been

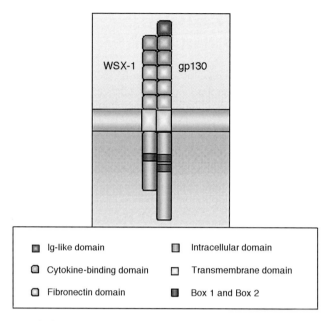

FIGURE 1. The IL-27 receptor complex. Schematic representation of the IL-27 receptor complex, comprising the WSX-1 and gp130 subunits. The WSX-1 chain has high affinity for IL-27 and signals through the gp130 chain. WSX-1 lacks an extracellular Ig domain but like gp130, WSX-1 contains two cytokine-binding motifs and three fibronectin domains. The cytoplasmic domains of WSX-1 and gp130 contain a membrane proximal Box 1 motif but no obvious Box 2 motif is present in WSX-1.

linked to the different biological effects that IL-27 exerts on different cell types. Mice nullizygous for WSX-1 had been generated prior to the discovery of the ligand and showed impaired Th1 development and IFN-γ production in response to antigen stimulation (Chen *et al.*, 2000; Yoshida *et al.*, 2001). In fact, most of the biology of IL-27 has been uncovered through the study of both WSX-1 and EBI3 deficient mice. Because of its homology with IL-12, IL-27 was initially studied for its capacity to induce the proliferation of naïve T cells. In fact, this is one of the effects that IL-27 can exert and, in combination with IL-12, it promotes IFN-γ production therefore inducing Th1 polarization. This is achieved by activating STAT1 and promoting the expression of the Th1 transcription factor T-bet and consequently regulating the expression of the *IL-12Rβ2* and *IFN-γ* genes.

2. Interleukin-27 Biological Activity

Several studies have suggested a proinflammatory role for IL-27. Overexpression of IL-27 in mice results in increased numbers of CD8 T cells and augmented IFN-γ production (Takeda *et al.*, 2005). The potential

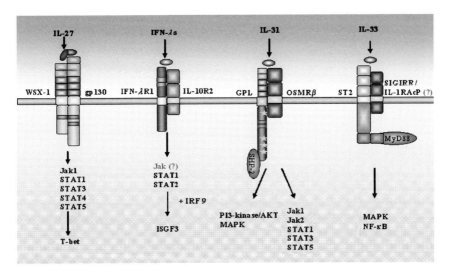

FIGURE 2. The new interleukins: receptor signaling. Schematic representation of the signaling events that follow ligand binding to the IL-27, IFN-λs, IL-31, and IL-33 receptor complexes.

proinflammatory role of IL-27 has also been suggested by experiments on adjuvant-induced arthritis in rats and experimental autoimmune encephalomyelitis (EAE) in mice. In these studies it was shown that the severity of the disease can be reduced by using IL-27-neutralizing antibodies (Goldberg et al., 2004a,b). This could be explained by the increased expression of WSX-1 in the CNS and lymph nodes during EAE induction (Li et al., 2005).

The suggestion that IL-27 could be an important cytokine in the mounting proper cell-mediated immunity was in accordance with what had been previously reported for WSX-1-deficient mice. T cells from these mice produce lower levels of IFN-γ when stimulated in vitro. As a consequence of this, WSX-1$^{-/-}$ mice have increased susceptibility to intracellular pathogens like Listeria monocytogenes and an increased production of IL-4 and augmented Th2 response. A similar situation has been observed during Leishmania infections, although this deficiency is transient, after some time mice started developing a Th1 response and were able to control the infection. Taking into account the fact that the IL-27 receptor is downregulated on T cell activation, it appears that the role of IL-27 in the development of Th1 response is transient and may function as a "kick-start" but IL-12 remains the major player in the mounting of an appropriate Th1 response.

Besides affecting Th1 development, disruption of the WSX-1 gene also resulted in changes in the pathology associated with the MRL/lpr mice. Absence of the IL-27 receptor resulted in a disease similar to the human membranous glomerulonephritis. These animals also had reduced levels of

IFN-γ and increased IL-4 expression. The loss of WSX-1 therefore resulted in a change of the disease from a Th1 autoimmune disease to a Th2 autoimmune response (Shimizu *et al.*, 2005).

Support for a role for IL-27 as a Th1 cytokine came from the generation of EBI3-deficient mice. These mice have normal numbers of T cells and B cells, but markedly decreased numbers of invariant NKT cells. These animals showed decreased IL-4 production after alphaGalCer stimulation and a transiently increased IFN-γ production. Accordingly, EBI3$^{-/-}$ mice did not develop oxazolone-induced colitis, which is normally mediated by Th2 cytokines whereas another model of colitis was unaltered.

The loss of responsiveness to IL-27, however, appears to be dependent on the pathogenic context in which it is analyzed. Mice injected with the T cell mitogen Concavalin A or infected with *Toxoplasma gondii* showed a normal Th1 response. In contrast, *Listeria* and *Leishmania* infection resulted in increased T cell proliferation, increased numbers of activated CD4 and CD8 T cells, and augmented IL-2 and IFN-γ production. The mice eventually succumbed as a result of the T cell–dependent inflammatory disease. Similar results were obtained after infection with *Trypanosoma cruzii* which leads to the development of liver necrosis due to excessive IFN-γ, tumor necrosis factor (TNF)-α, and IL-6 production. This phenotype is similar to that previously observed in *T. gondii*-infected STAT1-deficient mice where the T cells were found to be activated, hyperproliferating and an augmented production of IFN-γ was observed. Therefore, the pathogenic activation of the Th1-mediated response observed in these models suggests that IL-27 may have an inhibitory effect on T cell responses (Chen *et al.*, 2000; Yoshida *et al.*, 2001). However, IL-27 shows both pro- and anti-inflammatory effects since T cell functions can be augmented or inhibited by IL-27. In support of this suggestion is the fact that *Mycobacterium tuberculosis* infection of WSX1-deficient mice results in diminished bacterial load and more severe lung damage (Holscher *et al.*, 2005; Pearl *et al.*, 2004). In contrast, infection of WSX1-deficient mice with the parasitic nematode *Trichuris muris* produced an augmented Th2 response and improved control of larval worms (Artis *et al.*, 2004; Bancroft *et al.*, 2004). It therefore appears that powerful stimulations result in IL-27 production, which suppresses inflammatory cytokine release, increases the production of Th2 cytokines, and reduces effector T cell proliferation.

Natural killer cells express reasonable levels of the IL-27 receptor and IL-27 induces IFN-γ production in NK cells but the opposite effect is exerted on NKT cells thus supporting the dual role of pro- and anti-inflammatory cytokine. The IL-27 receptor is also expressed in monocytes, macrophages, and mast cells, and IL-27 can stimulate the production of IL-1 and TNF in these cells (Pflanz *et al.*, 2004). Whereas, in the absence of IL-27 receptor the production of inflammatory cytokines by these cells is increased (Artis *et al.*, 2004; Hamano *et al.*, 2003; Yamanaka *et al.*, 2004). In all these cell types although, the molecular mechanisms by which IL-27 exerts its effects are still unclear. Because of this peculiarity of IL-27 at this time it is difficult to envisage a strategy involving IL-27 manipulation *in vivo* for therapeutic purposes.

B. IL-28A, IL-28B, AND IL-29: THE IFN-λS

As already seen for IL-27, computational analysis of the human genome has enabled the identification of previously uncharacterized families of proteins. The novel IL-10 related cytokines, the IFN-λ family, have been identified using this approach (Kotenko *et al.*, 2003; Sheppard *et al.*, 2003). This group of cytokines has been classified as interleukins, but also as IFNs because they activate IFN-stimulated response elements (ISRE) and induce antiviral activity. There are three members of the family, IFN-λ1, 2, and 3, also known as IL-29, IL-28A, and IL-28B, respectively. IL-28A and IL-28B are virtually identical sharing 96% amino acid identity whereas IL-29 has 81% homology to IL-28. The IFN-λs have low homology to IL-10 and IL-22 (11–19%) and IFN-α (16%), however, the conserved cysteine pattern and amphipathic profile of the IFN-λs suggests that they belong to the helical cytokine family. The IFN-λs, therefore, appear to represent an evolutionary link between IL-10 and type I IFNs.

The genes encoding IL-28 and IL-29 are located on chromosome 19q13.13. Unlike the genes for other type I IFN family members, which are clustered on chromosome 9 and encoded within a single exon, the genes encoding IL-28 and IL-29 are contained within five exons (Kotenko *et al.*, 2003). It is the gene structure of the IFN-λs that supports their classification as interleukins since the genes for interleukins are typically encoded within multiple exons.

IFN-λs are expressed at low levels in human blood, brain, lung, ovary, pancreas, pituitary gland, placenta, prostate, and testis. They are coexpressed with IFN-α and IFN-β in virally infected cells (Kotenko *et al.*, 2003; Sheppard *et al.*, 2003). Virtually all cells are capable of expressing IFN-λs. However, the main producers of IFN-λs are antigen-presenting cells, such as DCs and macrophages. These cells have been shown to produce and secrete IFN-λs following stimulation with Toll-like receptor (TLR) agonists (Coccia *et al.*, 2004; Siren *et al.*, 2005). IFN-λs are produced following TLR3 and TLR4 ligation, weak expression is induced by TLR2 antagonists, whereas TLR7 stimulation fails to induce any IFN-λ expression. The expression of IFN-λ following TLR stimulation mirrors TLR-induced IFN-α expression. In addition, IFN-α has a positive regulatory effect on the expression of IFN-λs. This was clearly demonstrated by Siren *et al.* (2005), where pretreatment with IFN-α was shown to enhance the production of IFN-λs by macrophages stimulated with TLR3 and TLR4 agonists. It is therefore hypothesized that IFN-λ genes are regulated in a similar manner to IFN-α and β genes (Siren *et al.*, 2005).

1. IFN-λ Receptor and Signaling

Like other IFNs, the IFN-λs are secreted proteins that exert their cellular activity through binding to a unique heterodimeric receptor. The IFN-λR complex is composed of IFN-λR1 (also designated CRF2–12) and a common second chain IL-10R2 (also designated CRF2–4). IFN-λR is a member of the class II cytokine receptor family. Other members of this family of receptors include the receptors for IL-10 related cytokines and receptors for type I and type II interferons. IFN-λR1 is expressed in a wide variety of tissues, with the highest levels observed in the pancreas, thyroid, skeletal muscle, heart, prostate, and testis. The receptors for IFN-λ do not appear to be present on leukocytes.

There are three different isoforms of IFN-λR1 mRNA, IFN-λR1 V1, V2, and V3, which are thought to arise from alternative splicing and encode three different forms of the receptor. The extracellular domain of IFN-λR1 contains a cytokine-binding domain with two fibronectin domains. These regions are in all three variants of the receptor. The IFN-λR1 V3 consists of only the extracellular regions and although its function is still unknown it is thought to be a soluble form of the receptor. On the other hand, V1 and V2 possess both a transmembrane region and an intracellular domain. The V2 isoform of the receptor has a 29 amino acid deletion in the intracellular domain (Fig. 3) (Sheppard *et al.*, 2003).

The IFN-λR1 chain and the IL-10R2 chain of the IFN-λR complex are both required for ligand binding and signal transduction (Kotenko *et al.*, 2003). Ligation of the IFN-λR results in receptor heterodimerization, signaling via the JAK-STAT signal-transduction pathway, activation of ISRE-regulated gene expression, and upregulation of expression of major histocompatibility complex (MHC) class I antigen and antiviral proteins (Fig. 2).

Signaling through other class II family receptor complexes, for example, the IL-10R and IL-22R complexes, results primarily in the activation of STAT3. However, IFN-λ, signaling causes the phosphorylation of STAT1 and STAT2 which, together with the accessory factor IFN regulatory factor 9 (IRF9), forms the IFN-stimulated gene factor 3 transcription complex (ISGF3). Activation of ISGF3 and STAT2 are functions characteristic of type I IFN responses. A common tyrosine-based motif in the C terminus of the intracellular domain of the IFN-αR and IFN-λR complexes is thought to be responsible for STAT2 phosphorylation, and may be responsible for the overlap between the signaling pathways of the two cytokines and their similar biological activities (Dumoutier *et al.*, 2004; Kotenko *et al.*, 2003). Signaling through the IFN-λR complex results in the activation of many of the genes that are induced by signaling via IFN-α/βRs, which mostly encode

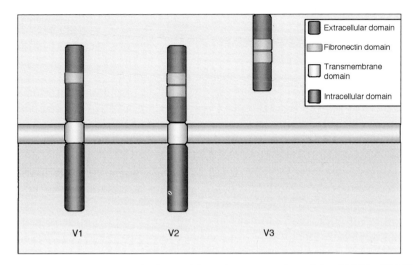

FIGURE 3. The IFN-λR1 isoforms. Schematic representation of the IFN-λR. IFN-λR1 has three splice variants, V1, V2, and V3. All isoforms have an extracellular domain containing two fibronectin domains. Unlike V1 and V2, the V3 isoform does not contain a transmembrane or intracellular domain and is thought to be a soluble version of the receptor. The V2 variant has a 29 amino acid deletion in the intracellular domain.

proteins with antiviral activity. Brand *et al.* (2005) demonstrated that IFN-λ induced the expression of the antiviral proteins myxovirus resistance-A (MxA) and 2′,5′-oligoadenylate synthase 1 (2′,5′-OAS), two proteins which are also produced in response to IFN-α (Kuhen *et al.*, 1998).

2. IFN-λs Biological Activities

Despite having been discovered more than three years ago, the importance of the IFN-λs remains to be fully elucidated. However, it is clear that they behave like weak type I IFNs. Receptors for type I IFNs are present on almost all somatic cells including lymphocytes and monocytes. In contrast, receptors for IFN-λ have a more restricted expression and are absent on leukocytes.

Surprisingly, animal models with deficiency in either IFN-λs or IFN-λRs have not yet been reported. Type I IFNs, in particular IFN-α, are often used in the treatment of various cancers, multiple sclerosis and, chronic hepatitis B and C (Gutterman, 1994). Treatment with IFN-α results in myelosuppression which is a common side-effect associated with type I IFN therapy. Therefore, since the receptor for IFN-λ is not present on leukocytes, the IFN-λs may serve as an alternative therapeutic choice to type I IFNs and reduce the adverse side-effects of type I IFN therapy. Nonetheless, further studies regarding the specific biological activities of IL-28A/B and IL-29 and their receptor will be required before their use in the clinical setting.

C. INTERLEUKIN-31

IL-31 belongs to the gp130/IL-6 family of cytokines, which are required for a variety of fundamental processes, such as neuronal growth, bone maintenance, cardiac development, and immune regulation. The IL-6 family encompasses, IL-6, the viral IL-6, IL-11, IL-27, leukemia inhibitory factor (LIF), oncostatin M (OSM), ciliary neurotrophic factor, cardiotrophin-1, and cardiotrophin-like cytokine. All family members share the common gp130 chain in their multimeric receptors that propagate intracellular signaling (Diveu et al., 2003; Taga and Kishimoto, 1997).

Members of the gp130/IL-6 cytokine family share very little sequence homology and consequently the identification of novel family members has proved challenging. The receptors for this family of cytokines are type I receptors and they share a number of common structural motifs, such as the cytokine-binding domain with two pairs of conserved cysteine residues and a WSXWS sequence motif in the extracellular domain. Novel receptors are therefore more readily identified and they have been utilized as a means to discover new members of the gp130/IL-6 family of cytokines. IL-31 was identified following the discovery of its receptor, the gp130-like receptor (GPL) (Ghilardi et al., 2002). The cognate ligand for this receptor was subsequently identified by a functional cloning technique based on the proliferation of cells bearing the novel GPL receptor and other known receptors of the gp130 family and the new ligand was subsequently designated IL-31 (Dillon et al., 2004).

1. Structural Features and Tissue Expression of IL-31

The gene encoding human IL-31 is located on chromosome 12q24.31 and the mouse IL-31 gene is situated in a syntenic region of chromosome 5 (Dillon et al., 2004). The IL-31 cDNA is composed of an open reading frame encoding a 164 amino acid precursor and a mature polypeptide of 138 amino acids. The gene structure of IL-31 is similar to that of LIF, oncostatin M, and cardiotrophin (Gross and Sprecher, 2003). IL-31 was suggested to belong to the short-chain cytokine group, which either have short cytoplasmic tails or lack an immunoglobulin (Ig) domain but have long cytoplasmic tails (Boulay et al., 2003). However, IL-31 lacks apparent homology to the other well-defined four-helical-bundle cytokines.

IL-31 cDNA was originally isolated from an activated T cell library (Gross and Sprecher, 2003). IL-31 mRNA is highly expressed in activated CD4+ T cells whereas lower expression was detected in activated CD8+ cells (Dillon et al., 2004). Further investigations have shown that IL-31 is linked with Th2 cells and expression of both mouse and human IL-31 mRNA was found to be higher in T cells activated in Th2-skewing conditions. IL-31 mRNA was also found in testis, bone marrow, skeletal muscle, kidney, colon, thymus, small intestine, and trachea (Dillon *et al.*, 2004), but its function in these tissues has not been investigated.

2. IL-31 Receptors

The novel cytokine receptor for IL-31 named GPL (also known as IL-31 RA) displays a 28% identity with the common receptor component shared by the IL-6 family of cytokines-gp130, but lacks the Ig-like domain present at the N terminus of gp130 (Diveu *et al.*, 2004; Ghilardi *et al.*, 2002). GPL has been shown to pair with another IL-6 receptor family member, the oncostatin M receptor β (OSMRβ), to form the receptor complex for IL-31 (Dillon *et al.*, 2004; Dreuw *et al.*, 2004). Hence, IL-31 receptor is classified into the G-CSF/IL-6/gp130 receptor family.

The genomic structure of GPL is organized within 15 exons on chromosome 5q11.2, only 24kb downstream of gp130. In mouse, GPL and gp130 are separated by only 19kb in a syntenic region on mouse chromosome 13. Human and mouse GPL are remarkably similar, displaying 73% homology (Ghilardi *et al.*, 2002).

Constitutive expression of GPL has been reported in epithelium from skin, lung, and prostate tissue, as well as skin fibroblasts. Monocytes and DCs also express GPL whereas B cells and NK cells do not (Gross and Sprecher, 2003). GPL expression is upregulated in human monocytes and DCs in response to IFN-γ suggesting a role for GPL in Th1 immune responses (Dillon *et al.*, 2004; Diveu *et al.*, 2003).

IL-31 does not appear to play a role in normal development, since GPL-deficient mice have no apparent abnormalities and have normal tissue and organ histopathology. Immune cell subsets were also found to develop normally. This is in contrast to gp130-deficient mice which display embryonic lethality (Dillon et al., 2004).

To date, four membrane-spanning splice variants of the GPL have been identified GPL$_{560}$, GPL$_{610}$, GPL$_{626}$, and GPL$_{745}$ (Dillon *et al.*, 2004; Diveu *et al.*, 2003). The extracellular domain starts with a signal peptide, followed by a cytokine-binding domain with two pairs of conserved cysteine residues and a WSXWS signature motif found in all type I cytokine receptors, and three fibronectin type III domain repeats (GPL$_{560}$ has only one fibronectin domain) (Dreuw *et al.*, 2004; Ghilardi *et al.*, 2002). GPL$_{610}$, GPL$_{626}$, and GPL$_{745}$ have identical transmembrane domains but their intracellular regions differ greatly with the exception of the Box 1 region, which is required for binding of JAKs (Dillon *et al.*, 2004; Dreuw *et al.*, 2004) (Fig. 4).

The absence of an Ig-like domain in GPL suggests that a second signaling receptor is required. Through the use of chimeric receptor constructs it was shown that the intracellular regions of GPL can interact with OSMRβ to transduce a functional signal in response to IL-31 stimulation (Diveu *et al.*, 2003; Dreuw *et al.*, 2004). IL-31 signals through the GPL/OSMRβ heterodimeric receptors via activation of JAK1, JAK2, STAT1, STAT3, and

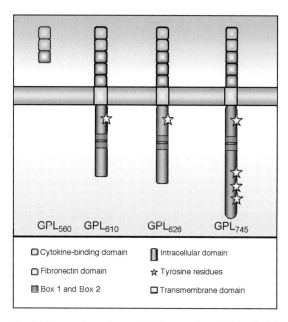

GPL$_{560}$ GPL$_{610}$ GPL$_{626}$ GPL$_{745}$

☐ Cytokine-binding domain   ▊ Intracellular domain

☐ Fibronectin domain   ☆ Tyrosine residues

▪ Box 1 and Box 2   ☐ Transmembrane domain

FIGURE 4. The IL-31 receptor—the gp130-like receptor (GPL). Model of the four GPL receptor variants. The GPL receptor has four variants, GPL$_{560}$, GPL$_{610}$, GPL$_{626}$, and GPL$_{745}$. The extracellular motifs of the GPL receptor all contain a cytokine-binding domain and fibronectin domains. The GPL$_{560}$ contains one fibronectin domain whereas the other three variants have three fibronectin domains. GPL$_{560}$ is the smallest isoform and has no transmembrane or intracellular domain and it is thought to be a soluble form of GPL. The other forms of the GPL receptor possess an intracellular domain which has Box 1 and Box 2 signaling motifs and also multiple tyrosine phosphorylation sites.

STAT5. The IL-31 receptor complex also recruits SHP-2, leading to the activation of the PI3-kinase/Akt and the MAPK pathway (Diveu *et al.*, 2004) (Fig. 2). Furthermore, STAT3 and STAT5 activation requires the phosphorylation of key tyrosine residues [721]YLKN and [652]YVTC in the cytoplasmic tail of GPL, which are only present in GPL$_{745}$ (Dreuw *et al.*, 2004). In contrast, the shortest form of GPL has been shown to behave as a dominant negative receptor, antagonizing the signaling cascade (Diveu *et al.*, 2004).

3. Biological Activity of IL-31

Target cells for IL-31 activity are those expressing both the GPL and OSMR receptors, however, the precise biological functions mediated by IL-31 are still unclear. Regulation of expression of the IL-31 receptor on human monocytes and DCs by IFN-γ and CD40L treatment has led people to hypothesize that IL-31 may act as a regulator of antigen presentation during an immune response (Dillon *et al.*, 2004).

IL-31 has also been shown to promote the chemotaxis of inflammatory cells. Indeed, IL-31 induces the expression of several chemokine genes such as those encoding GRO1α (CXCL1), TARC (CCL17), MIP3β (CCL19), MDC (CCL22), MIP-3 (CCL23), MIP-1β (CCL4), and I-309. Consistent with this finding, administration of IL-31 to mice resulted in enhanced infiltration of polymorphonuclear cells and mononuclear cells at the site of injection resulting in the thickening of the epidermis and acanthosis (Dillon et al., 2004).

Several studies now support a role for IL-31 in dermatitis and epithelial pathologies, such as psoriasis and both atopic and nonatopic dermatitis. Transgenic mice overexpressing IL-31 present with all the hallmarks of atopic dermatitis (Dillon et al., 2004; Leung and Bieber, 2003). Further support for this notion comes from studies on a mouse model of atopic dermatitis (NC/Nga mice) which develops a phenotype similar to human atopic dermatitis. NC/Nga mice develop dermatitis when raised under conventional conditions but not under pathogen free conditions (Suto et al., 1999). Under conventional conditions scratching behavior develops, resulting in the formation of skin-lesions. Serum IgE levels are also elevated in the NC/Nga mice and the dermatitis is more severe in male mice than in female mice. In these animals IL-31 mRNA expression was increased when dermatitis appeared (Takaoka et al., 2005).

Asthma is a Th2-mediated disorder which is linked to the development of atopic dermatitis. A possible role for IL-31 in asthma could be assumed by comparing the pathologic features of the patients with nonatopic dermatitis and the phenotype of transgenic mice overexpressing IL-31. Moreover, increased GPL mRNA expression has been observed in lung tissues and brochoalveolar lavage cells obtained from an animal model of asthma. However, it remains unclear whether IL-31 is directly or indirectly responsible for the pathologies associated with these conditions (Takaoka et al., 2005). Further studies could clarify the role of IL-31 in allergic disorders such as asthma and atopic dermatitis, but it is foreseeable that antagonizing this novel cytokine may prove successful in clinical studies for the treatment of these conditions.

D. INTERLEUKIN-32

IL-32 was originally described as NK transcript 4 (NK4) (Dahl et al., 1992) and was found to be highly expressed in human T cells and NK cells following stimulation with mitogens or IL-2. In addition, patients receiving high dose IL-2 therapy for treatment of metastatic melanoma were observed to have high NK4 transcript expression in PBMC (Panelli et al., 2002). Further investigations into the biological function of NK4 were later carried out by Kim and coworkers (Kim et al., 2005). In an attempt to determine IL-18 inducible genes they observed an upregulation of NK4 in response to IL-18 in

A459 cells transfected with IL-18Rβ chain. Recombinant NK4 protein was subsequently produced, it was found to possess typical cytokine activity and NK4 was renamed IL-32. The term NK4 is now used to refer to a variant of hepatocyte growth factor (Martin *et al.*, 2002).

1. Structural Features of IL-32

The gene encoding IL-32 is located on human chromosome 16p13.3 and organized into eight small exons. There are four splice variants: IL-32α, IL-32β, IL-32δ, and IL-32γ. IL-32γ is the variant reported in the original study by Dahl (Dahl *et al.*, 1992) as NK4. Translation initiation of IL-32 occurs at the ATG start codon which is located in exon 2 of all variants with the exception of IL-32δ in which the second exon is missing therefore the start codon is shifted to the third exon. IL-32α is the most abundant transcript, which has a 57 amino acid deletion in the C terminus as a result of splicing of exons 7 and 8 (Kim *et al.*, 2005).

IL-32 shares the highest degree of homology with equine IL-32β (31.8% identity) and displays some homology with bovine, ovine, and porcine IL-32 (Kim *et al.*, 2005). It would therefore appear that IL-32 is not very well conserved between species. IL-32 also shows very little homology with other cytokines and consequently has not yet been assigned to any family.

Northern blot analysis of human tissues has revealed low levels of IL-32 expression in thymus, prostate, colon, and small intestine. However, the most prominent IL-32 expression was observed in lymphocytes and spleen (Kim *et al.*, 2005). The IL-32 protein does not possess a typical hydrophobic signal peptide in its N terminus which is a typical feature of secreted cytokines. However, the protein contains predicted tyrosine sulphation sites which are a common posttranslational modification of secretory proteins. IL-32 has been identified as a soluble protein in tissue culture medium of A549 and Wish epithelial cells following treatment with IFN-γ and IL-1β (Dahl *et al.*, 1992; Kim *et al.*, 2005). The isoforms of IL-32 differ in their secretory capacity, with IL-32β being more readily released into culture medium than IL-32α. The observed variation in secretion of the IL-32 isoforms is reminiscent of IL-15, which has a long and short isoform. Both isoforms of IL-15 share the same receptor and biological function. However, the long isoform of IL-15 is more readily secreted, which is similar to IL-32β (Tagaya *et al.*, 1997). However, how IL-32 is secreted is still unclear since IL-32 not only lacks a signal peptide but also the caspase-1 proteolytic cleavage sites present in IL-1β and IL-18 for the generation of the mature secreted cytokine (Dahl *et al.*, 1992; Kim *et al.*, 2005).

2. Signaling Pathway of IL-32

Despite the reasonable amount of biochemical data that has been accumulated concerning IL-32 its receptor is still unknown and relatively little is known about the downstream signal transduction. However, it is clear that

IL-32 exerts its effects on highly differentiated cells such as the mouse macro-phage cell line RAW 264.7 and the human monocytic cell line THP1. The IL-32 specific receptor is therefore likely to be expressed by these differentiated cell types. Interaction of IL-32 with its receptor results in degradation of IκB and NFκB activation, as well as phosphorylation of p38 MAPK. Activation of these two pathways is characteristic of signaling cascades of proinflammatory cytokines.

The limited knowledge gathered to date regarding this novel cytokine suggests that IL-32 may play an important role in autoimmunity and inflam-matory diseases. IL-32 expression is induced by a number of proinflammatory cytokines. IFN-γ, in particular appears to play a significant role in the regulation of IL-32 suggesting that IL-32 may be important in the innate as well as the adaptive immune responses. IL-32 itself induces TNF-α expression which plays a significant role in a number of autoimmune disorders includ-ing rheumatoid arthritis and Crohn's disease, the symptoms of which are significantly ameliorated by TNF-α blockade (Suryaprasad and Prindiville, 2003).

IL-32 was shown to enhance the innate immune response to peptidogyl-can components, muropeptides, by specifically modulating the NOD1/NOD2 pathway (Netea et al., 2005a). In particular, IL-32γ was shown to specifically synergize with muropeptide leading to enhanced production of IL-1β and IL-6. This synergism is dependent on NOD1 and NOD2, which are intracellular recognition receptors for muropeptides. Since NOD2 is considered an important susceptibility gene for Crohn's disease (Netea et al., 2005b) and because IL-32 is expressed by intestinal mucosal epithelial cells, it is hypothesized that IL-32 may play a significant role in intestinal homeostasis and/or inflammation and the pathogenesis of Crohn's disease (Netea et al., 2005a).

It is clear that IL-32 may have therapeutic potential in autoimmune/inflammatory diseases. However, further studies are required to identify IL-32 receptor components, the regulation of IL-32 expression, and clarifi-cation of the molecular mechanisms of IL-32 function. In addition, the generation of IL-32 knockout or knock-in mouse models should provide insight into both its molecular mechanisms and the possibility of harnessing the IL-32 system as a therapeutic target.

E. INTERLEUKIN-33

Similar to the other cytokines described in this chapter, IL-33 was identi-fied by bioinformatics analysis of the human genome, its sequence is similar to those of IL-1 and fibroblast growth factor (Schmitz et al., 2005) and is now designated a novel member of the IL-1 family of cytokines, IL-1F11/IL-33. There are four members of the IL-1 family of cytokines, IL-1α/β, IL-1R, and IL-18 (Dinarello, 1997). The IL-33 protein contains the 12 core β strands that make up the characteristic β-trefoil fold of the IL-1 family cytokines and it is most closely related to IL-18 (Priestle *et al.*, 1988; Schmitz *et al.*, 2005).

IL-33 gene is mapped to human chromosome 9p24.1 site (19qC1 region in mouse), whereas the chromosome location of other members of the IL-1 family, with the exception of IL-18, is a gene cluster on chromosome 2. IL-33 cDNA encodes a peptide of 270 amino acids and 269 amino acids for human and mouse, respectively. The pro-IL-33 protein is 30 kDa in humans and 29 kDa in mouse and, like IL-1β and IL-18, it requires cleavage by caspase-1 to produce the mature, secreted 18 kDa form.

IL-1 family members are widely expressed in hematopoietic cells and play roles in inflammatory responses and host defense (Dinarello, 1997). However, the expression pattern of human IL-33 seems to be restricted to specific cell types. The mRNA for IL-33 has only been detected in epithelial cells from the bronchus and small airways, fibroblasts, and smooth muscle cells (Schmitz *et al.*, 2005). The expression profile of IL-33 suggests that it may be involved in the regulation of mucosal organ function.

1. IL-33 Receptor and Signaling

Receptors for the IL-1 cytokine family all possess a conserved protein sequence in their cytoplasmic domain called the Toll-IL-1 receptor (TIR) domain. The TIR domain is required for activation of common signaling pathways resulting in the activation of NF-κB and the MAP kinases p38, Jun kinase (JNK), and extracellular signal regulated kinase (ERK)1/2 following receptor ligation (Liew *et al.*, 2005; O'Neill, 2002). The TIR domain superfamily is divided into three subgroups, the first group is those containing an extracellular Ig domain such as IL-1 receptor and ST2, the second group is the TLRs, and the third group comprises the adaptor molecules, MyD88, Mal, and TRIF which are located in the cytoplasm and recruited to receptor TIR domains where they initiate signaling (Brint *et al.*, 2004; Liew *et al.*, 2005).

The receptor for IL-33 has yet to be fully characterized. The orphan IL-1 receptor ST2 has been shown to serve as the binding subunit for IL-33 and is therefore thought to make up one chain of the receptor (Schmitz *et al.*, 2005). However, the second chain of the complex, which usually has reduced-binding affinity but contributes to the signal transduction, has not yet been determined. Proposed candidates include the orphan IL-1 receptor SIGIRR and IL-1RAcP (Schmitz *et al.*, 2005; Towne *et al.*, 2004). The detected interaction of IL-33R with cytosolic proteins MyD88, IRAK, IRAK4, and TRAF6 suggests that these molecules may serve as key adaptors for IL-33 signal transduction (Schmitz *et al.*, 2005) (Fig. 5).

2. IL-33 Biological Activity

ST2 is expressed on mast cells and Th2 cells but not on Th1 cells and is essential for Th2 effector function (Lohning *et al.*, 1998). Exposure of cells to IL-33 leads to the production of Th2-associated cytokines, such as IL-5 and

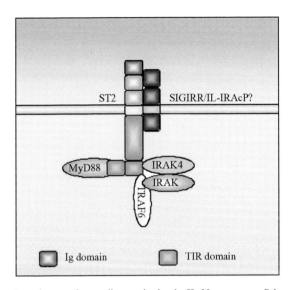

FIGURE 5. Recruitment of cytosolic proteins by the IL-33 coreceptor. Schematic representation of the IL-33 receptor complex. ST2 and SIGIRR or IL-1RAcP are thought to dimerize and form the IL-33 specific receptor. The ST2 receptor chain contains an extracellular domain with an immunoglobulin domain. The intracellular region of the receptor has a TIR domain to which cytosolic adaptor proteins are recruited. On IL-33 binding the adaptor protein MyD88, which also possesses a TIR domain, is recruited to the active receptor complex and interacts with the receptor through homotypic TIR domain interactions. IRAK and IRAK4 are then thought to be recruited to the complex followed by their interaction with TRAF6 leading to activation of the NF-κB transcription factors.

IL-13, and increased serum Ig levels and is dependent on the presence of ST2. These findings suggest a role for IL-33 and its receptor ST2 in sustaining Th2 effector functions. However, IL-33 is not thought to be involved in promoting Th2 cell development. In order to exert its effect on Th2 cells, IL-33 may initiate signals through IL-1 receptor ST2 complexed with SIGIRR or other coreceptors, followed by the recruitment of cytosolic proteins MyD88, IRAK, IRAK4, and TRAF6 to ST2, activating MAP kinases and the transcriptional factor NF-κB, and eventually turning on Th2 cytokine gene transcription (Schmitz et al., 2005) (Fig. 2).

In vivo analysis of IL-33 activity revealed that mice treated with IL-33 display profound pathological changes in the mucosal tissues including eosinophilia in the lung, esophagus, and intestines; splenomegaly; and enhanced levels of serum IgA and IgE (Schmitz et al., 2005). The Th2 cytokines IL-4 and IL-5 cause increased levels of IgE and the differentiation and release of eosinophils, respectively, therefore it is likely that they are responsible for the pathologies resulting from IL-33 treatment. Consequently, it appears that IL-33 may serve as a booster of Th2 immunity even though it does not directly control this type of response. In conclusion, the discovery of

IL-33 may provide novel insight into the allergic disorders caused by eosino-philic tissue damage such as asthma and makes it an attractive candidate for therapeutic intervention for these types of diseases (Chomarat and Banchereau, 1998; Pene *et al.*, 1988).

II. CONCLUSIONS

The mechanisms playing a role in the regulation of leukocyte function are quite complex and require the biological interaction of different cell types most of which are mediated by cytokines. Moreover, these soluble mediators are well known to synergize or to antagonize each other. In the past few years, extensive progress has been made in our understanding of how the immune system develops and maintains its functionality and of the role that interleukins play in these events. Nonetheless, a complete knowledge of the molecular players and their interactions is still incomplete.

The latest additions to the interleukin family are beginning to give us a more complete understanding of the fine tuning which is required for a normal immune response. For example, the discovery of IL-27 has greatly improved our understanding of how the Th1-Th2 balance is achieved and similarly, IL-31 appears to be an important regulator of the Th2 response. IL-28 and IL-29 are likely to be critical for a proper antiviral response and cytokines such as IL-32 and IL-33, albeit poorly characterized, are emerging as important components of the inflammatory response.

Mining of the human genome for additional interleukins may yet prove fruitful, however there are likely to be very few undiscovered cytokines at this point. Instead, it is possible that information about new immunoregulatory proteins with interleukin-like properties will come from studies of how viruses evade our immune response. Further discovery of new cytokines, their recep-tors, and characterization of their signaling cascades will undoubtedly provide us with a more in depth understanding of the normal immune system and will open up more possibilities for the treatment of human diseases.

ACKNOWLEDGMENTS

We would like to thank Alan Coffey and Verica Paunovic for insightful suggestions and critical reading of the chapter.

REFERENCES

Artis, D., Villarino, A., Silverman, M., He, W., Thornton, E. M., Mu, S., Summer, S., Covey, T. M., Huang, E., Yoshida, H., Koretzky, G., Goldschmidt, M., *et al.* (2004). The IL-27 receptor (WSX-1) is an inhibitor of innate and adaptive elements of type 2 immunity. *J. Immunol.* **173,** 5626–5634.

Bancroft, A. J., Humphreys, N. E., Worthington, J. J., Yoshida, H., and Grencis, R. K. (2004). WSX-1: A key role in induction of chronic intestinal nematode infection. *J. Immunol.* **172**, 7635–7641.

Boulay, J. L., O'Shea, J. J., and Paul, W. E. (2003). Molecular phylogeny within type I cytokines and their cognate receptors. *Immunity* **19**, 159–163.

Brand, S., Zitzmann, K., Dambacher, J., Beigel, F., Olszak, T., Vlotides, G., Eichhorst, S. T., Goke, B., Diepolder, H., and Auernhammer, C. J. (2005). SOCS-1 inhibits expression of the antiviral proteins 2′, 5′-OAS and MxA induced by the novel interferon-lambdas IL-28A and IL-29. *Biochem. Biophys. Res. Commun.* **331**, 543–548.

Brint, E. K., Xu, D., Liu, H., Dunne, A., McKenzie, A. N., O'Neill, L. A., and Liew, F. Y. (2004). ST2 is an inhibitor of interleukin 1 receptor and Toll-like receptor 4 signaling and maintains endotoxin tolerance. *Nat. Immunol.* **5**, 373–379.

Chen, Q., Ghilardi, N., Wang, H., Baker, T., Xie, M. H., Gurney, A., Grewal, I. S., and de Sauvage, F. J. (2000). Development of Th1-type immune responses requires the type I cytokine receptor TCCR. *Nature* **407**, 916–920.

Chomarat, P., and Banchereau, J. (1998). Interleukin-4 and interleukin-13: Their similarities and discrepancies. *Int. Rev. Immunol.* **17**, 1–52.

Coccia, E. M., Severa, M., Giacomini, E., Monneron, D., Remoli, M. E., Julkunen, I., Cella, M., Lande, R., and Uze, G. (2004). Viral infection and Toll-like receptor agonists induce a differential expression of type I and lambda interferons in human plasmacytoid and monocyte-derived dendritic cells. *Eur. J. Immunol.* **34**, 796–805.

Dahl, C. A., Schall, R. P., He, H. L., and Cairns, J. S. (1992). Identification of a novel gene expressed in activated natural killer cells and T cells. *J. Immunol.* **148**, 597–603.

Devergne, O., Hummel, M., Koeppen, H., Le Beau, M. M., Nathanson, E. C., Kieff, E., and Birkenbach, M. (1996). A novel interleukin-12 p40-related protein induced by latent Epstein-Barr virus infection in B lymphocytes. *J. Virol.* **70**, 1143–1153.

Devergne, O., Birkenbach, M., and Kieff, E. (1997). Epstein-Barr virus-induced gene 3 and the p35 subunit of interleukin 12 form a novel heterodimeric hematopoietin. *Proc. Natl. Acad. Sci. USA* **94**, 12041–12046.

Dillon, S. R., Sprecher, C., Hammond, A., Bilsborough, J., Rosenfeld-Franklin, M., Presnell, S. R., Haugen, H. S., Maurer, M., Harder, B., Johnston, J., Bort, S., Mudri, S., *et al.* (2004). Interleukin 31, a cytokine produced by activated T cells, induces dermatitis in mice. *Nat. Immunol.* **5**, 752–760.

Dinarello, C. A. (1997). Interleukin-1. *Cytokine Growth Factor Rev.* **8**, 253–265.

Diveu, C., Lelievre, E., Perret, D., Lak-Hal, A. H., Froger, J., Guillet, C., Chevalier, S., Rousseau, F., Wesa, A., Preisser, L., Chabbert, M., Gauchat, J. F., *et al.* (2003). GPL, a novel cytokine receptor related to GP130 and leukemia inhibitory factor receptor. *J. Biol. Chem.* **278**, 49850–49859.

Diveu, C., Lak-Hal, A. H., Froger, J., Ravon, E., Grimaud, L., Barbier, F., Hermann, J., Gascan, H., and Chevalier, S. (2004). Predominant expression of the long isoform of GP130-like (GPL) receptor is required for interleukin-31 signaling. *Eur. Cytokine Netw.* **15**, 291–302.

Dreuw, A., Radtke, S., Pflanz, S., Lippok, B. E., Heinrich, P. C., and Hermanns, H. M. (2004). Characterization of the signaling capacities of the novel gp130-like cytokine receptor. *J. Biol. Chem.* **279**, 36112–36120.

Dumoutier, L., Tounsi, A., Michiels, T., Sommereyns, C., Kotenko, S. V., and Renauld, J. C. (2004). Role of the interleukin (IL)-28 receptor tyrosine residues for antiviral and antiproliferative activity of IL-29/interferon-lambda 1: Similarities with type I interferon signaling. *J. Biol. Chem.* **279**, 32269–32274.

Ghilardi, N., Li, J., Hongo, J. A., Yi, S., Gurney, A., and de Sauvage, F. J. (2002). A novel type I cytokine receptor is expressed on monocytes, signals proliferation, and activates STAT-3 and STAT-5. *J. Biol. Chem.* **277**, 16831–16836.

Goldberg, R., Wildbaum, G., Zohar, Y., Maor, G., and Karin, N. (2004a). Suppression of ongoing adjuvant-induced arthritis by neutralizing the function of the p28 subunit of IL-27. *J. Immunol.* **173**, 1171–1178.

Goldberg, R., Zohar, Y., Wildbaum, G., Geron, Y., Maor, G., and Karin, N. (2004b). Suppression of ongoing experimental autoimmune encephalomyelitis by neutralizing the function of the p28 subunit of IL-27. *J. Immunol.* **173**, 6465–6471.

Gross, J. A., and Sprecher, C. (2003). A novel cytokine made by activated T cells, signals through a novel hetero-dimeric receptor complex expressed in skin. *Eur. Cytokine Netw.* **14**, 308.

Gutterman, J. U. (1994). Cytokine therapeutics: Lessons from interferon alpha. *Proc. Natl. Acad. Sci. USA* **91**, 1198–1205.

Hamano, S., Himeno, K., Miyazaki, Y., Ishii, K., Yamanaka, A., Takeda, A., Zhang, M., Hisaeda, H., Mak, T. W., Yoshimura, A., and Yoshida, H. (2003). WSX-1 is required for resistance to Trypanosoma cruzi infection by regulation of proinflammatory cytokine production. *Immunity* **19**, 657–667.

Holscher, C., Holscher, A., Ruckerl, D., Yoshimoto, T., Yoshida, H., Mak, T., Saris, C., and Ehlers, S. (2005). The IL-27 receptor chain WSX-1 differentially regulates antibacterial immunity and survival during experimental tuberculosis. *J. Immunol.* **174**, 3534–3544.

Kim, S. H., Han, S. Y., Azam, T., Yoon, D. Y., and Dinarello, C. A. (2005). Interleukin-32: A cytokine and inducer of TNFalpha. *Immunity* **22**, 131–142.

Kotenko, S. V., Gallagher, G., Baurin, V. V., Lewis-Antes, A., Shen, M., Shah, N. K., Langer, J. A., Sheikh, F., Dickensheets, H., and Donnelly, R. P. (2003). IFN-lambdas mediate antiviral protection through a distinct class II cytokine receptor complex. *Nat. Immunol.* **4**, 69–77.

Kuhen, K. L., Vessey, J. W., and Samuel, C. E. (1998). Mechanism of interferon action: Identification of essential positions within the novel 15-base-pair KCS element required for transcriptional activation of the RNA-dependent protein kinase *pkr* gene. *J. Virol.* **72**, 9934–9939.

Leung, D. Y., and Bieber, T. (2003). Atopic dermatitis. *Lancet* **361**, 151–160.

Li, J., Gran, B., Zhang, G. X., Rostami, A., and Kamoun, M. (2005). IL-27 subunits and its receptor (WSX-1) mRNAs are markedly up-regulated in inflammatory cells in the CNS during experimental autoimmune encephalomyelitis. *J. Neurol. Sci.* **232**, 3–9.

Liew, F. Y., Liu, H., and Xu, D. (2005). A novel negative regulator for IL-1 receptor and Toll-like receptor 4. *Immunol. Lett.* **96**, 27–31.

Lohning, M., Stroehmann, A., Coyle, A. J., Grogan, J. L., Lin, S., Gutierrez-Ramos, J. C., Levinson, D., Radbruch, A., and Kamradt, T. (1998). T1/ST2 is preferentially expressed on murine Th2 cells, independent of interleukin 4, interleukin 10, and interleukin 10, and important for Th2 effector function. *Proc. Natl. Acad. Sci. USA* **95**, 6930–6935.

Martin, T. A., Mansel, R. E., and Jiang, W. G. (2002). Antagonistic effect of NK4 on HGF/SF induced changes in the transendothelial resistance (TER) and paracellular permeability of human vascular endothelial cells. *J. Cell. Physiol.* **192**, 268–275.

Netea, M. G., Azam, T., Ferwerda, G., Girardin, S. E., Walsh, M., Park, J. S., Abraham, E., Kim, J. M., Yoon, D. Y., Dinarello, C. A., and Kim, S. H. (2005a). IL-32 synergizes with nucleotide oligomerization domain (NOD) 1 and NOD2 ligands for IL-1beta and IL-6 production through a caspase 1-dependent mechanism. *Proc. Natl. Acad. Sci. USA* **102**, 16309–16314.

Netea, M. G., Ferwerda, G., de Jong, D. J., Jansen, T., Jacobs, L., Kramer, M., Naber, T. H., Drenth, J. P., Girardin, S. E., Kullberg, B. J., Adema, G. J., and Van der Meer, J. W. (2005b). Nucleotide-binding oligomerization domain-2 modulates specific TLR pathways for the induction of cytokine release. *J. Immunol.* **174**, 6518–6523.

O'Neill, L. A. (2002). Signal transduction pathways activated by the IL-1 receptor/toll-like receptor superfamily. *Curr. Top. Microbiol. Immunol.* **270**, 47–61.

Panelli, M. C., Wang, E., Phan, G., Puhlmann, M., Miller, L., Ohnmacht, G. A., Klein, H. G., and Marincola, F. M. (2002). Gene-expression profiling of the response of peripheral blood mononuclear cells and melanoma metastases to systemic IL-2 administration. *Genome Biol.* **3**, research 0035, 1–17.

Pearl, J. E., Khader, S. A., Solache, A., Gilmartin, L., Ghilardi, N., deSauvage, F., and Cooper, A. M. (2004). IL-27 signaling compromises control of bacterial growth in mycobacteria-infected mice. *J. Immunol.* **173**, 7490–7496.

Pene, J., Rousset, F., Briere, F., Chretien, I., Paliard, X., Banchereau, J., Spits, H., and De Vries, J. E. (1988). IgE production by normal human B cells induced by alloreactive T cell clones is mediated by IL-4 and suppressed by IFN-gamma. *J. Immunol.* **141**, 1218–1224.

Pflanz, S., Hibbert, L., Mattson, J., Rosales, R., Vaisberg, E., Bazan, J. F., Phillips, J. H., McClanahan, T. K., de Waal Malefyt, R., and Kastelein, R. A. (2004). WSX-1 and glycoprotein 130 constitute a signal-transducing receptor for IL-27. *J. Immunol.* **172**, 2225–2231.

Priestle, J. P., Schar, H. P., and Grutter, M. G. (1988). Crystal structure of the cytokine interleukin-1 beta. *EMBO J.* **7**, 339–343.

Scheller, J., Schuster, B., Holscher, C., Yoshimoto, T., and Rose-John, S. (2005). No inhibition of IL-27 signaling by soluble gp130. *Biohem. Biophys. Res. Commun.* **3**, 724–728.

Schmitz, J., Owyang, A., Oldham, E., Song, Y., Murphy, E., McClanahan, T. K., Zurawski, G., Moshrefi, M., Qin, J., Li, X., Gorman, D. M., Bazan, J. F., *et al.* (2005). IL-33, an interleukin-1-like cytokine that signals via the IL-1 receptor-related protein ST2 and induces T helper type 2-associated cytokines. *Immunity,* **23**, 479–490.

Sheppard, P., Kindsvogel, W., Xu, W., Henderson, K., Schlutsmeyer, S., Whitmore, T. E., Kuestner, R., Garrigues, U., Birks, C., Roraback, J., Ostrander, C., Dong, D., *et al.* (2003). IL-28, IL-29 and their class II cytokine receptor IL-28R. *Nat. Immunol.* **4**, 63–68.

Shimizu, S., Sugiyama, N., Masutani, K., Sadanaga, A., Miyazaki, Y., Inoue, Y., Akahoshi, M., Katafuchi, R., Hirakata, H., Harada, M., Hamano, S., Nakashima, H., *et al.* (2005). Membranous glomerulonephritis development with Th2-type immune deviations in MRL/lpr mice deficient for IL-27 receptor (WSX-1). *J. Immunol.* **175**, 7185–7192.

Siren, J., Pirhonen, J., Julkunen, I., and Matikainen, S. (2005). IFN-alpha regulates TLR-dependent gene expression of IFN-alpha, IFN-beta, IL-28, and IL-29. *J. Immunol.* **174**, 1932–1937.

Suryaprasad, A. G., and Prindiville, T. (2003). The biology of TNF blockade. *Autoimmun. Rev.* **2**, 346–357.

Suto, H., Matsuda, H., Mitsuishi, K., Hira, K., Uchida, T., Unno, T., Ogawa, H., and Ra, C. (1999). NC/Nga mice: A mouse model for atopic dermatitis. *Int. Arch. Allergy Immunol.* **120** (Suppl. 1), 70–75.

Taga, T., and Kishimoto, T. (1997). Gp130 and the interleukin-6 family of cytokines. *Annu. Rev. Immunol.* **15**, 797–819.

Tagaya, Y., Kurys, G., Thies, T. A., Losi, J. M., Azimi, N., Hanover, J. A., Bamford, R. N., and Waldmann, T. A. (1997). Generation of secretable and nonsecretable interleukin 15 isoforms through alternate usage of signal peptides. *Proc. Natl. Acad. Sci. USA* **94**, 14444–14449.

Takaoka, A., Arai, I., Sugimoto, M., Yamaguchi, A., Tanaka, M., and Nakaike, S. (2005). Expression of IL-31 gene transcripts in NC/Nga mice with atopic dermatitis. *Eur. J. Pharmacol.* **516**, 180–181.

Takeda, A., Hamano, S., Shiraishi, H., Yoshimura, T., Ogata, H., Ishii, K., Ishibashi, T., Yoshimura, A., and Yoshida, H. (2005). WSX-1 over-expression in CD4(+) T cells leads to hyperproliferation and cytokine hyperproduction in response to TCR stimulation. *Int. Immunol.* **17**, 889–897.

Towne, J. E., Garka, K. E., Renshaw, B. R., Virca, G. D., and Sims, J. E. (2004). Interleukin (IL)-1F6, IL-1F8, and IL-1F9 signal through IL-1Rrp2 and IL-1RAcP to activate the pathway leading to NF-kappaB and MAPKs. *J. Biol. Chem.* **279,** 13677–13688.

Villarino, A. V., Larkin, J., III, Saris, C. J., Caton, A. J., Lucas, S., Wong, T., de Sauvage, F. J., and Hunter, C. A. (2005). Positive and negative regulation of the IL-27 receptor during lymphoid cell activation. *J. Immunol.* **174,** 7684–7691.

Yamanaka, A., Hamano, S., Miyazaki, Y., Ishii, K., Takeda, A., Mak, T. W., Himeno, K., Yoshimura, A., and Yoshida, H. (2004). Hyperproduction of proinflammatory cytokines by WSX-1-deficient NKT cells in concanavalin A-induced hepatitis. *J. Immunol.* **172,** 3590–3596.

Yoshida, H., Hamano, S., Senaldi, G., Covey, T., Faggioni, R., Mu, S., Xia, M., Wakeham, A. C., Nishina, H., Potter, J., Saris, C. J., and Mak, T. W. (2001). WSX-1 is required for the initiation of Th1 responses and resistance to L. major infection. *Immunity* **15,** 569–578.

9

THE INTERLEUKIN-1 RECEPTOR FAMILY

DIANA BORASCHI* AND ALDO TAGLIABUE[†]

*Institute of Biomedical Technologies
National Research Council, Pisa, Italy
[†]ALTA S.r.l., Siena, Italy

The cytokines IL-1 and IL-18 are key molecules both in the innate and in the adaptive immune response. Their activity is mediated by specific

0083-6729/06 $35.00
DOI: 10.1016/S0083-6729(06)74009-2

receptors present on the membrane of target cells. It has become apparent that these receptors are members of a larger family of related receptors, most of which are apparently involved in the mechanisms of host defense. Thus, the large Toll/IL-1R (TIR) superfamily encompasses the Ig domain family (IL-1 receptors, IL-18 receptors, and IL-1R-like receptors), the leucine-rich domain family [the Toll-like receptors (TLR) and similar receptors], and a series of TIR domain-containing intracellular adapter molecules. The TIR superfamily is defined by a common intracellular TIR domain, involved in the initiation of signaling. A group of TIR domain-containing adapters (MyD88, TIRAP, TRIF, and TRAM) are differentially recruited to the Toll/IL-1 receptors, contributing to the specificity of signaling. Recent studies have also begun to unravel the mechanisms of negative regulation of the Toll/IL-1 receptors. The orphan receptor TIR8/SIGIRR, a member of TIR superfamily, while unable to initiate signaling, can negatively modulate the TIR-mediated responses. Other negative regulators of the Toll/IL-1R family include T1/ST2, some soluble forms of TLR, and MyD88s. The coordinated positive and negative regulation of the TIR activation ensures the appropriate modulation of the innate and inflammatory responses and avoids the risk of pathological derangement. This chapter will consider in detail the characteristics and functional role of the Ig domain receptor subfamily in the regulation of host defense and their possible role in pathology. © 2006 Elsevier Inc.

I. INTRODUCTION

The family of interleukin-1 (IL-1) receptors is a large family of molecules of key importance in mediating the activation of innate immunity, the first line of defense against pathogenic microorganisms. Stimulation of the innate immune system through Toll-like receptors (TLR) induces the production of inflammatory cytokines, thereby activating the more specific and effective adaptive response. Cytokines produced, such as IL-1 and IL-18, activate target cells through receptors of the same family as TLR, inducing pronounced amplification of the immune response which, if not tightly controlled, can cause severe autoimmune and inflammatory diseases such as rheumatoid arthritis, lupus, and inflammatory bowel diseases. On the other hand, recognition of commensal bacteria through TLR occurs under normal steady-state conditions, and this interaction plays a crucial role in the maintenance of intestinal epithelial homeostasis (Rakoff-Nahoum et al., 2004). Likewise, IL-1 is apparently involved in homeostatic cell–cell communication (Dinarello, 1998). Therefore it is of critical importance to investigate the mechanisms by which the Toll/IL-1 receptors (TIR) recognize danger signals, mediate activation signaling, and are downregulated, with the long-term objective of understanding the pathogenic mechanisms of chronic inflammatory and autoimmune diseases in order to design effective therapeutic strategies.

The receptors of the TIR superfamily are defined by the presence of an intracellular TIR domain, which initiates the signaling cascade. TIR receptors can be divided into two main subgroups based on the extracellular domains, those containing an immunoglobulin (Ig)-like domain (Mitcham *et al.*, 1996), and those characterized by a leucine-rich repeat motif (LRR) (Medzhitov *et al.*, 1997) (Fig. 1). The Ig domain subgroup (Table I) includes the IL-1 receptor type I (IL-1RI) and its accessory protein (IL-1RAcP), the IL-18 receptors (IL-18Rα and IL-18Rβ), the regulatory receptors T1/ST2 and single immunoglobulin IL-1R related molecule (SIGIRR), and a series of other orphan receptors (TIGIRR-1, TIGIRR-2, and IL-1Rrp2). IL-1RII, although lacking a TIR domain, is considered part of this subgroup due to its high similarity to the IL-1RI. The best known ligand for the receptors of the Ig subgroup is IL-1. There are now 11 known members of the IL-1

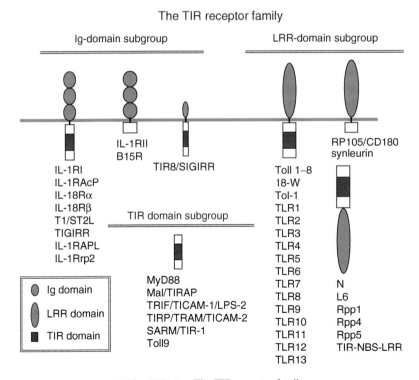

FIGURE 1.   The TIR receptor family.

TABLE 1. The IL-1 Receptor Family

Name	Ligand	Expression
IL-1RI (membrane and soluble form)	Initiates and amplifies the immune and inflammatory response upon binding the agonist ligands IL-1α and IL-1β; inhibited upon binding the antagonist ligand IL-1Ra; the soluble form binds IL-1F10	Expressed by all cells responsive to IL-1, predominant type of IL-1R on T cells, fibroblasts, epithelial and endothelial cells
IL-1RII (membrane and soluble form)	Binds IL-1β and less efficiently IL-1α and IL-1Ra; decoy receptor, unable to initiate signal transduction. Both membrane and soluble form have inhibitory activity	Expressed by many cell types, particularly abundant on B cells, mononuclear phagocytes, polymorphonuclear leukocytes, and bone marrow
IL-1RAcP (membrane and soluble form)	Coreceptor for IL-1RI responsible for signaling after binding IL-1α or IL-1β; can form inactive complexes with IL-1RII bound to IL-1; coreceptor for IL-1Rrp2 in activation by IL-1F6, IL-1F8, and IL-1F9	Expressed by all cells responsive to IL-1
IL-18Rα (IL-1Rrp1)	Binds IL-18 and IL-1F7	Mononuclear phagocytes, neutrophils, Th1 cells, NK cells, endothelial cells, smooth muscle cells
IL-18Rβ (AcPL)	Coreceptor for IL-18Rα responsible for signaling after binding of IL-18	Mononuclear phagocytes, neutrophils, Th1 cells, NK cells, endothelial cells, smooth muscle cells
T1/ST2 (membrane and soluble form)	Orphan receptor; negative regulator of IL-1R, TLR2, and TLR4	Th2 cells, mast cells, fibroblasts
TIGIRR (TIGIRR-1)	Orphan receptor	Skin; less in liver, placenta, fetal brain
IL-1RAPL (TIGIRR-2)	Orphan receptor; Ca²⁺-dependent inhibition of exocytosis; involved in X-linked mental retardation	Heart, brain, ovary, skin; less in tonsils, fetal liver, prostate, testis, small intestine, placenta, colon
IL-1Rrp2	Binds the agonists IL-1F6, IL-1F8, and IL-1F9, as well as IL-1F5 (antagonist of IL-1F9)	Lung, epididymis, lower levels in testis, and cerebral cortex (nonneuronal)
TIR8 (SIGIRR)	Orphan receptor; negative regulator of TLR/IL-1R signaling	Ubiquitous; highly expressed in intestinal epithelial cells

family, all of which share similar amino acid sequence, gene structure, and predicted three-dimensional fold (Table II). Of these, the best characterized are the three IL-1-like molecules (IL-1α, IL-1β, and the antagonist IL-1Ra) and IL-18, the first IL-1 homolog to be found (Bazan et al., 1996; Okamura et al., 1995).

IL-1 has been demonstrated to be a key orchestrator of the immune response playing roles in inflammatory and immune defense response, and involved in many inflammatory diseases (Dinarello, 1998). While IL-1 activates its signaling cascade upon binding to a receptor complex that includes IL-1RI and IL-1RAcP, IL-1RII serves as a negative regulator of IL-1 signaling by binding IL-1 and preventing its interaction with IL-1RI.

IL-18 is the major inducer of IFN-γ (it was originally defined as IGIF, IFN-γ-inducing factor), and plays an important role in promoting inflammatory Th1 and natural killer (NK) cell activation (Akira, 2000). For this role in inflammation, IL-18 is also involved in chronic inflammatory and autoimmune diseases (Boraschi and Dinarello, 2006; Bossù et al., 2003). As for IL-1, IL-18 activates cells upon binding to the complex IL-18Rα/ IL-18Rβ, while the soluble receptor-like molecule IL-18BP functions as decoy inhibitory binding protein (Kim et al., 2000; Novick et al., 1999).

T1/ST2 (Brint et al., 2004) and TIR8/SIGIRR (Garlanda et al., 2004; Wald et al., 2003) are receptors of the TIR superfamily which have been shown to function as negative regulators for TIR-mediated signaling. Other orphan receptors of this subgroup are still ill-characterized in their function.

The LRR subgroup consists of at least 13 TLR molecules in mammals (Chuang and Ulevitch, 2000; Hemmi et al., 2000; Medzhitov et al., 1997; Rock et al., 1998; Takeuchi et al., 1999b; Zandi et al., 1997). These receptors are structurally and functionally conserved in evolution and are present also in invertebrates (Toll was first indentified in insects; Lemaitre et al., 1996). Different TLR are activated by a limited array of microbial products/stress signals. While TLR4 is essential for the responses to lipopolysaccharide (LPS), a component of Gram-negative bacteria (Poltorak et al., 1998), and to a series of endogenous stress-related molecules, TLR2, associated either with TLR1 or with TLR6, responds to mycobacteria, yeast, Gram-positive bacteria, and lipoproteins (Ozinsky et al., 2000; Takeuchi et al., 1999a, 2000; Underhill et al., 1999a,b). TLR5 mediates the immune response to bacterial flagellins (Hayashi et al., 2001), TLR9 has been shown to recognize bacterial and viral DNA (Hemmi et al., 2000), TLR3 recognizes double-stranded RNA (dsRNA) (Alexopoulou et al., 2001), TLR7 and TLR8 are activated by ssRNA (Diebold et al., 2004; Heil et al., 2004; Lund et al., 2004), and TLR11 is involved in the recognition of uropathogenic bacteria (Zhang et al., 2004). The natural ligand for TLR10 is still unknown, while no information is available for TLR12 and -13. A summary of the TLR family of receptors (1–11) is reported in Table III.

TABLE II. The IL-1 Cytokine Family

Name	Previous	Expression	Features
IL-1F1	IL-1α	Ubiquitous	1. Binds to IL-1RI and forms complexes with IL-1RAcP; binds little to IL-1RII; does not bind to other IL-1R-like receptors 2. Membrane-bound form most common 3. Immunostimulating and inflammatory activities
IL-1F2	IL-1β	Ubiquitous	1. Binds to IL-1RI and forms complexes with IL-1RAcP; binds well to IL-1RII; does not bind to other IL-1R-like receptors 2. Soluble form 3. Immunostimulating and inflammatory activities
IL-1F3	IL-1Ra	Ubiquitous	1. Binds to IL-1RI but does not form complexes with IL-1RAcP; binds little to IL-1RII; does not bind to other IL-1R-like receptors 2. Soluble form and two intracellular forms 3. Antagonizes IL-1α and IL-1β
IL-1F4	IL-18, IGIF, IL-1γ	Monocytes, tissue macrophages, DC, Kupffer cells, osteoclasts, keratinocytes, epithelial cells, tumor cell lines	1. Binds to IL-18Rα and forms complexes with IL-18Rβ; binds to IL-18BP; does not bind other IL-1R-like receptors 2. Soluble form 3. Induction IFN-γ in Th1 and NK cells; induces TNF-α, GM-CSF, IL-8, IL-6, IL-1β, FasL expression in different cell types

IL-1F5	IL-1Hy1, FIL1δ, IL-1H3, IL-1RP3, IL-1L1, IL-1δ	Placenta, uterus, skin (also psoriatic), brain, heart, kidney, keratinocytes, monocytes, B cells, DC	1. Does not bind to IL-1RI, IL-1RAcP, IL-18R, AcPL, T1/ST2, TIGIRR, IL-1RAPL 2. Antagonizes IL-1F9 in activating NFκB through IL-1Rrp2
IL-1F6	FIL1ε	Spleen, lymph node, tonsil, leukocytes, bone marrow, fetal brain, monocytes, B cells, T cells	1. Does not bind to IL-1RI, IL-1RAcP, IL-18R, AcPL, T1/ST2, TIGIRR, IL-1RAPL 2. Binds to IL-1Rrp2 and forms complexes with IL-1RAcP, activating NF-κB
IL-1F7	FIL1ζ, IL-1H4, IL-1RP1, IL-1H	Lymph node, thymus, bone marrow, lung, testis, placenta, uterus, skin, colon, NK, monocytes, stimulated B cells, keratinocytes	1. Binds to IL-18Rα; binds to IL-18BP 2. Neither agonize nor antagonize IL-18 3. Enhances IL-18 inhibitory activity of IL-18BP possibly by sequestration of IL-18Rβ
IL-1F8	FIL1η, IL-1H2	Bone marrow, tonsil, heart, placenta, lung, testis, colon, monocytes, B cells	1. Does not bind to IL-1RI, IL-18R, AcPL, T1/ST2, TIGIRR, IL-1RAPL 2. Binds to IL-1Rrp2 and forms complexes with IL-1RAcP, activating NF-κB
IL-1F9	IL-1H1, IL-1RP2, IL-1ε	Placenta, stimulated keratinocytes, epithelial cells, squamous cell-epithelia of esophagus, psoriatic skin	1. Does not bind to IL-1RI, IL-18R, T1/ST2 2. Activates NFκB through IL-1Rrp2 together with IL-1RAcP 3. Expression upregulated during chronic contact hypersensitivity and HSV infection
IL-1F10	IL-1Hy2, FKSG75	Basal epithelia of skin, proliferating B cells in the tonsil	1. Binds to soluble IL-1RI
IL-1F11	IL-33	Dermal fibroblasts, smooth muscle cells, epithelial cells; low expression in lymphoid tissues	1. Binds to T1/ST2 2. Induces activation of NF-κB and MAP kinases 3. Induces Th-2-associated cytokine production and eosinophilia

TABLE III. TLR Receptors

Name	Ligand	Expression
TLR1	Coreceptor of TLR2	Leukocytes, lung, spleen
TLR2	Peptidoglycan, lipoteichoic acid, lipoarabinomannan, zymosan, bacterial lipoprotein, macrophage stimulatory lipopeptide 2, mannosylated soluble tuberculosis factor, modulin	Leukocytes, lung, spleen
TLR3	dsRNA	Dendritic cells, kidney, prostate, lung, small intestine, pancreas, spleen, placenta, testis
TLR4	Lipopolysaccharide, lipoteichoic acid, HSP60, taxol, fibronectin domain A, HSP70, RSV Protein F, HA fragments, β-defensin 2	Leukocytes, spleen, epithelial cells
TLR5	Flagellin	Ovary, kidney, PBL, prostate, lung, small intestine, pancreas, spleen, placenta, testis, thymus
TLR6	Coreceptor of TLR2	Leukocytes, spleen
TLR7	ssRNA, small antiviral compounds (guanine ribonucleoside analogs, imidazoquinolines)	Macrophages, lung, spleen, placenta
TLR8	ssRNA, small antiviral compounds (imidazoquinolines)	Leukocytes, lung, spleen, placenta
TLR9	Unmethylated CpG DNA	Leukocytes, ovary, spleen
TLR10	Unknown; genetic variations associated with asthma	Lymphoid tissues, B cells, plasmacytoid dendritic cells, lung
TLR11	Uropathogenic bacteria	Macrophages, epithelial cells of liver, kidney, and bladder

Part of the LLR subfamily can be considered another membrane molecule, CD180 or RP105, mainly expressed in B cells. The extracellular portion of RP105 is an LRR domain structurally similar to that of TLR, implying a role in pathogen sensing, in particular in mediating LPS effects on B cells (Miyake *et al.*, 1995; Ogata *et al.*, 2000) in concert with the accessory molecule MD-1 (Miura *et al.*, 1998). Very recent data indicate that RP105 can specifically downmodulate TLR4-mediated activation, by a mechanism dependent on its extracellular LRR domain (Divanovic *et al.*, 2005). In autoimmune patients with lupus, Sjögren's syndrome, and dermatomyositis, there is a significant increase in a population of RP105-negative B cells, which are responsible of autoantibody production (Kikuchi *et al.*, 2002; Koarada *et al.*, 2001).

A new class of intracellular pathogen-sensing molecules have been recently described, which share an LRR motif and a TIR domain with the TLR receptors. These molecules (generically defined TIR–NBS–LRR for their structure characteristics) include important defense mediators such as NOD/CARD and NALP sensors (Chamaillard *et al.*, 2003; Inohara and Nunez, 2001; Tschopp *et al.*, 2003). Mutations in NOD2/CARD15 and in NALP3 have been reported underlying severe inflammatory pathologies and autoimmunity (Aganna *et al.*, 2002; Behr *et al.*, 2004; Girardin *et al.*, 2003; Martinon and Tschopp, 2004). Evolutionarily, Toll-like intracellular molecules (such as N, L6, Rpp1, -4, -5) have been found in bacteria (where however a defense function has not been identified) and in plants where they are responsible of antiviral defense (Ausubel, 2005; Mushegian and Medzhitov, 2001) (Fig. 1).

Eventually, a series of TIR-containing intracellular adapters and signaling molecules have been described, which take part to the signaling pathway of the TIR superfamily membrane receptors. These include MyD88, Mal/TIRAP, TRIF and other recently identified molecules. Receptors of the IL-1R/IL-18R family and of the TLR family use some common adapters and some specific molecules within this group. A comprehensive analysis of the usage of adapters in the signal transduction of TIR receptors has been recently published (Akira and Takeda, 2004).

Negative regulation of TIR receptors takes place at several levels, and includes alternative forms of the active proteins, which can act as inactivating competitors. Among these there are MyD88s, and soluble forms of TLR and IL-1/IL-18 receptors, besides the already cited inhibitory receptor chains TIR8/SIGIRR, T1/ST2, and RP105 (Li and Qin, 2005; Liew *et al.*, 2005).

II. IL-1 RECEPTORS

The IL-1R is a complex of two chains, the IL-1R type I (IL-1RI) and the IL-1R accessory protein (IL-1RAcP). IL-1, the cytokine ligand of IL-1R, is a family of cytokines, which are encoded by distinct genes and are regulated independently. The agonist ligands of IL-1R are IL-1α and IL-1β, which share an overlapping spectrum of biological activities, although the latter is more abundantly expressed during the initial steps of the defense response and is one of the major effectors of inflammation (Dinarello, 1998). The third ligand is the IL-1 receptor antagonist (IL-1Ra), a molecule that resembles IL-1α and IL-1β in its amino acid sequence, three-dimensional folding pattern and gene structure (Eisenberg *et al.*, 1990; Nicklin *et al.*, 1994). IL-1Ra binds to IL-1RI but does not initiate signal transduction (Greenfeder *et al.*, 1995).

A. IL-1RI

The type I IL-1 receptor (IL-1RI) is the membrane receptor that binds the IL-1 ligands (Sims *et al.*, 1988). Its extracellular part comprises three Ig domains which contain the ligand-binding area. The cytoplasmic portion, of about 200 amino acids in length, is homologous to the cytoplasmic domains of the other members of the TIR family. IL-1RI was the first known receptor of the TIR family. The crystal structure of the extracellular portion of the IL-1RI bound to IL-1β has been solved to 2.5 Å resolution (Vigers *et al.*, 1997). It shows that the two N-terminal Ig domains of the receptor are in a quite rigid position because of an interdomain disulfide bond, whereas the third, membrane-proximal Ig domain is more flexibly connected to the other two. The receptor appears to wrap around the IL-1β molecule in such a way that IL-1 connects with the receptor in two places, a large area in the groove between the first and second domain, and a smaller area on the side of the third domain.

Binding of IL-1Ra to IL-1RI also occurs. Resolution of the X-ray crystal of the IL-1RI-IL-1Ra complex (Schreuder *et al.*, 1997) shows that IL-1Ra binds at the same site on IL-1RI as the main area of binding of IL-1β, that is, the groove between the first and second Ig domain. However, IL-1Ra fails to interact with the smaller area contacted by IL-1β in the third Ig domain. This leaves the structure of IL-1RI wrapping around IL-1Ra more extended and open as compared to that of the IL-1β-IL-1RI complex.

B. IL-1RACP

A second receptor chain is necessary for IL-1R signaling. This chain, known as the IL-1R accessory chain (IL-1RAcP), is a homolog of the IL-1RI (Cullinan *et al.*, 1998; Greenfeder *et al.*, 1995; Korherr *et al.*, 1997; Wesche *et al.*, 1997). IL-1RAcP does not bind to either IL-1α or IL-1β. However, once IL-1 has bound the IL-1RI chain, the IL-1RAcP is recruited to the ligand–receptor pair to form the high-affinity receptor complex. The approximation of the two intracellular domains of IL-1RI and IL-1RAcP consequent to the complex formation is the necessary and sufficient condition for initiation of signaling. While no experimental data are available describing the way in which IL-1RAcP binds to the IL-1–IL-1RI pair, a model for this interaction has been proposed, based on mutagenesis and antibody data (Boraschi *et al.*, 1995; Casadio *et al.*, 2001; D'Ettorre *et al.*, 1997). The model suggests that the IL-1RAcP wraps around the back surface of the IL-1RI which encloses IL-1, significantly limiting the potential areas of direct contact of the IL-1RAcP with the ligand. Thus, IL-1RAcP cannot contact either IL-1 or IL-1RI directly, but it can bind to areas of the interface IL-1–IL-1RI.

In the same modeling study, IL-1RAcP could not interact IL-1Ra–IL-1RI pair, which is structurally more relaxed than the IL-1–IL-1RI complex. This is in agreement with the finding that receptor-bound IL-1Ra cannot recruit IL-1RAcP, thus failing to form the signaling complex (Greenfeder *et al.*, 1995). The receptor antagonist action of IL-1Ra is therefore based on its ability to occupy the IL-1-binding site on IL-1RI, preventing binding of agonist IL-1α and IL-1β, and on failing to form the signaling complex with IL-1RAcP.

The presence in biological fluids of a soluble form of IL-1RAcP has been reported, which is encoded by an alternatively spliced mRNA (Greenfeder *et al.*, 1995). It can be hypothesized that the soluble IL-1RAcP could act as a negative regulator of IL-1RI activation, by forming an inactive complex with membrane IL-1RI bound to IL-1. This hypothesis was tested by Jensen *et al.* (2000), who however could demonstrate the inhibitory capacity of soluble IL-1RAcP only by artificially anchoring it in the cell membrane. However, a clear-cut inhibitory role has been described for sIL-1RAcP in synergy with the soluble form of IL-1RII (Smith *et al.*, 2003), as it will be described in more detail in the following section.

C. IL-1RII

Another receptor for IL-1 has been described, which however is unable to initiate signaling. This second receptor is called the type II IL-1R (IL-1RII) (Colotta *et al.*, 1994; McMahan *et al.*, 1991). IL-1RII is highly homologous to IL-1RI in the extracellular domain and can efficiently bind IL-1, but its cytoplasmic domain is very short, it does not contain a TIR domain, and is incapable of initiating signal transduction. The membrane receptor can be cleaved from the cell surface through the action of a specific metalloprotei-nase, releasing a soluble form of IL-1RII (sIL-1RII) (Cui *et al.*, 2003; Orlando *et al.*, 1997). The membrane IL-1RII captures IL-1 on the cell surface, while sIL-1RII uptakes IL-1 in the microenvironment, and both divert it from binding to IL-1RI on the cell surface, thus inhibiting its biological activity (Kollewe *et al.*, 2000; Neumann *et al.*, 2000). For this reason, IL-1RII has been dubbed "decoy" receptor (Colotta *et al.*, 1993, 1994). IL-1RII has a high affinity for IL-1β, but a much lower affinity for IL-1α and IL-1ra.

The high affinity for the inflammatory IL-1 and the low affinity for the IL-1 inhibitor allow IL-1RII to act as IL-1 inhibitor in coordination with IL-1Ra, without interfering with its inhibitory activity. Once bound to IL-1, the membrane form of IL-1RII can recruit IL-1RAcP into a non-signaling complex (Lang et $al.$, 1998; Malinowsky et $al.$, 1998). Thus, IL-1RII has an additional way of inhibiting IL-1 action, that is, the subtraction of the signaling chain IL-1RAcP from forming the signaling complex with IL-1RI, a mechanism called "co-receptor competition" (Lang et $al.$, 1998). This sequestration of IL-1RAcP greatly increases the inhibitory potency of IL-1RII. Indeed, whereas inhibition of IL-1β by IL-1RII could be easily overcome by increasing the ligand concentration, sequestration of the signaling chain would be more difficult to correct, as the levels of surface-expressed IL-1RAcP do not readily change. Thus, the ratio between IL-1RII and IL-1RAcP can determine the responsiveness to IL-1. In fact, overexpression of IL-1RII in IL-1-responsive cells (which express both IL-1RI and IL-1RAcP) can make them unresponsive to IL-1 (Bossù et $al.$, 1995; Re et $al.$, 1996).

A regulatory role for the soluble form of the IL-1RAcP has been proposed in forming complexes with soluble IL-1RII. The binding affinity of sIL-1RII for the agonist ligands IL-1α and IL-1β is increased by a factor 100 by sIL-1RAcP, whereas the very low affinity for the inhibitor IL-1Ra is not affected (Smith et $al.$, 2003). Thus, sIL-1RAcP greatly enhances the inhibitory capacity of sIL-1RII, functioning as an additional negative regulator of IL-1 activity.

III. IL-18 RECEPTORS

A. IL-18Rα AND IL-18Rβ

In agreement with the close relationship between IL-1 and IL-18, the receptor complex for IL-18 is remarkably similar to that for IL-1. IL-18 binds on the cell membrane to the binding receptor chain IL-18Rα, a molecule highly homologous to IL-1RI, which had been originally dubbed IL-1Rrp1 (IL-1 receptor related protein 1; Table II) (Parnet et $al.$, 1996; Torigoe et $al.$, 1997). Initial binding of IL-18 to IL-18Rα is characterized by a relatively low affinity (with a K_d around 50 nM), which however is increased over 100-fold upon recruitment of the receptor accessory protein IL-18Rβ into the receptor complex. The accessory protein of the IL-18R complex is another IL-1R homolog, initially called AcPL (Born et $al.$, 1998). Similarly to the IL-1R complex, both IL-18R chains are required for IL-18 signal transduction (Born et $al.$, 1998; Debets et $al.$, 2000). As already mentioned, IL-18Rα and IL-18Rβ are members of the Ig domain subgroup of TIR receptors (Table II), with an extracellular domain comprising three

Ig-like domains and with a TIR-containing intracellular segment responsible for signal transduction. The ligand binding chain IL-18Rα is expressed on the surface of Th1 lymphocytes and NK cells, and on a variety of other cells including macrophages and B cells, neutrophils and basophils, endothelial cells, smooth muscle cells, synovial fibroblasts, chondrocytes, and epithelial cells (Gerdes *et al.*, 2002; Gutzmer *et al.*, 2003; Yoshimoto *et al.*, 1998). After binding of IL-18 to the IL-18Rα, the accessory chain IL-18Rβ is recruited into a signaling complex (Debets *et al.*, 2000; Kim *et al.*, 2001). Signal transduction is initiated by the approximation of the TIR domains present in the intracellular segment of the receptor chains (O'Neill, 2000). The signaling pathway, shared with other receptors of the TIR superfamily, involves recruitment of the adapter molecule MyD88 and of the kinase IRAK, followed by interaction with TRAF6. Activation of IKK causes degradation of IκB and subsequent activation of NF-κB (Bowie and O'Neill, 2000; Dunne and O'Neill, 2003). Expression of chains of the IL-18R complex is upregulated by cytokines, such as IL-12 and IL-2, and inhibited by IL-4 (Neumann and Martin, 2001; Yoshimoto *et al.*, 1998). In particular, it has been shown that IL-12 can modulate cell response to IL-18 by upregulating expression of the accessory chain IL-18Rβ. True synergism of IL-12 and other cytokines with IL-18 for IFN-γ production can be mainly attributed to upregulation of IL-18Rβ (Neumann and Martin, 2001; Strengell *et al.*, 2002).

A truncated splice variant of the mRNA coding for IL-18Rβ has been detected in different brain areas and in liver, encoding for a soluble protein encompassing the first Ig domain of the receptor (Andre *et al.*, 2003). This soluble IL-18Rβ form is upregulated by LPS, but the functional activity of the encoded protein has not been described so far. A downregulatory role could be hypothesized for it, in analogy to that proposed for the soluble form of IL-1RAcP.

B. IL-18BP

Despite the similarities in the receptor complex and initiation of signaling, regulation of IL-18 action is different from that of IL-1. There is no true receptor antagonist similar to IL-1Ra, nor soluble forms of the IL-18Rα and IL-18Rβ have been yet described as having regulatory activity. Conversely, IL-18 regulation is apparently carried out by a soluble IL-18-binding protein (IL-18BP), which binds IL-18 preventing its interaction with the membrane IL-18R (Novick *et al.*, 1999). IL-18BP is a naturally occurring secreted protein, with high affinity specific binding to mature IL-18 (it does not bind the IL-18 precursor). With the exception of IL-1F7 (Bufler *et al.*, 2002), IL-18BP does not bind to other members of the IL-1 family nor to any of several cytokines tested. IL-18BP is not a soluble form of the membrane bound IL-18Rα, although it has many characteristics of a soluble receptor similar to the IL-1RII decoy receptor. Unlike most members of the IL-1 receptor family, which have three Ig-like domains in the extracellular receptor segment, IL-18BP has only one Ig-like domain. The only amino acid identity between IL-18BP and IL-18Rα is found in the third Ig domain of the α chain (Kim *et al.*, 2002). There are four isotypes of human IL-18BP and two isotypes of murine IL-18BP, formed by alternate mRNA splicing of the respective genes (Kim *et al.*, 2000). The four isotypes of human IL-18BP are termed IL-18BPa, b, c, and d. Only IL-18BPa and IL-18BPc have the intact Ig domain and neutralize IL-18 (Kim *et al.*, 2000). The isoforms IL-18BPb and IL-18BPd do not bind and do not neutralize IL-18, and their functional role is at present unknown.

IL-18BP gene expression is regulated by IFN-γ (Paulukat *et al.*, 2001). Therefore, in a Th1 response the IL-18-dependent production of IFN-γ contributes to the suppression of IFN-γ by increasing the production of IL-18BP in a self-regulating feedback loop. Elevated IL-18BP has been described in several chronic inflammatory and autoimmune diseases including rheumatoid arthritis (Bresnihan *et al.*, 2002; Kawashima *et al.*, 2001; Moller *et al.*, 2001).

Another putative regulator of IL-18 activity via binding to IL-18BP has been described, that is, the member of the IL-1 family IL-1F7. Among the several isoforms of IL-1F7, present exclusively in the human genome (Taylor *et al.*, 2002), the splice variant IL-1F7b can be cleaved by caspase-1 to give rise to a mature protein able to bind to IL-18Rα with low affinity (Kumar *et al.*, 2002). Possibly due to such low affinity, binding of IL-1F7b to IL-18Rα does not induce recruitment of the accessory chain IL-18Rβ, nor cell activation in terms of IFN-γ production. Likewise, IL-1F7b does not antagonize the IFN-γ-inducing capacity of IL-18 (Kumar *et al.*, 2002). It has been shown that IL-1F7 can bind also to IL-18BP, leading to the amplification of the capacity of IL-18BP to inhibit IL-18 (Bufler *et al.*, 2002). This can be explained by the fact that, similarly to what occurs with IL-1 bound to soluble IL-1RII (Lang *et al.*, 1998), the IL-1F7 bound to IL-18BP can form a complex with the accessory chain IL-18Rβ and subtract it from forming a functional receptor complex (Bufler *et al.*, 2002). A possible agonist activity (IL-12- and IFN-γ-dependent antitumor activity) has been also proposed for IL-1F7, based on results of *in vivo* gene transfer in the mouse (Gao *et al.*, 2003).

IV. RECEPTORS THAT DOWNREGULATE SIGNALING

A. TIR8/SIGIRR

TIR8/SIGIRR is a unique receptor of the IL-1R/IL-18R superfamily which, at variance with other members of the family, encompasses a single

Ig-like domain in its extracellular portion (Thomassen *et al.*, 1999). The intracellular domain of TIR8/SIGIRR has the highest similarity to the intracellular adapter MyD88 among members of the TIR superfamily (Du *et al.*, 2000). TIR8/SIGIRR does not interact with IL-1α, IL-1β, or IL-1Ra, and its intracellular domain is unable to transduce signal (Thomassen *et al.*, 1999). On the other hand, TIR8/SIGIRR apparently plays a central role in the downregulation of inflammation mediated by TIR receptors. TIR8/SIGIRR-deficient mice and cells are more susceptible to stimulation with IL-1, IL-18, and TLR agonists (LPS, CpG oligonucleotides), whereas TIR8/SIGIRR-overexpressing cells are less susceptible to IL-1 and IL-18 stimulation (Garlanda *et al.*, 2004; Wald *et al.*, 2003). TIR8/SIGIRR expression is ubiquitous; however, it is abundantly expressed by epithelial cells (kidney, gut, liver) and is possibly involved in the control of intestinal inflammation (Polentarutti *et al.*, 2003; Garlanda *et al.*, 2004). On the other hand, expression of TIR8/SIGIRR is poor in leukocytes and cannot be induced by a series of inflammatory/anti-inflammatory stimuli (Polentarutti *et al.*, 2003). Notably, expression of TIR8/SIGIRR in the mouse is significantly decreased in every organ/cell by *in vivo* administration of LPS (Polentarutti *et al.*, 2003). The mechanism by which TIR8/SIGIRR downregulates TIR receptor-mediated activation is based on the ability of the TIR-containing intracellular domain of TIR8/SIGIRR to compete for the signaling intermediates IRAK1 and TRAF6, thus subtracting them from the signal transduction pathway of TLR/IL-1R (Wald *et al.*, 2003).

B. T1/ST2

T1/ST2 is a receptor of the Ig-domain subgroup which, at variance with other receptors but similarly to TIR8/SIGIRR, does not induce an inflammatory response (Trajkovic *et al.*, 2004; Yanagisawa *et al.*, 1993). T1/ST2 was found unable to bind members of the IL-1 family such as IL-1 and IL-18 (Dunn *et al.*, 2001; Gayle *et al.*, 1996). A putative ligand of T1/ST2 has been identified, a membrane protein which however does not trigger receptor-mediated TIR-dependent NF-κB activation (Gayle *et al.*, 1996). Recently, the newly identified member of the IL-1 family IL-33 (or IL-1F11) was shown to bind to T1/ST2 and to trigger Th2-associated responses (Schmitz *et al.*, 2005). Besides the membrane form of the receptor (ST2L), two alternatively spliced forms have been identified, the soluble ST2, corresponding to the extracellular domain of the membrane receptor (Li *et al.*, 2000), and the membrane-anchored ST2V protein (Tago *et al.*, 2001). T1/ST2 is preferentially expressed by fibroblasts, mast cells, and Th2 cells (as opposed to Th1 cells which selectively express the IL-18R) (Lohning *et al.*, 1998; Xu *et al.*, 1998), and is involved in Th2 anti-inflammatory/allergic effector function (Coyle *et al.*, 1999; Lohning *et al.*, 1998; Schmitz *et al.*, 2005;

Townsend *et al.*, 2000). T1/ST2 has regulatory functions as it can down-regulate TLR2, TLR4, TLR9, and IL-1RI signaling, but not the MyD88-independent TLR3 signal transduction, based on the capacity of sequestering the adapters MyD88 and Mal through the intracellular TIR domain (Brint *et al.*, 2004; Sweet *et al.*, 2001). It could be therefore hypothesized that all signaling pathways involving MyD88 and/or Mal can be downregulated by T1/ST2. In addition, T1/ST2 can down-regulate TLR- and IL-1R-dependent inflammatory activation indirectly, by stimulating production of anti-inflammatory Th2-associated cytokines (Schmitz *et al.*, 2005). Physiological-ly, T1/ST2 is induced by inflammatory stimuli and is apparently involved in the late control of the inflammatory response (which explains its function in anti-inflammatory Th2 cells), including endotoxin tolerance (Brint *et al.*, 2004; Sweet *et al.*, 2001). In human pathologies, expression of T1/ST2 in human breast tumors is predictive of relapse-free survival (Prechtel *et al.*, 2001). Soluble T1/ST2, which is also an inhibitor of inflammation by un-known mechanisms (Leung *et al.*, 2004; Sweet *et al.*, 2001), was found at increased levels in serum of patients with pulmonary inflammation (Tajima *et al.*, 2003), heart failure (Weinberg *et al.*, 2003), and autoimmune lupus (Kuroiwa *et al.*, 2001).

V. OTHER IL-1R-LIKE RECEPTORS

Other members of the Ig-domain subgroup of the TIR family are some orphan receptors mainly identified by sequence similarity with known members of the family, and whose function is still a matter of investigation. These are TIGIRR, IL-1RAPL, and IL-1Rrp2.

A. TIGIRR

TIGIRR (also known as TIGIRR-1) was identified by sequence searches (Born *et al.*, 2000; Jin *et al.*, 2000; Sana *et al.*, 2000). It is highly similar to IL-1RAPL (about 63% amino acid identity) and both are encoded by very large genes on the X chromosome (TIGIRR on Xq, IL-1RAPL on Xp). No ligand has been identified for TIGIRR, whose extracellular domain is unable to bind any of the IL-1 family molecules (Sana *et al.*, 2000; Smith *et al.*, 2000). Likewise, the intracellular domain of TIGIRR (as demonstrated with chimeric constructs with the extracellular domain of IL-1R) is unable to mediate signaling.

B. IL-1RAPL

The IL-1RAPL molecule (or TIGIRR-2) was also discovered in a search of DNA sequence databases, while seeking the gene responsible for hereditary nonsyndromic mental retardation linked to chromosome region Xp22.1-21.3, that was identified as the IL-1RAPL (Born *et al.*, 2000; Carrié *et al.*, 1999; Jin *et al.*, 2000). IL-1RAPL is abundantly expressed in brain structures involved in the hippocampal memory system (hippocampus, dentate gyrus, entorhinal cortex), leading to hypothesize its possible role in brain development and/or memory and learning function (Carrié *et al.*, 1999). As for TIGIRR, no immune-related functions can be ascribed to this receptor so far, as no IL-1 family ligand, nor IL-1R-like signaling capacity has been identified (Born *et al.*, 2000; Smith *et al.*, 2000). The link of IL-1RAPL to brain homeostasis seems to suggest that mammalian TIR proteins, as it occurs in *Drosophila*, may take part in development, in addition to host defense, in different stages of the life cycle (Carrié *et al.*, 1999).

C. IL-1RRP2

The function of another receptor of the Ig-domain subgroup, IL-1Rrp2 (IL-1 receptor-related protein 2), is beginning to be clarified. Cells hyperexpressing IL-1Rrp2 can be activated (NF-κB activation) upon exposure to IL-1F9, a novel member of the IL-1 cytokine family (Debets *et al.*, 2001) and also to the other IL-1-like molecules IL-1F6 and IL-1F8 (Towne *et al.*, 2004). NF-κB activation takes place only with the cooperation of IL-1RAcP, which acts as coreceptor. IL-1Rrp2-transfected cells are not activated by another member of the IL-1 cytokine family, IL-1F5, which however can inhibit IL-1F9-dependent IL-1Rrp2-mediated activation. Thus, it appears that IL-1F9 and IL-1F5 act as agonist and antagonist ligands for IL-1Rrp2, similarly to the competitive binding of IL-1 and IL-1Ra to IL-1RI.

VI. CONCLUSIONS

The TIR superfamily is a group of structurally homologous receptor proteins of key importance in the mechanisms of host innate defense against infection, inflammation, injury, and stress (Bowie and O'Neill, 2000; O'Neill, 2000; O'Neill and Greene, 1998). The TIR proteins are characterized by the presence of an ancient intracellular Toll/IL-1R (TIR) domain that initiates signaling via a common pathway shared by invertebrates and vertebrates (Fallon *et al.*, 2001). Indeed, the protein Toll, after which is named the TIR domain, is an antifungal defense receptor of *Drosophila melanogaster* (Gay and Keith, 1991). Most TIR-domain–containing proteins are membrane receptors, but several are intracellular proteins including some adapters (e.g., MyD88) involved in the signaling pathway of the membrane TIR receptors, while others are intracellular sensing molecules that function as receptors in recognizing danger signals and in initiating activation. Several plant TIR proteins and the mammalian NOD/CARD proteins belong to this subclass of TIR molecules. TIR domains apparently are highly conserved in evolution, as TIR-containing proteins have been identified in mammals, birds, bony fish, tunicates, insects, nematodes, and plants. Besides the defense function, some TIR proteins (e.g., the *Drosophila* Toll, and in general invertebrate TIR-containing proteins) have an additional role in differentiation during embryonal life (e.g., dorsal-ventral polarization for Toll) (Anderson *et al.*, 1985a,b; Lemaitre *et al.*, 1996). A Toll homolog identified in *C. elegans*, tol-1, is important both for development and in pathogen recognition (where it participates to the danger avoidance behavior) (Pujol *et al.*, 2001). The same occurs in plants, where the TIR proteins have both developmental and defense functions (Hulbert *et al.*, 2001). On the other hand, fish, avian, and mammalian TIR proteins (such as IL-1R and TLR) have principally if not solely a defense function against microbial agents and during inflammation. The presence of TIR domain-containing receptors across taxanomic kingdoms suggests the importance of activating defense responses both in plants and animals (Johnson *et al.*, 2003). Tolls appeared about 1000 million years ago (Kimbrell and Beutler, 2001), long after separation of animals and plants (dating back another 1000 million years), with present Toll and vertebrate TLR molecules probably derived from a single ancestor (Luo and Zheng, 2000). That animal Tolls derive from plant TIR-containing receptors is unclear. If, from one side, the TIR conservation could be due to their key role in host defense against danger, on the other hand it is well possible that plant and animal TIR-containing genes have evolved separately, structural convergence being due to the common function to which they are devoted, implying that the TIR structure is the best defense effector possible (Ausubel, 2005).

IL-1R/IL-18R molecules are much more recent than Tolls, as the IL-1 molecules are also defense effectors present exclusively in vertebrates. Besides mammals, IL-1 has been identified and cloned in birds (Weining *et al.*, 1998), amphibians (Zou *et al.*, 2000), bony (Zou *et al.*, 1999) and cartilaginous fish (Bird *et al.*, 2002). Likewise, IL-1RI has been cloned in birds (Guida *et al.*, 1992), and both IL-1RI and IL-1RII in bony fish (Sangrador-Vegas *et al.*, 2000; Subramaniam *et al.*, 2002). Very few and indirect evidence seems to suggest the possible presence of IL-1-like molecules in invertebrates (Beck *et al.*, 2000; Ottaviani *et al.*, 1995).

Thus, it appears that the IL-1 receptor family (the Ig-domain subgroup of the TIR receptors) is a relatively new and more specific defense mechanism that has evolved quite recently from Toll/TLR. Its function, closely linked to the appearance in higher vertebrates of adaptive immunity (immunoglobulins), is that of bridging immediate nonspecific innate responses to the later, highly specific and potent adaptive immunity.

REFERENCES

Aganna, E., Martinon, F., Hawkins, P. N., Ross, J. B., Swan, D. C., Booth, D. R., Lachmann, H. J., Bybee, A., Gaudet, R., Woo, P., et al. (2002). Association of mutations in the NALP3/CIAS1/PYPAF1 gene with a broad phenotype including recurrent fever, cold sensitivity, sensorineural deafness, and AA amyloidosis. Arthritis Rheum. **46**, 2445–2452.

Akira, S. (2000). The role of IL-18 in innate immunity. Curr. Opin. Immunol. **12**, 59–63.

Akira, S., and Takeda, K. (2004). Toll-like receptor signalling. Nat. Rev. Immunol. **4**, 499–511.

Alexopoulou, L., Holt, A. C., Medzhitov, R., and Flavell, A. (2001). Recognition of double-stranded RNA and activation of NF-κB by Toll-like receptor 3. Nature **413**, 732–738.

Anderson, K. V., Bokla, L., and Nusslein-Volhard, C. (1985a). Establishment of dorsal-ventral polarity in the Drosophila embryo: The induction of polarity by the Toll gene product. Cell **42**, 791–798.

Anderson, K. V., Jurgens, G., and Nusslein-Volhard, C. (1985b). Establishment of dorsal-ventral polarity in the Drosophila embryo: Genetic studies on the role of the Toll gene product. Cell **42**, 779–789.

Andre, R., Wheeler, R. D., Collins, P. D., Luheshi, G. N., Pickering-Brown, S., Kimber, I., Rothwell, N. J., and Pinteaux, E. (2003). Identification of a truncated IL-18Rβ mRNA: A putative regulator of IL-18 expressed in rat brain. J. Neuroimmunol. **145**, 40–45.

Ausubel, F. M. (2005). Are innate immune signaling pathways in plants and animals conserved? Nat. Immunol. **6**, 973–979.

Bazan, J. F., Timans, J. C., and Kastelein, R. A. (1996). A newly defined interleukin-1? Nature **379**, 591.

Beck, G., Ellis, T. W., and Truong, N. (2000). Characterization of an IL-1 receptor from Asterias forbesi coelomocytes. Cell. Immunol. **203**, 66–73.

Behr, M. A., Semret, M., Poon, A., and Schurr, E. (2004). Crohn's disease, mycobacteria, and NOD2. Lancet Infect. Dis. **4**, 136–137.

Bird, S., Wang, T., Zou, J., Cunningham, C., and Secombes, C. J. (2002). The first cytokine sequence within cartilaginous fish: IL-1β in the small spotted catshark (Scyliorhinus canicula). J. Immunol. **168**, 3329–3340.

Boraschi, D., and Dinarello, C. A. (2006). IL-18 in autoimmunity. Eur. Cytokine Netw. in press.

Boraschi, D., Bossù, P., Ruggiero, P., Tagliabue, A., Bertini, R., Macchia, G., Gasbarro, C., Pellegrini, L., Melillo, G., Ulisse, E., Visconti, U., Bizzarri, C., et al. (1995). Mapping of receptor binding sites on IL-1β by reconstruction of IL-1ra-like domains. J. Immunol. **155**, 4719–4725.

Born, T. L., Thomassen, E., Bird, T. A., and Sims, J. E. (1998). Cloning of a novel receptor subunit, AcPL, required for interleukin-18 signaling. J. Biol. Chem. **273**, 29445–29450.

Born, T. L., Smith, D. E., Garka, K. E., Renshaw, B. R., Bertles, J. S., and Sims, J. E. (2000). Identification and characterization of two members of a novel class of the interleukin-1 receptor (IL-1R) family. Delineation of a new class of IL-1R-related proteins based on signaling. J. Biol. Chem. **275**, 29946–29954.

Bossù, P., Visconti, U., Ruggiero, P., Macchia, G., Muda, M., Bertini, R., Bizzarri, C., Colagrande, A., Sabbatini, V., Maurizi, G., Del Grosso, E., Tagliabue, A., et al. (1995). Transfected IL-1R$_{II}$ impairs responsiveness of human keratinocytes to IL-1. Am. J. Pathol. **147**, 1852–1861.

Bossù, P., Neumann, D., Del Giudice, E., Ciaramella, A., Gloaguen, I., Fantuzzi, G., Dinarello, C. A., Di Carlo, E., Musiani, P., Meroni, P. L., Caselli, G., Ruggiero, P., et al. (2003). IL-18 cDNA vaccination protects mice from spontaneous lupus-like autoimmune disease. Proc. Natl. Acad. Sci. USA **100**, 14181–14186.

Bowie, A., and O'Neill, L. A. (2000). The interleukin-1 receptor/Toll-like receptor superfamily: Signal generators for pro-inflammatory interleukins and microbial products. J. Leukoc. Biol. **67**, 508–514.

Bresnihan, B., Roux-Lombard, P., Murphy, E., Kane, D., FitzGerald, O., and Dayer, J. M. (2002). Serum interleukin 18 and interleukin 18 binding protein in rheumatoid arthritis. *Ann. Rheum. Dis.* **61,** 726–729.

Brint, E. K., Xu, D., Liu, H., Dunne, A., McKenzie, A. N., O'Neill, L. A., and Liew, F. Y. (2004). ST2 is an inhibitor of interleukin 1 receptor and Toll-like receptor 4 signaling and maintains endotoxin tolerance. *Nat. Immunol.* **5,** 373–379.

Bufler, P., Azam, T., Gamboni-Robertson, F., Reznikov, L. L., Kumar, S., Dinarello, C. A., and Kim, S. H. (2002). A complex of the IL-1 homologue IL-1F7b and IL-18-binding protein reduces IL-18 activity. *Proc. Natl. Acad. Sci. USA* **99,** 13723–13728.

Carrié, A., Jun, L., Bienvenu, T., Vinet, M. C., McDonell, N., Couvert, P., Zemni, R., Cardona, A., Van Buggenhout, G., Frints, S., Hamel, B., Moraine, C., *et al.* (1999). A new member of the IL-1 receptor family highly expressed in hippocampus and involved in X-linked mental retardation. *Nat. Genet.* **23,** 25–31.

Casadio, R., Frigimelica, E., Bossù, P., Neumann, D., Martin, M. U., Tagliabue, A., and Boraschi, D. (2001). Model of interaction of the IL-1 receptor accessory protein IL-1RAcP with the IL-1β/IL-1R(I) complex. *FEBS Lett.* **499,** 65–68.

Chamaillard, M., Girardin, S. E., Viala, J., and Philpott, D. J. (2003). Nods, Nalps and Naip: Intracellular regulators of bacterial-induced inflammation. *Cell. Microbiol.* **5,** 581–592.

Chuang, T. H., and Ulevitch, R. J. (2000). Cloning and characterization of a sub-family of human toll-like receptors: hTLR7, hTLR8 and hTLR9. *Eur. Cytokine Netw.* **11,** 372–378.

Colotta, F., Re, F., Muzio, M., Bertini, R., Polentarutti, N., Sironi, M., Giri, J. G., Dower, S. K., Sims, J. E., and Mantovani, A. (1993). Interleukin-1 type II receptor: A decoy target for IL-1 that is regulated by IL-4. *Science* **261,** 472–475.

Colotta, F., Dower, S. K., Sims, J. E., and Mantovani, A. (1994). The type II 'decoy' receptor: A novel regulatory pathway for interleukin 1. *Immunol. Today* **15,** 562–566.

Coyle, A. J., Lloyd, C., Tian, J., Nguyen, T., Erikkson, C., Wang, L., Ottoson, P., Persson, P., Delaney, T., Lehar, S., Lin, S., Poisson, L., *et al.* (1999). Crucial role of the interleukin 1 receptor family member T1/ST2 in T helper cell type 2-mediated lung mucosal immune responses. *J. Exp. Med.* **190,** 895–902.

Cui, X., Rouhani, F. N., Hawari, F., and Levine, S. J. (2003). Shedding of the type II IL-1 decoy receptor requires a multifunctional aminopeptidase, aminopeptidase regulator of TNF receptor type 1 shedding. *J. Immunol.* **171,** 6814–6819.

Cullinan, E. B., Kwee, L., Nunes, P., Shuster, D. J., Ju, G., McIntyre, K. W., Chizzonite, R. A., and Labow, M. A. (1998). IL-1 receptor accessory protein is an essential component of the IL-1 receptor. *J. Immunol.* **161,** 5614–5620.

Debets, R., Timans, J. C., Churakowa, T., Zurawski, S., de Waal Malefyt, R., Moore, K. W., Abrams, J. S., O'Garra, A., Bazan, J. F., and Kastelein, R. A. (2000). IL-18 receptors, their role in ligand binding and function: Anti-IL-1RAcPL antibody, a potent antagonist of IL-18. *J. Immunol.* **165,** 4950–4956.

Debets, R., Timans, J. C., Homey, B., Zurawski, S., Sana, T. R., Lo, S., Wagner, J., Edwards, G., Clifford, T., Menon, S., Bazan, J. F., and Kastelein, R. A. (2001). Two novel IL-1 family members, IL-1δ and IL-1ε, function as an antagonist and agonist of NF-κB activation through the orphan IL-1 receptor-related protein 2. *J. Immunol.* **167,** 1440–1446.

D'Ettorre, C., De Chiara, G., Casadei, R., Boraschi, D., and Tagliabue, A. (1997). Functional epitope mapping of human interleukin 1β by surface plasmon resonance. *Eur. Cytokine Netw.* **8,** 161–171.

Diebold, S. S., Kaisho, T., Hemmi, H., Akira, S., and Reis e Sousa, C. (2004). Innate antiviral responses by means of TLR7-mediated recognition of single-stranded RNA. *Science* **303,** 1529–1531.

Dinarello, C. A. (1998). Interleukin-1, interleukin-1 receptors and interleukin-1 receptor antagonist. *Int. Rev. Immunol.* **16,** 457–499.

Divanovic, S., Trompette, A., Atabani, S. F., Madan, R., Golenbock, D. T., Visintin, A., Finberg, R. W., Tarakhovsky, A., Vogel, S. N., Belkaid, J., Kurt-Jones, E. A., and Karp, C. L. (2005). Negative regulation of Toll-like receptor 4 signaling by the Toll-like receptor homolog RP105. *Nat. Immunol.* **6,** 571–578.

Du, X., Poltorak, A., Wei, Y., and Beutler, B. (2000). Three novel mammalian toll-like receptors: Gene structure, expression, and evolution. *Eur. Cytokine Netw.* **11,** 362–371.

Dunn, E., Sims, J. E., Nicklin, M. J., and O'Neill, L. A. (2001). Annotating genes with potential roles in the immune system: Six new members of the IL-1 family. *Trends Immunol.* **22,** 533–536.

Dunne, A., and O'Neill, L. A. (2003). The interleukin-1 receptor/Toll-like receptor superfamily: Signal transduction during inflammation and host defense. *Sci. STKE* **2003,** re3.

Eisenberg, S. P., Evans, R. J., Arend, W. P., Verderber, E., Brewer, M. T., Hannum, C. H., and Thompson, R. C. (1990). Primary structure and functional expression from complementary DNA of a human interleukin-1 receptor antagonist. *Nature* **343,** 341–346.

Fallon, P. G., Allen, R. L., and Rich, T. (2001). Primitive Toll signaling: Bugs, flies, worms and man. *Trends Immunol.* **22,** 63–66.

Gao, W., Kumar, S., Lotze, M. T., Hanning, C., Robbins, P. D., and Gambotto, A. (2003). Innate immunity mediated by the cytokine IL-1 homologue 4 (IL-1H4/IL-1F7) induces IL-12-dependent adaptive and profound antitumor immunity. *J. Immunol.* **170,** 107–113.

Garlanda, C., Riva, F., Polentarutti, N., Buracchi, C., Sironi, M., De Bortoli, M., Muzio, M., Bergottini, R., Scanziani, E., Vecchi, A., Hirsch, E., and Mantovani, A. (2004). Intestinal inflammation in mice deficient in Tir8, an inhibitory member of the IL-1 receptor family. *Proc. Natl. Acad. Sci. USA* **101,** 3522–3526.

Gay, N. J., and Keith, F. J. (1991). *Drosophila* Toll and IL-1 receptor. *Nature* **351,** 355–356.

Gayle, M. A., Slack, J. L., Bonnert, T. P., Renshaw, B. R., Sonoda, G., Taguchi, T., Testa, J. R., Dower, S. K., and Sims, J. E. (1996). Cloning of a putative ligand for the T1/ST2 receptor. *J. Biol. Chem.* **271,** 5784–5789.

Gerdes, N., Sukhova, G. K., Libby, P., Reynolds, R. S., Young, J. L., and Schonbeck, U. (2002). Expression of interleukin (IL)-18 and functional IL-18 receptor on human vascular endothelial cells, smooth muscle cells, and macrophages: Implications for atherogenesis. *J. Exp. Med.* **195,** 245–257.

Girardin, S. E., Hugot, J. P., and Sansonetti, P. J. (2003). Lessons from Nod2 studies: Towards a link between Crohn's disease and bacterial sensing. *Trends Immunol.* **24,** 652–658.

Greenfeder, S. A., Nunes, P., Kwee, L., Labow, M., Chizzonite, R. A., and Ju, G. (1995). Molecular cloning and characterization of a second subunit of the interleukin 1 receptor complex. *J. Biol. Chem.* **270,** 13757–13765.

Guida, S., Heguy, A., and Melli, M. (1992). The chicken IL-1 receptor: Differential evolution of the cytoplasmic and extracellular domains. *Gene* **111,** 239 243.

Gutzmer, R., Langer, K., Mommert, S., Wittmann, M., Kapp, A., and Werfel, T. (2003). Human dendritic cells express the IL-18R and are chemoattracted to IL-18. *J. Immunol.* **171,** 6363–6371.

Hayashi, F., Smith, K. D., Ozinsky, A., Hawn, T. R., Yi, E. C., Goodlett, D. R., Eng, J. K., Akira, S., Underhill, D. M., and Aderem, A. (2001). The innate immune response to bacterial flagellin is mediated by Toll-like receptor 5. *Nature* **410,** 1099–1103.

Heil, F., Hemmi, H., Hochrein, H., Ampenberger, F., Kirschning, C., Akira, S., Lipford, G., Wagner, H., and Bauer, S. (2004). Species-specific recognition of single-stranded RNA via Toll-like receptor 7 and 8. *Science* **303,** 1526–1529.

Hemmi, H., Takeuchi, O., Kawai, T., Kaisho, T., Sato, S., Sanjo, H., Matsumoto, M., Hoshino, K., Wagner, H., Takeda, K., and Akira, S. (2000). A Toll-like receptor recognizes bacterial DNA. *Nature* **408,** 740–745.

Hulbert, S. H., Webb, C. A., Smith, S. M., and Sun, Q. (2001). Resistance gene complexes: Evolution and utilization. *Annu. Rev. Phytopathol.* **39,** 285–312.

Inohara, N., and Nunez, G. (2001). The NOD: A signaling module that regulates apoptosis and host defense against pathogens. *Oncogene* **20**, 6473–6481.

Jensen, L. E., Muzio, M., Mantovani, A., and Whitehead, A. S. (2000). IL-1 signaling cascade in liver cells and the involvement of a soluble form of the IL-1 receptor accessory protein. *J. Immunol.* **164**, 5277–5286.

Jin, H., Gardner, R. J., Viswesvaraiah, R., Muntoni, F., and Roberts, R. G. (2000). Two novel members of the interleukin-1 receptor gene family, one deleted in Xp22. 1–Xp21. 3 mental retardation. *Eur. J. Hum. Genet.* **8**, 87–94.

Johnson, G. B., Brunn, G. J., Tang, A. H., and Platt, J. L. (2003). Evolutionary clues to the functions of the Toll-like family as surveillance receptors. *Trends Immunol.* **24**, 19–24.

Kawashima, M., Yamamura, M., Taniai, M., Yamauchi, H., Tanimoto, T., Kurimoto, M., Miyawaki, S., Amano, T., Takeuchi, T., and Makino, H. (2001). Levels of interleukin-18 and its binding inhibitors in the blood circulation of patients with adult-onset Still's disease. *Arthritis Rheum.* **44**, 550–560.

Kikuchi, Y., Koarada, S., Tada, Y., Ushiyama, O., Morito, F., Suzuki, N., Ohta, A., Miyake, K., Kimoto, M., Horiuchi, T., and Nagasawa, K. (2002). RP105-lacking B cells from lupus patients are responsible for the production of immunoglobulins and autoantibodies. *Arthritis Rheum.* **46**, 3259–3265.

Kimbrell, D. A., and Beutler, B. (2001). The evolution and genetics of innate immunity. *Nat. Rev. Genet.* **2**, 256–267.

Kim, S. H., Eisenstein, M., Reznikov, L., Fantuzzi, G., Novick, D., Rubinstein, M., and Dinarello, C. A. (2000). Structural requirements of six naturally occurring isoforms of the IL-18 binding protein to inhibit IL-18. *Proc. Natl. Acad. Sci. USA* **97**, 1190–1195.

Kim, S. H., Reznikov, L. L., Stuyt, R. J., Selzman, C. H., Fantuzzi, G., Hoshino, T., Young, H. A., and Dinarello, C. A. (2001). Functional reconstitution and regulation of IL-18 activity by the IL-18Rβ chain. *J. Immunol.* **166**, 148–154.

Kim, S. H., Azam, T., Novick, D., Yoon, D. Y., Reznikov, L. L., Bufler, P., Rubinstein, M., and Dinarello, C. A. (2002). Identification of amino acid residues critical for biological activity in human interleukin-18. *J. Biol. Chem.* **277**, 10998–11003.

Koarada, S., Tada, Y., Kikuchi, Y., Ushiyama, O., Suzuki, N., Ohta, A., and Nagasawa, K. (2001). CD180 (RP105) in rheumatic diseases. *Rheumatology* **40**, 1315–1316.

Kollewe, C., Neumann, D., and Martin, M. U. (2000). The first two N-terminal immunoglobulin-like domains of soluble human IL-1 receptor type II are sufficient to bind and neutralize IL-1β. *FEBS Lett.* **29**, 189–193.

Korherr, C., Hofmeister, R., Wesche, H., and Falk, W. (1997). A critical role for interleukin-1 receptor accessory protein in interleukin-1 signaling. *Eur. J. Immunol.* **27**, 262–267.

Kumar, S., Hanning, C. R., Brigham-Burke, M. R., Rieman, D. J., Lehr, R., Khandekar, S., Kirkpatrick, R. B., Scott, G. F., Lee, J. C., Lynch, F. J., Gao, W., Gambotto, A., *et al.* (2002). Interleukin-1F7B (IL-1H4/IL-1F7) is processed by caspase-1 and mature IL-1F7B binds to the IL-18 receptor but does not induce IFN-γ production. *Cytokine* **18**, 61–71.

Kuroiwa, K., Arai, T., Okazaki, H., Minota, S., and Tominaga, S. (2001). Identification of human ST2 protein in the sera of patients with autoimmune diseases. *Biochem. Biophys. Res. Commun.* **284**, 1104–1108.

Lang, D., Knop, J., Wesche, H., Raffetseder, U., Kurrle, R., Boraschi, D., and Martin, M. U. (1998). The type II interleukin-1 receptor interacts with the interleukin-1 receptor accessory protein: A novel mechanism of regulation of the interleukin-1 responsiveness. *J. Immunol.* **161**, 6871–6877.

Lemaitre, B., Nicolas, E., Michaut, L., Reichhart, J. M., and Hoffmann, J. A. (1996). The dorsoventral regulatory gene cassette spatzle/Toll/cactus controls the potent antifungal response in *Drosophila* adults. *Cell* **86**, 973–983.

Leung, B. P., Xy, D., Culshaw, S., McInnes, I. B., and Liew, F. Y. (2004). A novel therapy of murine collagen-induced arthritis with soluble T1/ST2. *J. Immunol.* **173**, 145–150.

Li, H., Tago, K., Io, K., Kuroiwa, K., Arai, T., Iwahana, H., Tominaga, S., and Yanagisawa, K. (2000). The cloning and nucleotide sequence of human ST2L cDNA. *Genomics* **67**, 284–290.

Li, X., and Qin, J. (2005). Modulation of Toll-interleukin 1 receptor mediated signaling. *J. Mol. Med.* **83**, 258–266.

Liew, F. Y., Xu, D., Brint, E. K., and O'Neill, L. A. J. (2005). Negative regulation of Toll-like receptor-mediated immune responses. *Nat. Rev. Immunol.* **5**, 446–458.

Lohning, M., Stroehmann, A., Coyle, A. J., Grogan, J. L., Lin, S., Gutierrez-Ramos, J. C., Levinson, D., Radbruch, A., and Kamradt, T. (1998). T1/ST2 is preferentially expressed on murine Th2 cells, independent of interleukin 4, interleukin 5, and interleukin 10, and important for Th2 effector function. *Proc. Natl. Acad. Sci. USA* **95**, 6930–6935.

Lund, J., Alexopoulou, M. L., Sato, A., Karow, M., Adams, N. C., Gale, N. W., Iwasaki, A., and Flavell, R. A. (2004). Recognition of single-stranded RNA viruses by Toll-like receptor 7. *Proc. Natl. Acad. Sci. USA* **101**, 5598–5603.

Luo, C., and Zheng, L. (2000). Independent evolution of Toll and related genes in insects and mammals. *Immunogenetics* **51**, 92–98.

Malinowsky, D., Lundkvist, J., Laye, S., and Bartfai, T. (1998). Interleukin-1 receptor accessory protein interacts with the type II interleukin-1 receptor. *FEBS Lett.* **429**, 299–302.

Martinon, F., and Tschopp, J. (2004). Inflammatory caspases: Linking an intracellular innate immune system to autoinflammatory diseases. *Cell* **117**, 561–574.

McMahan, C. J., Slack, J. L., Mosley, B., Cosman, D., Lupton, S. D., Brunton, L. L., Grubin, C. E., Wignall, J. M., Jenkins, N. A., Brannan, C. I., Copeland, N. G., Huebner, K., *et al.* (1991). A novel IL-1 receptor, cloned from B cells by mammalian expression, is expressed in many cell types. *EMBO J.* **10**, 2821–2832.

Medzhitov, R., Preston-Hurlburt, P., and Janeway, C. A., Jr. (1997). A human homologue of the *Drosophila* Toll protein signals activation of adaptive immunity. *Nature* **388**, 394–397.

Mitcham, J. L., Parnet, P., Bonnert, T. P., Garka, K. E., Gerhart, M. J., Slack, J. L., Gayle, M. A., Dower, S. K., and Sims, J. E. (1996). T1/ST2 signaling establishes it as a member of an expanding interleukin-1 receptor family. *J. Biol. Chem.* **271**, 5777–5783.

Miura, Y., Shimazu, R., Miyake, K., Akashi, S., Ogata, H., Yamashita, Y., Narisawa, Y., and Kimoto, M. (1998). RP105 is associated with MD-1 and transmits an activation signal in human B cells. *Blood* **92**, 2815–2822.

Miyake, K., Yamashita, Y., Ogata, M., Sudo, T., and Kimoto, M. (1995). RP105, a novel B cell surface molecule implicated in B cell activation, is a member of the leucine-rich repeat protein family. *J. Immunol.* **154**, 3333–3340.

Moller, B., Kukoc-Zivojnov, N., Kessler, U., Rehart, S., Kaltwasser, J. P., Hoelzer, D., Kalina, U., and Ottmann, O. G. (2001). Expression of interleukin-18 and its monokine-directed function in rheumatoid arthritis. *Rheumatology (Oxford)* **40**, 302–309.

Mushegian, A., and Medzhitov, R. (2001). Evolutionary perspective on innate immune recognition. *J. Cell Biol.* **155**, 705–710.

Neumann, D., and Martin, M. U. (2001). Interleukin-12 upregulates the IL-18Rβ chain in BALB/c thymocytes. *J. Interferon Cytokine Res.* **21**, 635–642.

Neumann, D., Kollewe, C., Martin, M. U., and Boraschi, D. (2000). The membrane form of the type II IL-1 receptor accounts for inhibitory function. *J. Immunol.* **165**, 3350–3357.

Nicklin, M. J., Weith, A., and Duff, G. W. (1994). A physical map of the region encompassing the human interleukin-1α, interleukin-1β, and interleukin-1 receptor antagonist genes. *Genomics* **19**, 382–384.

Novick, D., Kim, S. H., Fantuzzi, G., Reznikov, L. L., Dinarello, C. A., and Rubinstein, M. (1999). Interleukin-18 binding protein: A novel modulator of the Th1 cytokine response. *Immunity* **10**, 127–136.

Ogata, H., Su, I., Miyake, K., Nagai, Y., Akashi, S., Mecklenbrauker, I., Rajewsky, K., Kimoto, M., and Tarakhovsky, A. (2000). The toll-like receptor protein RP105 regulates lipopolysaccharide signaling in B cells. *J. Exp. Med.* **192**, 23–29.

Okamura, H., Tsutsui, H., Komatsu, T., Yutsudo, M., Hakura, A., Tanimoto, T., Torigoe, K., Okura, T., Nukada, Y., Hattori, K., Akita, K., Namba, M., *et al.* (1995). Cloning of a new cytokine that induces IFN-γ production by T cells. *Nature* **378,** 88–91.

O'Neill, L. A. (2000). The Toll/interleukin-1 receptor domain: A molecular switch for inflammation and host defence. *Biochem. Soc. Trans.* **28,** 557–563.

O'Neill, L. A., and Greene, C. (1998). Signal transduction pathways activated by the IL-1 receptor family: Ancient signaling machinery in mammals, insects, and plants. *J. Leukoc. Biol.* **63,** 650–657.

Orlando, S., Sironi, M., Bianchi, G., Drummond, A. H., Boraschi, D., Yabes, D., and Mantovani, A. (1997). Role of metalloproteases in the release of the IL-1 type II decoy receptor. *J. Biol. Chem.* **272,** 31764–31769.

Ottaviani, E., Franchini, A., Cassanelli, S., and Genedani, S. (1995). Cytokines and invertebrate immune responses. *Biol. Cell.* **85,** 87–91.

Ozinsky, A., Underhill, D. M., Fontenot, J. D., Hajjar, A. M., Smith, K. D., Wilson, C. B., Schroeder, L., and Aderem, A. (2000). The repertoire for pattern recognition of pathogens by the innate immune system is defined by cooperation between toll-like receptors. *Proc. Natl. Acad. Sci. USA* **97,** 13766–13771.

Parnet, P., Garka, K. E., Bonnert, T. P., Dower, S. K., and Sims, J. E. (1996). IL-1Rrp is a novel receptor-like molecule similar to the type I interleukin-1 receptor and its homologues T1/ST2 and IL-1R AcP. *J. Biol. Chem.* **271,** 3967–3970.

Paulukat, J., Bosmann, M., Nold, M., Garkisch, S., Kampfer, H., Frank, S., Raedle, J., Zeuzem, S., Pfeilschifter, J., and Muhl, H. (2001). Expression and release of IL-18 binding protein in response to IFN-γ. *J. Immunol.* **167,** 7038–7043.

Polentarutti, N., Penton Rol, G., Muzio, M., Bosisio, D., Camnasio, M., Riva, F., Zoja, C., Benigni, A., Tomasoni, S., Vecchi, A., Garlanda, C., and Mantovani, A. (2003). Unique pattern of expression and inhibition of IL-1 signaling by the IL-1 receptor family member TIR8/SIGIRR. *Eur. Cytokine Netw.* **14,** 211–218.

Poltorak, A., He, X., Smirnova, I., Liu, M. Y., Huffel, C. V., Du, X., Birdwell, C., Alejos, E., Silva, M., Galanos, C., Freudenberg, M., Ricciardi-Castagnoli, P., *et al.* (1998). Defective LPS signaling in C3H/HeJ and C57BL/10ScCr mice: Mutations in Tlr4 gene. *Science* **282,** 2085–2088.

Prechtel, D., Harbeck, N., Berger, U., Hofler, H., and Werenskiold, A. K. (2001). Clinical relevance of T1-S, an oncogene-inducible, secreted glycoprotein of the immunoglobulin superfamily, in node-negative breast cancer. *Lab. Invest.* **81,** 159–165.

Pujol, N., Link, E. M., Liu, L. X., Kurz, C. L., Alloing, G., Tan, M.-W., Ray, K. P., Solari, R., Johnson, C. D., and Ewbank, J. J. (2001). A reverse genetic analysis of components of the Toll signaling pathway in *Caenorhabditis elegans. Curr. Biol.* **11,** 809–821.

Rakoff-Nahoum, S., Paglino, J., Eslami-Varzaneh, F., Edberg, S., and Medzhitov, S. (2004). Recognition of commensal microflora by toll-like receptors is required for intestinal homeostasis. *Cell* **118,** 229–241.

Re, F., Sironi, M., Muzio, M., Matteucci, C., Introna, M., Orlando, S., Penton-Rol, G., Dower, S. K., Sims, J. E., Colotta, F., and Mantovani, A. (1996). Inhibition of interleukin-1 responsiveness by type II receptor gene transfer: A surface 'receptor' with anti-interleukin-1 function. *J. Exp. Med.* **183,** 1841–1850.

Rock, L., Hardiman, G., Timans, J. C., Kastelein, R. A., and Bazan, J. F. (1998). A family of human receptors structurally related to *Drosophila* Toll. *Proc. Natl. Acad. Sci. USA* **95,** 588–593.

Sana, T. R., Debets, R., Timans, J. C., Bazan, J. F., and Kastelein, R. A. (2000). Computational identification, cloning, and characterization of IL-1R9, a novel interleukin-1 receptor-like gene encoded over an unusually large interval of human chromosome Xq22. 2–q22. 3. *Genomics* **69,** 252–262.

Sangrador-Vegas, A., Martin, S. A., O'Dea, P. G., and Smith, T. J. (2000). Cloning and characterization of the rainbow trout (*Oncorhynchus mykiss*) type II interleukin-1 receptor cDNA. *Eur. J. Biochem.* **267,** 7031–7037.

Schmitz, J., Owyang, A., Oldham, E., Song, Y., Murphy, E., McClanahan, T. K., Zurawski, G., Moshrefi, M., Qin, J., Li, X., Gorman, D. M., Bazan, J. F., *et al.* (2005). IL-33, an interleukin-1-like cytokine that signals via the IL-1 receptor-related protein ST2 and induces T helper type 2-associated cytokines. *Immunity* **23,** 479–490.

Schreuder, H., Tardif, C., Trump-Kallmeyer, S., Soffientini, A., Sarubbi, E., Akeson, A., Bowlin, T., Yanofsky, S., and Barrett, R. W. (1997). A new cytokine-receptor binding mode revealed by the crystal structure of the IL-1 receptor with an antagonist. *Nature* **386,** 194–200.

Sims, J. E., March, C. J., Cosman, D., Widmer, M. B., MacDonald, H. R., McMahan, C. J., Grubin, C. E., Wignall, J. M., Jackson, J. L., Call, S. M., Friend, D., Alpert, A. R., *et al.* (1988). cDNA expression cloning of the IL-1 receptor, a member of the immunoglobulin superfamily. *Science* **241,** 585–589.

Smith, D. E., Renshaw, B. R., Ketchem, R. R., Kubin, M., Garka, K. E., and Sims, J. E. (2000). Four new members expand the interleukin-1 superfamily. *J. Biol. Chem.* **275,** 1169–1175.

Smith, D. E., Hanna, R., Friend, D., Moore, H., Chen, H., Farese, A. M., MacVittie, T. J., Virca, G. D., and Sims, J. E. (2003). The soluble form of IL-1 receptor accessory protein enhances the ability of soluble type II IL-1 receptor to inhibit IL-1 action. *Immunity* **18,** 87–96.

Strengell, M., Sareneva, T., Foster, D., Julkunen, I., and Matikainen, S. (2002). IL-21 up-regulates the expression of genes associated with innate immunity and Th1 response. *J. Immunol.* **169,** 3600–3605.

Subramaniam, S., Stansberg, C., Olsen, L., Zou, J., Secombes, C. J., and Cunningham, C. (2002). Cloning of a *Salmo salar* interleukin-1 receptor-like cDNA. *Dev. Comp. Immunol.* **26,** 415–431.

Sweet, M. J., Leung, B. P., Kang, D., Sogaard, M., Schulz, K., Trajkovic, V., Campbell, C. C., Xu, D., and Liew, F. Y. (2001). A novel pathway regulating lipopolysaccharide-induced shock by ST2/T1 via inhibition of Toll-like receptor 4 expression. *J. Immunol.* **166,** 6633–6639.

Tago, K., Noda, T., Hayakawa, M., Iwahana, H., Yanagisawa, K., Yashiro, T., and Tominaga, S. (2001). Tissue distribution and subcellular localization of a variant form of the human ST2 gene product, ST2V. *Biochem. Biophys. Res. Commun.* **285,** 1377–1383.

Tajima, S., Oshikawa, K., Tominaga, S., and Sugiyama, Y. (2003). The increase in serum soluble ST2 protein upon acute exacerbation of idiopathic pulmonary fibrosis. *Chest* **124,** 1206–1214.

Takeuchi, O., Hoshino, K., Kawai, T., Sanjo, H., Takada, H., Ogawa, T., Takeda, K., and Akira, S. (1999a). Differential roles of TLR2 and TLR4 in recognition of gram-negative and gram-positive bacterial cell wall components. *Immunity* **11,** 443–451.

Takeuchi, O., Kawai, T., Sanjo, H., Copeland, N. G., Gilbert, D. J., Jenkins, N. A., Takeda, K., and Akira, S. (1999b). TLR6: A novel member of an expanding toll-like receptor family. *Gene* **231,** 59–65.

Takeuchi, O., Kaufmann, A., Grote, K., Kawai, K., Hoshino, K., Morr, M., Muhlradt, P. F., and Akira, S. (2000). Cutting edge: Preferentially the R-stereoisomer of the mycoplasmal lipopeptide macrophage-activating lipopeptide-2 activates immune cells through a toll-like receptor 2– and MyD88-dependent signaling pathway. *J. Immunol.* **164,** 554–557.

Taylor, S. L., Renshaw, B. R., Garka, K. E., Smith, D. E., and Sims, J. E. (2002). Genomic organization of the interleukin-1 locus. *Genomics* **79,** 726–733.

Thomassen, E., Renshaw, B. R., and Sims, J. E. (1999). Identification and characterization of SIGIRR, a molecule representing a novel subtype of the IL-1R superfamily. *Cytokine* **11,** 389–399.

Torigoe, K., Ushio, S., Okura, T., Kobayashi, S., Taniai, M., Kunikata, T., Murakami, T., Sanou, O., Kojima, H., Fujii, M., Ohta, T., Ikeda, M., *et al.* (1997). Purification and characterization of the human interleukin-18 receptor. *J. Biol. Chem.* **272,** 25737–25742.

Towne, J. E., Garka, K. E., Renshaw, B. R., Virca, G. D., and Sims, J. E. (2004). Interleukin
    (IL)-1F6, IL-1F8, and IL-1F9 signal through IL-1Rrp2 and IL-1RAcP to activate the
    pathway leading to NF-κB and MAPKs. *J. Biol. Chem.* **279**, 13677–13688.

Townsend, M. J., Fallon, P. G., Matthews, D. J., Jolin, H. E., and McKenzie, A. N. (2000).
    T1/ST2-deficient mice demonstrate the importance of T1/ST2 in developing primary T
    helper cell type 2 responses. *J. Exp. Med.* **191**, 1069–1076.

Trajkovic, V., Sweet, M. J., and Xu, D. (2004). T1/ST2-an IL-1 receptor-like modulator of
    immune responses. *Cytokine Growth Factor Rev.* **15**, 87–95.

Tschopp, J., Martinon, F., and Burns, K. (2003). NALPs: A novel protein family involved in
    inflammation. *Nat. Rev. Mol. Cell. Biol.* **4**, 95–104.

Underhill, D. M., Ozinsky, A., Hajjar, A. M., Stevens, A., Wilson, C. B., Bassetti, M., and
    Aderem, A. (1999a). The Toll-like receptor 2 is recruited to macrophage phagosomes and
    discriminates between pathogens. *Nature* **401**, 811–815.

Underhill, D. M., Ozinsky, A., Smith, K. D., and Aderem, A. (1999b). Toll-like receptor-
    2 mediates mycobacteria-induced proinflammatory signaling in macrophages. *Proc. Natl.
    Acad. Sci. USA* **96**, 14459–14463.

Vigers, G. P., Anderson, L. J., Caffes, P., and Brandhuber, B. J. (1997). Crystal structure of the
    type-I interleukin-1 receptor complexed with interleukin-1β. *Nature* **386**, 190–194.

Wald, D., Qin, J., Zhao, Z., Qian, Y., Naramura, M., Tian, L., Towne, J., Sims, J. E., Stark,
    G. R., and Li, X. (2003). SIGIRR, a negative regulator of Toll-like receptor-interleukin 1
    receptor signaling. *Nat. Immunol.* **4**, 920–927.

Weinberg, E. O., Shimpo, M., Hurwitz, S., Tominaga, S., Rouleau, J. L., and Lee, R. T. (2003).
    Identification of serum soluble ST2 receptor as a novel heart failure biomarker. *Circulation*
    107, 721–726.

Weining, K. C., Sick, C., Kaspers, B., and Staeheli, P. (1998). A chicken homolog of
    mammalian interleukin-1β: cDNA cloning and purification of active recombinant protein.
    Eur. J. Biochem. **258**, 994–1000.

Wesche, H., Korherr, C., Kracht, M., Falk, W., Resch, K., and Martin, M. U. (1997). The
    interleukin-1 receptor accessory protein (IL-1RAcP) is essential for IL-1-induced activation
    of interleukin-1 receptor-associated kinase (IRAK) and stress-activated protein kinases
    (SAP kinases). *J. Biol. Chem.* **272**, 7727–7731.

Xu, D., Chan, W. L., Leung, B. P., Hunter, D., Schulz, K., Carter, R. W., McInnes, I. B.,
    Robinson, J. H., and Liew, F. Y. (1998). Selective expression and functions of interleukin 18
    receptor on T helper (Th) type 1 but not Th2 cells. *J. Exp. Med.* **188**, 1485–1492.

Yanagisawa, K., Takagi, T., Tsukamoto, T., Tetsuka, T., and Tominaga, S. (1993). Presence of
    a novel primary response gene ST2L, encoding a product highly similar to the interleukin 1
    receptor type 1. *FEBS Lett.* **318**, 83–87.

Yoshimoto, T., Takeda, K., Tanaka, T., Ohkusu, K., Kashiwamura, S., Okamura, H., Akira, S.,
    and Nakanishi, K. (1998). IL-12 up-regulates IL-18 receptor expression on T cells, Th1
    cells, and B cells: Synergism with IL-18 for IFN-γ production. *J. Immunol.* **161**, 3400–3407.

Zandi, E., Rothwarf, D. M., Delhase, M., Hayakawa, M., and Karin, M. (1997). The IκB
    kinase complex (IKK) contains two kinase subunits, IKKα and IKKβ, necessary for IκB
    phosphorylation and NF-κB activation. *Cell* **91**, 243–252.

Zhang, D., Zhang, G., Hayden, M. S., Greenblatt, M. B., Bussey, C., Flavell, R. A., and
    Ghosh, S. (2004). A toll-like receptor that prevents infection by uropathogenic bacteria.
    Science **303**, 1522–1526.

Zou, J., Grabowski, P. S., Cunningham, C., and Secombes, C. J. (1999). Molecular cloning of
    interleukin 1β from rainbow trout *Oncorhynchus mykiss* reveals no evidence of an ice cut
    site. *Cytokine* **11**, 552–560.

Zou, J., Bird, S., Minter, R., Horton, J., Cunningham, C., and Secombes, C. J. (2000).
    Molecular cloning of the gene for interleukin-1β from *Xenopus laevis* and analysis of
    expression *in vivo* and *in vitro*. *Immunogenetics* **51**, 332–338.

10

THE IL-17
CYTOKINE FAMILY

SARAH L. GAFFEN,*,† JILL M. KRAMER,*
JEFFREY J. YU,† AND FANG SHEN*

*Department of Oral Biology, School of Dental Medicine
University at Buffalo, SUNY, Buffalo, New York 14214
†Department of Microbiology and Immunology
School of Medicine and Biomedical Sciences
University at Buffalo, SUNY, Buffalo, New York 14214

IL-17A and its receptor are the founding members of a recently
described cytokine family, with unique sequences and functions in the

0083-6729/06 $35.00
DOI: 10.1016/S0083-6729(06)74010-9

immune system and elsewhere. Consisting of six ligands (IL-17A–F) and five receptors (IL-17RA–IL-17RE) in mammals, these molecules have distinct primary amino acid structures with only minimal homology to other cytokine families. By far the best studied of these cytokines to date are IL-17A and its receptor, IL-17RA. IL-17A is produced primarily by T cells, and is the hallmark cytokine of a newly defined T helper cell subset that appears to be involved in generation of autoimmunity. Despite its production by the adaptive immune system, IL-17A exhibits proinflammatory activities similar to innate immune cytokines such as IL-1β and TNF-α and appears to play important and nonredundant roles in regulating granulocytes *in vivo*. As a result, IL-17A also plays key roles in host defense. In contrast to the restricted expression of IL-17A, the IL-17RA receptor is ubiquitously expressed, and thus most cells are potential physiological targets of IL-17A. This chapter describes the major molecular properties, biological activities, and known signaling pathways of the IL-17 family, with an emphasis on IL-17A and IL-17RA. © 2006 Elsevier Inc.

I. OVERVIEW OF THE IL-17 FAMILY

The completion of human and rodent genome sequencing has revealed the "parts list" of genes required to control the many complex physiological processes required for survival. However, the daunting task remains to assign roles to each gene product in its physical and functional context. Cytokines, in a sense, represent a microcosm of this task, with approximately 200 cytokines together with their cognate receptors responsible for coordinating virtually every aspect of immunity, as well as other biological processes such as bone remodeling, nervous system function, and so on.

Understanding cytokine function requires an understanding of receptor signal transduction, and receptor structure is often predictive of function. Cytokines have been subdivided into families based primarily on receptor structure (Ozaki and Leonard, 2002), and the newest subfamily with unique structures to be described is the interleukin (IL)-17[1] family (Aggarwal and Gurney, 2002; Moseley *et al.*, 2003). Although first identified over a decade ago, this enigmatic family has recently received considerable attention for its

---

[1]Abbreviations: C/EBP, CCAAT/enhancer-binding protein; CIA, collagen-induced arthritis; COX, cyclooxygenase; DC, dendritic cells; EAE, experimental autoimmune encephalomyelitis; G-CSF, granulocyte colony-stimulating factor; GM-CSF, granulocyte-macrophage colony-stimulating factor; IL-, interleukin; iNOS, inducible nitric oxide synthase; JAK, Janus kinase; LIX, LPS-inducible CXC chemokine; MMP, matrix metalloproteinase; PI 3-K, phosphatidy-linositol-3′ kinase; RA, rheumatoid arthritis; SEF, similar expression to FGF receptor genes; STAT, signal transducer and activator of transcription; TNF, tumor necrosis factor.

role as a hallmark cytokine produced by a novel T helper subset (Wynn, 2005). The following sections review structural and functional aspects of the IL-17 family, with an emphasis on the prototypical and best understood of these, IL-17A.

II. MOLECULAR AND STRUCTURAL ASPECTS OF THE IL-17 FAMILY

A. IL-17 FAMILY LIGANDS

Originally cloned from a rodent T cell hybridoma library screen and termed CTLA-8 (Rouvier *et al.*, 1993), **IL-17A** (often called simply IL-17) is the founding member of a novel family of cytokines, termed IL-17A through IL-17F (Table I) (Aggarwal and Gurney, 2002). Family members share the highest degree of similarity in their C-terminal portions, with 20–30% amino acid identity and strict conservation of four cysteine residues (Lee *et al.*, 2001). IL-17A has a molecular weight of approximately 17 kDa and three potential N-linked glycosylation sites. Biochemically, IL-17A migrates as a dimer, apparently through cysteine bond interactions (Fossiez *et al.*, 1996). X-ray crystallography studies revealed an unexpected structural homology between IL-17 family members and neurotrophins such as nerve growth factor (NGF) (see IL-17F in a later section) (Hymowitz *et al.*, 2001). As will be described in detail in subsequent sections, IL-17A is produced almost exclusively by activated T cells, and is definitive of a new T cell subset that is distinct from Th1 or Th2 (Harrington *et al.*, 2005; Park *et al.*, 2005; Wynn, 2005). Although produced by the adaptive immune system, IL-17A is clearly a proinflammatory cytokine with potent effects on numerous cells of the innate immune system, particularly the granulocyte lineage.

TABLE I.   IL-17 Family Ligands[a]

Family member	Alternate names	Chromosome	Receptor(s)
IL-17A	CTLA-8, IL-17	6p12	IL-17RA, IL-17RC
IL-17B	CX1	5q32–34	IL-17RB
IL-17C	CX2	16g24	Not determined
IL-17D		13q12.11	Not determined
IL-17E	IL-25	14q11.2	IL-17RB
IL-17F	ML-1	6p12	IL-17RA, IL-17RC
vIL-17	ORF13	N/A[b] (*H. Saimiri*)	IL-17RA

[a]Additional information on nomenclature in Eberl (2002).
[b]N/A: Not applicable.

Compared to IL-17A, little is known about other members of the IL-17 family, most of which were first identified by homology searches to IL-17A. In contrast to IL-17A and other IL-17 family members, size exclusion chromatography demonstrated that **IL-17B** appears to be a nondisulfide-linked dimer. Also unlike IL-17A, its expression is quite widespread; Northern blot analyses showed strong signals in spinal cord, small intestine, brain, heart, and testis. *In vivo* studies revealed that IL-17B causes a dose-dependent recruitment of neutrophils to the peritoneal cavity following injection of IL-17B into this site (Shi *et al.*, 2000). **IL-17C** is expressed at very low levels, and is only detectable in adult prostate and fetal kidney libraries. Although they are both proinflammatory, the functions of IL-17B and C are clearly distinct from those of IL-17A, because IL-17A but not IL-17B or IL-17C induce secretion of IL-6 in human fibroblasts. In addition, IL-17B and IL-17C induce the release of TNF-α and IL-1β from the monocytic cell line THP-1, whereas IL-17A has only a minor effect on these cells (Li *et al.*, 2000). However, the mechanisms involved in IL-17B and IL-17C signaling are still poorly understood, and little is known about the major biological roles for these cytokines.

IL-17D shares the most sequence homology with IL-17B, with 27% sequence identity, and is found in skeletal muscle, brain, adipose tissue, heart, lung, and pancreas. Like IL-17A, IL-17D stimulation triggers the secretion of IL-6, IL-8, and GM-CSF in target cells, and thus appears to be proinflammatory. In addition, IL-17D suppresses the proliferation of myeloid progenitor cells in colony formation assays. It is postulated that in addition to its proinflammatory activities, IL-17D plays a role in the anemia of chronic disease, as IL-17D secretion appears to decrease hematopoiesis (Starnes *et al.*, 2002). Again, much remains to be learned about this cytokine *in vivo*.

IL-17E (more commonly referred to as IL-25) was also cloned by a homology search, and has a 25–35% identity with other IL-17 family members (Fort *et al.*, 2001; Kim *et al.*, 2002). IL-25 transcripts are expressed in a variety of tissues, and high levels are present in testis and polarized Th2 cells. Numerous studies have borne out the observation that IL-25 drives a Th2-type response. For example, parenteral administration of IL-25 or overexpression by transgenesis induces expression of Th2-type cytokines, such as IL-4, IL-5, and IL-13, together with Th2-type pathologies (Hurst *et al.*, 2002; Kim *et al.*, 2002; Pan *et al.*, 2001). Transgenic mice overexpressing human IL-25 under a promoter that directs secretion from liver showed dramatic hematopoietic changes, such as splenomegaly and lymphadenopathy. Strikingly, these mice also exhibited a 50-fold increase in eosinophils, along with smaller but significant increases in lymphocytes and neutrophils. In addition, these studies revealed a role for IL-25 in lymphocyte development and B cell trafficking (Kim *et al.*, 2002). Corroborative data were obtained from mice transgenic for the murine IL-25 gene under the control of the systemic myosin L-chain promoter, which also showed growth retardation and jaundiced skin (Pan *et al.*, 2001). Data also support a role for IL-25 in autoimmunity and parasitic infections, as IL-25-deficient mice show accelerated onset of experimental autoimmune encephalomyelitis (EAE) as well as increased susceptibility to the parasitic worm *Trichuris muris* (Owyang *et al.*, 2005).

The most recently discovered IL-17 family member, **IL-17F**, resembles IL-17A most closely, both in terms of homology and function. IL-17F has 58% sequence identity with IL-17A at the protein level, and both bind to the same receptor (see Section II.B). IL-17A and IL-17F are potent inducers of G-CSF and numerous CXC chemokines in a variety of cell types, and a synergistic enhancement of signaling is observed when these cytokines are combined with TNF-α. In addition, both IL-17A and IL-17F play important roles in neutrophil recruitment, particularly in lung (Kolls and Linden, 2004). Furthermore, both IL-17A and IL-17F are demonstrated to play important inflammatory roles in the pathogenesis of cystic fibrosis (McAllister *et al.*, 2005). IL-17A and IL-17F are linked on chromosome 6p12 and may be coordinately regulated at the transcriptional level (Table I). Recent work has demonstrated that, in addition to NFAT, the STAT3 transcription factor plays an important role in regulating these genes (Chen *et al.*, 2006). IL-17F is also the only IL-17 family member whose crystal structure has been solved. This study revealed that IL-17F adopts a cysteine knot fold, which is characterized by three sets of disulfide linkages. Importantly, IL-17F forms an unusually large cavity by residues in the dimer interface, which is suggestive of a region that may bind another molecule (Hymowitz *et al.*, 2001). Based on sequence analysis, an analogous cavity is predicted to exist for other IL-17 family members, which could provide clues to specific amino acids in the cytokine that are critical for receptor interactions. Identification of such contact points may provide valuable targets for rationally designed therapeutics aimed at mitigating IL-17 signaling.

Another intriguing aspect of the IL-17 family is the existence of a viral homolog of IL-17A encoded in the T cell–tropic gamma herpesvirus, *Herpesvirus saimiri* (Rouvier *et al.*, 1993). Termed **vIL-17**, the biological significance of its presence in this viral genome is unclear. However, the vIL-17 gene (ORF13) is not required for viral replication or pathogenicity in susceptible primates, or T cell transformation *in vitro* (Knappe *et al.*, 1998). Since vIL-17 is agonistic for the same receptor subunit that binds IL-17A and IL-17F, it may contribute to viral persistence in the squirrel monkey, its natural host (Fossiez *et al.*, 1996; Yao *et al.*, 1995).

B. IL-17 FAMILY RECEPTORS

The IL-17 receptor family also comprises a unique class of cytokine receptors (Table II). The founding member of the family was identified on the basis of binding to IL-17A. Originally termed IL-17R, it is now known as **IL-17RA**, and bears almost no homology to other known cytokine receptors (Yao *et al.*, 1995, 1997). It was also shown that IL-17RA binds another IL-17

TABLE II. IL-17 Receptor Family Members

Family member	Alternate names	Ligand(s)	Chromosome	Splice variants?
IL-17RA	IL-17R	IL-17A, IL-17F	22q11.1	No
IL-17RB	IL-17Rh1	IL-17B, IL-17E/IL-25	3p21.1	Yes
IL-17RC	IL-17RL	IL-17F, IL-17A	3p25.3	Yes
IL-17RD	SEF	FGF?	3p21.2	Yes
IL-17RE		Not determined	3p25.3	Yes

family ligand, IL-17F (Hymowitz et al., 2001), albeit with 10- to 30-fold reduced affinity compared to IL-17A (S. Levin, personal communication). In contrast to the tissue-specific expression of IL-17A (Fossiez et al., 1996), IL-17RA is expressed essentially ubiquitously (Yao et al., 1995). It is a type I transmembrane glycoprotein receptor, containing an extracellular domain of 293 amino acids, a transmembrane domain of 21 amino acids, and a cytoplasmic domain of 525 amino acids. The IL-17RA has a molecular weight of 128–132 kDa, but usually migrates at larger sizes due to extensive and variable glycosylation (Yao et al., 1997; J. M. Kramer, unpublished data).

Surprisingly, the composition and stoichiometry of the IL-17A-binding complex has still not been completely defined. It is certain that IL-17RA is an essential subunit, as cells from IL-17RA knockout mice fail to bind IL-17A. However, IL-17A binds its receptor complex with a relatively low affinity, with reported K_a values ranging from $2 \times 10^7/M$ to $2 \times 10^8/M$, whereas much lower doses of IL-17A (5 ng/ml) are able to elicit biological responses in target cells (Yao et al., 1997). These data hint that another subunit may be present in the IL-17RA signaling complex. Indeed, very recent work has demonstrated that IL-17RC may be this elusive second subunit (Toy et al., 2006). In this regard, all known cytokine receptors contain multiple subunits, and since IL-17A forms a homodimer, it was long assumed that the receptor was also homodimeric. Accordingly, fluorescence resonance energy transfer (FRET) analyses showed that the IL-17RA complex contains at least two identical subunits (Kramer et al., 2006). Notably, this interaction is observed in the absence of ligand, suggesting that the receptor complex is preassembled in the membrane, a phenomenon that has been observed for other cytokine receptors, particularly erythropoietin and TNF family receptors (Chan et al., 2000; Remy et al., 1999). Strikingly, addition of ligand (IL-17A or IL-17F) causes a loss of FRET, indicating that a conformational change occurs and/or that an additional protein is recruited to the receptor complex, thereby increasing the distance between IL-17RA monomers (Kramer et al., 2006). Since other IL-17 family cytokines are also homo-dimers, this may be a typical mode of IL-17 receptor interactions.

The IL-17RA receptor constitutes the founding member of a family composed of at least four other distantly related receptors (Table II). **IL-17RB** (also known as Evi-27 or IL-17rh-1), binds to IL-17B with a relatively high affinity of 7.6 nM (Shi *et al.*, 2000). This receptor also binds to IL-17E, although direct affinity measurements were not reported (Lee *et al.*, 2001). The IL-17RB protein has 19.2% and 18.2% protein sequence identity to the human and murine IL-17RA sequences, respectively. Unlike IL-17RA, several alternatively spliced forms of IL-17BR with different extracellular domains exist (Moseley *et al.*, 2003; Shi *et al.*, 2000), suggesting the intriguing likelihood of soluble "decoy" receptors and multiple potential ligands for this receptor (Tian *et al.*, 2000). IL-17RB mRNA is present in several endocrine tissues, and is highly expressed in fetal and adult liver, kidney, pancreas, small intestine, and colon. The receptor is absent or at least poorly expressed in peripheral blood leukocytes and lymphoid organs (Lee *et al.*, 2001; Shi *et al.*, 2000). The IL-17RB locus is also a common site of retroviral integration in certain murine myeloid leukemias and thus may contribute to malignancy (Tian *et al.*, 2000).

IL-17RC, first named IL-17 receptor like protein (IL-17RL), was also identified through database searches of human expressed sequence tags (ESTs) (Haudenschild *et al.*, 2002). This protein is 22% identical and 34% similar to the human IL-17RA. The cytoplasmic domains of these proteins are most highly conserved, with 25% identity and 41% similarity. IL-17RC expression is quite ubiquitous, being highest in prostate, liver, kidney, muscle, and heart. This receptor has several splice variants, as four exons are frequently spliced out in various combinations, resulting in at least 12 possible proteins. The receptor is reported to have multiple molecular weights, ranging from 33–60 kDa, which corresponds with the high number of predicted splice variants. It was demonstrated that one splice variant of IL-17RC binds IL-17F with quite high affinity, both in humans and mice (S. Levin, personal communication). IL-17RC expression is reduced in prostate cancer compared to normal prostate, and expression correlates with Gleason grade. Therefore, redistribution of IL-17RC may indicate dysregulation of expression or signaling in prostate cancer (Haudenschild *et al.*, 2002; Moseley *et al.*, 2003). As indicated, at least one splice variant of IL-17RC appears to be an essential part of the IL-17A binding complex as well (Toy *et al.*, 2006).

IL-17RD reveals a striking relationship between the IL-17R family and evolutionarily conserved molecules involved in embryonic development. First described as an inhibitor of fibroblast growth factor (FGF) signaling in zebrafish (Tsang *et al.*, 2002), *s*imilar *e*xpression to *f*ibroblast growth factor genes (SEF) and its mammalian counterparts (hSEF and mSEF in human and mouse, respectively) share sequence homology primarily with the intracellular domain of IL-17R family members (Yang *et al.*, 2003). The extracellular domain of human SEF/IL-17RD shares seven potential sites for N-linked glycosylation, and eight cysteine residues are conserved among the extracellular domains of human, mouse, and zebrafish SEF homologs.

This receptor is found in numerous cell types, with especially high expression in ovary, breast, kidney, heart, skeletal muscle, and colon. Similar to its role in zebrafish and *Xenopus laevis*, hSEF coimmunoprecipitates with human FGF receptor 1 and inhibits FGF-dependent signaling through Ras-mitogen-activated protein (MAP) kinase (MAPK) pathways (Tsang and Dawid, 2004; Xiong *et al.*, 2003; Yang *et al.*, 2003). The ligand(s) for IL-17RD are not known; in fact, the extracellular domain of SEF is dispensable for its ability to inhibit FGF signal transduction (Tsang *et al.*, 2002).

IL-17RE was identified by bioinformatics efforts to identify receptor proteins (Clark *et al.*, 2003), but nothing is presently known about its ligand specificity or biological functions. In addition, IL-17R homologs have been reported in sea lamprey (Pancer *et al.*, 2004), dog, cow, and chicken (NCBI nucleotide database).

Interactions among IL-17 family cytokines and receptors are emerging as a complex story (Table II). Both IL-17A and IL-17F interact with IL-17RA, although the IL-17F affinity is one to two orders of magnitude less than that of IL-17A (Hymowitz *et al.*, 2001). IL-17A also binds to IL-17RC (Toy *et al.*, 2006). Further studies demonstrate that IL-17F binds to IL-17RC (S. Levin, personal communication). Similarly, IL-17B and IL-17E/IL-25 both bind IL-17RB. No receptors are identified for IL-17C and IL-17D (Aggarwal and Gurney, 2002), and no ligand has been found for SEF or IL-17RE (Clark *et al.*, 2003; Kolls and Linden, 2004). Understanding interactions among IL-17 and IL-17R family members is perhaps valuable in understanding and treating a wide variety of disease ranging from cancer to cystic fibrosis.

III. IL-17A *IN VIVO*

A. TH17, A NEW T CELL SUBSET

Shortly after its discovery, it became clear that IL-17A was secreted primarily, if not exclusively by activated T lymphocytes in response to stimulation through the T cell receptor (Fossiez *et al.*, 1996). Because these T cells were CD62L-CD44+CD45RO+, they were classified as effector memory cells (Shin *et al.*, 1999). However, efforts to assign IL-17 to a Th1 or Th2 subset were largely unsuccessful. A major advance in understanding IL-17A biology was made with the appreciation that the IL-12 family cytokine, IL-23, drives IL-17A expression in a CD4+ T cell subset, termed "Th17" (Aggarwal *et al.*, 2002; Ghilardi *et al.*, 2004; Happel *et al.*, 2003; Liu *et al.*, 2005). Recent developments have modified this model, showing that it is actually TGFβ and IL-6 that drive Th17 development, whereas IL-23 is important for expanding this population (Bettelli *et al.*, 2006; Mangan *et al.*, 2006; Veldhoen *et al.*, 2006). This "pathological" T cell population produces IL-17A as well as IL-17F, TNF-α, IL-6, and increased expression of numerous chemokines and chemokine receptors. This population is postulated to arise as a unique T helper cell subset (Bettelli and Kuchroo, 2005; Langrish *et al.*, 2005). Strikingly, IL-17A-producing cells are sufficient to drive pathology in an EAE model (Langrish *et al.*, 2005). Consistent with this, IL-23-driven T cells produce IL-17A but not IFN-γ, whereas IL-12-driven Th1 cells produce IFN-γ but not IL-17A, suggesting a stage of T cell differentiation independent of Th1. Two studies have confirmed and extended these findings, showing that differentiation to the Th17 lineage can be generated in STAT4$^{-/-}$ and STAT6$^{-/-}$ mice. Moreover, IFN-γ and IL-4 both suppress development of the Th17 population, further supporting its existence as a unique subset (Harrington *et al.*, 2005; Park *et al.*, 2005). Finally, some studies have shown that IL-15 also appears to trigger IL-17A production in T cells (Ziolkowska *et al.*, 2000). Most interestingly, Th17 cells appear to develop in opposition to suppressive "Tregulatory" cells, suggesting another reason for the role of IL-17A in autoimmunity (Bettelli *et al.*, 2006).

The major source of IL-23 driving Th$_{IL-17}$ differentiation appears to be bone marrow derived dendritic cells (DCs) and macrophages (Aggarwal *et al.*, 2002; Liu *et al.*, 2005), although it has also been reported in fibroblasts (Zhang *et al.*, 2005). IL-23 and IL-17 are part of a homeostatic feedback loop regulating granulopoiesis. Specifically, phagocytosis of apoptotic neutrophils inhibits IL-23 secretion by macrophages and dendritic cells, which in turn reduces levels of IL-17A-secreting T cells (Stark *et al.*, 2005). IL-17A is a major stimulator of neutrophil-activating chemokines as well as G-CSF and GM-CSF (Linden *et al.*, 2005). Consequently, in mice that lack leukocyte adhesion molecules or other neutrophil-trafficking defects, apoptotic neutrophils cannot migrate into tissues to be phagocytosed, and thus IL-17A secretion is not restricted. As a result, these mice have elevated granulopoiesis and excessive numbers of circulating neutrophils (Stark *et al.*, 2005). Consistent with this, IL-17A receptors are downregulated on human polymorpho nuclear cells (PMNs) during apoptosis (Kobayashi *et al.*, 2003).

While IL-23 is clearly important for maximal expression of IL-17A *in vivo* (Happel *et al.*, 2003), signals from the T cell receptor are also critical (Liu *et al.*, 2004, 2005), and production of IL-17A can be completely blocked with the immunosuppressant cyclosporine A (Liu *et al.*, 2004; Ziolkowska *et al.*, 2000). Consistent with this, characterization of the human IL-17A proximal promoter has identified two essential nuclear factor of activated T cells (NFAT)–binding sites required for transcriptional activation of a linked reporter (Liu *et al.*, 2004). The murine IL-17A promoter is surprisingly divergent from the human promoter, although NFAT sites are also present upstream of the transcriptional start site and it is also sensitive to cyclosporine A (Liu *et al.*, 2004, 2005; X. K. Liu, unpublished observations). In this regard, the role of T cell costimulation in regulating IL-17A expression is somewhat confusing. In human cells, costimulation of the T cell receptor (CD3) through CD28 signaling leads to strongly enhanced IL-17A production, similar to the hallmark T cell cytokine, IL-2. Moreover, human cells with a defective CD28-signaling pathway fail to show any costimulation of the IL-17A promoter (Liu *et al.*, 2004). It is known that CD28 costimulation of the IL-2 gene requires activation of the NF-κB pathway, and there is a key NF-κB-binding site in the IL-2 promoter that responds to these signals (Lin and Wang, 2004). However, there is no apparent NF-κB target site in the human IL-17A proximal promoter (Liu *et al.*, 2004). Moreover, the mouse IL-17A gene is neither enhanced in a substantive way by costimulatory signals from CD28 (Liu *et al.*, 2005) nor is there evidence for a functional NF-κB element in the mouse IL-17A proximal promoter. However, mice deficient in another CD28-related costimulatory molecule, inducible costimulator (ICOS), are defective in IL-17A production, and these mice are also highly resistant to autoimmune conditions such as collagen-induced arthritis (Dong and Nurieva, 2003). In the same regard, the TNFα receptor (TNFR) family costimulator, OX40, has also been implicated in IL-17A expression *in vivo* (Nakae *et al.*, 2003b). Surprisingly, studies *in vitro* did not find a noteworthy costimulatory effect of ICOS or OX40 (or several other costimulators) on IL-17A production in murine T cells (Liu *et al.*, 2005). Therefore, the means by which IL-17A expression is controlled in T cells remains an important area of inquiry.

B. IL-17A IN AUTOIMMUNE/INFLAMMATORY DISEASES

The proinflammatory functions of IL-17A have been examined in many contexts. *In vitro*, IL-17A has been shown to augment the activities of several classic inflammatory cytokines, such as TNF-α, IL-1β, and IFN-γ (Albanesi *et al.*, 1999; Chabaud *et al.*, 1998; Miossec, 2003; Shen *et al.*, 2005). IL-17A in humans has been associated with pathology in numerous autoimmune and inflammatory conditions, including rheumatoid arthritis (Kotake *et al.*, 1999; Van Bezooijen *et al.*, 1999), systemic lupus erythematosis (Wong *et al.*, 2000), multiple sclerosis (Matusevicius *et al.*, 1999), psoriasis (Arican *et al.*, 2005; Teunissen *et al.*, 1998), asthma (Laan *et al.*, 1999), cystic fibrosis (McAllister *et al.*, 2005), and Crohn's disease (Fujino *et al.*, 2003; Yen *et al.*, 2006). Particular attention has been paid to the role of IL-17A in arthritis in animal models, both collagen-induced arthritis (CIA) (Dong and Nurieva, 2003; Gaffen, 2004; Kolls and Linden, 2004; Lubberts *et al.*, 2003; Nakae *et al.*, 2003a) and streptococcal cell wall–induced arthritis (Koenders *et al.*, 2005; Lubberts *et al.*, 2005b). These studies and many others have shown an association with IL-17A signaling and upregulation of joint destructive factors (Fig. 1) (Lubberts *et al.*, 2005a).

Considerable emerging evidence shows that IL-17A plays an essential, nonredundant role in neutrophil activation, maturation, and homeostasis (Kolls and Linden, 2004), but how this relates to arthritis pathology is still unclear. Several studies have linked the neutrophil recruitment activity of

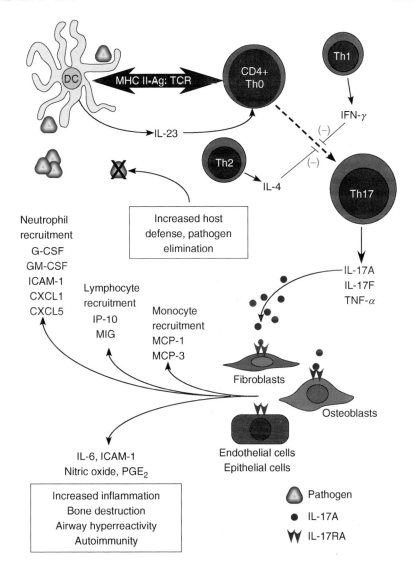

FIGURE 1. IL-17A in inflammation and disease. Dendritic cells (DCs) produce IL-23, which drives development of the "Th17" subset of T cells that secrete IL-17A, IL-17F, and TNF-α. IL-17A (and, to a lesser extent, IL-17F) bind to the IL-17RA on numerous target cells, including fibroblasts, osteoblasts, and epithelial/endothelial cells. Signals from IL-17RA lead to expression of a variety of inflammatory genes, particularly chemokines and cytokines that promote granulocyte hematopoiesis and recruitment. Depending on context, these inflammatory signals can be pathogenic (as in RA and EAE) or protective (as in various infectious diseases).

IL-17A to bone and joint destruction. Based on microarray data, IL-17A, particularly in concert with TNF-α, significantly upregulates neutrophil-attracting chemokines such as LPS-inducible CXC chemokine, CXCL5 (LIX) and keratinocyte-derived chemokine, CXCL1 or Groα (KC) in osteo-blast and bone marrow stromal cells (Shen *et al.*, 2005). In light of the strong association of IL-17A with RA, and the presence of extensive neutrophil populations in synovium of arthritic joints, it has been suggested that IL-17A plays a direct role in recruiting neutrophils to synovium and mediating joint destruction through release of reactive oxygen and nitrogen species (Liew and McInnes, 2005).

Because IL-17A drives bone-resorptive activities in the context of arthritis, some studies have examined IL-17A as a potential mediator of inflammatory bone pathology in periodontal disease (Takahashi *et al.*, 2005). Consistent with this, IL-17A mRNA has been found in gingival crevicular fluid of some patients with severe periodontal disease (Johnson *et al.*, 2004), but a direct mechanistic link to pathology has not yet been established. Conversely, neutrophils play an undisputed protective role in host defense against periodontal infection (Kantarci *et al.*, 2003), and the profound effects of IL-17A on promoting neutrophil activity may prove to be more important than its bone resorptive activity in the context of periodontal disease (J. J. Yu *et al.*, unpublished data).

C. IL-17A IN INFECTIOUS DISEASE

Despite its apparent pathologic role in autoimmunity and some inflammatory conditions, IL-17 plays a protective role in many infectious settings. Studies of bacterial infections [*Klebsiella pneumonia* (Ye *et al.*, 2001), *Porphyromonas gingivalis* (J. J. Yu *et al.*, unpublished data), parasitic infections (*Toxoplasma gondii*) (Kelly *et al.*, 2005), and fungal infections (*Candida albicans*) (Huang *et al.*, 2004)] have revealed that a deficiency in IL-17A signaling in IL-17RA-deficient mice results in a more severe disease course than in wild-type animals (Ye *et al.*, 2001). In most cases, this has been linked to a failure to expand and/or recruit neutrophils rather than an inherent defect in neutrophil function. For example, in mice infected with *K. pneumoniae* or *C. albicans*, an IL-17RA-deficiency caused reduced production of neutrophil-attractive CXC chemokines as well as granulopoietic cytokines (Kelly *et al.*, 2005; Ye *et al.*, 2001). Similarly, in *P. gingivalis*-infected IL-17RKO mice, neutrophils failed to be recruited to the site of infected gingiva, apparently due to reduced LIX/CXCL5 and KC/CXCL1 expression (J. J. Yu, unpublished observations). In some cases, contributions of IL-17A have been inferred through studies of IL-23. For example, in *Mycobacterium tuberculosis* infection, pulmonary IL-23 administration enhanced protective immunity by driving IL-17A production from lung T cells; moreover, IL-23-deficient mice show a reduction in both IL-17A-producing

M. tuberculosis-specific T cells and IL-12p70-independent protection from infection (Happel *et al.*, 2005; Khader *et al.*, 2005).

Notably, IL-17A does not play a defensive role in all infectious diseases. For example, in murine schistosomiasis, hepatic granuloma formation was linked to high levels of IL-17A. Moreover, neutralizing IL-17A antibody treatment reduced granuloma size (Rutitzky *et al.*, 2005). Consistent with this, IL-17RA-deficient mice show a reduced worm burden on *Schistosoma mansoni* infection (C. Carvalho-Queiroz, P. T. Loverde, and S. L. Gaffen, unpublished observations). The underlying mechanism for the role of IL-17A (and perhaps IL-17F) in this disease is not understood. Therefore, these findings warrant examination of IL-17A in other infections that rely on nonneutrophil-mediated immunity.

D. IL-17A IN CANCER

IL-17A has been linked with the pathogenesis of several malignancies, particularly those associated with production of inflammatory molecules. For example, a human cervical carcinoma cell line transfected with IL-17A caused significantly larger tumors in nude mice than untransfected cells (Tartour *et al.*, 1999). It was subsequently shown that, in addition to its ability to upregulate proangiogenic factors in target cells, IL-17A itself was proangiogenic (Numasaki *et al.*, 2003). Moreover, IL-17A selectively augments secretion of angiogenic CXC chemokines but not angiostatic chemokines in the context of non-small cell lung cancer implanted in SCID mice (Numasaki *et al.*, 2005). In humans, elevated levels of IL-17A are found in patients with ovarian cancer (Kato *et al.*, 2001), Hodgkin's lymphoma (Maggio *et al.*, 2002), benign prostatic hyperplasia and prostatic carcinoma (Steiner *et al.*, 2003), and cutaneous T cell lymphomas such as mycosis fungoides and Sézary syndrome (Ciree *et al.*, 2004).

Conversely, the proinflammatory action of IL-17A has also been considered to be a protective factor in some cancer settings via augmentation of antitumor immunity. For example, murine Meth-A fibrosarcoma cells transfected with IL-17A were readily rejected by immunocompetent mice, whereas untransfected cells were not. The increased rejection was associated with increased MHC class I and class II expression in transfected cells (Hirahara *et al.*, 2001). Similarly, some hematopoietic tumors transfected with IL-17A exhibited impaired growth, associated with increased generation of cytotoxic T lymphocytes specific for tumor antigens (Benchetrit *et al.*, 2002). Finally, preincubation of U-2 OS osteosarcoma cells with IL-17A increased NK cell-mediated cytotoxicity through increased expression of fibronectin (Honorati *et al.*, 2003). Thus, like many aspects of the immune system, IL-17 can have both pro- and antineoplastic effects, depending on the immunogenicity of the tumor cell, as well as the mechanism of tumorigenesis that is unique to each tumor type.

IV. GENE TARGETS AND SIGNAL
TRANSDUCTION

While considerable information regarding the biological roles of IL-17A and its receptor has been obtained, surprisingly little is known about the molecular mechanics of IL-17RA-mediated signal transduction. Even less is known about signaling by other IL-17R family members, so the following sections will deal only with IL-17RA-mediated events. However, as these become elucidated for IL-17RA, they are likely to apply to other IL-17R family members as well.

A. MAJOR GENE TARGETS

The endpoint of most signaling pathways is specific gene transcription. Many genes have been defined as specific targets of IL-17RA signaling, the majority of which are inflammatory in nature. One of the earliest IL-17A target genes identified was **IL-6** (Yao *et al.*, 1995), which is still the standard bioassay for IL-17A activity. This cytokine is induced by IL-17A in numerous cell types, and it is regulated both at the transcriptional level and by mRNA stability. Moreover, IL-17A and TNF-α exhibit potent synergy in regulation of IL-6 expression. The mechanism(s) by which synergy occurs are still not completely defined, but evidence for cooperation at the transcriptional and mRNA stability level have been reported (Hata *et al.*, 2002; Henness *et al.*, 2004; Hwang *et al.*, 2004; Ruddy *et al.*, 2004b; Shimada *et al.*, 2002).

IL-17A is an important regulator of granulocyte generation and neutrophil trafficking. In this regard, other cytokines regulated by IL-17A include G-CSF and GM-CSF, which drive expansion and survival of the granulocyte and macrophage lineages. G-CSF can be induced by IL-17 in numerous cells, including human bronchial epithelial cells (Kolls and Linden, 2004; McAllister *et al.*, 2005). *In vivo*, local costimulation with mouse IL-17A together with TNF-α caused a potentiation of neutrophil accumulation of in bronchoalveolar lavage fluid from mouse airways, and this effect could be blocked by a neutralizing anti-GM-CSF antibody (Laan *et al.*, 2003). In addition, adenovirus-mediated gene transfer of murine IL-17A in liver results in a transiently transgenic phenotype, with dramatic effects on granulopoiesis (Schwarzenberger *et al.*, 1998). Another interesting study revealed that in mice with neutrophil-trafficking defects, levels of G-CSF and IL-17A were elevated in proportion to the neutrophilia seen in these mice, regardless of the underlying mutation. Moreover, blocking IL-17A or G-CSF function significantly reduced neutrophil counts in severely neutrophilic mice. Thus, peripheral blood neutrophil numbers are regulated by a feedback loop involving G-CSF and IL-17A (Forlow *et al.*, 2001; Stark *et al.*, 2005).

IL-17A also induces expression of various chemokines, particularly those involved in neutrophil recruitment. CXCL8 (IL-8) was identified early as a human gene target of IL-17A, and CXCL1 (KC, Groα), CXCL2 (MIP2), and CXCL5 (LIX) were also subsequently identified as important targets in mice, both *in vitro* and *in vivo* (Kolls and Linden, 2004; Ruddy *et al.*, 2004a; Ye *et al.*, 2001). Specifically, in many IL-17RA-deficient mouse infection models, failures in host defense have been linked to reduction in chemokine production and neutrophil recruitment to infected sites. Consistent with this, ICAM-1, an adhesion molecule important for granulocyte recruitment and inflammation, is also induced strongly by IL-17A (Albanesi *et al.*, 1999; Schwandner *et al.*, 2000). Several studies have shown that CCL5 (RANTES), a chemokine primarily involved in recruiting T cells, monocytes, basophils, and eosinophils, is actually suppressed by IL-17A, either alone or in combination with TNF-α (Andoh *et al.*, 2002; Maertzdorf *et al.*, 2002; Shen *et al.*, 2005). However, the significance of this finding is not clear, although it may relate to the decreased sensitivity of IL-17RA-deficient mice to murine Schistosomiasis (Rutitzky *et al.*, 2005).

A variety of other inflammatory genes are induced by IL-17A. For example, several studies showed that IL-17A enhances prostaglandin E_2 production via upregulation of cyclooxygenase-2 (COX-2) (Fossiez *et al.*, 1996; LeGrand *et al.*, 2001; Shalom-Barak *et al.*, 1998). IL-17A induction of COX-2 gene expression is initiated ATF2/CREB transactivation of the proximal promoter and stabilized by the stress-activated protein kinase 2/p38 MAPK cascade. Adding IL-17A to cells stabilized COX-2 mRNA, a process compromised by MAPK inhibitors (Faour *et al.*, 2003). Nitric oxide (NO) is another important signaling molecule in inflammation, and pathogenic NO is produced mainly by inducible NO synthase (iNOS) during inflammatory events. IL-17A triggers a dose- and time-dependent increase in the level of NO in various cell types, and iNOS is induced by IL-17A in chondrocytes (Martel-Pelletier *et al.*, 1999), mouse and rat primary astrocytes (Trajkovic *et al.*, 2001), and menisci from patients with osteoarthritis (LeGrand *et al.*, 2001). The iNOS gene is regulated by NF-κB and MAPK pathways (Martel-Pelletier *et al.*, 1999; Shalom-Barak *et al.*, 1998) but may also be partly regulated through IRF-1 activation (Miljkovic and Trajkovic, 2004; Miljkovic *et al.*, 2005). IL-17A-mediated enhancement of NO is independent of IL-1β, as a soluble IL-1 receptor cannot block IL-17A-induced NO production (Attur *et al.*, 1997).

Considerable data implicates IL-17A as a bone destructive factor in arthritis (Gaffen, 2004). The matrix metalloproteinases (MMPs) are potent mediators of tissue damage in arthritis, and MMP-3 and MMP-13 are induced by IL-17A in bovine chondrocytes (Liacini *et al.*, 2005b), subepithelial myofibroblasts (Bamba *et al.*, 2003), fetal mouse metatarsals (Van Bezooijen *et al.*, 2002), and human synovial fibroblasts (Liacini *et al.*, 2005a). IL-17A also increases concentrations of biologically active MMP-9 and MMP-1

(Chabaud *et al.*, 2000; Jovanovic *et al.*, 2000; Prause *et al.*, 2004). Moreover, IL-17A was also shown to stimulate a dose-dependent release of proteoglycan and type II collagen from cartilage explants via increased MMP-1, MMP-3, and MMP-13 expression, which was completely inhibited by tissue inhibitor of metalloproteinase (TIMP)-1 or BB-94, a synthetic metalloproteinase inhibitor (Koshy *et al.*, 2002). As with many other IL-17RA target genes, the NF-κB and MAPK pathways appear to be involved in MMP gene regulation. For example, IL-17A-induced MMP-9 expression is dependent on both MAPK and NF-κB (Jovanovic *et al.*, 2000), while IL-17-inducible AP-1 DNA-binding activity is essential for both basal and cytokine-induced MMP-13 promoter activity. IL-17A also increases the concentration of biologically active MMP-9 and MMP-1 (Chabaud *et al.*, 2000; Jovanovic *et al.*, 2000; Prause *et al.*, 2004).

A number of other genes with inflammatory activities are induced by IL-17A, alone or combination with other inflammatory cytokines such as TNF-α or IL-1β. For example, the acute phase protein 24p3/lipocalin 2 is strongly enhanced by IL-17A in osteoblasts and bone marrow stromal cells (Shen *et al.*, 2005, 2006). 24p3 exhibits potent antibacterial functions by competing with bacterial siderophores to limit concentrations of free iron in blood, and thus may be involved in IL-17A-mediated host defense to certain types of bacterial infections (Flo *et al.*, 2004). IL-17A also enhances expression of β-defensins (Kao *et al.*, 2004), IκBζ (Shen *et al.*, 2005) and C/EBP family transcription factors (Ruddy *et al.*, 2004b) (see Section IV.B). Although the entire spectrum of IL-17A target genes has probably not been completely defined, it is clear that the major function of IL-17A *in vivo* is to promote inflammation, which is reflected in the genes it regulates.

B. MAJOR SIGNALING PATHWAYS

On its discovery, IL-17RA shared no apparent homology with other known receptor proteins, making it impossible to predict signaling function on the basis of receptor primary structure. However, early studies showed that IL-17A activated the NF-κB pathway (Yao *et al.*, 1995), a classic inflammatory signaling pathway activated by diverse stimuli including antigen receptors, inflammatory cytokines, Toll-like receptors, and UV light (Lin and Wang, 2004). Although the means by which IL-17RA signaling leads to NF-κB activation is still poorly understood, a bioinformatics analysis has proposed that IL-17R family members contain a region within the intracellular tail that appears to be homologous to the TIR domain, a functional motif present in *T*LR and *I*L-1 *r*eceptors. The TIR domain is a site of interaction for other TIR-containing molecules such as MyD88 (Novatchkova *et al.*, 2003), which in turn initiate intracellular signaling cascades leading to NF-κB activation. However, the functionality of this putative signaling motif in IL-17RA has not been verified experimentally. Its homology with the TIR domain suggests that IL-17RA may activate signaling components common to TIR-domain containing receptors such as the IL-1R. Consistent with this, IL-17A-induced NF-κB activation is dependent on the molecule TRAF6 (Awane *et al.*, 1999; Schwandner *et al.*, 2000), which is also recruited by IL-1β and TLRs. However, there are no obvious TRAF6-binding domains within IL-17RA (Pullen *et al.*, 1999), and therefore, it is likely that TRAF6 does not bind IL-17RA directly, but rather bridges it through MyD88 or a related adaptor. Moreover, the downstream effectors of TRAF6 in the IL-17RA signaling pathway have not been defined, and it remains to be seen if IL-17A, IL-1β, or TLR ligands activate the same signaling pathways. Also consistent with a key role for NF-κB, the majority of IL-17A target genes contain NF-κB sites in their proximal promoters, and in some cases it has been shown directly that these sites are indeed essential for IL-17A-mediated transcription (Ruddy *et al.*, 2004b). Although it is certainly clear that IL-17A activates NF-κB, in many cell types NF-κB activation is considerably lower than the level of activation induced by other inflammatory stimuli such as LPS or TNF-α, even at very high concentrations of IL-17A (Hwang *et al.*, 2004; Ruddy *et al.*, 2004b). Therefore, given the powerful *in vivo* effects of IL-17, it is likely that this cytokine activates additional signaling pathways.

While NF-κB is one essential transcription factor activated by IL-17A, microarray studies examining IL-17A-induced target genes revealed that members of the C/EBP family [also known as the NF-IL6 transcription factors (Ramji and Foka, 2002)] were also involved in IL-17A signal transduction (Fig. 2). Specifically, treatment of various cell types with IL-17A and/ or TNF-α lead to upregulation of expression of C/EBPδ and C/EBPβ mRNA (Shen *et al.*, 2005). In the IL-6 promoter, the NF-κB site and C/EBP sites are both essential for IL-17A/TNF-α-mediated promoter activation. Moreover, C/EBP-deficient cells fail to induce IL-6 in response to IL-17A, and overexpression of C/EBPβ or C/EBPδ can partly substitute for IL-17A-mediated signal transduction (Ruddy *et al.*, 2004b). Strikingly, many other IL-17A-induced genes such as COX2, 24p3, and CXCL1 also contain conserved C/EBP and NF-κB promoter elements in their minimal promoters, suggesting a common pathway by which IL-17A may activate transcription of target genes through both NF-κB and C/EBP (Shen *et al.*, 2006). C/EBP protein expression and activities are regulated both transcriptionally and by post-transcriptional events. For example, phosphorylation of C/EBPβ has been suggested to be required for its nuclear localization (Piwien Pilipuk *et al.*, 2003; Ramji and Foka, 2002). In this regard, a number of kinases have been implicated in phosphorylation of C/EBPβ, including MAPK and glycogen synthase kinase 3β (GSK3β) (Tang *et al.*, 2005). The C/EBPδ gene is also capable of autoregulation, as its own promoter contains a functional C/EBP DNA-binding site (Yamada *et al.*, 1998). Since C/EBP family members are

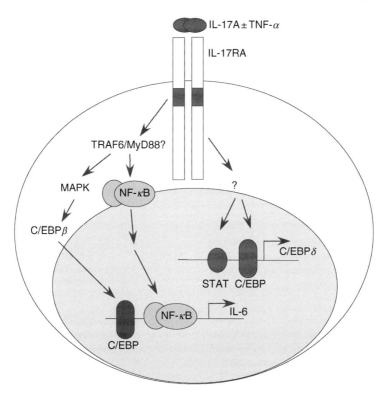

FIGURE 2. Role of C/EBP in IL-17RA-mediated signal transduction. Treatment of target cells with IL-17A and/or TNF-α leads to activation of the NF-κB and MAPK pathways, probably through the adaptors MyD88 and TRAF6. These signals lead to transcriptional upregulation of various C/EBP isoforms, especially C/EBPδ, as well as posttranscriptional modification (e.g., phosphorylation) of C/EBPβ. In addition, critical C/EBP DNA-binding sites are present in the promoters of both the C/EBPδ and IL-6 genes, leading to further enhancement of C/EBP-dependent gene activation.

also transcriptional targets of IL-17A signaling, this suggests a positive reinforcement of IL-17A signaling mediated via C/EBP expression (Fig. 2).

Considerable evidence supports a role for the MAP kinases ERK1, ERK2, JNK, and p38 in IL-17A receptor signaling. Numerous studies using kinase-specific inhibitors showed blunted IL-17A activation of MAPKs and inhibited expression of respective target genes (Laan *et al.*, 2001; Martel-Pelletier *et al.*, 1999; Shalom-Barak *et al.*, 1998). Although never proven directly, it is likely that the MAPK pathway is downstream of TRAF6 (Schwandner *et al.*, 2000), as it is in TLR-signaling pathways. One key function of IL-17A-induced MAPK activation may be to regulate mRNA stability. For example, IL-17 increased COX-2 reporter gene mRNA stability and protein synthesis via distal regions of the 3′-untranslated region.

This response was mediated entirely by p38 MAPK cascade (Faour *et al.*, 2003). Other genes such as IL-6 are probably also regulated by mRNA stability through the MAPK pathway (Henness *et al.*, 2004). MAPK signaling probably also activates the AP1 transcription factor complex, which is classically composed of c-fos (induced by the p38 MAPK pathway) and c-Jun (activated by the JNK pathway). Numerous IL-17A target genes contain important AP1 DNA-binding elements, and are probably the endpoints of MAPK-signaling pathways. It has also been suggested that the MAPK pathway is another point of synergy between IL-17A and TNF-α signaling (Tokuda *et al.*, 2004).

Additional kinase pathways may also be involved in IL-17RA signaling. For example, a specific src kinase inhibitor was shown to reduce IL-6, IL-8, and MCP-1 mRNA expression stimulated by IL-17A in a dose-dependent manner (Hsieh *et al.*, 2002). Although some reports have suggested that the JAK-STAT pathway may be involved in IL-17A-mediated signaling, none of the data are especially convincing (Subramaniam *et al.*, 1999); moreover, a report showed that IL-17A treatment increased IL-6 expression in STAT1-deficient fibroblasts, thus indicating that STAT1 activation and subsequent IRF-1 transcription are not required for induction of IL-6 (Samardzic *et al.*, 2001). It has also been suggested that IL-17A also activates the phosphatidylinositol-3 kinase (PI-3K)/Akt signaling pathway and that this event is upstream of IL-6 and IL-8 gene expression (Hwang *et al.*, 2004). If true, PI-3K signaling may intersect the NF-κB pathway, analogous to signals in the T cell receptor system (Kane *et al.*, 1999). In summary, there remains much to be learned about the mechanisms of IL-17RA signal transduction, and elucidation of such pathways may eventually be the basis for rational drug design for diseases involving this cytokine.

V. CONCLUDING REMARKS

The genomics era has revealed the existence of many new cytokines. The IL-17 family of cytokines and receptors remain enigmatic in their ligand–receptor relationships, functions, and signaling mechanisms, but their biological significance is rapidly becoming appreciated.

ACKNOWLEDGMENT

SLG was supported by the NIH (AR050458) and the Arthritis Foundation. JMK was supported by an individual predoctoral training grant (DE01483) and JJY was supported by the Medical Scientist Training Program at the University at Buffalo and an Oral Biology training grant (DE007034). We thank Dr. Steven Levin of Zymogenetics for sharing unpublished information and Dr. Matthew Ruddy for critical reading of the chapter.

REFERENCES

Aggarwal, S., Ghilardi, N., Xie, M. H., De Sauvage, F. J., and Gurney, A. L. (2002). Interleukin 23 promotes a distinct CD4 T cell activation state characterized by the production of interleukin 17. *J. Biol. Chem.* **3,** 1910–1914.

Aggarwal, S., and Gurney, A. L. (2002). IL-17: A prototype member of an emerging family. *J. Leukoc. Biol.* **71,** 1–8.

Albanesi, C., Cavani, A., and Girolomoni, G. (1999). IL-17 is produced by nickel-specific T lymphocytes and regulates ICAM-1 expression and chemokine production in human keratinocytes: Synergistic or antagonistic effects with IFN-γ and TNF-α. *J. Immunol.* **162,** 494–502.

Andoh, A., Fujino, S., Bamba, S., Araki, Y., Okuno, T., Bamba, T., and Fujiyama, Y. (2002). IL-17 selectively down-regulates TNF-alpha-induced RANTES gene expression in human colonic subepithelial myofibroblasts. *J. Immunol.* **169,** 1683–1687.

Arican, O., Aral, M., Sasmaz, S., and Ciragil, P. (2005). Serum Levels of TNF-alpha, IFN-gamma, IL-**6,** IL-**8,** IL-**12,** IL-**17,** and IL-18 in patients with active psoriasis and correlation with disease severity. *Mediators Inflamm.* **2005,** 273–279.

Attur, M. G., Patel, R. N., Abramson, S. B., and Amin, A. R. (1997). Interleukin-17 up-regulation of nitric oxide production in human osteoarthritis cartilage. *Arthritis Rheum.* **40,** 1050–1053.

Awane, M., Andres, P. G., Li, D. J., and Reinecker, H. C. (1999). NF-kappa B-inducing kinase is a common mediator of IL-17-, TNF-alpha-, and IL-1 beta-induced chemokine promoter activation in intestinal epithelial cells. *J. Immunol.* **162,** 5337–5344.

Bamba, S., Andoh, A., Yasui, H., Araki, Y., Bamba, T., and Fujiyama, Y. (2003). Matrix metalloproteinase-3 secretion from human colonic subepithelial myofibroblasts: Role of interleukin-17. *J. Gastroenterol.* **38,** 548–554.

Benchetrit, F., Ciree, A., Vives, V., Warnier, G., Gey, A., Sautes-Fridman, C., Fossiez, F., Haicheur, N., Fridman, W. H., and Tartour, E. (2002). Interleukin-17 inhibits tumor cell growth by means of a T-cell-dependent mechanism. *Blood* **99,** 2114–2121.

Bettelli, E., and Kuchroo, V. K. (2005). IL-12- and IL-23-induced T helper cell subsets: Birds of the same feather flock together. *J. Exp. Med.* **201,** 169–171.

Bettelli, E., Carrier, Y., Gao, W., Korn, T., Strom, T. B., Oukka, M., Weiner, H. L., and Kuchroo, V. J. (2006). Reciprocal developmental pathways for the generation of pathogenic effector T$_H$17 and regulatory T cells. *Nature* **441,** 235–238.

Chabaud, M., Fossiez, F., Taupin, J. L., and Miossec, P. (1998). Enhancing effect of IL-17 on IL-1-induced IL-6 and leukemia inhibitory factor production by rheumatoid arthritis, synoviocytes and its regulation by Th2 cytokines. *J. Immunol.* **161,** 409–414.

Chabaud, M., Garnero, P., Dayer, J. M., Guerne, P. A., Fossiez, F., and Miossec, P. (2000). Contribution of interleukin 17 to synovium matrix destruction in rheumatoid arthritis. *Cytokine* **12,** 1092–1099.

Chan, F. K., Chun, H. J., Zheng, L., Siegel, R. M., Bui, K. L., and Lenardo, M. J. (2000). A domain in TNF receptors that mediates ligand-independent receptor assembly and signaling. *Science* **288,** 2351–2354.

Chen, A., Laurence, A., Kanno, Y., Pacher-Zavisin, M., Zhu, B.-M., Tato, C., Yoshimura, A., Hennighausen, L., and O'Shea, J. J. (2006). Selective regulatory function of Socs3 in the formation of IL-17-secreting cells. *Proc. Natl. Acad. Sci. USA* **103,** 8137–8142.

Ciree, A., Michel, L., Camilleri-Broet, S., Jean Louis, F., Oster, M., Flageul, B., Senet, P., Fossiez, F., Fridman, W. H., Bachelez, H., and Tartour, E. (2004). Expression and activity of IL-17 in cutaneous T-cell lymphomas (mycosis fungoides and Sezary syndrome). *Int. J. Cancer* **112,** 113–120.

Clark, H. F., Gurney, A. L., Abaya, E., Baker, K., Baldwin, D., Brush, J., Chen, J., Chow, B., Chui, C., Crowley, C., Currell, B., Deuel, B., *et al.* (2003). The secreted protein discovery initiative (SPDI), a large-scale effort to identify novel human secreted and transmembrane proteins: A bioinformatics assessment. *Genome Res.* **13,** 2265–2270.

Dong, C., and Nurieva, R. I. (2003). Regulation of immune and autoimmune responses by ICOS. *J. Autoimmunity* **21,** 255–260.

Eberl, M. (2002). Don't count your interleukins before they've hatched. *Trends Immunol.* **23,** 341–342.

Faour, W. H., Mancini, A., He, Q. W., and Di Battista, J. A. (2003). T-cell-derived interleukin-17 regulates the level and stability of cyclooxygenase-2 (COX-2) mRNA through restricted activation of the p38 mitogen-activated protein kinase cascade: Role of distal sequences in the 3'-untranslated region of COX-2 mRNA. *J. Biol. Chem.* **278,** 26897–26907.

Flo, T. H., Smith, K. D., Sato, S., Rodriguez, D. J., Holmes, M. A., Strong, R. K., Akira, S., and Aderem, A. (2004). Lipocalin 2 mediates an innate immune response to bacterial infection by sequestrating iron. *Nature* **432,** 917–921.

Forlow, S. B., Schurr, J. R., Kolls, J. K., Bagby, G. J., Schwarzenberger, P. O., and Ley, K. (2001). Increased granulopoiesis through interleukin-17 and granulocyte colony-stimulating factor in leukocyte adhesion molecule-deficient mice. *Blood* **98,** 3309–3314.

Fort, M. M., Cheung, J., Yen, D., Li, J., Zurawski, S. M., Lo, S., Menon, S., Clifford, T., Hunte, B., Lesley, R., Muchamuel, T., Hurst, S. D., *et al.* (2001). IL-25 induces IL-4, IL-5, and IL-13 and Th2–associated pathologies *in vivo*. *Immunity* **15,** 985–995.

Fossiez, F., Djossou, O., Chomarat, P., Flores-Romo, L., Ait-Yahia, S., Maat, C., Pin, J.-J., Garrone, P., Garcia, E., Saeland, S., Blanchard, D., Gaillard, C., *et al.* (1996). T cell interleukin-17 induces stromal cells to produce proinflammatory and hematopoietic cytokines. *J. Exp. Med.* **183,** 2593–2603.

Fujino, S., Andoh, A., Bamba, S., Ogawa, A., Hata, K., Araki, Y., Bamba, T., and Fujiyama, Y. (2003). Increased expression of interleukin 17 in inflammatory bowel disease. *Gut* **52,** 65–70.

Gaffen, S. L. (2004). Interleukin-17: A unique inflammatory cytokine with roles in bone biology and arthritis. *Arth. Res. Ther.* **6,** 240–247.

Ghilardi, N., Kljavin, N., Chen, Q., Lucas, S., Gurney, A., and de Sauvage, F. J. (2004). Compromised humoral and delayed-type hypersensitivity responses in IL-23–deficient mice. *J. Immunol.* **172,** 2827–2833.

Happel, K. I., Lockhart, E. A., Mason, C. M., Porretta, E., Keoshkerian, E., Odden, A. R., Nelson, S., and Ramsay, A. J. (2005). Pulmonary interleukin-23 gene delivery increases local T-cell immunity and controls growth of *Mycobacterium tuberculosis* in the lungs. *Infect. Immun.* **73,** 5782–5788.

Happel, K. I., Zheng, M., Young, E., Quinton, L. J., Lockhart, E., Ramsay, A. J., Shellito, J. E., Schurr, J. R., Bagby, G. J., Nelson, S., and Kolls, J. K. (2003). Cutting Edge: Roles of Toll-like receptor 4 and IL-23 in IL-17 expression in response to *Klebsiella pneumoniae* Infection. *J. Immunol.* **170,** 4432–4436.

Harrington, L. E., Hatton, R. D., Mangan, P. R., Turner, H., Murphy, T. L., Murphy, K. M., and Weaver, C. T. (2005). Interleukin 17–producing CD4+ effector T cells develop via a lineage distinct from the T helper type 1 and 2 lineages. *Nat. Immunol.* **6,** 1123–1132.

Hata, K., Andoh, A., Shimada, M., Fujino, S., Bamba, S., Araki, Y., Okuno, T., Fujiyama, Y., and Bamba, T. (2002). IL-17 stimulates inflammatory responses via NF-kappaB and MAP kinase pathways in human colonic myofibroblasts. *Am. J. Physiol. Gastrointest. Liver Physiol.* **282,** G1035–G1044.

Haudenschild, D., Moseley, T., Rose, L., and Reddi, A. H. (2002). Soluble and transmembrane isoforms of novel interleukin-17 receptor-like protein by RNA splicing and expression in prostate cancer. *J. Biol. Chem.* **277,** 4309–4316.

Henness, S., Johnson, C. K., Ge, Q., Armour, C. L., Hughes, J. M., and Ammit, A. J. (2004). IL-17A augments TNF-alpha-induced IL-6 expression in airway smooth muscle by enhancing mRNA stability. *J. Allergy Clin. Immunol.* **114,** 958–964.

Hirahara, N., Nio, Y., Sasaki, S., Minari, Y., Takamura, M., Iguchi, C., Dong, M., Yamasawa, K., and Tamura, K. (2001). Inoculation of human interleukin-17 gene-transfected Meth-A fibrosarcoma cells induces T cell-dependent tumor-specific immunity in mice. *Oncology* **61**, 79–89.

Honorati, M. C., Neri, S., Cattini, L., and Facchini, A. (2003). IL-17 enhances the susceptibility of U-2 OS osteosarcoma cells to NK cell lysis. *Clin. Exp. Immunol.* **133**, 344–349.

Hsieh, H. G., Loong, C. C., and Lin, C. Y. (2002). Interleukin-17 induces src/MAPK cascades activation in human renal epithelial cells. *Cytokine* **19**, 159–174.

Huang, W., Na, L., Fidel, P. L., and Schwarzenberger, P. (2004). Requirement of interleukin-17A for systemic anti-Candida albicans host defense in mice. *J. Infect. Dis.* **190**, 624–631.

Hurst, S. D., Muchamuel, T., Gorman, D. M., Gilbert, J. M., Clifford, T., Kwan, S., Menon, S., Seymour, B., Jackson, C., Kung, T. T., Brieland, J. K., Zurawski, S. M., *et al.* (2002). New IL-17 family members promote Th1 or Th2 responses in the lung: *In vivo* function of the novel cytokine IL-25. *J. Immunol.* **169**, 443–453.

Hwang, S. Y., Kim, J. Y., Kim, K. W., Park, M. K., Moon, Y., Kim, W. U., and Kim, H. Y. (2004). IL-17 induces production of IL-6 and IL-8 in rheumatoid arthritis synovial fibroblasts via NF-kappaB- and PI3-kinase/Akt-dependent pathways. *Arthritis Res. Ther.* **6**, R120–128.

Hymowitz, S. G., Filvaroff, E. H., Yin, J. P., Lee, J., Cai, L., Risser, P., Maruoka, M., Mao, W., Foster, J., Kelley, R. F., Pan, G., Gurney, A. L., *et al.* (2001). IL-17s adopt a cystine knot fold: Structure and activity of a novel cytokine, IL-17F, and implications for receptor binding. *EMBO J.* **20**, 5332–5341.

Johnson, R. B., Wood, N., and Serio, F. G. (2004). Interleukin-11 and IL-17 and the pathogenesis of periodontal disease. *J. Periodontol.* **75**, 37–43.

Jovanovic, D. V., Martel-Pelletier, J., Di Battista, J. A., Mineau, F., Jolicoeur, F.-C., Benderdour, M., and Pelletier, J.-P. (2000). Stimulation of 92-kD gelatinase (matrix metalloproteinase 9) production by interleukin-17 in human monocyte/macrophages. *Arthritis Rheum.* **43**, 1134–1144.

Kane, L. P., Shapiro, V. S., Stokoe, D., and Weiss, A. (1999). Induction of NF-kappaB by the Akt/PKB kinase. *Curr. Biol.* **9**, 601–604.

Kantarci, A., Oyaizu, K., and Van Dyke, T. E. (2003). Neutrophil-mediated tissue injury in periodontal disease pathogenesis: Findings from localized aggressive periodontitis. *J. Periodontol.* **74**, 66–75.

Kao, C. Y., Chen, Y., Thai, P., Wachi, S., Huang, F., Kim, C., Harper, R. W., and Wu, R. (2004). IL-17 markedly up-regulates beta-defensin-2 expression in human airway epithelium via JAK and NF-kappaB signaling pathways. *J. Immunol.* **173**, 3482–3491.

Kato, T., Furumoto, H., Ogura, T., Onishi, Y., Irahara, M., Yamano, S., Kamada, M., and Aono, T. (2001). Expression of IL-17 mRNA in ovarian cancer. *Biochem. Biophys. Res. Commun.* **282**, 735–738.

Kelly, M. N., Kolls, J. K., Happel, K., Schwartzman, J. D., Schwarzenberger, P., Combe, C., Moretto, M., and Khan, I. A. (2005). Interleukin-17/interleukin-17 receptor-mediated signaling is important for generation of an optimal polymorphonuclear response against *Toxoplasma gondii* infection. *Infect. Immun.* **73**, 617–621.

Khader, S. A., Pearl, J. E., Sakamoto, K., Gilmartin, L., Bell, G. K., Jelley-Gibbs, D. M., Ghilardi, N., deSauvage, F., and Cooper, A. M. (2005). IL-23 compensates for the absence of IL-12p70 and is essential for the IL-17 response during tuberculosis but is dispensable for protection and antigen-specific IFN-gamma responses if IL-12p70 is available. *J. Immunol.* **175**, 788–795.

Kim, M. R., Manoukian, R., Yeh, R., Silbiger, S. M., Danilenko, D. M., Scully, S., Sun, J., DeRose, M. L., Stolina, M., Chang, D., Van, G. Y., Clarkin, K., *et al.* (2002). Transgenic overexpression of human IL-17E results in eosinophilia, B-lymphocyte hyperplasia, and altered antibody production. *Blood* **100**, 2330–2340.

Knappe, A., Hiller, C., Niphuis, H., Fossiez, F., Thurau, M., Wittmann, S., Kuhn, E. M., Lebecque, S., Banchereau, J., Rosenwirth, B., Fleckenstein, B., Heeney, J., *et al.* (1998). The interleukin-17 gene of herpesvirus saimiri. *J. Virol.* **72**, 5797–5801.

Kobayashi, S. D., Voyich, J. M., Braughton, K. R., and DeLeo, F. R. (2003). Down-regulation of proinflammatory capacity during apoptosis in human polymorphonuclear leukocytes. *J. Immunol.* **170**, 3357–3368.

Koenders, M. I., Kolls, J. K., Oppers-Walgreen, B., van den Bersselaar, L., Joosten, L. A., Schurr, J. R., Schwarzenberger, P., van den Berg, W. B., and Lubberts, E. (2005). Interleukin-17 receptor deficiency results in impaired synovial expression of interleukin-1 and matrix metalloproteinases 3, 9, and 13 and prevents cartilage destruction during chronic reactivated streptococcal cell wall-induced arthritis. *Arthritis Rheum.* **52**, 3239–3247.

Kolls, J. K., and Linden, A. (2004). Interleukin-17 family members and inflammation. *Immunity* **21**, 467–476.

Koshy, P. J., Henderson, N., Logan, C., Life, P. F., Cawston, T. E., and Rowan, A. D. (2002). Interleukin 17 induces cartilage collagen breakdown: Novel synergistic effects in combination with proinflammatory cytokines. *Ann. Rheum. Dis.* **61**, 704–713.

Kotake, S., Udagawa, N., Takahashi, N., Matsuzaki, K., Itoh, K., Ishiyama, S., Saito, S., Inoue, K., Kamatani, N., Gillespie, M. T., Martin, T. J., and Suda, T. (1999). IL-17 in synovial fluids from patients with rheumatoid arthritis is a potent stimulator of osteoclastogenesis. *J. Clin. Invest.* **103**, 1345–1352.

Kramer, J., Yi, L., Shen, F., Maitra, A., Jiao, X., Jin, T., and Gaffen, S. (2006). Cutting edge: Evidence for ligand-independent multimerization of the IL-17 receptor. *J. Immunol.* **176**, 711–715.

Laan, M., Cui, A.-H., Hoshino, H., Lötvall, J., Sjöstrand, M., Gruenert, D. C., Skoogh, B.-E., and Lindén, A. (1999). Neutrophil recruitment by human IL-17 via C-X-C chemokine release in the airways. *J. Immunol.* **162**, 2347–2352.

Laan, M., Lotvall, J., Chung, K. F., and Linden, A. (2001). IL-17–induced cytokine release in human bronchial epithelial cells *in vitro*: Role of mitogen-activated protein (MAP) kinases. *Br. J. Pharmacol.* **133**, 200–206.

Laan, M., Prause, O., Miyamoto, M., Sjostrand, M., Hytonen, A. M., Kaneko, T., Lotvall, J., and Linden, A. (2003). A role of GM-CSF in the accumulation of neutrophils in the airways caused by IL-17 and TNF-alpha. *Eur. Respir. J.* **21**, 387–393.

Langrish, C. L., Chen, Y., Blumenschein, W. M., Mattson, J., Basham, B., Sedgwick, J. D., McClanahan, T., Kastelein, R. A., and Cua, D. J. (2005). IL-23 drives a pathogenic T cell population that induces autoimmune inflammation. *J. Exp. Med.* **201**, 233–240.

Lee, J., Ho, W. H., Maruoka, M., Corpuz, R. T., Baldwin, D. T., Foster, J. S., Goddard, A. D., Yansura, D. G., Vandlen, R. L., Wood, W. I., and Gurney, A. L. (2001). IL-17E, a novel proinflammatory ligand for the IL-17 receptor homolog IL-17Rh1. *J. Biol. Chem.* **276**, 1660–1664.

LeGrand, A., Fermor, B., Fink, C., Pisetsky, D. S., Weinberg, J. B., Vail, T. P., and Guilak, F. (2001). Interleukin-1, tumor necrosis factor alpha, and interleukin-17 synergistically up-regulate nitric oxide and prostaglandin E2 production in explants of human osteoarthritic knee menisci. *Arthritis Rheum.* **44**, 2078–2083.

Li, H., Chen, J., Huang, A., Stinson, J., Heldens, S., Foster, J., Dowd, P., Gurney, A. L., and Wood, W. I. (2000). Cloning and characterization of IL-17B and IL-17C, two new members of the IL-17 family. *Proc. Natl. Acad. Sci. USA* **97**, 773–778.

Liacini, A., Sylvester, J., Li, W. Q., and Zafarullah, M. (2005a). Mithramycin downregulates proinflammatory cytokine-induced matrix metalloproteinase gene expression in articular chondrocytes. *Arthritis Res. Ther.* **7**, R777–R783.

Liacini, A., Sylvester, J., and Zafarullah, M. (2005b). Triptolide suppresses proinflammatory cytokine-induced matrix metalloproteinase and aggrecanase-1 gene expression in chondrocytes. *Biochem. Biophys. Res. Commun.* **327**, 320–327.

Liew, F. Y., and McInnes, I. B. (2005). A fork in the pathway to inflammation and arthritis. *Nat. Med.* **11**, 601–602.

Lin, X., and Wang, D. (2004). The roles of CARMA1, Bcl10, and MALT1 in antigen receptor signaling. *Semin. Immunol.* **16**, 429–435.

Linden, A., Laan, M., and Anderson, G. (2005). Neutrophils, interleukin-17A and lung disease. *Eur. Respir. J.* **25**, 159–172.

Liu, X., Lin, X., and Gaffen, S. L. (2004). Crucial role for nuclear factor of activated T cells (NFAT) in T cell receptor-mediated regulation of the human interleukin-17 gene. *J. Biol. Chem.* **279**, 52762–52771.

Liu, X. K., Clements, J. L., and Gaffen, S. L. (2005). Signaling through the murine T cell receptor induces IL-17 production in the absence of costimulation, IL-23 or dendritic cells. *Mol. Cells* **20**, 329–337.

Lubberts, E., van den Bersselaar, L., Oppers-Walgreen, B., Schwarzenberger, P., Coenen-de Roo, C. J., Kolls, J. K., Joosten, L. A., and van den Berg, W. B. (2003). IL-17 promotes bone erosion in murine collagen-induced arthritis through loss of the receptor activator of NF-kappa B ligand/osteoprotegerin balance. *J. Immunol.* **170**, 2655–2662.

Lubberts, E., Koenders, M. I., and van den Berg, W. B. (2005a). The role of T cell interleukin-17 in conducting destructive arthritis: Lessons from animal models. *Arthritis Res. Ther.* **7**, 29–37.

Lubberts, E., Schwarzenberger, P., Huang, W., Schurr, J. R., Peschon, J. J., van den Berg, W. B., and Kolls, J. K. (2005b). Requirement of IL-17 receptor signaling in radiation-resistant cells in the joint for full progression of destructive synovitis. *J. Immunol.* **175**, 3360–3368.

Maertzdorf, J., Osterhaus, A. D., and Verjans, G. M. (2002). IL-17 expression in human herpetic stromal keratitis: Modulatory effects on chemokine production by corneal fibroblasts. *J. Immunol.* **169**, 5897–5903.

Maggio, E., van den Berg, A., Diepstra, A., Kluiver, J., Visser, L., and Poppema, S. (2002). Chemokines, cytokines and their receptors in Hodgkin's lymphoma cell lines and tissues. *Ann. Oncol.* **13**(Suppl. 1), 52–56.

Mangan, P. R., Harrington, L. E., O'Quinn, D. B., Helms, W. S., Bullard, D. C., Elson, C. O., Hatton, R. D., Wahl, S. M., Schoe, T. R., and Weaver, C. T. (2006). Transforming growth factor-β induces development of the $T_H 17$ lineage. *Nature* **441**, 231–234.

Martel-Pelletier, J., Mineau, F., Jovanovic, D., Di Battista, J. A., and Pelletier, J. P. (1999). Mitogen-activated protein kinase and nuclear factor kappaB together regulate interleukin-17–induced nitric oxide production in human osteoarthritic chondrocytes: Possible role of transactivating factor mitogen-activated protein kinase-activated protein kinase (MAP-KAPK). *Arthritis Rheum.* **42**, 2399–2409.

Matusevicius, D., Kivisakk, P., He, B., Kostulas, N., Ozenci, V., Fredrikson, S., and Link, H. (1999). Interleukin-17 mRNA expression in blood and CSF mononuclear cells is augmented in multiple sclerosis. *Mult. Scler.* **5**, 101–104.

McAllister, F., Henry, A., Kreindler, J. L., Dubin, P. J., Ulrich, L., Steele, C., Finder, J. D., Pilewski, J. M., Carreno, B. M., Goldman, S. J., Pirhonen, J., and Kolls, J. K. (2005). Role of IL-17A, IL-17F, and the IL-17 receptor in regulating growth-related oncogene-alpha and granulocyte colony-stimulating factor in bronchial epithelium: Implications for airway inflammation in cystic fibrosis. *J. Immunol.* **175**, 404–412.

Miljkovic, D., and Trajkovic, V. (2004). Inducible nitric oxide synthase activation by interleukin-17. *Cytokine Growth Factor Rev.* **15**, 21–32.

Miljkovic, D., Cvetkovic, I., Momcilovic, M., Maksimovic-Ivanic, D., Stosic-Grujicic, S., and Trajkovic, V. (2005). Interleukin-17 stimulates inducible nitric oxide synthase-dependent toxicity in mouse beta cells. *Cell. Mol. Life Sci.* **62**, 2658–2668.

Miossec, P. (2003). Interleukin-17 in rheumatoid arthritis: If T cells were to contribute to inflammation and destruction through synergy. *Arthritis Rheum.* **48**, 594–601.

Moseley, T. A., Haudenschild, D. R., Rose, L., and Reddi, A. H. (2003). Interleukin-17 family and IL-17 receptors. *Cytokine Growth Factor Rev.* **14**, 155–174.

Nakae, S., Nambu, A., Sudo, K., and Iwakura, Y. (2003a). Suppression of immune induction of collagen-induced arthritis in IL-17–deficient mice. *J. Immunol* **171**, 6173–6177.

Nakae, S., Saijo, S., Horai, R., Sudo, K., Mori, S., and Iwakura, Y. (2003b). IL-17 production from activated T cells is required for the spontaneous development of destructive arthritis in mice deficient in IL-1 receptor antagonist. *Proc. Natl. Acad. Sci. USA* **100**, 5986–5990.

Novatchkova, M., Leibbrandt, A., Werzowa, J., Neubuser, A., and Eisenhaber, F. (2003). The STIR-domain superfamily in signal transduction, development and immunity. *Trends Biochem. Sci.* **28**, 226–229.

Numasaki, M., Fukushi, J., Ono, M., Narula, S. K., Zavodny, P. J., Kudo, T., Robbins, P. D., Tahara, H., and Lotze, M. T. (2003). Interleukin-17 promotes angiogenesis and tumor growth. *Blood* **101**, 2620–2627.

Numasaki, M., Watanabe, M., Suzuki, T., Takahashi, H., Nakamura, A., McAllister, F., Hishinuma, T., Goto, J., Lotze, M. T., Kolls, J. K., and Sasaki, H. (2005). IL-17 enhances the net angiogenic activity and *in vivo* growth of human non-small cell lung cancer in SCID mice through promoting CXCR-2–dependent angiogenesis. *J. Immunol.* **175**, 6177–6189.

Owyang, A., Schmitz, J., McClanahan, T., Artis, D., Kastelein, R., and Cua, D. (2005). IL-25 is required for the regulation of autoimmunity and immunity to parasites. Paper presented at Keystone Symposia: Cytokines, Disease and Therapeutic Intervention (Santa Fe, NM).

Ozaki, K., and Leonard, W. J. (2002). Cytokine and cytokine receptor pleiotropy and redundancy. *J. Biol. Chem.* **277**, 29355–29358.

Pan, G., French, D., Mao, W., Maruoka, M., Risser, P., Lee, J., Foster, J., Aggarwal, S., Nicholes, K., Guillet, S., Schow, P., and Gurney, A. L. (2001). Forced expression of murine IL-17E induces growth retardation, jaundice, a Th2–biased response, and multiorgan inflammation in mice. *J. Immunol.* **167**, 6559–6567.

Pancer, Z., Mayer, W. E., Klein, J., and Cooper, M. D. (2004). Prototypic T cell receptor and CD4–like coreceptor are expressed by lymphocytes in the agnathan sea lamprey. *Proc. Natl. Acad. Sci. USA* **101**, 13273–13278.

Park, H., Li, Z., Yang, X. O., Chang, S. H., Nurieva, R., Wang, Y. H., Wang, Y., Hood, L., Zhu, Z., Tian, Q., and Dong, C. (2005). A distinct lineage of CD4 T cells regulates tissue inflammation by producing interleukin 17. *Nat. Immunol.* **6**, 1133–1141.

Piwien Pilipuk, G., Galigniana, M. D., and Schwartz, J. (2003). Subnuclear localization of C/EBP beta is regulated by growth hormone and dependent on MAPK. *J. Biol. Chem.* **278**, 35668–35677.

Prause, O., Bozinovski, S., Anderson, G. P., and Linden, A. (2004). Increased matrix metalloproteinase-9 concentration and activity after stimulation with interleukin-17 in mouse airways. *Thorax* **59**, 313–317.

Pullen, S. S., Dang, T. T., Crute, J. J., and Kehry, M. R. (1999). CD40 signaling through tumor necrosis factor receptor-associated factors (TRAFs). Binding site specificity and activation of downstream pathways by distinct TRAFs. *J. Biol. Chem.* **274**, 14246–14254.

Ramji, D. P., and Foka, P. (2002). CCAAT/enhancer-binding proteins: Structure, function and regulation. *Biochem. J.* **365**, 561–575.

Remy, I., Wilson, I. A., and Michnick, S. W. (1999). Erythropietin receptor activation by a ligand-induced conformation change. *Science* **283**, 990–993.

Rouvier, E., Luciani, M.-F., Mattei, M.-G., Denizot, F., and Golstein, P. (1993). CTLA-**8,** cloned from an activated T cell, bearing AU-rich messenger RNA instability sequences, and homologous to a *Herpesvirus Saimiri* gene. *J. Immunol.* **150**, 5445–5456.

Ruddy, M. J., Shen, F., Smith, J., Sharma, A., and Gaffen, S. L. (2004a). Interleukin-17 regulates expression of the CXC chemokine LIX/CXCL5 in osteoblasts: Implications for inflammation and neutrophil recruitment. *J. Leukoc. Biol.* **76**, 135–144.

Ruddy, M. J., Wong, G. C., Liu, X. K., Yamamoto, H., Kasayama, S., Kirkwood, K. L., and Gaffen, S. L. (2004b). Functional cooperation between interleukin-17 and tumor necrosis factor-α is mediated by CCAAT/enhancer-binding protein family members. *J. Biol. Chem.* **279**, 2559–2567.

Rutitzky, L. I., Lopes da Rosa, J. R., and Stadecker, M. J. (2005). Severe CD4 T cell-mediated immunopathology in murine schistosomiasis is dependent on IL-12p40 and correlates with high levels of IL-17. *J. Immunol.* **175**, 3920–3926.

Samardzic, T., Jankovic, V., Stosic-Grujicic, S., and Trajkovic, V. (2001). STAT1 is required for iNOS activation, but not IL-6 production in murine fibroblasts. *Cytokine* **13**, 179–182.

Schwandner, R., Yamaguchi, K., and Cao, Z. (2000). Requirement of tumor necrosis factor-associated factor (TRAF) 6 in interleukin 17 signal transduction. *J. Exp. Med.* **191**, 1233–1239.

Schwarzenberger, P., La Russa, V., Miller, A., Ye, P., Huang, W., Zieske, A., Nelson, S., Bagby, G. J., Stoltz, D., Mynatt, R. L., Spriggs, M., and Kolls, J. K. (1998). IL-17 stimulates granulopoiesis in mice: Use of an alternate, novel gene therapy-derived method for *in vivo* evaluation of cytokines. *J. Immunol.* **161**, 6383–6389.

Shalom-Barak, T., Quach, J., and Lotz, M. (1998). Interleukin-17–induced gene expression in articular chondrocytes is associated with activation of mitogen-activated protein kinases and NF-kappaB. *J. Biol. Chem.* **273**, 27467–27473.

Shen, F., Ruddy, M. J., Plamondon, P., and Gaffen, S. L. (2005). Cytokines link osteoblasts and inflammation: Microarray analysis of interleukin-17- and TNF-alpha-induced genes in bone cells. *J. Leukoc. Biol.* **77**, 388–399.

Shen, F., Hu, Z., Goswami, J., and Gaffen, S. L. (2006). Identification of common transcriptional regulatory elements in interleukin-17 target genes. *J. Biol. Chem.,* in press.

Shi, Y., Ullrich, S. J., Zhang, J., Connolly, K., Grzegorzewski, K. J., Barber, M. C., Wang, W., Wathen, K., Hodge, V., Fisher, C. L., Olsen, H., Ruben, S. M., *et al.* (2000). A novel cytokine receptor-ligand pair. Identification, molecular characterization, and *in vivo* immunomodulatory activity. *J. Biol. Chem.* **275**, 19167–19176.

Shimada, M., Andoh, A., Hata, K., Tasaki, K., Araki, Y., Fujiyama, Y., and Bamba, T. (2002). IL-6 secretion by human pancreatic periacinar myofibroblasts in response to inflammatory mediators. *J. Immunol.* **168**, 861–868.

Shin, H. C., Benbernou, N., Esnault, S., and Guenounou, M. (1999). Expression of IL-17 in human memory CD45RO+ T lymphocytes and its regulation by protein kinase A pathway. *Cytokine* **11**, 257–266.

Stark, M. A., Huo, Y., Burcin, T. L., Morris, M. A., Olson, T. S., and Ley, K. (2005). Phagocytosis of apoptotic neutrophils regulates granulopoiesis via IL-23 and IL-17. *Immunity* **22**, 285–294.

Starnes, T., Broxmeyer, H. E., Robertson, M. J., and Hromas, R. (2002). Cutting edge: IL-17D, a novel member of the IL-17 family, stimulates cytokine production and inhibits hemopoiesis. *J. Immunol.* **169**, 642–646.

Steiner, G. E., Newman, M. E., Paikl, D., Stix, U., Memaran-Dagda, N., Lee, C., and Marberger, M. J. (2003). Expression and function of pro-inflammatory interleukin IL-17 and IL-17 receptor in normal, benign hyperplastic, and malignant prostate. *Prostate* **56**, 171–182.

Subramaniam, S. V., Cooper, R. S., and Adunyah, S. E. (1999). Evidence for the involvement of JAK/STAT pathway in the signaling mechanism of interleukin-17. *Biochem. Biophys. Res. Commun.* **262**, 14–19.

Takahashi, K., Azuma, T., Motohira, H., Kinane, D. F., and Kitetsu, S. (2005). The potential role of interleukin-17 in the immunopathology of periodontal disease. *J. Clin. Periodontol.* **32**, 369–374.

Tang, Q. Q., Gronborg, M., Huang, H., Kim, J. W., Otto, T. C., Pandey, A., and Lane, M. D. (2005). Sequential phosphorylation of CCAAT enhancer-binding protein beta by MAPK and glycogen synthase kinase 3beta is required for adipogenesis. *Proc. Natl. Acad. Sci. USA* **102**, 9766–9771.

Tartour, E., Fossiez, F., Joyeux, I., Galinha, A., Gey, A., Claret, E., Sastre-Garau, X., Couturier, J., Mosseri, V., Vives, V., Banchereau, J., Fridman, W. H., *et al.* (1999). Interleukin 17, a T–cell-derived cytokine, promotes tumorigenicity of human cervical tumors in nude mice. *Cancer Res.* **59**, 3698–3704.

Teunissen, M. B., Koomen, C. W., de Waal Malefyt, R., Wierenga, E. A., and Bos, J. D. (1998). Interleukin-17 and interferon-γ synergize in the enhancement of proinflammatory cytokine production by human keratinocytes. *J. Invest. Dermatol.* **111**, 645–649.

Tian, E., Sawyer, J. R., Largaespada, D. A., Jenkins, N. A., Copeland, N. G., and Shaughnessy, J. D. (2000). *Evi27* encodes a novel membrane protein with homology to the IL-17 receptor. *Oncogene* **19,** 2098–2109.

Tokuda, H., Kanno, Y., Ishisaki, A., Takenaka, M., Harada, A., and Kozawa, O. (2004). Interleukin (IL)-17 enhances tumor necrosis factor-alpha-stimulated IL-6 synthesis via p38 mitogen-activated protein kinase in osteoblasts. *J. Cell. Biochem.* **91,** 1053–1061.

Toy, D., Kugler, D., Wolfson, M., Bos, T. V., Gurgel, J., Tocker, J., and Peschon, J. (2006). Cutting Edge: IL-17 signals through a heteromeric receptor complex. *J. Immunol.* **117,** 136–139.

Trajkovic, V., Stosic-Grujicic, S., Samardzic, T., Markovic, M., Miljkovic, D., Ramic, Z., and Mostarica Stojkovic, M. (2001). Interleukin-17 stimulates inducible nitric oxide synthase activation in rodent astrocytes. *J. Neuroimmunol.* **119,** 183–191.

Tsang, M., and Dawid, I. (2004). Promotion and attenuation of FGF signaling through the Ras-MAPK pathway. *Sci. STKE* **228,** PE17.

Tsang, M., Friesel, R., Kudoh, T., and Dawid, I. (2002). Identification of Sef, a novel modulator of FGF signalling. *Nat. Cell. Biol.* **4,** 165–169.

Van Bezooijen, R. L., Farih-Sips, H. C. M., Papapoulos, S. E., and Löwik, C. W. G. M. (1999). Interleukin-17: A new bone acting cytokine *in vitro. J. Bone Min. Res.* **14,** 1513–1521.

Van Bezooijen, R. L., Van Der Wee-Pals, L., Papapoulos, S. E., and Lowik, C. W. (2002). Interleukin 17 synergises with tumour necrosis factor alpha to induce cartilage destruction *in vitro. Ann. Rheum. Dis.* **61,** 870–876.

Veldhoen, M., Hocking, R. J., Atkins, C. J., Locksley, R. M., and Stockinger, B. (2006). TGFβ in the context of an inflammatory cytokine milieu supports de novo differentiation of IL-17-producing T cells. *Immunity* **24,** 179–189.

Wong, C. K., Ho, C. Y., Li, E. K., and Lam, C. W. (2000). Elevation of proinflammatory cytokine (IL-18, IL-17, IL-12) and Th2 cytokine (IL-4) concentrations in patients with systemic lupus erythematosus. *Lupus* **9,** 589–593.

Wynn, T. A. (2005). T(H)-17: A giant step from T(H)1 and T(H)2. *Nat. Immunol.* **6,** 1069–1070.

Xiong, S., Zhao, Q., Rong, Z., Huang, G., Huang, Y., Chen, P., Zhang, S., Liu, L., and Chang, Z. (2003). hSef inhibits PC-12 cell differentiation by interfering with Ras-mitogen-activated protein kinase MAPK signaling. *J. Biol. Chem.* **278,** 50273–50282.

Yamada, T., Tsuchiya, T., Osada, S., Nishihara, T., and Imagawa, M. (1998). CCAAT/enhancer-binding protein δ gene expression is mediated by autoregulation through downstream binding sites. *Biochem. Biophys. Res. Commun.* **242,** 88–92.

Yang, R. B., Ng, C. K., Wasserman, S. M., Komuves, L. G., Gerritsen, M. E., and Topper, J. N. (2003). A novel interleukin-17 receptor-like protein identified in human umbilical vein endothelial cells antagonizes basic fibroblast growth factor-induced signaling. *J. Biol. Chem.* **278,** 33232–33238.

Yao, Z., Fanslow, W. C., Seldin, M. F., Rousseau, A.-M., Painter, S. L., Comeau, M. R., Cohen, J. I., and Spriggs, M. K. (1995). Herpesvirus Saimiri encodes a new cytokine, IL-17, which binds to a novel cytokine receptor. *Immunity* **3,** 811–821.

Yao, Z., Spriggs, M. K., Derry, J. M. J., Strockbine, L., Park, L. S., VandenBos, T., Zappone, J., Painter, S. L., and Armitage, R. J. (1997). Molecular characterization of the human interleukin-17 receptor. *Cytokine* **9,** 794–800.

Ye, P., Rodriguez, F. H., Kanaly, S., Stocking, K. L., Schurr, J., Schwarzenberger, P., Oliver, P., Huang, W., Zhang, P., Zhang, J., Shellito, J. E., Bagby, G. J., *et al.* (2001). Requirement of interleukin 17 receptor signaling for lung CXC chemokine and granulocyte colony-stimulating factor expression, neutrophil recruitment, and host defense. *J. Exp. Med.* **194,** 519–527.

Yen, D., Cheung, J., Scheeres, H., Poulet, F., McClanahan, T., Mckenzie, B., Kleinschek, M. A., Owyang, A., Mattson, J., Blumenschein, W., Murphy, E., Sathe, M., Cua, D. J., Kastelein,

R. A., and Rennick, D. (2006). IL-23 is essential for T cell-mediated colitis and promotes inflammation via IL-17 and IL-6. *J. Clin. Invest.* **116,** 1310–1316.

Zhang, Z., Andoh, A., Yasui, H., Inatomi, O., Hata, K., Tsujikawa, T., Kitoh, K., Takayanagi, A., Shimizu, N., and Fujiyama, Y. (2005). Interleukin-1beta and tumor necrosis factor-alpha upregulate interleukin-23 subunit p19 gene expression in human colonic subepithelial myofibroblasts. *Int. J. Mol. Med.* **15,** 79–83.

Ziolkowska, M., Koc, A., Luszczukiewicz, G., Ksiezopolksa-Pietrzak, K., Klimczak, E., Chwalinska-Sadowska, H., and Maslinski, W. (2000). High levels of IL-17 in rheumatoid arthritis patients: IL-15 triggers *in vitro* IL-17 production via cyclosporin A-sensitive mechanism. *J. Immunol.* **164,** 2832–2838.

11

NF-κB AND CYTOKINES

DAGMAR KULMS* AND THOMAS SCHWARZ[†]

*Department of Cell Biology and Immunology, University of Stuttgart
D-70569 Stuttgart, Germany
†Department of Dermatology, University of Kiel
D-24105 Kiel, Germany

Cytokines represent a heterogeneous group of soluble mediators which are involved in almost any physiological and pathological process. The release of many cytokines and numerous of their biological activities are mediated by nuclear factor-κB (NF-κB). NF-κB is a ubiquitous transcription factor which is crucially involved in many biological processes, including tissue development and maintenance of tissue homeostasis. NF-κB also controls apoptotic cell death of both normal and malignant

0083-6729/06 $35.00
DOI: 10.1016/S0083-6729(06)74011-0

cells. Thus, it is a challenging target for anticancer and anti-inflammatory strategies. However, it has been recognized that NF-κB does not only influence many biological processes but also under certain conditions the activities of NF-κB can be altered as well, for example, by cytokines. This cross talk needs to be taken into account when developing strategies targeting NF-κB for anticancer therapy. © 2006 Elsevier Inc.

I. THE CYTOKINE FAMILY

Two types of immune responses are differentiated, the innate and the adaptive. The classical immune response is the adaptive which is characterized by specificity due to the creation of immunological memory (specific immunity) (Parkin and Cohen, 2001). The innate immune response is a more primitive defense system which acts in a rapid but nonspecific way (Medzhitov and Janeway, 2000). In both types of immune reactions cytokines are critically involved.

The term cytokines comprises a large family of heterogeneous low-molecular-weight messenger substances which play a crucial role in intercellular communication. Cytokines are secreted by almost any cell; they can therefore act in an autocrine, paracrine, or endocrine manner. Cytokines exert their various biological activities via binding to specific cell surface receptors (Thomson, 1996). The vast majority of cytokines occur in soluble form, some can be membrane-bound which makes the differentiation between cytokine and receptor difficult. Cytokines influence the proliferation, differentiation, and activation of cells. Each cytokine exhibits multiple activities, a fact which does not allow strict categorization.

The cytokine nomenclature has to be seen and can only be understood in a historic perspective. Cytokines which were produced by leukocytes and exerted effects preferentially on other white cells were called interleukins (IL), although it is known today that these mediators are also produced by and act on many other cells than leukocytes. The cytokine tumor necrosis factor (TNF), for example, has been designated according to its biological activity. Although TNF is released also by leukocytes and acts on leukcytes, its name has never been changed into an interleukin. The term colony-stimulating factors (CSF) comprises those mediators which induce differentiation and proliferation of hematopoietic progenitor cells. The term interferons (IFN) refers to mediators which interfere with viral replication. Cytokines that have chemoattractant activity and play a crucial role in leukocyte migration are termed chemokines. Two main subgroups are differentiated according to the position of two cysteine (C) residues compared with the other amino acids (X), CXC-, or α-chemokines and CC- or β-chemokines (Cyster, 1999). Chemokines which recruit leukocytes are termed inflammatory chemokines, those which regulate trafficking within lymphoid tissues lymphoid chemokines.

During an innate immune response, mostly cytokines with inflammatory (e.g., IL-1, IL-6, TNF-α, and inflammatory chemokines) and antiviral (IFN-α, IFN-β) capacities are involved. Induction of an adaptive immune response is critically dependent on cytokines with immunomodulatory capacities (e.g., IL-2, IL-4, IL-10, IL-12, IL-13, IL-18, and IFN-γ, lymphoid chemokines). However, since most of these mediators exhibit multiple and sometimes overlapping activities, a strict separation into inflammatory and immunologic cytokines is not possible.

Because of the numerous cytokines described—the list is still increasing—and because of their multiple activities and the overlap in activities the cytokine field is a very complex one. This refers also to the question how the release of cytokines is regulated and how cytokines exert their biological effects. It become quite rapidly clear that transcription factors are critically involved in these processes. Nuclear factor-kappa B (NF-κB) turned out not only to be one of these ubiquitous factors which frequently participates both in the regulation of the release of cytokines but also in mediating the biological effects of a variety of these mediators.

II. NUCLEAR FACTOR-κB

NF-κB was discovered in 1986 by Sen and Baltimore, as a nuclear factor that binds to the enhancer of the kappa light chain of immunoglobin in B cells (Sen and Baltimore, 1986). NF-κB was found to be activated in response to bacterial lipopolysaccharide (LPS), indicating its role in immune responses. In addition, NF-κB has been found to interfere in the balance between proliferation and programmed cell death (apoptosis), thereby crucially influencing tissue homeostasis and immune development and responses. Because of the ability to modulate such essential processes it is obvious the NF-κB also plays an important role in disease development. Thus, NF-κB is one of the most frequently and extensively investigated transcription factors.

NF-κB is crucially involved in the regulation of genes–encoding cytokines [e.g., IL-1, IL-2, IL-6, IL-12, TNF-α, lymphotoxin (LT)-α, LTβ, and granulocyte-macrophage (GM)-CSF], chemokines (e.g., IL-8, MIP-1α, MCP-1, and RANTES), antimicrobial peptides, MHC proteins, and costimulatory molecules. Thus, it plays an essential role in coordinating innate and adaptive immune responses. It is also essential for antiviral responses through induction of IFNs. Furthermore, NF-κB controls overall tissue differentiation and homeostasis by regulating the expression of anti- (c-IAP1/2, x-IAP, FLIP, Bcl-X_L) and proapoptotic (Fas ligand) as well as of cell cycle genes (c-myc, cyclin D1) (Bonizzi and Karin, 2004; Gosh and Karin, 2002; Pöppelmann et al., 2005).

Since NF-κB is an inducible transcription factor responsible for the regulation of multiple genes involved in a variety of cellular responses, its activity needs to be controlled by endogenous mechanisms. Therefore, NF-κB induces the transcription of inhibitory proteins which in a negative feedback loop terminate NF-κB activity (Evans et al., 2004; Jono et al., 2004; Verma and Stevenson, 1997; Wertz et al., 2004). When these regulatory systems are impaired, uncontrolled NF-κB activity may contribute to the development of diseases. Accordingly, constitutive activation of NF-κB has been predominantly linked to transformation, proliferation, apoptosis suppression, invasion, angiogenesis, and metastasis (Aggarwal, 2004). Consequently, inappropriate regulation of NF-κB is claimed to be directly responsible for a wide range of human disorders including certain types of cancers, neurodegenerative diseases, ataxia-telangiectasia, arthritis, asthma, inflammatory bowel diseases, multiple sclerosis, and psoriasis, just to mention a few ones (Aggarwal, 2004; Barnes and Adcock, 1998; Foxwell et al., 1998; Grilli and Memo, 1999; Laque and Gelinas, 1997). Moreover, NF-κB activation has been reported to be responsible for conferring chemo- and radioresistance in cancer treatment (Tergaonkar et al., 2002; Wang et al., 1999). However, there is evidence that under certain conditions NF-κB can even act as a tumor suppressor by supporting proapoptotic pathways (Perkins, 2004; Pöppelmann et al., 2005). This indicates the many faces of NF-κB, making it an attractive but also delicate target for intervention.

Taken together, NF-κB plays a crucial role in tissue development and homeostasis but once out of control contributes to the development and maintenance of diseases. Therefore, targeting NF-κB pathways with inhibitory drugs are attractive strategies both for cancer treatment and anti-inflammatory therapies. However, this requires careful analysis because of the many faces of NF-κB, which may be associated with undesired and unexpected side effects. The present chapter will focus on the interplay between cytokines and NF-κB, with a special emphasis on how the proinflammatory cytokines IL-1 and TNF-α influence NF-κB with regard to its effects on apoptosis.

III. NF-κB/REL FAMILY MEMBERS

NF-κB activity is inducible in all cell types leading to a variety of different cellular responses. The NF-κB family of transcription factors comprises five structurally related members: p50/p105 (NF-κB 1), p52/p100 (NF-κB 2), p65 (RelA), c-Rel, and RelB; all of which exist within the cell as homo- and heterodimers. The most abundant and best studied form of NF-κB/Rel is the heterodimer consisting of p50/p65 (Thanos and Maniatis, 1995). However, functional distribution of subunits is cell type dependent and is influenced by their recognition properties. All NF-κB/Rel family members are characterized by an N-terminal Rel homology domain (RHD) responsible for DNA binding, dimerization, nuclear translocation, interaction with inhibitory proteins (IκBs), and transcriptional regulation. p65 (RelA), c-Rel, and RelB are transcriptional activators through interaction of their C-terminal transactivation domains (TAD) with various components of the basal transcription machinery (Verma et al., 1995). In turn, homo- or heterodimers of p50 and p52 serve as transcriptional repressors since they lack the transactivation domain. However, they still can bind to κB-consensus sites and therefore compete with other transcriptionally active NF-κB dimers (Fujita et al., 1992). RelB exhibits a greater regulatory flexibility and can function as an activator as well as a repressor of transcription upon interaction with either p50 or p52 (Ruben et al., 1992; Ryseck et al., 1992).

Two pathways leading to translocation of NF-κB members from the cytoplasm into the nucleus exist: the common canonical one mediated by IKKβ-dependent IκBα degradation and the alternative one, namely noncanonical, engaging IKKα as the RelB/p52 activator. The independence of the two pathways was confirmed by studying IKKβ$^{-/-}$ and IKKγ$^{-/-}$ cells in which the integrity of the noncanonical IKKα-mediated pathway remained unaffected (Claudio et al., 2002; Dejardin et al., 2002).

A. THE CANONICAL PATHWAY

The canonical pathway is triggered by proinflammatory cytokines and pathogen-associated molecular patterns (PAMP) that are conserved among microorganisms. This is achieved via activation of different receptors belonging to the TNF receptor, Toll-like receptor (TLR), or IL-1 receptor superfamilies (Bonizzi and Karin, 2004). It has an important function in innate immunity, resulting basically in activation of RelA/p50 heterodimers which mediate secondary inflammatory as well as antiapoptotic responses of the cell. Under resting conditions, NF-κB dimers containing p65 or c-Rel are retained in the cytoplasm by interaction with inhibitors of NF-κB (IκBs). The most important inhibitory proteins are IκBα, IκBβ, and IκBε which bind the RHD, thereby masking the nuclear localization signal (NLS) of NF-κB and avoiding nuclear translocation of the respective dimers (Bauerle and Baltimore, 1996). Nuclear translocation of RelA/p50 requires activation of the multisubunit IκB kinase (IKK) complex. This consists of the IKKα/IKK1 and IKKβ/IKK2 catalytic subunits and the IKKγ/NEMO regulatory subunit (Brown et al., 1995; DiDonato et al., 1997). The activated IKK complex catalyzes the phosphorylation of IκBα at Ser32 and Ser36 in an IKKγ- and IKKβ-dependent manner. Subsequently, the upstream E2 ubiquitin ligases TNF-associated proteins TRAF-2 and TRAF-6 polyubiquitinate the Lys21 and Lys22 residues which finally designates IκBα to proteolytic degradation via the 26S proteasome (Bauerle and Baltimore, 1988; Palombella et al., 1994). The activity of NF-κB is strictly regulated by NF-κB-dependent resynthesis of a number of inhibitory proteins including IκBs, A20, and cylindromatosis (CYLD). While IκBs sequester NF-κB in the cytoplasm, A20 and CYLD act as ubiquitin proteases, leading to disruption of the activating signaling pathway. Whereas A20 prevents association of the IKK complex with upstream signaling molecules like receptor interacting protein (RIP), CYLD causes disassembly of the IKK complex by deubiquitination of IKK-γ (Evans et al., 2004; Wertz et al., 2004).

B. THE NONCANONICAL PATHWAY

The noncanonical pathway instead is triggered by certain members of the TNF cytokine family including BAFF, CD40L, as well as TLbR but not by TNF-α (Dejardin et al., 2002). It is mostly involved in adaptive immunity (Bonizzi and Karin, 2002). Here, p52/RelB or p50/RelB do not associate with IκBs but are retained in the cytoplasm by p100 and p105, respectively (Dobrzanski et al., 1995). Thus, NF-κB1 (p105) and NF-κB2 (p100) can function as IκB-like proteins. Upon phosphorylation by homodimerized IKKα (Senftleben et al., 2001), the C-terminal domains of the precursor proteins are removed by ubiquitin-dependent proteasomal processing releasing mature p50 and p52, respectively (Betts and Nabel, 1996).

Another unusual member of the IκB family is Bcl-3 which interacts specifically with p50 and p52 homodimers, consequently inducing p50- and p52-mediated expression of κB regulated genes (Dechend et al., 1999). For illustration see Fig. 1.

IV. IMMUNE DEVELOPMENT, INFLAMMATORY RESPONSE, AND DISEASE

The coordinated function of innate immunity depends on classical pathways involving mostly RelA/p50 heterodimers which are responsible for the induction of proinflammatory cytokines and inhibitors of apoptosis. Thus, deficiencies in RelA or IKKβ result in susceptibility to infections, provided the embryonic lethality usually associated with these deficiencies is prevented (Alcamo et al., 2001; Li et al., 1999). Activation of NF-κB in intestinal epithelial cells and macrophages occurs in response to injury, bacterial infection, or invasion of parasites leading to the release of cytokines (TNF-α, IL-1, IL-6) and chemokines (MCP-1, IL-8) and to the expression of adhesion molecules (ICAM-1, VCAM-1, ELAM). Appearance of those substances serves as a signal for recruitment of inflammatory and phagocytic cells which in turn can activate an adaptive response on presentation of antigens in

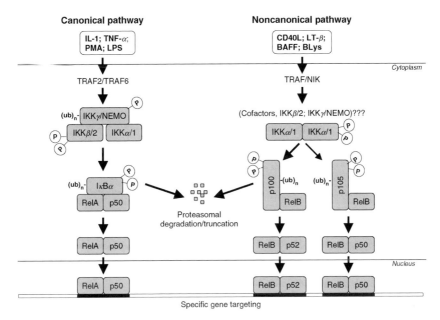

FIGURE 1. Scheme displaying the canonical and noncanonical pathway triggered by different cytokines, all resulting in activation of different NF-κB isoforms.

secondary lymphoid organs (Elewaut *et al.*, 1999). Analysis of macrophage populations from c-Rel[-/-] or RelB[-/-] mice identified several functional disorders, in particular impaired production of some cytokines (e.g., TNF-α) or overproduction of others (e.g., GM-CSF, IL-6). This documents the importance of other NF-κB subunits for an effective defense against infections (Grigoriadis *et al.*, 1996). Although, NF-κB is not required for lymphocyte development, it is crucial for suppressing lymphocyte apoptosis during early development or in response to TNF-α. Thus, another important aspect of the innate function of the classical NF-κB signaling pathway is maintaining the survival of professional immune cells during bacterial infections or acute inflammation.

The importance of NF-κB-mediated pathways in tissue development and maintaining healthy conditions was extensively studied in skin. Observations that inhibition of NF-κB caused hyperproliferation of epidermal cells evoked intensive studies with mice lacking particular components of the NF-κB-signaling pathway. Transgenic mice deficient in functional IKKβ in the epidermis suffer from severe inflammatory skin disease which is caused by a TNF-mediated, T cell–independent inflammatory response (Pasparakis *et al.*, 2002). A study revealed that RelA and c-Rel are essential for normal skin development, in particular for embryonic basal keratinocyte division and epidermal cell differentiation as well as for suppression of innate immune-mediated epidermal inflammation in postembryonic environment. The phenotype of *rela*$^{-/-}$ *c-rel*$^{-/-}$ *tnfα*$^{-/-}$ in fetal skin resembled the phenotype of a human genetic disorder termed hypohidrotic ectodermal dysplasia which is characterized by hair, nail, teeth, and sweat gland defects. In contrast, on grafting of mutant skin graft into wild-type hosts basal cells, hyperplasia and immune-mediated inflammation was observed. A similar skin phenotype has been described in female *ikkγ* $^{-/-}$ mice, an animal model for the human X-linked disorder incontinentia pigmenti (Gugasyan *et al.*, 2004; Makris *et al.*, 2000). Germline mutations in genes encoding molecules involved in NF-κB activation cause primary immunodeficiencies in humans with impaired response to a large variety of stimuli including TLR agonists. Anhidrotic ectodermal dysplasia with an immunodeficient phenotype (EDA-ID) is associated with X-linked recessive mutations in IKKγ or autosomal dominant mutations in IκBα. EDA-ID patients show developmental anomalies of skin appendages and are sensitive towards a broad spectrum of infectious diseases (Ku *et al.*, 2005). Taken together, the canonical NF-κB-signaling pathway seems to be essential for the maintenance of the balanced interplay between epidermis, dermis, and immune system.

The noncanonical pathway instead plays an important role in adaptive immunity. It is activated by certain members of the TNF cytokine family namely BAFF, CD40 ligand, and TLβR but not by TNF-α and displays much slower kinetics than the canonical track. Analysis of knockout mice with targeted disruption of individual NF-κB subunits suggested distinct roles for different family members in the spleen (Weih *et al.*, 1994). B cell proliferation, selection, maturation, and death during antibody responses are impaired in *Nf-κb2*$^{-/-}$ or *RelB*$^{-/-}$ mice (Sha *et al.*, 1995; Weih *et al.*, 2001). Formation of germinal centers with secondary B cells and splenic organization was impaired in *Ikkα*$^{-/-}$ mutants or *Ikkα*$^{A/A}$ (Ser32/36Ala) knockin mice as well as in *aly/aly* mice expressing an inactive form of NF-κB-inducing kinase (NIK) (Senftleben *et al.*, 2001; Shinkura *et al.*, 1999). Furthermore, macrophage development in the splenic marginal zone was shown to be dependent on functional p52 and Bcl-3. Several other mutant mouse strains such as *Nf-κB2*$^{-/-}$ and *RelB*$^{-/-}$ display defective splenic microarchitecture. The same applies also for mice with targeted disruption of the genes encoding TNF-α, LTα, LTβ, TNF-R1, LTβR, and NIK which lack organized germinal centers and follicular dendritic cells (Bonizzi and Karin, 2004). A defective microarchitecture of the spleen has been reported also in mice deficient in Bcl-3.

Collectively, the major function of IKKα in the immune system appears to be related to the development and organization of secondary lymphoid organs and B cell maturation, whereas IKKβ is essential for activation of innate immune responses and for maintaining survival of immune cells.

The observation that *IKKα*$^{AA/AA}$ mice have exacerbated inflammatory responses to infections which enhances bacterial clearance but provokes septic shock indicates a new role of IKKα in the negative regulation of macrophage activation and inflammation. Suppression of NF-κB activity by an accelerated turnover of RelA and c-Rel may cause their rapid removal from proinflammatory gene promoters. This discovery may offer new therapeutic opportunities for IKKα inhibitors in treatment of complicated infections caused by antibiotic resistance or impaired host immunity (Lawrence *et al.*, 2005). Selective IKKα inhibitors were thought to be useful also for preventing B cell–mediated autoimmune diseases (Karin *et al.*, 2004).

NF-κB also plays a critical role in Th2 cell differentiation and is therefore involved in the induction of allergic airway inflammation. NF-κB inhibition was shown to be associated with strong attenuation of allergic lung inflammation, airway hyperresponsiveness and local production of mucus, and release of IL-5, IL-13, and eotaxin. This indicates that selective inhibition of NF-κB in the lung may have a therapeutic potential in the control of pulmonary allergy (Desmet *et al.*, 2004).

One of the major functions of the NF-κB defense response is its antiviral activity via induction of interferon genes. Due to their adaptation potential many viruses, including human immunodeficiency virus type-1 (HIV-1) and human T-lymphotropic virus type-1 (HTLV-1) which do not induce interferon production, exploit NF-κB to activate their own genes and to stimulate the survival and proliferation of lymphoid cells in which they replicate (Bex and Gaynor, 1998; Roulston *et al.*, 1995). For example, the Tax protein of HTLV-1 directly interacts with IKKγ to activate IKK complex and NF-κB (Sun and Ballard, 1999). Conclusively, inactivation of the NF-κB-signaling pathway may also have a beneficial role in fighting defined viral infections.

V. CYTOKINES AND NF-κB IN TUMORIGENESIS AND APOPTOSIS

Apoptosis is a programed cell death that can be induced by a variety of different stimuli, such as growth factor deprivation (Cornelis *et al.*, 2005), ionizing radiation (Konemann *et al.*, 2005), chemotherapeutic drugs (Sordet *et al.*, 2003), ultraviolet (UV) radiation (Kulms and Schwarz, 2002a), and activation of cell death receptors (Wajant *et al.*, 2005). Despite the fact that proapoptotic signals trigger a cascade of complex events and activate a variety of signal transduction pathways, all converge at the state of execution of apoptosis accompanied with activation of cystein proteases (caspases) and endonucleases. Membrane blebbing, cytosolic condensation, and breakdown of nuclear DNA with subsequent nucleosomal fragmentation characterize cells dying in an apoptotic fashion. Well-enclosed apoptotic bodies are removed by phagocytic cells without causing inflammation. Thus, host (or viral) DNA can be efficiently degraded without causing damage to neighboring cells (Fiers et al., 1999). Because of its non-inflammatory features apoptotic cell death does not only serve as a protective mechanism removing damaged or altered cells and tissues but also represents an interesting target for anticancer therapy. Apoptosis can be induced by extrinsic stimuli including ligand-dependent death receptor activation or by intrinsic stimuli including genotoxic and oxidative stress.

Death receptor–induced apoptosis requires binding of Fas-associated protein with death domain (FADD) to the activated intracellular death domain of the death receptor. This forms the death-inducing signaling complex (DISC) upon recruitment of the initiator procaspase-8 into the complex. Autocatalytically activated caspase-8 either directly activates downstream effector caspases via proteolytic cleavage or truncates the proapoptotic Bcl-2 family member Bid (Scaffidi et al., 1998). Truncated Bid (t-Bid) targets the mitochondrial outer membrane where it induces activation of Bax and Bak proteins, resulting in loss of the mitochondrial membrane potential and release of cytochrome c into the cytoplasm. Cytoplasmic cytochrome c together with Apaf-1 and the initiator procaspase-9 forms the apoptosome. This causes caspase-9 activation in an ATP-dependent manner. Caspase-9 is now able to proteolytically activate effector caspases, resulting in cleavage of death substrates and execution of cell death (Wang, 2001). Death receptor–induced apoptosis can efficiently be blocked by recruitment of FLICE inhibitory protein (FLIP) to the DISC. Two splicing variants, the p55 $FLIP_L$ and the p28 $FLIP_S$ exist within the cell, both of which interfere with procaspase-8 activation (Irmler et al., 1997; Tschopp et al., 1998). Among the death receptors described TNF-R1 represents an exception, since the outcome of receptor activation depends critically on the adapter proteins recruited to the activated death domain. On the one hand, recruitment of FADD results in the induction of the apoptotic pathway, whereas on the other hand, recruitment of TNF receptor-associated factor (TRAF)-1 and TRAF-2 leads to activation of NF-κB which finally mediates cell survival signals (Micheau and Tschopp, 2003).

Besides its important role in controlling immune function, cell proliferation, and differentiation, NF-κB has mainly been described to induce the expression of antiapoptotic genes like c-IAP, FLIP, survivin, Bcl-2 family members, and so on (La Casse et al., 1998; Micheau et al., 2001; Wang et al., 1998; Zong et al., 1999). Therefore, NF-κB has been regarded as a tumor-promoting molecule which antagonizes apoptosis induced by chemotherapeutic drugs, ionizing radiation, and death ligands (Kothny-Wilkes et al., 1998; Wang et al., 1996). Correspondingly, the development and progression of a number of cancer types is supported by constitutive NF-κB activation. NF-κB was even found to be a mediator of malignant transformation of tumors deriving from chronic inflammation (Cao and Karin, 2003; Li et al., 2005). For these reasons the signal transduction pathways activating NF-κB are in major focus for the development of new anticancer strategies. In this context, IKK2 has been suggested as a good target for chemoprevention since inhibition of IKK2 sensitizes tumor cells towards TNF-α-induced apoptosis (Maeda *et al.*, 2003).

The potential of different substances to trigger apoptosis has been exploited to kill cancer cells. Among inducers of apoptosis used widely in anticancer therapy, chemotherapeutic drugs and ionizing radiation are the predominant ones. They induce cell death via induction of DNA damage and activation of the mitochondrial pathway. Ultraviolet radiation exerts also potent proapoptotic activity and thus is used with and without photosensitizers in phototherapy to treat several skin disorders including cutaneous T cell lymphoma (Nisticò *et al.*, 2004; Stadler, 2002). Apart from systemic treatment with interferons and/or cytokines applied to stimulate tumor immune responses, TNF-related apoptosis-inducing ligand (TRAIL/ Apo2L) has been considered as a promising candidate for anticancer therapy because of its initially described potential to selectively induce apoptosis in tumor cells (Walczak *et al.*, 1999; Wiley *et al.*, 1995). However, it has to be taken into account that tumor cells are generally surrounded by immune and inflammatory cells which constantly release proinflammatory cytokines like IL-1. Therefore, IL-1-mediated activation of NF-κB may represent a pathway by which tumor cells can escape the cytotoxic effect of TRAIL. Accordingly, activation of NF-κB by IL-1 resulted in inhibition of TRAIL-induced apoptosis in transformed keratinocytes and coincided with upregulation of antiapoptotic proteins FLIP, c-IAP1, and c-IAP2 (Kothny-Wilkes *et al.*, 1998; Pöppelmann *et al.*, 2005). The same effect was observed for CD95-induced apoptosis, supporting the assumption that NF-κB protects from apoptosis universally (Kothny-Wilkes *et al.*, 1998). The antiapoptotic activity of NF-κB depends on the expression of a variety of endogenous inhibitors of apoptosis. These include caspase inhibitors such as c-IAPs, X-IAP, c-FLIP, membrane-stabilizing proteins like Bcl-2 or adapter molecules which trigger antiapoptoic instead of proapoptoic pathways on death receptor activation (Chen and Goeddel, 2002). c-IAPs and x-IAP directly bind and inhibit different effector caspases and can therefore inhibit apoptosis induced by both death receptors and the mitochondrial pathway (Deveraux *et al.*, 1998; Harlin *et al.*, 2001). Although, c-IAPs cannot directly bind to caspase-8, their interaction with TRAF-2 and recruitment to TNF-R1-signaling complex may mediate inhibition of apoptosis via NF-κB activation (Wang *et al.*, 1998). c-FLIP also interacts with TRAF-2 and RIP which are both responsible for JNK and IKK activation via the TNF-R1 complex. This implies that the antiapoptotic effect of c-FLIP may also be due to enhanced NF-κB activation (Karin and Lin, 2002). Apoptotic pathways involved are illustrated in Fig. 2.

Many tumors of lymphoid or epithelial origin harbor constitutively activated NF-κB. NF-κB-deficient epithelial cells show not only marked increase in their susceptibility to TNF-α−induced apoptosis but also

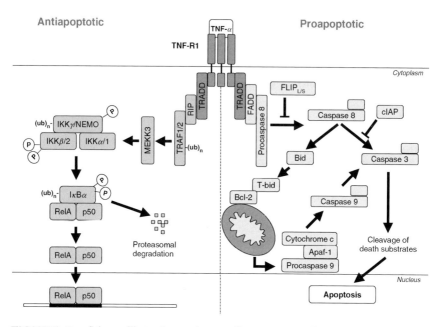

FIGURE 2. Scheme illustrating anti- as well as proapoptotic pathways triggered by activation of TNF-R1. Upon receptor activation by the cognate ligand binding of the initial adapter TRADD builds the platform for recruitment of different adapter proteins. Binding of RIP and TRAF induces activation of NF-κB, resulting in mediation of antiapoptotic effects. In contrast, recruitment of FADD and procaspase-8 to TRADD mediates execution of cell death. The balance between pro- and antiapoptotic pathways can furthermore be influenced by the expression of antiapoptotic proteins like cIAP and FLIP which inhibit caspase activation.

increased sensitivity to a variety of DNA-damaging chemotherapeutic drugs and ionizing radiation (Baldwin, 2001). P53 is the major tumor suppressor being activated in response to genotoxic stress like DNA damage as well as to oncogene activation. The same stimuli are known to activate NF-κB (Karin and Lin, 2002). Whereas p53 mediates cell cycle arrest followed by induction of apoptosis, induction of NF-κB is usually associated with resistance against apoptosis and cell proliferation. This indicates the existence of a cross talk between the two divergent pathways. A study described UV-induced NF-κB activation which resulted in the transcriptional upregulation of the transcription factor Egr-1. Egr-1 activated GADD 45a/b which is involved in the nucleotide excision repair. GADD 45a/b consequently modulated the action of p53 in a way to promote apoptosis instead of inducing cell cycle arrest and DNA repair in epidermal cells (Thyss et al., 2005). Thus, this study provides some evidence that NF-κB can also act as a tumor suppressor instead of a tumor promoter in response to genotoxic stress.

The proapoptotic function of NF-κB is considered to coincide with the repression of antiapoptotic genes rather than the expression of proapoptotic genes. Actually, apoptosis induced by UVB radiation was shown to be significantly enhanced on IL-1-mediated NF-κB activation and was found to coincide with a pronounced release of TNF-α (Kothny-Wilkes *et al.*, 1999). To allow additional induction of apoptosis through autocrine activation of TNF-R1, major changes of the intracellular protein content are required and were shown to be initiated by NF-κB as well. Besides the NF-κB-dependent enhancement of TNF-α transcription, NF-κB-dependent repression of c-IAP and FLIP genes as well as TRAF-1, TRAF-2, and TRAF-6 genes was observed (Pöppelmann *et al.*, 2005). Repression of TRAF proteins allows the FADD-dependent proapoptotic-signaling branch to be activated upon engagement of TNF-R1. Additionally, downregulation of inhibitory cIAP and FLIP proteins accelerates apoptosis triggered by TNF-R1, thereby finally enhancing the apoptosis rate (Pöppelmann *et al.*, 2005). Thus, repression of genes by NF-κB, which NF-κB usually activates, appears to be a mechanism by which it can exceptionally enhance apoptosis. Accordingly, NF-κB-dependent repression of the antiapoptotic $bcl-x_L$ gene can promote anti-CD3-mediated apoptosis in CD4+, CD8+ double positive thymocytes. This effect was inhibited in transgenic mice expressing a superinhibitory mutant of IκBα (Hettmann *et al.*, 1999). Although the mechanisms underlying NF-κB-dependent transcriptional repression still need to be clarified, evidence exists that the tumor suppressor phosphatase PTEN (Mayo *et al.*, 2002) and the cell cycle inhibitor INK4 (Wolff and Naumann, 1999) might play a role. In addition, association of the NF-κB p65 subunit with the gene silencer histone deacetylase 1 (Campbell *et al.*, 2004) and alternative phosphorylation of NF-κB p65 subunit (Rocha *et al.*, 2005) appear to be involved as well. Overexpression of a c-Jun dominant-negative phosphorylation mutant was shown to inhibit UV-induced transactivation of NF-κB as well as of AP-1 due to protein–protein interactions (Cooper *et al.*, 2005). Therefore, it is tempting to propose that NF-κB generally exerts its proapoptotic effect through repression of those antiapoptotic genes which it usually activates. On the one hand, results from our laboratory confirmed that IL-1-mediated enhancement of UV-induced apoptosis is dependent on NF-κB-dependent repression of antiapoptotic genes but on the other, it was shown to be as critically dependent on prolonged NF-κB-mediated transcription of TNF-α (Pöppelmann *et al.*, 2005). NF-κB-mediated enhancement of TNF-α expression and secretion enhances apoptosis induced by base modifications in genomic DNA but not in response to induction of DNA strand breaks (Strozyk *et al.*, 2006). Taken together, the different pathways and components that may convert NF-κB from an inhibitor of apoptosis into a promoter of apoptosis are quite versatile and complex. Cytokines are certainly one trigger which can influence this process.

VI. CONCLUSIONS

NF-κB is a ubiquitous transcription factor which is involved in the signal transduction of numerous physiological and pathological processes. Among its many activities NF-κB also controls the release of a variety of cytokines. However, in turn NF-κB can be influenced by cytokines. The switch from an antiapoptoic into a proapoptotic factor by IL-1 on UV radiation is just one example. Because of its involvement in carcinogenesis and inflammation, NF-κB represents an attractive target for pharmacologic intervention. This applies in particular for anticancer and anti-inflammatory strategies which mostly utilize NF-κB inhibitors. However, one has to bear in mind that under certain conditions NF-κB can change its activities dramatically. Cytokines can contribute to this phenomenon essentially. These observations should carefully be taken into account when designing new treatment concepts, especially those targeting the inhibition of NF-κB.

REFERENCES

Aggarwal, B. B. (2004). Nuclear factor-κB: The enemy within. *Cancer Cell* **6**, 203–208.

Alcamo, E., Mizgerd, J. P., Horwitz, B. H., Bronson, R., Beg, A. A., Scott, M., Doerschuk, C. M., Hynes, R. O., and Baltimore, D. (2001). Targeted mutation of TNF receptor I rescues the RelA-deficient mouse and reveals a critical role for NF-κB in leukocyte recruitment. *J. Immunol.* **167**, 1592–1600.

Baldwin, A. S. (2001). Control of oncogenesis and cancer therapy resistance by the transcription factor NFκB. *J. Clin. Invest.* **107**, 241–246.

Barnes, P. J., and Adcock, I. M. (1998). Transcription factors and asthma. *Eur. Resp. J.* **12**, 221–234.

Bauerle, P. A., and Baltimore, D. (1988). IκB: A specific inhibitor of the NF-kappa B transcription factor. *Science* **242**, 540–546.

Bauerle, P. A., and Baltimore, D. (1996). NF-κB: Ten years after. *Cell* **87**, 13–20.

Betts, J. C., and Nabel, G. J. (1996). Differential regulation of NF-κB2 (p100) processing and control by amino-terminal sequences. *Mol. Cell. Biol.* **16**, 6363–6371.

Bex, F., and Gaynor, R. B. (1998). Regulation of gene expression by HTLV-1 Tax protein. *Methods* **16**, 83–94.

Bonizzi, G., and Karin, M. (2004). The two NF-κB activation pathways and their role in innate and adoptive immunity. *Trends Immunol.* **25**, 280–288.

Brown, K., Gerstberger, S., Carlson, L., Franzoso, G., and Siebenlist, U. (1995). Control of IκBα proteolysis by site specific, signal-induced phosphorylation. *Science* **267**, 1485–1488.

Campbell, K. J., Rocha, S., and Perkins, N. D. (2004). Active repression of antiapoptotic gene expression by RelA(p65) NFkappaB. *Mol. Cell* **13**, 853–865.

Cao, Y., and Karin, M. (2003). NFkappaB in mammary gland development and breast cancer. *J. Mammary Gland Biol. Neoplasia* **8**, 215–223.

Chen, G., and Goeddel, D. V. (2002). TNFR1 signalling: A beautiful pathway. *Science* **296**, 1634–1635.

Claudio, E., Brown, K., Park, S., Wang, H., and Siebenlist, U. (2002). BAFF-induced NEMO-independent processing of NF-κβ2 in maturing B cells. *Nat. Immunol.* **3**, 958–965.

Cooper, S., Ranger-Moore, J., and Bowden, T. G. (2005). Differential inhibition of UVB-induced AP-1 and NFkappaB transactivation by components of the jun bZIP domain. *Mol. Carcinogen* **43**, 108–116.

Cornelis, S., Bruynooghe, Y., Van Loo, G., Saelens, X., Vandenbeele, P., and Bayaert, R. (2005). Apoptosis of hematopoietic cells induced by growth factor withdrawal is associated with caspase-9 mediated cleavage of Raf-1. *Oncogene* **24**, 1552–1562.

Cyster, J. G. (1999). Chemokines and cell migration in secondary lymphoid organs. *Science* **286**, 2098–2102.

Dechend, R., Hirano, F., Lehmann, K., Heissmeyer, V., Ansieau, S., Wulczyn, F. G., Scheidreit, C., and Leutz, A. (1999). The Bcl-3 oncoprotein acts as a bridging factor between NF-κB/Rel and nuclear co-regulators. *Oncogene* **18**, 3316–3323.

Dejardin, E., Droin, N. M., Delhase, M., Haas, E., Cao, Y., Makris, C., Li, Z. W., Karin, M., Ware, C. F., and Green, D. R. (2002). The lympho-toxin-β receptor induces different patterns of gene expression via two NF-κB pathways. *Immunity* **17**, 525–535.

Desmet, C., Gosset, P., Pajak, B., Cataldo, D., Bentires-Alj, M., Lekeux, P., and Bureau, F. (2004). Selective blockade of NF-kappa B activity in airway immune cells inhibits the effector phase of experimental asthma. *J. Immunol.* **173**, 5766–5775.

Deveraux, Q. L., Roy, N., Stennicke, H. R., Van Arsdale, T., Zhou, Q., Srinivasula, S. M., Alnemri, E. S., Salvesen, G. S., and Reed, J. C. (1998). IAPs block apoptotic events induced by caspase-8 and cytochrome c by direct inhibition of distinct caspases. *EMBO J.* **17**, 2215–2223.

DiDonato, J. A., Hayakawa, M., Rothwarf, D. M., Zandi, E., and Karin, M. (1997). A cytokine responsive IκB kinase that activates the transcription factor NFκB. *Nature* **388**, 548–554.

Dobrzanski, P., Ryseck, R. P., and Bravo, R. (1995). Specific inhibition of RelB/p52 transcriptional activity by the C-terminal domain of p100. *Oncogene* **10**, 1003–1007.

Elewaut, D., DiDonato, J. A., Kim, J. M., Truong, F., Eckmann, L., and Kagnoff, M. F. (1999). NF-κB is a central regulator of the intestinal epithelial cell innate immune response induced by infection with enteroinvasive bacteria. *J. Immunol.* **163**, 1457–1466.

Evans, P. C., Ovaa, H., Hamon, M., Kilshaw, P. J., Hamm, S., Bauer, S., Ploegh, H. L., and Smith, T. S. (2004). Zinc-finger protein A20, a regulator of inflammation and cell survival, has de-uiquitin activity. *Biochem. J.* **378**, 727–734.

Fiers, W., Beyaert, R., Declerq, W., and Vandenabeele, P. (1999). More than one way to die: Apoptosis, necrosis and reactive oxygen damage. *Oncogene* **18**, 7719–7730.

Foxwell, B., Browne, K., Bondeson, J., Clarke, C., Martin, R., Brennan, F., and Feldmann, M. (1998). Efficient adenoviral infection with IκB reveals that macrophage tumor necrosis factor alpha production in rheumatoid arthritis is NF-κB dependent. *Proc. Natl. Acad. Sci. USA* **95**, 8211–8215.

Fujita, T., Nolan, G. P., Ghosh, S., and Baltimore, D. (1992). Independent modes of transcriptional activation by the p50 and p65 subunits of NF-kappa B. *Genes Dev.* **6**, 775–787.

Gosh, S., and Karin, M. (2002). Missing pieces in the NF-κB puzzle. *Cell* **109**, 81–96.

Grigoriadis, G., Zhan, Y., Grumont, R. J., Metcalf, D., Handman, E., Cheers, C., and Gerondakis, S. (1996). The Rel subunit of NF-κB-like transcription factors is a positive and negative regulator of macrophage gene expression: Distinct roles for Rel in different macrophage populations. *EMBO J.* **15**, 7099–7107.

Grilli, M., and Memo, M. (1999). NF-κB/Rel proteins: A point of convergence of signalling pathways relevant in neuronal function and dysfunction. *Biochem. Pharmacol.* **57**, 1–7.

Gugasyan, R., Voss, A., Varigos, G., Thomas, T., Grumont, R. J., Kaur, P., Grigoriadis, G., and Gerondakis, S. (2004). The transcription factors c-rel and RelA control epidermal development and homeostasis in embryonic and adult skin via distinct mechanisms. *Mol. Cell. Biol.* **24**, 5733–5745.

Harlin, H., Reffey, S. B., Duckett, C. S., Lindsten, T., and Thompson, C. B. (2001). Characterisation of XIAP-deficient mice. *Mol. Cell. Biol.* **21**, 3604–3608.

Hettmann, T., DiDonato, J., Karin, M., and Leiden, J. M. (1999). An essential role for nuclear factor κB in promoting double positive thymocyte apoptosis. *J. Exp. Med.* **189**, 145–157.

Irmler, M., Thome, M., Hahne, M., Schneider, P., Hofmann, K., Steiner, V., Bodmer, J. L., Schroter, M., Burns, K., Mattmann, C., Rimoldi, D., French, L. E., *et al.* (1997). Inhibition of death receptor signals by cellular FLIP. *Nature* **388**, 190–195.

Jono, H., Lim, J. H., Chen, L.-F., Xu, H., Trompouki, E., Pan, Z. K., Mosialos, G., and Li, J.-D. (2004). NF-κB ss essential for induction of CYLD, the negative regulator of NF-κB. *J. Biol. Chem.* **279**, 36171–36174.

Karin, M., and Lin, A. (2002). NFκB at the crossroads of life and death. *Nat. Imunol.* **3**, 221–227.

Karin, M., Yamamoto, Y., and Wang, Q. M. (2004). The IKK NF-κB system: A treasure trove for drug development. *Nat. Rev. Drug Discov.* **3**, 17–26.

Konemann, S., Bolling, T., Kolkmeyer, A., Riesenbeck, D., Hesselmann, S., Vormoor, J., Willich, N., and Schuck, S. (2005). Heterogeneity of radiation induced apoptosis in Ewing Tumor cell lines characterized on a single cell level. *Apoptosis* **10**, 177–184.

Kothny-Wilkes, G., Kulms, D., Pöppelmann, B., Luger, T. A., Kubin, M., and Schwarz, T. (1998). Interleukin-1 protects transformed keratinocytes from tumor necrosis factor-related apoptosis-inducing ligand. *J. Biol. Chem.* **273**, 29247–29253.

Kothny-Wilkes, G., Kulms, D., Luger, T. A., Kubin, M., and Schwarz, T. (1999). Interleukin-1 protects transformed keratinocytes from tumor necrosis factor-related apoptosis-inducing ligand- and CD95-induced apoptosis but not from ultraviolet radiation-induced apoptosis. *J. Biol. Chem.* **274**, 28916–28921.

Ku, C. L., Yang, K., Bustamante, J., Puel, A., von Bermuth, H., Santos, O. F., Lawrence, T., Chang, H. H., Al-Mousa, H., Picard, C., and Casanova, J. L. (2005). Inherited disorders of human Toll-like receptor signaling: Immunological implications. *Immunol. Rev.* **203**, 10–20.

Kulms, D., and Schwarz, T. (2002a). Independent contribution of three different pathways to ultraviolet-B-induced apoptosis. *Biochem. Pharmacol.* **64**, 837–841.

La Casse, E. C., Baird, S., Korneluk, R. G., and MacKenzie, A. E. (1998). The inhibitors of apoptosis (IAPs) and their emerging role in cancer. *Oncogene* **17**, 3247–3259.

Laque, I., and Gelinas, C. (1997). Rel/NFκB and IκB factors in oncogenesis. *Semin. Cancer Biol.* **8**, 103–111.

Lawrence, T., Bebien, M., Liu, G. Y., Nizet, V., and Karin, M. (2005). IKKα limits macrophage NF-κB activation and contributes to resolution of inflammation. *Nature* **434**, 1138–1143.

Li, Q., Van Antwerp, D., Mercurio, F., Lee, K. F., and Verma, I. M. (1999). Severe liver degradation in mice lacking the IκB kinase 2. *Science* **284**, 321–325.

Li, Q., Withoff, S., and Verma, I. M. (2005). Inflammation-associated cancer: NFκB is the lynchpin. *Trends Immunol.* **26**, 318–325.

Maeda, S., Chang, L., Li, Z. W., Luo, J. L., Leffert, H., and Karin, M. (2003). IKKbeta is required for prevention of apoptosis mediated by cell-bound but not by circulating TNFalpha. *Immunity* **19**, 725–737.

Makris, C., Godfrey, V. L., Krahn-Senftleben, G., Takahashi, T., Roberts, J. L., Schwarz, T., Feng, L., Johnson, R. S., and Karin, M. (2000). Female mice heterozygous for IKK gamma/NEMO deficiencies develop a dermatopathy similar to the human X-linked disorder incontinentia pigmenti. *Mol. Cell* **6**, 969–979.

Mayo, M. W., Madrid, L. V., Westerheide, S. D., Jones, D. R., Yuan, X. J., Baldwin, A. S., Jr., and Whang, Y. E. (2002). PTEN blocks tumor necrosis factor-induced NFkappa B-dependent transcription by inhibiting the transactivation potential of the p65 subunit. *J. Biol. Chem.* **277**, 1116–1125.

Medzhitov, R., and Janeway, C., Jr. (2000). Innate immunity. *N. Engl. J. Med.* **343**, 338–344.

Micheau, O., and Tschopp, J. (2003). Induction of TNF receptor I-mediated apoptosis via two sequential signaling complexes. *Cell* **114**, 181–190.

Micheau, O., Lens, S., Gaide, O., Alevizopoulos, K., and Tschopp, J. (2001). NFκB signals induce the expression of c-FLIP. *Mol. Cell. Biol.* **21**, 5299–5305.

Nisticò, S., Costanzo, A. R., Saraceno, R., and Chimenti, S. (2004). Efficacy of monochromatic excimer laser radiation (308 nm) in the treatment of early stage mycosis fungoides. *Br. J. Dermatol.* **151**, 877–879.

Palombella, V. J., Rando, O. J., Goldberg, A. L., and Maniatis, T. (1994). The ubiquitin-proteasome pathway is required for processing the NF-κB1 precursor protein and the activation of NF-κB. *Cell* **78**, 773–785.

Parkin, J., and Cohen, B. (2001). An overview of the immune system. *Lancet* **357**, 1777–1789.

Pasparakis, M., Courtois, G., Hafner, M., Schmidt-Supprian, M., Nenci, A., Toksoy, A., Krampert, M., Goebeler, M., Gillitzer, R., Israel, A., Krieg, T., Rajewsky, K., *et al.* (2002). TNF-mediated inflammatory skin disease in mice with epidermis-specific deletion of IKK2. *Nature* **417**, 861–866.

Perkins, N. D. (2004). NF-κB: Tumor promoter or suppressor? *Trends Immunol.* **14**, 64–69.

Pöppelmann, B., Klimmek, K., Strozyk, E., Voss, R., Schwarz, T., and Kulms, D. (2005). NFκB-dependent down-regulation of tumor necrosis factor receptor-associated proteins contributes to interleukin-1-mediated enhancement of ultraviolet B-induced apoptosis. *J. Biol. Chem.* **280**, 15635–16643.

Rocha, S., Garrett, M. D., Campbell, K. J., Schumm, K., and Perkins, N. D. (2005). Regulation of NFkappaB and p53 through activation of ATR and Chk1 by the ARF tumor suppressor. *EMBO J.* **24**, 1157–1169.

Roulston, A., Lin, R., Beauparlant, P., Wainberg, M. A., and Hiscott, J. (1995). Regulation of human immunodeficiency virus type 1 and cytokine gene expression in myeloid cells by NFκB/Rel transcription factors. *Microbiol. Rev.* **59**, 481–505.

Ruben, S. M., Klement, J. F., Coleman, T. A., Maher, M., Chen, C. H., and Rosen, C. A. (1992). I-Rel: A novel rel-related protein that inhibits NF-kappa B transcriptional activity. *Genes Dev.* **6**, 745–760.

Ryseck, R. P., Bull, P., Takamiya, M., Bours, V., Siebenlist, U., Dobrzanski, P., and Bravo, R. (1992). RelB, a new Rel family transcription activator that can interact with p50-NF-kappa B. *Mol. Cell. Biol.* **12**, 674–684.

Scaffidi, C., Fulda, S., Srinivasan, A., Friesen, C., Li, F., Tomaselli, K. J., Debatin, K. M., Krammer, P. H., and Peter, M. E. (1998). Two CD95 (APO-1/Fas) signaling pathways. *EMBO J.* **17**, 1675–1687.

Sen, R., and Baltimore, D. (1986). Multiple nuclear factors interact with the immunoglobulin enhancer sequences. *Cell* **46**, 705–716.

Senftleben, U., Cao, Y., Xia, O. G., Greten, F. R., Krahn, G., Bonizzi, G., Chen, Y., Hu, Y., Fong, A., Sun, S. C., and Karin, M. (2001). Activation by IKKalpha of a second, evolutionary conserved, NF-kappa B signaling pathway. *Science* **293**, 1495–1499.

Sha, W. C., Liou, H. C., Tuomanen, E. I., and Baltimore, D. (1995). Targeted disruption of the p50 subunit of NF-kappa B leads to multifocal defects in immune responses. *Cell* **80**, 321–330.

Shinkura, R., Kitada, K., Matsuda, F., Tashiro, K., Ikuta, K., Suzuki, M., Kogishi, K., Serikawa, T., and Honjo, T. (1999). Alymphoplasia is caused by a point mutation in the mouse gene encoding NF-kappa B-inducing kinase. *Nat. Genet.* **22**, 74–77.

Sordet, O., Khan, Q. A., Kohn, K. W., and Pommier, Y. (2003). Apoptosis induced by topoisomerase inhibitors. *Curr. Med. Chem.* **3**, 271–290.

Stadler, R. (2002). Treatment of cutaneous T cell lymphoma. *Skin Pharmacol. Appl. Skin Physiol.* **15**, 139–146.

Strozyk, E., Pöppelman, B., Schwarz, T., and Kulms, D. (2006). Differential effects of NF-kappaB on apoptosis induced by DNA-damaging agents: The type of DNA damage determines the final outcome. *Oncogene,* online.

Sun, S. C., and Ballard, D. W. (1999). Persistent activation of NF-κB by the tax transforming protein of HTLV-1: Hijacking cellular IκBkinases. *Oncogene* **18**, 6948–6958.

Tergaonkar, V., Pando, M., Vafa, O., Wahl, G., and Verma, I. (2002). p53 stabilisation is decreased upon NKκB activation: A role for NKκB in acquisition of resistance to chemotherapy. *Cancer Cell* **1**, 493–503.

Thanos, D., and Maniatis, T. (1995). NF-κB: A lesson in family values. *Cell* **80**, 529–532.

Thomson, A. W. (1996). "The Cytokine Handbook," 2nd ed. Academic Press, London.

Thyss, R., Virolle, V., Imbert, V., Peyron, J. F., Aberdam, D., and Virolle, T. (2005). NFκB/Egr-1/Gadd45 are sequentially activated upon UVB irradiation to mediate epidermal cell death. *EMBO J.* **24**, 128–137.

Tschopp, J., Irmler, M., and Thome, M. (1998). Inhibition of Fas death signals by FLIPs. *Curr. Opin. Immunol.* **10**, 552–558.

Verma, I. M., and Stevenson, J. (1997). IκB kinase: Beginning, not the end. *Proc. Natl. Acad. Sci. USA* **94**, 11758–11760.

Verma, I. M., Stevenson, J. K., Schwarz, E. M., Van Antwerp, D., and Miyamoto, S. (1995). Rel/NF-κB/IκB family: Intimate tales of association and dissociation. *Genes Dev.* **9**, 2723–2735.

Wajant, H., Gerspach, J., and Pfizenmaier, K. (2005). Tumor therapeutics by design: Targeting and activation of death receptors. *Cytokine Growth Factor Rev.* **16**, 55–76.

Walczak, H., Miller, R. E., Ariail, K., Gliniak, B., Griffith, T. S., Kubin, M., Chin, W , Jones, J., Woodward, A., Le, T., Smith, C., Smolak, P., *et al.* (1999). Tumoricidal activity of tumor necrosis factor-related apoptosis-inducing ligand *in vivo. Nat. Med.* **5**, 157–163.

Wang, C. Y., Mayo, M. W., and Baldwin, A. S., Jr. (1996). TNF and cancer therapy-induced apoptosis: Potentiation by inhibition of NFkappaB. *Science* **274**, 784–787.

Wang, C. Y., Mayo, M. W., Korneluk, R. G., Goeddel, D. V., and Baldwin, A. S., Jr. (1998). NFkappaB antiapoptosis: Induction of TRAF1 and TRAF2 and c-IAP1 and c-IAP2 to suppress caspase 8 activation. *Science* **281**, 1680–1683.

Wang, C. Y., Cusack, J. C., Jr., Liu, R., and Baldwin, A. S., Jr. (1999). Control of inducible chemoresistance: Enhanced anti-tumor therapy through increased apoptosis by inhibition of NF-κB. *Nat. Med.* **5**, 412–417.

Wang, X. (2001). The expanding role of mitochondria in apoptosis. *Genes Dev.* **15**, 2922–2933.

Weih, D. S., Yilmaz, Z. B., and Weih, F. (2001). Essential role of RelB in germinal center and marginal zone formation and proper expression of homing chemokines. *J. Immunol.* **167**, 1909–1919.

Weih, F., Carrasco, D., and Bravo, R. (1994). Constitutive and inducible Rel/NF-kappa B activities in mouse thymus and spleen. *Oncogene* **9**, 3289–3297.

Wertz, I. E., O'Rourke, K. M., Zhou, H., Eby, M., Aravind, L., Seshagiri, S., Wu, P., Wiesmann, C., Baker, R., Boone, D. L., Ma, A., Koonin, E. V., *et al.* (2004). De-ubiquitination and ubiquitin ligase domains of A20 downregulate NF-κB-signalling. *Nature* **430**, 694–699.

Wiley, S. R., Schooley, K., Smolak, P. J., Din, W. S., Huang, C. P., Nicholl, J. K., Sutherland, G. R., Smith, T. D., Rauch, C., and Smith, C. A., and Goodwin, R. G. (1995). Identification and characterization of a new member of the TNF family that induces apoptosis. *Immunity* **3**, 673–682.

Wolff, B., and Naumann, M. (1999). INK4 cell cycle inhibitors direct transcriptional inactivation of NFkappaB. *Oncogene* **18**, 2663–2666.

Zong, W. X., Edelstein, L. C., Chen, C., Bash, J., and Gelinas, C. (1999). The prosurvival Bcl-2 homolog Bfl-1/A1 is a direct transcriptional target of NFkappaB that blocks TNFalpha-induced apoptosis. *Genes Dev.* **13**, 382–387.

12

IκB-ζ: An Inducible Regulator of Nuclear Factor-κB

Tatsushi Muta

Department of Molecular and Cellular Biochemistry
Graduate School of Medical Sciences, Kyushu University, Fukuoka 812-8582, Japan

The innate immune system responds to various microbial substances to elicit production of cytokines, chemokines, and costimulatory molecules that regulate activation of the acquired immune system. Although the transcription factor nuclear factor (NF)[1]-κB plays central roles in the induction, it remains to be clarified how appropriate genes are selectively activated with appropriate timing and duration by the multifunctional transcription factor after integration of signals activated by invasion of

[1]The abbreviations used are: ARE, AU-rich element; IL, interleukin; LPS, lipopolysaccharide; NF, nuclear factor; TAK, transforming growth factor-activated kinase; TIR, Toll/IL-1 receptor; TLR, Toll-like receptor; TNF, tumor necrosis factor; TRAF, TNF receptor-associated factor.

Vitamins and Hormones, Volume 74
0083-6729/06 $35.00
DOI: 10.1016/S0083-6729(06)74012-2

various pathogens. IκB-ζ is barely detectable in resting cells and is strongly induced upon stimulation of the innate immune system. The induced IκB-ζ associates with the NF-κB subunit in the nucleus and regulates its transcriptional activity both positively and negatively depending on genes. Thus, the innate immune system utilizes NF-κB as a major transcription factor and modulates its activity in a gene-specific manner by the regulatory factor IκB-ζ, which is specifically induced upon stimulation of the innate immune system. This multistep regulation of the transcription would be fundamental in selective expression of genes upon cell activation. © 2006 Elsevier Inc.

I. INTRODUCTION

To maintain the integrity of multicellular organisms consisting of cells with a single genome, the innate immune system detects and responds to invading microorganisms with different genomes (Janeway, 1989). Even in mammals with adaptive immunity, the innate immune system controls activation of the adaptive immune systems through production of cytokines and costimulatory molecules upon recognition of microbes (Medzhitov and Janeway, 1999). Intensive studies in the last decade have revealed that the innate immune system responds to various types of microbial and viral constituents, such as lipopolysaccharide (LPS), peptidoglycan, and unmodified nucleic acids (Janeway and Medzhitov, 2002; Takeda *et al.*, 2003).

Once cells recognize the microbial ligands, the transcription factor nuclear factor (NF)-κB and MAP kinases are activated by kinase cascades in the cells, which culminate in the induction of many inflammatory genes. This series of reactions is essential for the defense against invading microbes, but simultaneously, these reactions need precise regulation; otherwise excessive reactions lead to life-threatening symptoms represented by septic shock.

LPS on Gram-negative bacteria is one of the strongest activators of the innate immune system (Ulevitch and Tobias, 1999). Upon stimulation with LPS of macrophages, robust induction of various inflammatory genes is elicited. The genes include antimicrobial substances, cytokines, chemokines, costimulatory molecules, and cell adhesion molecules, which directly act on microbes to kill them or control activation of the adaptive immune system in concert. Another important group of the induced genes functions in the regulation of the system, which comprises positive- and negative-feedback loops, which determine strength and duration of the induction, and involved in selection of genes to be induced. In this chapter, I would like to review one such inducible gene with the regulatory functions, which was recently identified and named IκB-ζ.

II. STRUCTURE OF IκB-ζ

IκB-ζ was identified by subtractive hybridization screening as a gene that is strongly induced upon LPS stimulation of macrophages (Yamazaki *et al.*, 2001). It was named because of its structural and functional similarities with the IκB family proteins, which harbor multiple copies of the ankyrin-repeat at its COOH-terminus and associate with the NF-κB subunit (Fig. 1). The same gene was independently identified by two other groups as a gene with unknown function that is induced in response to LPS or interleukin (IL)-1β, and, therefore, was called molecule possessing ankyrin-repeats induced by lipopolysaccharide (MAIL) (Kitamura *et al.*, 2000) or IL-1-inducible nuclear protein (INAP) (Haruta *et al.*, 2001).

The structure of IκB-ζ is shown in Fig. 1 in comparison with the other IκB family proteins. IκB-α, β, and ε are the most typical IκB proteins, which have been actively investigated (Karin and Ben-Neriah, 2000). These cytosolic IκB proteins bind to the Rel domains of the NF-κB subunits via their ankyrin-repeats and inhibit their nuclear translocation and DNA-binding activities. Upon stimulation, two specific serine residues at their NH₂-terminal region are phosphorylated. The phosphorylation subsequently induces

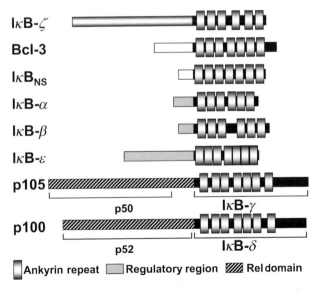

FIGURE 1. Structures of the IκB family proteins. All IκB proteins harbor the ankyrin-repeats at its COOH-terminal region. The NH₂-terminal regulatory regions of IκB-α, β, and ε contain specific sequences that are phosphorylated and ubiquitinated. p105 and p100 are precursor of the NF-κB p50 and p52 subunits, respectively, with the Rel-homology domains. The COOH-terminal regions correspond to IκB-γ and -δ. The NH₂-terminal region of IκB-ζ exhibit no homology to known proteins. See text for details.

ubiquitination of specific lysine residues near the phosphorylation sites. The ubiquitinated IκB proteins are rapidly degraded by proteasome and liberated NF-κB translocates into the nucleus, where it engages the transcription of the target genes. NF-κB consists of homo- or heterodimer of the Rel family proteins, Rel A, Rel B, and c-Rel with a transactivation domain, and p50 and p52, which lack the domain. NF-κB1 (p105) and NF-κB2 (p100) are precursors for the p50 and p52 subunits of NF-κB, respectively. The COOH-terminal portions with the ankyrin-repeats are believed to inhibit the activities of the NH_2-terminal region intramolecularly. IκB-γ and IκB-δ are derived from the COOH-terminal regions of NF-κB1 and NF-κB2, respectively, either by alternative transcription initiation or posttranslational modification (Dobrzanski et al., 1995; Inoue et al., 1992). The ankyrin-repeats of IκB-ζ exhibits highest similarity with bcl-3 (Ohno et al., 1990) and $IκB_{NS}$ (Fiorini et al., 2002). These IκB family members belong to the nuclear IκB protein family as IκB-ζ, which are likely directly to regulate the transcriptional activity of NF-κB in the nucleus. In contrast to the COOH-terminal ankyrin-repeats, the NH_2-terminal region of IκB-ζ does not show any homology with other known proteins.

The IκB-ζ gene spanning ~30 kb harbors 14 exons encoding IκB-ζ(L) (Shiina et al., 2001). Several exon–intron junctions in the region encoding the ankyrin-repeats are conserved with other IκB proteins. An alternative splicing variant, IκB-ζ(S), is generated by skipping the third exon (Kitamura et al., 2000; Yamazaki et al., 2001). Furthermore, another splicing variant, IκB-ζ(D), is present as a minor form, with a large deletion in the central region by an additional splicing in the seventh exon (Motoyama et al., 2005).

III. INDUCTION OF IκB-ζ BY STIMULATION OF THE INNATE IMMUNE SYSTEM

The Northern blotting of LPS-stimulated macrophages indicates that IκB-ζ is barely detectable in the unstimulated cells but is rapidly induced upon stimulation with LPS as low as 0.1–1 ng/ml (Kitamura et al., 2000; Yamazaki et al., 2001). The induction peaked at 1 h after stimulation and then gradually decreased but was sustained even 48 h after the stimulation. As suggested by the rapid kinetics, the induction of IκB-ζ mRNA does not depend on de novo protein synthesis as the induction was not inhibited by cycloheximide treatment. On intraperitoneal administration of LPS, the induction of IκB-ζ is observed in various tissues including lung, heart, liver, kidney, and testis, as well as spleen, lymph node, and thymus (Kitamura et al., 2000).

Among alternative splicing variants of IκB-ζ, IκB-ζ(L) is predominantly expressed on LPS stimulation (Kitamura et al., 2003; Yamazaki et al., 2005). Expression of IκB-ζ(S) is detected on both mRNA and protein levels as a minor species (Yamazaki *et al.*, 2005). IκB-ζ(D) mRNA is detected in LPS-stimulated macrophages, but the corresponding protein has not been detected (Motoyama *et al.*, 2005).

Not only LPS, a ligand for the Toll-like receptor (TLR)4/MD-2, but also other TLR ligands elicit robust induction of IκB-ζ, which include peptidoglycan, bacterial and mycoplasmal lipopeptides, flagellin, an imidazoquinoline-derivative (R-848), and CpG oligonucleotide, ligands for TLR2, 5, 7, and 9 (Eto *et al.*, 2003; Yamamoto *et al.*, 2004b).

The potent inflammatory cytokine IL-1β, which activates an intracellular signaling pathway shared with TLRs, also elicits strong induction of IκB-ζ (Eto *et al.*, 2003; Haruta *et al.*, 2001; Yamazaki *et al.*, 2001, 2005). However, the induction of IκB-ζ is not observed with another inflammatory cytokine tumor necrosis factor (TNF)-α although it activates both NF-κB and MAP kinases as TLR ligands or IL-1β does (Eto *et al.*, 2003; Haruta *et al.*, 2001; Yamazaki *et al.*, 2001, 2005).

IV. MOLECULAR FUNCTIONS OF IκB-ζ

Since all of the ankyrin-repeats in the IκB family proteins shown in Fig. 1 interact with NF-κB, IκB-ζ was suspected to regulate the NF-κB activity. NF-κB reporter analyses indicated that overexpressed IκB-ζ dose-dependently inhibited the activity of NF-κB stimulated by LPS-treatment of macrophages (Yamazaki *et al.*, 2001). This effect was not specific to NF-κB activities elicited by LPS: IκB-ζ inhibited the NF-κB activity stimulated by the inflammatory cytokine IL-1β or TNF-α. Moreover, IκB-ζ inhibited the NF-κB activity that is activated by transfection of the p65 subunit of NF-κB as well as IκB kinase (IKK)-β, indicating that it directly inhibits the NF-κB itself rather than its signaling pathway activating the transcription factor.

When subcellular localization of IκB-ζ was examined, a striking difference from the typical IκB proteins was observed (Yamazaki *et al.*, 2001). Whereas IκB-α, a most popular IκB protein, distributes throughout cells, IκB-ζ was found to localize exclusively in the nucleus. As expected from the subcellular localization, expression of IκB-ζ did not affect the nuclear translocation of NF-κB stimulated by TNF-α, which is effectively inhibited by IκB-α.

Thus, IκB-ζ localizes in nuclei and does not affect the nuclear translocation of NF-κB. Does IκB-ζ bind to NF-κB in the nucleus? In fact, immunoprecipitation analyses indicated that transfected IκB-ζ strongly associates with the p50 subunit of NF-κB (Yamazaki *et al.*, 2001). The association of the endogenous IκB-ζ and the p50 subunit was also detected in LPS-stimulated macrophages (Yamamoto *et al.*, 2004b). The association of IκB-ζ with the p65 subunits is much weaker but was detected by overexpression of both proteins (Yamazaki *et al.*, 2001). The preferential binding to the p50 subunit rather than the p65 subunit of NF-κB also has been reported in bcl-3

(Wulczyn *et al.*, 1992) and IκB$_{NS}$ (Fiorini *et al.*, 2002; Hirotani *et al.*, 2005), both of which harbor the ankyrin-repeats that are most homologous to those of IκB-ζ.

The DNA-binding activity of the p65/p50 heterodimer of NF-κB as well as the p50 homodimer was inhibited by a recombinant IκB-ζ protein when examined by an electrophoretic mobility shift assay using a probe harboring a canonical NF-κB binding sequence (Yamazaki *et al.*, 2001). The COOH-terminal ankyrin-repeats of IκB-ζ was sufficient for the inhibition (Fig. 2). The effect of IκB-ζ on the DNA-binding activity of NF-κB, however, should be carefully evaluated by using various DNA sequences, as IκB-ζ exhibits two opposite activities on NF-κB depending on the promoters of different genes as discussed in a later section.

The NH$_2$-terminal region of IκB-ζ is much larger than most of the other IκB family proteins (Fig. 1). As mentioned previously, this region of IκB-ζ does not show any significant sequence similarity to other proteins. A bipartite nuclear localization signal with a sequence of -K-R-X$_{12}$-K-R- was identified in the region of amino acids 163–178 (Motoyama *et al.*, 2005) (Fig. 2). When truncated mutants were transfected, the COOH-terminal ankyrin-repeats of IκB-ζ, which lacks the nuclear localization signal, localized in the cytosol and effectively inhibited NF-κB as IκB-α did (Yamazaki *et al.*, 2001).

Despite the nuclear localization signal, the function of most of the large NH$_2$-terminal region had remained unknown. An artificial experimental system using a fusion protein with the DNA-binding domain of the yeast transcription factor GAL4 provided evidence that this region has potential activity of transcriptional activation: the GAL4-fusion protein of the NH$_2$-terminal region of IκB-ζ activated transcription on a reporter with a GAL4-binding sequence in the promoter (Motoyama *et al.*, 2005). Further analyses with truncation mutants revealed that a central portion (amino acids 329–402) of the region is responsible for the activity (Fig. 2). The corresponding portion of human IκB-ζ also exhibited the similar activities, while

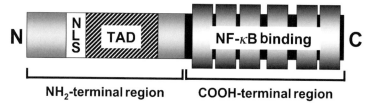

FIGURE 2.   Gross structures of IκB-ζ. The COOH-terminal region of IκB-ζ harbor the ankyrin-repeats, which is responsible for the NF-κB binding. The NH$_2$-terminal region contains a nuclear localization signal (NLS) and a transcriptional activation domain (TAD). See text for details.

this portion is less conserved between the species. It is tempting to speculate that this region might have been an intron of an ancestral IκB protein that evolved to a transactivation domain acquiring unique characteristics of IκB-ζ. This region is spliced out in the alternative splicing variant IκB-ζ(D) as discussed later.

It was found, however, that no transcriptional activity was detected with the fusion protein of the full-length protein of IκB-ζ(L) or (S) (Motoyama et al., 2005). These results suggest that the COOH-terminal region with the ankyrin-repeats inhibits the activity in the NH₂-terminal region. Because the COOH-terminal ankyrin-repeats had been known to bind the NF-κB p50 subunit, the activity of the complex of the p50 subunit and IκB-ζ was evaluated by using a GAL4-p50 subunit fusion protein. Although the GAL4-p50 fusion protein or IκB-ζ alone did not show the transcriptional activation activity on the GAL4-reporter, coexpression of the GAL4-p50 subunit fusion protein and the full-length IκB-ζ(L) or (S) resulted in the expression of significant activity, indicating that the complex had the transcriptional activation activity (Motoyama et al., 2005). The p50 subunit could be replaced with the Rel domain of the p65 subunit of NF-κB in this experimental system. The activity requires both NH₂-terminal and COOH-terminal regions of IκB-ζ, which contain the active site for the transcriptional activity and the binding site for the Rel domain, respectively. Thus, IκB-ζ possesses the latent transcriptional activation activity that is masked by the COOH-terminal ankyrin-repeats. The activity is unmasked by a conformational change that would be induced upon the complex formation with the p50 subunit of NF-κB via the ankyrin-repeats.

In addition to the artificial reporter system, IκB-ζ was shown to stimulate transcription of endogenous genes. Forced expression of IκB-ζ in macrophages (Motoyama et al., 2005) or fibroblasts (Kitamura et al., 2000; Motoyama et al., 2005) augments IL-6 production in response to LPS. This effect is on the transcriptional level because similar augmentation was observed with IL-6 mRNA. Both IκB-ζ(L) and (S) isoforms exhibited the stimulating activity. Interestingly, the effect of IκB-ζ is gene specific; expression of IκB-ζ inhibited the LPS-mediated TNF-α production in macrophages (Motoyama et al., 2005).

Another isoform, IκB-ζ(D), has a large deletion in the central portion (amino acids 236–429) responsible for the transcriptional activation activity (Motoyama et al., 2005). As expected, the deletion abolishes the transactivation activity on the GAL4-reporter system, and IκB-ζ(D) did not stimulate IL-6 production upon LPS stimulation. Nevertheless, IκB-ζ(D) exhibited the inhibitory activity on the NF-κB reporter system. Although IκB-ζ(D) is a minor population that has not been detected on the protein level, its function is intriguing if it is induced in specific physiological or pathological situations because it has distinct properties from IκB-ζ(L) or (S).

V. PHYSIOLOGICAL ROLES FOR IκB-ζ

IκB-ζ-deficient mice have been generated by gene targeting (Shiina et al., 2004; Yamamoto et al., 2004b). The number of homozygotes of IκB-ζ-deficient mice obtained by heterozygous intercrosses is much lower than that expected from the Mendelian ratio. Approximately 90% of the IκB-ζ-deficient embryo die in utero (Shiina et al., 2004). Ten percent of the IκB-ζ-deficient mice are born and grow normally with a normal composition of B and T lymphocytes until 4–5 weeks after birth (Yamamoto et al., 2004b). By 10 weeks after birth, all IκB-ζ-deficient mice develop atopic dermatitis-like skin lesions with acanthosis and lichenoid changes with infiltration of inflammatory cells (Shiina et al., 2004; Yamamoto et al., 2004b). IκB-ζ-deficient mice exhibit chronic inflammation in ocular surface as well. Histological analyses indicated pathological changes in the submucosa of the conjunctival epithelia of the mutant mice with heavy infiltration of lymphocytes, mainly CD45R/B220$^+$ cells and CD4$^+$ cells (Ueta et al., 2005; Yamamoto et al., 2004b). Because of the heavy inflammation in the conjunctiva, almost all goblet cells are lost in IκB-ζ-deficient mice (Ueta et al., 2005; Yamamoto et al., 2004b), as observed in human ocular surface disorders such as Stevens-Jonson syndrome and ocular cicatricial pemphigoid (Faraj and Hoang-Xuan, 2001). Constitutive expression of IκB-ζ was found in the skin, especially in the keratinocytes, and a variety of mucosal tissues of wild-type mice (Shiina et al., 2004; Ueta et al., 2005). Thus, IκB-ζ is expressed on the exposed surfaces of the body that contact resident microbiota and appears to negatively regulate the activation of inflammatory cells.

Peritoneal macrophages from IκB-ζ-deficient mice exhibited apparently normal production of TNF-α and nitric oxide (NO) upon LPS stimulation. However, IL-6 production in response to LPS was completely abolished (Yamamoto et al., 2004b). Although LPS-induced activations of NF-κB and MAP kinases appeared normal, the induction of IL-6 mRNA was not detected in IκB-ζ-deficient macrophages, indicating that IκB-ζ is essential for the LPS-induced transcription on the IL-6 gene. The essential role for IκB-ζ in IL-6 production is not specific to LPS-mediated induction: IL-6 production was abolished or severely impaired in the mutant cells in response to other stimuli that induce IκB-ζ, such as peptidoglycan, bacterial and mycoplasmal lipopeptides, CpG DNA, R-848, and IL-1β. On the other hand, IL-6 is normally produced in IκB-ζ-deficient embryonic fibroblasts in response to TNF-α, which does not provoke IκB-ζ induction.

As mentioned earlier, IκB-ζ was suggested to activate transcription via complex formation with the p50 subunit of NF-κB (Motoyama et al., 2005). Consistent with this notion, severe impairments of IL-6 production were observed with the NF-κB1 (the gene encoding the NF-κB p50 subunit)-deficient macrophages in response to above-mentioned stimulants that induce

IκB-ζ (Yamamoto *et al.*, 2004b). Furthermore, *NF-κB1*-deficient embryonic fibroblasts produce TNF-α but not IL-6 in response to LPS.

The target genes for IκB-ζ-mediated transcription are not restricted to IL-6. DNA microarray analysis indicated that LPS-mediated induction of a subset of genes, such as IL-12, GM-CSF, and M-CSF, was abolished or severely impaired in *IκB-ζ*-deficient mice (Yamamoto *et al.*, 2004b). A list of the genes is in Table I. *IκB-ζ*-deficient splenocytes exhibited defective proliferation in response to LPS but not to anti-CD40 or IL-4 and anti-IgM antibody (Yamamoto *et al.*, 2004b), strongly suggesting that one of the target genes of IκB-ζ-mediated transcription is involved in LPS-induced proliferation of B cells. Thus, IκB-ζ plays essential roles in transcriptional activation of a subset of inflammatory genes in concert with the p50 subunit of NF-κB.

In vivo analyses of *IκB-ζ*-deficient mice have revealed more complicated regulation of cytokine induction. Serum IL-12 concentrations after

TABLE I.   Genes that Require IκB-ζ for the LPS-Mediated Induction[a]

Category	Gene
Cytokine	IL-6[b], IL-12 p40 subunit[b], IL-18, granulate-macrophage colony stimulating factor (GM-CSF), granulocyte colony-stimulating factor (G-CSF)[b], growth-differentiation factor (GDF) 15, Epstein-Barr virus-induced gene (EBI) 3
Chemokine	CXC chemokine ligand (CXCL)5, CXCL13, CC chemokine ligand (CCL)7, CCL17
Enzyme	Histidine decarboxylase, caspase 11, inositol polyphosphate-5-phosphatase B, deltex 2B, glutathione reductase, guanylate nucleotide–binding protein (GBP) 1
Receptor	Formyl peptide receptor 1, macrophage receptor with collagenous structure (MARCO)
Biological active peptide	Endothelin 1[b], ghrelin
Transcription factor	Basic leucine zipper transcription factor (BATF), CCAAT/enhancer-binding protein (C/EBP)-δ^2
Antimicrobial substance	Lipocalin 2/neutrophil gelatinase-associated lipocalin (NGAL)
Others	Tax1-binding protein, extracellular proteinase inhibitor, solute carrier family 11 member 2 (Slc11a2), Src-like adaptor protein (SLAP), immunoglobulin heavy chain, immunoglobulin light chain, membrane-spanning 4-domains (MS4A1), thrombospondin 1, immediate early response 3 (IER3/IEX1), disabled-2

[a]Genes whose impaired LPS-mediated induction in IκB-ζ-deficient macrophages was shown by DNA microarray analysis (Yamamoto *et al.*, 2004b).
[b]Confirmed by Northern blotting.

intraperitoneal injection of LPS were significantly lower in $I\kappa B$-ζ-deficient mice than those of wild-type mice as expected from the studies on isolated macrophages (Yamamoto *et al.*, 2004b). However, serum IL-6 levels following LPS injection did not appear to differ significantly from those of wild-type mice. In contrast to IL-12 and IL-6, TNF-α production in response to LPS injection was considerably upregulated in $I\kappa B$-ζ-deficient mice. In wild-type mice, TNF-α in serum is detected transiently after LPS injection: it appears 1.5 h after the injection but is rapidly cleared and is not detected in the serum after 3 h. The serum TNF-α levels in $I\kappa B$-ζ-deficient mice were higher than that of wild-type mice at 1.5 h after the injection and were sustained for much longer time: it is detected even 6 h after the injection (Yamamoto *et al.*, 2004b). The apparent normal IL-6 production in $I\kappa B$-ζ-deficient mice is at least in part due to this upregulated TNF-α production. By neutralizing TNF-α by an anti-TNF-α antibody, the LPS-induced IL-6 production in $I\kappa B$-ζ-deficient mice were significantly reduced and became lower than those of wild-type mice (Yamamoto *et al.*, 2004b). Thus, the defect in the LPS-induced IL-6 production in $I\kappa B$-ζ-deficient mice is likely compensated by secondary IL-6 production induced by augmented TNF-α production.

VI. MECHANISMS OF THE INDUCTION OF IκB-ζ

$I\kappa B$-ζ is strongly induced by various microbial substances that stimulate TLRs and IL-1β but not by TNF-α (Eto *et al.*, 2003; Yamazaki *et al.*, 2001, 2005). The cytoplasmic tails of TLRs and IL-1 receptors exhibit sequence homology and is hence called the Toll/IL-1 receptor (TIR) domain. As expected from the homology, except for TLR3, they share common signaling pathways initiated by an adaptor protein MyD88. $I\kappa B$-ζ is not induced by stimulation of TLR3, which utilized another adapter molecule named TRIF/TICAM1 (Oshiumi *et al.*, 2003; Yamamoto *et al.*, 2002, 2003). As expected from the specificity, the induction of $I\kappa B$-ζ depends on MyD88 as the induction was not observed in *MyD88*-deficient cells (Yamamoto *et al.*, 2004b).

Upon receptor ligation by TLR ligands, clustering the TIR domains induce recruitment of the adapter MyD88, which subsequently activates interleukin receptor-associated kinase (IRAK) 1 and 4 as well as TNF receptor-associated factor (TRAF) 6 (Yamamoto *et al.*, 2004a). The activation of the ubiquitin ligase TRAF6 leads to activation of transforming growth factor-activated kinase (TAK) 1. TAK1 bifurcates the signal; NF-κB and MAP kinase are activated via IKKβ and MKK7, respectively (Irie *et al.*, 2000; Ninomiya-Tsuji *et al.*, 1999). TNF-α signaling utilizes TRAF2 instead of TRAF6 and activates both NF-κB and MAP kinases (Wallach *et al.*, 1999). The fact that TNF-α does not induce $I\kappa B$-ζ indicates that activation of NF-κB and/or MAP kinases are not sufficient for the induction of IκB-ζ, and it requires a specific signal(s) that come from MyD88.

Analyses using various inhibitors indicated that different types of NF-κB inhibitors, such as pyrrolidinedithiocarbamate (PDTC), acetylsalicylic acid, and proteasome inhibitors, inhibited the induction of IκB-ζ (Eto *et al.*, 2003). Furthermore, the induction was suppressed in cells overexpressing IκB-β, one of the natural cytosolic inhibitors of NF-κB. On the other hand, specific inhibitors of MAP kinases, Erk, JNK, and p38, or its activators did not inhibit the induction, indicating that the three types of MAP kinases are dispensable. A promoter region of *IκB-ζ* gene harbors three NF-κB binding site within 300-bp upstream of the transcription initiation site (Shiina *et al.*, 2001; Yamazaki *et al.*, 2005). Reporter analyses of the promoter indicated that the distal two NF-κB binding sites, which are completely conserved between the mouse and human genes, are essential for the LPS-mediated induction of IκB-ζ (Ito *et al.*, 2004; Yamazaki *et al.*, 2005).

All these data indicate that NF-κB is essential for the induction of IκB-ζ. However, activation of NF-κB alone is not sufficient for the induction of IκB-ζ, as exemplified by defective induction of IκB-ζ on TNF-α stimulation. In fact, transfection of any of the five subunits of NF-κB or their combinations did not elicit induction of IκB-ζ although strong NF-κB activation was observed by the transfection (Eto *et al.*, 2003).

Extensive reporter analyses on the sequence of the promoter and the introns of the *IκB-ζ* gene failed to identify any enhancer elements that allows the stimuli-specific induction (Yamazaki *et al.*, 2005). Furthermore, nuclear run-on analysis on IκB-ζ gene showed that transcriptional activity on the *IκB-ζ* gene was similarly activated upon stimulation with TNF-α as well as LPS or IL-1β (Yamazaki *et al.*, 2005). These data led to the idea that IκB-ζ induction might be regulated posttranscriptionally. One of the well-known posttranscriptional mechanisms of gene expression is the regulation of mRNA stability (Mitchell and Tollervey, 2000). The IκB-ζ mRNA stability was examined with an artificial gene in which the full-length mRNA was driven by the chicken β-actin promoter, whose transcription is unaffected by the stimuli (Yamazaki *et al.*, 2005). The stability of mRNA was examined by chasing its decay after terminating transcription by actinomycin D treatment. The IκB-ζ mRNA was found to be unstable with a half life of approximately 30 min. On stimulation with LPS or IL-1β, however, significant stabilization of the IκB-ζ mRNA was observed. In contrast, the stability of the IκB-ζ mRNA did not change by TNF-α stimulation. mRNA for IκB-α is also unstable, but the stimulation-dependent stabilization was not observed (Yamazaki *et al.*, 2005). Several AU-rich elements (AREs), which are known to destabilize mRNA, is present in the 3'-untranslated region of IκB-ζ mRNA. However, mutational analyses did not provide any indications that these AREs are involved in the stimuli-specific stabilization (Yamazaki *et al.*, 2005). Furthermore, overexpression of HuR (Myer *et al.*, 1997) or

Apobec-1 (Anant and Davidson, 2000), a transacting factor that binds ARE to stabilize mRNA, did not affect the stability of IκB-ζ mRNA.

Not only LPS and IL-1β, but also IL-17 (Kolls and Linden, 2004), secreted from activated T cells, was found to stabilize the IκB-ζ mRNA. Although TNF-α or IL-17 alone does not elicit IκB-ζ, costimulation with thesetwocytokines resulted in the induction ofIκB-ζ, suggesting that NF-κB-mediated transcription and specific stabilization of IκB-ζ mRNA, activated by TNF-α and IL-17, respectively, are sufficient to elicit the induction of IκB-ζ (Yamazaki et al., 2005). Considering active roles for TNF-α and IL-17 in inflammatory and autoimmune diseases, induction of IκB-ζ might be critically involved in these pathological conditions.

VII. CONCLUSIONS

Upon inflammatory stimuli, the transcription factor NF-κB is playing critical roles in the subsequent transcriptional activation. When LPS or other TLR ligands stimulates cells, the cytosolic inhibitors IκB-α and -β are phosphorylated and degraded, which allows nuclear translocation of NF-κB. The nuclear NF-κB activates a subset of inflammatory genes (genes A in Fig. 3).

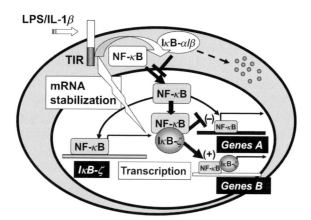

FIGURE 3.   Roles for IκB-ζ in inflammatory response. Activation of the TIR-containing receptors by LPS or IL-1β elicits phosphorylation and ubiquitination-induced degradation of the cytosolic IκB-α/β, which allows nuclear translocation of NF-κB. NF-κB, then, activates transcription of a subset of genes (Genes A) including IκB-ζ. The expression of IκB-ζ requires a specific mRNA stabilization signal that come from the TIR-containing receptors as well as activation of NF-κB. The expressed IκB-ζ associates with NF-κB, and the complex engages transcription of another subset of genes (Genes B). Simultaneously, IκB-ζ inhibits the transcription of the genes A. See text for details.

Simultaneously, NF-κB activates transcription of IκB-ζ. However, NF-κB is not sufficient for the induction of IκB-ζ and posttranslational regulation, such as specific mRNA stabilization, is necessary for the induction. The induced IκB-ζ associates with NF-κB and the complex activates another subset of inflammatory genes (genes B in Fig. 3). Simultaneously, IκB-ζ inhibits the transcription of the inflammatory genes A.

The studies on IκB-ζ-deficient mice demonstrated the roles for IκB-ζ as a positive and negative regulator of the NF-κB-mediated transcription. IκB-ζ is an indispensable component for the LPS-induced transcriptional complex for the genes represented by IL-6. However, the transcription complex on the same gene appears to be different depending on stimuli. Upon TNF-α stimulation, IκB-ζ is not required for IL-6 production; therefore, some unknown factor, possibly induced by TNF-α, is playing a role for IκB-ζ. The role for IκB-ζ as the negative regulator was not evident in the isolated cells, probably because of redundant negative regulators of NF-κB. Its inhibitory roles on NF-κB-mediated transcription, however, are critical in a fine tuning to balance inflammatory reactions to maintain homeostasis *in vivo*. Such roles for IκB-ζ are exemplified in the mutant mice by the higher and prolonged expression of TNF-α upon innate immune stimulation, which might lead to chronic inflammation of skin and eyes.

Determinants that distinguish genes that are inhibited or activated by IκB-ζ appear to be present in the promoter of each gene. Our preliminary studies have indicated that in addition to an NF-κB binding site, another element is required for the IκB-ζ-mediated transcriptional activation. IκB-ζ acts as a negative regulator on the promoters harboring canonical NF-κB binding sequences alone. Since the transcriptional activation activity of IκB-ζ on the GAL4-reporter system is much weaker than that of the NF-κB p65 subunit, another transcription factor(s) may be necessary for efficient IκB-ζ-mediated transcription. Alternatively, IκB-ζ may also have activities to modify chromatin structures. Because the ankyrin-repeats of IκB-ζ are most homologous to that of bcl-3 and IκB$_{NS}$, these nuclear IκB family proteins may act as a competitor for IκB-ζ, or vice versa. In fact, IκB$_{NS}$ has been reported to inhibit LPS-induced IL-6 production (Hirotani et al., 2005).

The studies on IκB-ζ provided evidence for multistep regulation of inflammatory responses (Fig. 4). Upon activation, primary responses are carried out by rapid activation of the major transcription factors, represented by NF-κB, which is activated through posttranslational modifications, such as phosphorylation, without *de novo* protein synthesis. During this period, transcriptional regulators, such as IκB-ζ, are induced via stimuli-specific mechanisms. By combinations of the major transcription factors and the inducible regulators, secondary responses are activated, and primary responses are gradually diminished. Since the genes that are activated via secondary responses also include other transcription factors, stimulus-specific transcriptional

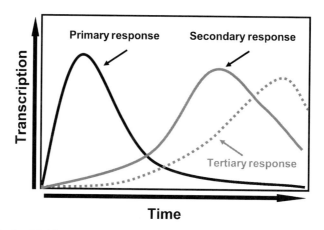

FIGURE 4. Multistep regulation of transcriptional activation during inflammatory responses. Upon inflammatory stimulation, primary responses are activated by the major transcription factors, such as NF-κB and AP-1. The secondary responses are mediated by transcriptional complexes of the major transcription factors and the regulatory factors including IκB-ζ, which is induced during the primary response. During the secondary responses, other transcription factors are synthesized, which constitute the tertiary response. See text for details.

activation would proceed in a multistep fashion along with the time after the stimulation.

As described in this chapter, IκB-ζ have dual and opposite, that is, positive and negative, roles to regulate NF-κB-mediated transcription. If directions of cellular reactions are already committed, as trains on rail tracks, the reactions can be controlled basically with just an accelerator and a brake. Cells that are directed to proliferation or apoptosis may be controlled like a train. However, if cells initiate inflammation or differentiation, in other words, if there are several ways to go, an accelerator and a brake are not enough. When one drives a car, one needs a steering wheel to determine the directions to go, in addition to an accelerator and a brake. NF-κB and IκB-α correspond to the accelerator and the brake, respectively, and IκB-ζ would play a role as the steering wheel. The steering wheels should be specifically induced upon different stimuli. LPS/IL-1β and TNF-α induce similar sets of genes in the early phases, and IκB-ζ is one of the genes that is differentially expressed in the earliest phase (T. Muta, unpublished data).

Not only IκB-ζ, cells should be equipped with several steering wheels that are used on different stimuli. Appropriate cellular responses are regulated by controlling precise balances of the accelerators, the brakes, and the steering wheels to maintain homeostasis upon environmental change. Identification of other steering wheels and analysis on the molecular mechanisms for their specific induction will further advance our understanding of regulation of inflammatory responses.

ACKNOWLEDGMENTS

The author would like to express sincere thanks to Koichiro Takeshige, Soh Yamazaki, and all other collaborators. The author's works were supported in part by grants-in-aid for Scientific Research from the Ministry of Education, Science, Sports, and Culture of Japan, and grants from Sumitomo Foundation, the Mochida Memorial Foundation for Medical and Pharmaceutical Research, the Naito Foundation, and the Kaibara Foundation.

REFERENCES

Anant, S., and Davidson, N. O. (2000). An AU-rich sequence element (UUUN[A/U]U) downstream of the edited C in apolipoprotein B mRNA is a high-affinity binding site for Apobec-1: Binding of Apobec-1 to this motif in the 3′ untranslated region of c-myc increases mRNA stability. *Mol. Cell Biol.* **20,** 1982–1992.

Dobrzanski, P., Ryseck, R. P., and Bravo, R. (1995). Specific inhibition of RelB/p52 transcriptional activity by the C-terminal domain of p100. *Oncogene* **10,** 1003–1007.

Eto, A., Muta, T., Yamazaki, S., and Takeshige, K. (2003). Essential roles for NF-κB and a Toll/IL-1 receptor domain-specific signal(s) in the induction of IκB-ζ. *Biochem. Biophys. Res. Commun.* **301,** 495–501.

Faraj, H. G., and Hoang-Xuan, T. (2001). Chronic cicatrizing conjunctivitis. *Curr. Opin. Ophthalmol.* **12,** 250–257.

Fiorini, E., Schmitz, I., Marissen, W. E., Osborn, S. L., Touma, M., Sasada, T., Reche, P. A., Tibaldi, E. V., Hussey, R. E., Kruisbeek, A. M., Reinherz, E. L., and Clayton, L. K. (2002). Peptide-induced negative selection of thymocytes activates transcription of an NF-κB inhibitor. *Mol. Cell* **9,** 637–648.

Haruta, H., Kato, A., and Todokoro, K. (2001). Isolation of a novel interleukin-1-inducible nuclear protein bearing ankyrin-repeat motifs. *J. Biol. Chem.* **276,** 12485–12488.

Hirotani, T., Lee, P. Y., Kuwata, H., Yamamoto, M., Matsumoto, M., Kawase, I., Akira, S., and Takeda, K. (2005). The nuclear IκB protein IκBNS selectively inhibits lipopolysaccharide-induced IL-6 production in macrophages of the colonic lamina propria. *J. Immunol.* **174,** 3650–3657.

Inoue, J., Kerr, L. D., Kakizuka, A., and Verma, I. M. (1992). IκBγ, a 70 kd protein identical to the C-terminal half of p110 NF-κB: A new member of the IκB family. *Cell* **68,** 1109–1120.

Irie, T., Muta, T., and Takeshige, K. (2000). TAK1 mediates an activation signal from toll-like receptor(s) to nuclear factor-κB in lipopolysaccharide-stimulated macrophages. *FEBS Lett.* **467,** 160–164.

Ito, T., Morimatsu, M., Oonuma, T., Shiina, T., Kitamura, H., and Syuto, B. (2004). Transcriptional regulation of the MAIL gene in LPS-stimulated RAW264 mouse macrophages. *Gene* **342,** 137–143.

Janeway, C. A., Jr. (1989). Approaching the asymptote? Evolution and revolution in immunology. *Cold Spring Harb. Symp. Quant. Biol.* **54**(Pt.1), 1–13.

Janeway, C. A., Jr., and Medzhitov, R. (2002). Innate immune recognition. *Annu. Rev. Immunol.* **20,** 197–216.

Karin, M., and Ben-Neriah, Y. (2000). Phosphorylation meets ubiquitination: The control of NF-κB activity. *Annu. Rev. Immunol.* **18,** 621–663.

Kitamura, H., Kanehira, K., Okita, K., Morimatsu, M., and Saito, M. (2000). MAIL, a novel nuclear IκB protein that potentiates LPS-induced IL-6 production. *FEBS Lett.* **485,** 53–56.

Kitamura, H., Kanehira, K., Shiina, T., Morimatsu, M., Jung, B. D., Akashi, S., and Saito, M. (2002). Bacterial lipopolysaccharide induces mRNA expression of an IκB MAIL through toll-like receptor 4. *J. Vet. Med. Sci.* **64,** 419–422.

Kitamura, H., Matsushita, Y., Iwanaga, T., Mori, K., Kanehira, K., Fujikura, D., Morimatsu, M., and Saito, M. (2003). Bacterial lipopolysaccharide-induced expression of the IκB protein MAIL in B-lymphocytes and macrophages. *Arch. Histol. Cytol.* **66,** 53–62.

Kolls, J. K., and Linden, A. (2004). Interleukin-17 family members and inflammation. *Immunity* **21**, 467–476.

Medzhitov, R., and Janeway, C. A., Jr. (1999). Innate immune induction of the adaptive immune response. *Cold Spring Harb. Symp. Quant. Biol.* **64**, 429–435.

Mitchell, P., and Tollervey, D. (2000). mRNA stability in eukaryotes. *Curr. Opin. Genet. Dev.* **10**, 193–198.

Motoyama, M., Yamazaki, S., Eto-Kimura, A., Takeshige, K., and Muta, T. (2005). Positive and negative regulation of nuclear factor-kappaB-mediated transcription by IkappaB-zeta, an inducible nuclear protein. *J. Biol. Chem.* **280**, 7444–7451.

Myer, V. E., Fan, X. C., and Steitz, J. A. (1997). Identification of HuR as a protein implicated in AUUUA-mediated mRNA decay. *EMBO J.* **16**, 2130–2139.

Ninomiya-Tsuji, J., Kishimoto, K., Hiyama, A., Inoue, J., Cao, Z., and Matsumoto, K. (1999). The kinase TAK1 can activate the NIK-IκB as well as the MAP kinase cascade in the IL-1 signalling pathway. *Nature* **398**, 252–256.

Ohno, H., Takimoto, G., and McKeithan, T. W. (1990). The candidate proto-oncogene bcl-3 is related to genes implicated in cell lineage determination and cell cycle control. *Cell* **60**, 991–997.

Oshiumi, H., Matsumoto, M., Funami, K., Akazawa, T., and Seya, T. (2003). TICAM-1, an adaptor molecule that participates in Toll-like receptor 3-mediated interferon-beta induction. *Nat. Immunol.* **4**, 161–167.

Shiina, T., Morimatsu, M., Kitamura, H., Ito, T., Kidou, S., Matsubara, K., Matsuda, Y., Saito, M., and Syuto, B. (2001). Genomic organization, chromosomal localization, and promoter analysis of the mouse Mail gene. *Immunogenetics* **53**, 649–655.

Shiina, T., Konno, A., Oonuma, T., Kitamura, H., Imaoka, K., Takeda, N., Todokoro, K., and Morimatsu, M. (2004). Targeted disruption of MAIL, a nuclear IκB protein, leads to severe atopic dermatitis-like disease. *J. Biol. Chem.* **279**, 55493–55498.

Takeda, K., Kaisho, T., and Akira, S. (2003). Toll-like receptors. *Annu. Rev. Immunol.* **21**, 335–376.

Ueta, M., Hamuro, J., Yamamoto, M., Kaseda, K., Akira, S., and Kinoshita, S. (2005). Spontaneous ocular surface inflammation and goblet cell disappearance in I kappa B zeta gene-disrupted mice. *Invest. Ophthalmol. Vis. Sci.* **46**, 579–588.

Ulevitch, R. J., and Tobias, P. S. (1999). Recognition of Gram-negative bacteria and endotoxin by the innate immune system. *Curr. Opin. Immunol.* **11**, 19–22.

Wallach, D., Varfolomeev, E. E., Malinin, N. L., Goltsev, Y. V., Kovalenko, A. V., and Boldin, M. P. (1999). Tumor necrosis factor receptor and Fas signaling mechanisms. *Annu. Rev. Immunol.* **17**, 331–367.

Wulczyn, F. G., Naumann, M., and Scheidereit, C. (1992). Candidate proto-oncogene bcl-3 encodes a subunit-specific inhibitor of transcription factor NF-κB. *Nature* **358**, 597–599.

Yamamoto, M., Sato, S., Mori, K., Hoshino, K., Takeuchi, O., Takeda, K., and Akira, S. (2002). Cutting edge: A novel Toll/IL-1 receptor domain-containing adapter that preferentially activates the IFN-β promoter in the Toll-like receptor signaling. *J. Immunol.* **169**, 6668–6672.

Yamamoto, M., Sato, S., Hemmi, H., Hoshino, K., Kaisho, T., Sanjo, H., Takeuchi, O., Sugiyama, M., Okabe, M., Takeda, K., and Akira, S. (2003). Role of adaptor TRIF in the MyD88-independent toll-like receptor signaling pathway. *Science* **301**, 640–643.

Yamamoto, M., Takeda, K., and Akira, S. (2004a). TIR domain-containing adaptors define the specificity of TLR signaling. *Mol. Immunol.* **40**, 861–868.

Yamamoto, M., Yamazaki, S., Uematsu, S., Sato, S., Hemmi, H., Hoshino, K., Kaisho, T., Kuwata, H., Takeuchi, O., Takeshige, K., Saitoh, T., Yamaoka, S., Yamamoto, N., Yamamoto, S., Muta, T., Takeda, K., and Akira, S. (2004b). Regulation of Toll/IL-1-receptor-mediated gene expression by the inducible nuclear protein IkBz. *Nature* **430**, 218–222.

Yamazaki, S., Muta, T., and Takeshige, K. (2001). A novel IkappaB protein, IκB-ζ, induced by proinflammatory stimuli, negatively regulates nuclear factor-κB in the nuclei. *J. Biol. Chem.* **276**, 27657–27662.

Yamazaki, S., Muta, T., Matsuo, S., and Takeshige, K. (2005). Stimulus-specific induction of a novel nuclear factor-κB regulator, IκB-ζ, via Toll/Interleukin-1 receptor is mediated by mRNA stabilization. *J. Biol. Chem.* **280**, 1678–1687.

13

THE INHIBITORY EFFECTS OF INTERLEUKIN-1 ON GROWTH HORMONE ACTION DURING CATABOLIC ILLNESS

ROBERT N. COONEY*,† AND MARGARET SHUMATE*

*Department of Surgery
The Pennsylvania State University–College of Medicine
Hershey, Pennsylvania 17033
†Department of Cellular and Molecular Physiology
The Pennsylvania State University–College of Medicine
Hershey, Pennsylvania 17033

0083-6729/06 $35.00
DOI: 10.1016/S0083-6729(06)74013-4

XIV. Inhibition of GH-Inducible Gene Expression
    by Cytokines (IL-1)
XV. Conclusions
    References

Growth hormone (GH) induces the expression of the anabolic genes
responsible for growth, metabolism, and differentiation. Normally, GH
stimulates the synthesis of circulating insulin-like growth factor-I (IGF-I)
by liver, which upregulates protein synthesis in many tissues. The
development of GH resistance during catabolic illness or inflammation
contributes to loss of body protein, resulting in multiple complications
that prolong recovery and cause death. In septic patients, increased levels
of proinflammatory cytokines and GH resistance are commonly observed
together. Numerous studies have provided evidence that the inhibitory
effects of cytokines on skeletal muscle protein synthesis during sepsis and
inflammation are mediated indirectly by changes in the GH/IGF-I system.
Interleukin (IL)-1, a member of the family of proinflammatory cytokines,
interacts with most cell types and is an important mediator of the
inflammatory response. Infusion of a specific IL-1 receptor antagonist
(IL-1Ra) ameliorates protein catabolism and GH resistance during
systemic infection. This suggests that IL-1 is an important mediator of GH
resistance during systemic infection or inflammation. Consequently, a
better understanding of the interaction between GH, IL-1, and the
regulation of protein metabolism is of great importance for the care of the
patient. © 2006 Elsevier Inc.

I. INTRODUCTION

The host response to injury or infection is characterized by a series of
physiologic and metabolic adaptations which are commonly referred to
as the systemic inflammatory response syndrome (SIRS) (Marshall, 2000;
Wilmore, 2000). The signs and symptoms of SIRS include: fever, tachycardia,
tachypnea, and elevated white blood cell (WBC) count (Marshall, 2000). The
host response to SIRS is characterized by significant alterations in metabolism including increased oxygen consumption, increased CO_2 production,
reprioritization of hepatic protein synthesis, and the catabolism of muscle
protein (Marshall, 2000). The catabolism of muscle during sepsis is caused by
both an increase in protein degradation and reductions in protein synthesis
(Rennie, 1985; Vary and Kimball, 1992). While the catabolism of muscle may
provide substrate for intermediary metabolism in other tissues, it can only be
attenuated (but not prevented) by the provision of adequate nutrition support

(Cerra *et al.*, 1980). This suggests that mechanisms other than simple starvation are responsible for the loss of lean body mass that is observed during systemic inflammation (Cooney *et al.*, 1997).

Although the pathophysiology of protein catabolism is complex, several observations suggest that the inflammatory cytokines tumor necrosis factor (TNF) and interleukin-1 (IL-1) act as indirect mediators of muscle catabolism via their inhibitory actions on the growth hormone (GH)/insulin-like growth factor-I (IGF-I) axis (Cooney *et al.*, 1999b; Fong *et al.*, 1989; Lang *et al.*, 1996). First, sepsis is associated with increased cytokine production and studies performed using incubated muscle preparations have been unable to demonstrate a direct effect of either recombinant IL-1 or TNF on protein synthesis or degradation (Guirao and Lowry, 1996; Moldawer *et al.*, 1987). Second, during systemic infection, the increase in circulating GH and reductions in plasma IGF-I that are observed are reproduced by TNF-α or IL-1β administration (Fan *et al.*, 1995a, 1996; Lang *et al.*, 1997). Third, the administration of specific TNF and IL-1 antagonists significantly attenuates the sepsis-induced alterations in the IGF-I system and prevents the catabolism of muscle protein (Cooney *et al.*, 1999b; Lang *et al.*, 1996; Yumet *et al.*, 2002; Zamir *et al.*, 1992). Finally, the role of IGF-I as a mediator of muscle protein synthesis in septic rats has been confirmed in isolated hind limb perfusions (Jurasinski and Vary, 1995). In these studies, increasing the concentration of IGF-I in the perfusate produced a dose-dependent increase in muscle protein synthesis. In summary, the results of these and other studies suggest that the inhibitory effects of TNF and IL-1 on muscle protein synthesis are mediated indirectly by changes in the GH/IGF-I system.

The goal of this chapter is to review the interactions between IL-1 and the GH/IGF-I system. First, we will discuss the IL-1 family of proteins, the regulation of IL-1 expression and bioactivity. This will be followed by an overview of the physiologic effects of IL-1 administration and the role of IL-1 in disease. Then, we will discuss the regulation of GH secretion and activity, GH signaling pathways, and gene expression, followed by a summary of the effects of IL-1 on GH activity.

II. THE INTERLEUKIN-1 FAMILY

The term IL-1 refers to a family of structurally related, multifunctional proteins which influence most cell types and are important mediators of the inflammatory response (Dinarello *et al.*, 1984). The IL-1 family is made up of three distinct genes: IL-1α, IL-1β, and IL-1 receptor antagonist (IL-1-Ra) which are located on chromosome 2 (Webb *et al.*, 1986). The IL-1 genes demonstrate significant homology in nucleotide sequence (45%) and gene structure (7 exons) suggesting evolution from a common gene (March *et al.*, 1985). IL-1α and IL-1β demonstrate significant structural homology

(26% amino acid sequence) and act as agonists by initiating intracellular signaling on binding to IL-1 receptors (March *et al.*, 1985). In contrast, IL-1Ra binds to the same receptors as IL-1α and IL-1β, but does not initiate cell signaling, thereby inhibiting IL-1 biologic activity (Arend *et al.*, 1990; Granowitz *et al.*, 1991).

Despite their structural similarities, the IL-1 proteins demonstrate significant differences in their regulatory mechanisms of gene expression, peptide synthesis, posttranslational modification, and secretion (Auron and Webb, 1994; March *et al.*, 1985; Martin and Wesche, 2002). Although their promoter regions are different (March *et al.*, 1985), both IL-1α and IL-1β are transcribed in response to various inflammatory stimuli including: lipopolysaccharide (LPS), hypoxia, substance P, coagulation, and complement proteins (Dinarello, 1991; Dunne and O'Neill, 2003). The regulation of IL-1 peptide synthesis is also important as IL-1 mRNA may either accumulate or be translated into mature protein under different conditions (Schindler *et al.*, 1990). Additionally, IL-1α and -β are both synthesized as propeptides which lack signal sequences and accumulate in the cytoplasm until maturation and secretion occur. Both Pro-IL-1α and IL-1α are biologically active and may function in an autocrine fashion in the cytoplasm by regulating cell differentiation (Hauser *et al.*, 1986) or in a paracrine fashion at the cell membrane (Dinarello, 1991; Hauser *et al.*, 1986; Stevenson *et al.*, 1992). In contrast, pro-IL-1β is neither biologically active nor secreted until it is cleaved by the "IL-1β converting enzyme" (ICE) (Cerretti *et al.*, 1992). Secreted IL-1β may act locally or systemically on various cells by activating the transmembrane IL-1 receptor-type I (IL-1RI) and IL-1 receptor accessory protein (IL-1R-AcP) complex.

The production of IL-1Ra, the last member of the IL-1 family, is induced by inflammatory stimuli like LPS as well as anti-inflammatory cytokines (IL-4, IL-10, IL-13) (Dinarello, 2000; Roux-Lombard, 1998). However, maximal expression of IL-1Ra is typically delayed several hours relative to IL-1β (Arend *et al.*, 1991; Vannier *et al.*, 1992). Unlike IL-1α or -β, the IL-1Ra gene contains a signal sequence that facilitates protein secretion. Once secreted, IL-1Ra binds the IL-1RI receptor with the same affinity as either IL-1α or -β, but lacks the binding site for IL-1R-AcP required for activation of cell signaling (Arend, 1991). Because IL-1Ra is unable to activate IL-1 signaling, it acts as a competitive antagonist for extracellular IL-1α and -β.

III. REGULATION OF IL-1 SYNTHESIS

Under normal conditions, plasma concentrations of IL-1 are usually undetectable. However, the synthesis of IL-1 (by mononuclear and other cells) is stimulated following their exposure to microbial products or inflammation.

IL-1 synthesis is also induced by neuroactive and inflammatory substances, cell matrix proteins, clotting factors, lipids, cytokines, and other biologic materials (Dinarello, 1991). Environmental stressors, such as hypoxia, ischemia, gamma radiation, and thermal injury may also stimulate IL-1 production (Dinarello, 1996). Consequently, elevations in plasma IL-1β are most commonly seen in patients with severe infection, injury, or associated inflammatory conditions (Cannon et al., 1992; Casey et al., 1993; Eastgate et al., 1988; Roubenoff et al., 1994). In fact, plasma IL-1 concentrations appear to correlate with both the severity of inflammation and mortality in patients with sepsis, trauma, and burn injury (Cannon et al., 1992; Casey et al., 1993; Eastgate et al., 1988; Roubenoff et al., 1994). Despite the association of increased plasma IL-1 with the severity of inflammation, the relative importance of circulating IL-1 remains controversial. Studies suggest that plasma IL-1 levels are frequently below the range of detection by routine technology (Casey et al., 1993; Dinarello, 1996, 2005). Very little IL-1 (a few nanograms per kilogram) is needed to activate the IL-1 receptor and initiate IL-1-mediated effects (Dinarello, 1991, 1996, 2005; Smith et al., 1990). Consequently, studies examining tissue levels of IL-1 and the biological effects of IL-1 blockade have become important in understanding the pathophysiologic role of IL-1 in disease.

IV. IL-1 BIOACTIVITY: RECEPTORS AND CELL SIGNALING

The regulation of IL-1 bioactivity involves not only the synthesis and secretion of IL-1 but also the production of IL-1 antagonists, the relative abundance of IL-1 receptors, the activation of IL-1-signaling pathways, and IL-1 mediated gene expression. Three different IL-1 receptors have been described: IL-1RI, IL-1RII, and IL-1R-AcP (Dinarello, 1997; Greenfeder et al., 1995; Sims et al., 1994). IL-1RI is a transmembrane molecule with no intrinsic kinase activity that participates in transmitting the IL-1 signal (Freshney et al., 1994; Sims et al., 1994). IL-IRI is constitutively expressed in numerous cell types (lymphocytes, endothelial cells, fibroblasts, and so on), most commonly in relatively low abundance (50–200 receptors per cell). IL-1R-AcP is also widely expressed and interacts with both IL-1 and IL-1RI to form an activated receptor complex. IL-1R-AcP is also required for IL-1-mediated cell signaling (Greenfeder et al., 1995; Sims et al., 1994). Both IL-1RI and IL-1R-AcP contain a cytosolic Toll-IL-1R (TIR) domain which provides an important docking site for the MyD88 adaptor protein and IL-1 receptor associated kinase (IRAK)-signaling proteins (Akira and Takeda, 2004). In contrast, IL-1RII which lacks a cytoplasmic TIR domain does not appear to participate in IL-1 signaling, acting instead as a "decoy receptor" (Auron and Webb, 1994; Colotta *et al.*, 1993; Dinarello, 1997; Dinarello and Wolff, 1993; Sims *et al.*, 1994).

IL-1 bioactivity is also regulated by both the soluble IL-1 receptor and the receptor antagonist (IL-1Ra). The soluble receptor consists of the extracellular portion of the naturally occurring type II receptor which is generated by proteolytic cleavage. This molecule specifically binds IL-1 and prevents it from binding to cell-surface receptors. (Dinarello and Wolff, 1993; Symons *et al.*, 1991). Low concentrations of the soluble receptor are found in the circulation of normal subjects, while levels are increased during reactivation of certain inflammatory conditions (i.e., rheumatoid arthritis) (Dinarello and Wolff, 1993). As previously mentioned, IL-1Ra also binds to IL-1 receptors, thereby preventing the binding of IL-1 to the same receptors (Arend, 1991). Thus, the biologic activity of IL-1 is tightly controlled by the synthesis and secretion of IL-1, as well as soluble receptors and receptor antagonists which regulate IL-1 mediated inflammation by blocking the binding of IL-1 to its cell-surface receptors (Granowitz *et al.*, 1991).

V. BIOLOGIC ACTIVITIES OF IL-1

As discussed in numerous reviews by Dinarello and associates (Dinarello, 1991, 1996; Dinarello and Wolff, 1993), IL-1α and -β interact with a wide variety of cell types and are involved in regulating numerous physiological activities including the immune response, hematopoiesis, appetite, and bone metabolism (Bagby, 1989; Smith *et al.*, 1990; Tatakis, 1993). In a variety of studies, administration of IL-1 to healthy animals or humans has been shown to induce fever, sleep, and hypotension (Fischer *et al.*, 1991; Okusawa *et al.*, 1988; Smith *et al.*, 1990). IL-1 stimulates the production of prostaglandins, decreasing the threshold of pain. IL-1 has also been implicated in autoimmune-related inflammation (i.e., arthritis and colitis) and development of atherosclerotic plaques (Bistrian *et al.*, 1992). IL-1 participates in host defense by stimulating T and B lymphocytes and reduces the mortality from bacterial and fungal infections in animals (Van der Meer *et al.*, 1988). However, the therapeutic utility of IL-1 in patients is limited by dose-dependent side effects including fever, gastrointestinal disturbances, myalgia, arthralgia, and hypotension (Smith *et al.*, 1990). Consequently, there is a fine line between the beneficial versus the detrimental aspects of IL-1 action to the host.

VI. IL-1 IN DISEASE

IL-1 has a pathogenic role in infections, the septic syndrome, trauma, and autoimmune disorders such as rheumatoid arthritis, inflammatory bowl disease, insulin-dependent diabetes mellitus, atherosclerosis, and others (Bistrian *et al.*, 1992). Clinicians have correlated the presence of circulating cytokines

(TNF, IL-1, and IL-6) with the survival in critically ill patients with the sepsis syndrome (Casey *et al.*, 1993). Proinflammatory cytokines are also elevated in disorders characterized by muscle wasting and weakness (Eastgate *et al.*, 1988; Saxne *et al.*, 1988). Studies examining the relationship between *in vitro* cytokine production (IL-1 and TNF) and metabolism in adults with rheumatoid arthritis (RA) demonstrate that cytokine production in RA is associated with altered energy metabolism and loss of body cell mass (Roubenoff *et al.*, 1994). When peripheral monocytes from patients with RA were stimulated with endotoxin, IL-1β production was increased when compared with healthy controls. Cytokine production was directly associated with resting energy expenditure in patients with RA, thus linking the presence of IL-1β to hypermetabolism and loss of body cell mass. While elevated levels of IL-1β have been observed in patients with active disease, it has been nearly impossible to detect IL-1β when the disease process is quiescent (Eastgate *et al.*, 1988; Roubenoff *et al.*, 1990; Saxne *et al.*, 1988).

VII. IL-1 AND PROTEIN CATABOLISM

The systemic administration of IL-1 to otherwise healthy animals has been used as an experimental technique to characterize the biologic effects of specific cytokines *in vivo*. The physiologic effects of IL-1β administration in healthy individuals (fever, neutrophilia, thrombocytosis, induction of IL-6, and acute phase protein synthesis) resemble the metabolic abnormalities observed in patients with catabolic diseases, like sepsis, burn injury, and so on (Dinarello, 1996). IL-1 administration also reproduces the effects of LPS administration on the GH/IGF-I system, specifically decreased levels of IGF-I in blood, liver, and muscle (Fan *et al.*, 1996; Lang *et al.*, 1998a). Chronic IL-1 administration is also associated with negative nitrogen balance, decreased synthesis of skeletal muscle proteins, and the loss of lean body mass (Cooney *et al.*, 1999a). Administration of specific IL-1Ra prevents the sepsis-induced reductions in plasma and muscle IGF-I and attenuates the catabolism of muscle protein (Lang *et al.*, 1996). Collectively, these observations suggest that IL-1 is an important mediator of inflammation-induced changes in the GH/IGF-I system and the catabolism of muscle protein. Before the specific interactions between IL-1 and the GH/IGF-I system are addressed, we will provide an overview of the GH/IGF-I system.

VIII. GROWTH HORMONE: PHYSIOLOGIC AND METABOLIC ACTIVITIES

Growth hormone is synthesized by the anterior pituitary gland and secreted into the bloodstream in a pulsatile fashion. Growth hormone releasing hormone (arcuate nucleus) and ghrelin (stomach) promote GH secretion, while somatostatin (periventricular nucleus) inhibits it. Sleep, exercise, diet, IGF-I, adrenal, and gonadal steroids also influence the secretion of GH by the pituitary. At the cellular level, GH responsiveness is determined by the presence of the transmembrane GH receptor (GHR) which is expressed in most tissues (Carter-Su *et al.*, 1996; Kopchick and Andry, 2000; Matthews *et al.*, 1989).

The biologic actions of GH are predominantly anabolic including stimulation of cell growth, energy, and protein metabolism (Carter-Su *et al.*, 1996; Flores-Morales *et al.*, 2005; Kopchick and Andry, 2000). GH plays a critical role in regulating normal growth during childhood with deficiency resulting in short stature (Le Roith *et al.*, 2001). In adults, GH induces protein synthesis and metabolism resulting in decreased fat and increased lean body mass (Davidson, 1987; Le Roith *et al.*, 2001; Woelfle *et al.*, 2005). GH also stimulates lipolysis in adipose tissue resulting in increased plasma fatty acids (FAs), regulates the immune system (Jeay *et al.*, 2002; Touw *et al.*, 2000), cardiac development and function (Lombardi *et al.*, 1997; Touw *et al.*, 2000), affects brain activity related to emotion and behavior (Coculescu, 1999) and stress responses (Yoshizato *et al.*, 1998), and impacts aging and longevity (Tatar *et al.*, 2003; Woelfle *et al.*, 2005).

Many of GHs' important activities are mediated via the induction of IGF-I, another important anabolic hormone with significant homology (50% of amino acids) to insulin (Lang *et al.*, 1998b). IGF-I gene transcription is rapidly activated in most tissues following GH administration in healthy animals. The somatomedin hypothesis proposes that circulating IGF-I is synthesized by the liver in response to GH and is responsible for the effects of GH on postnatal growth and development (Bichell *et al.*, 1992; Le Roith *et al.*, 2001). However, mice with liver-specific IGF-I gene deletions demonstrate essentially normal growth suggesting the synthesis of IGF-I in peripheral tissues is more important than previously thought (Le Roith *et al.*, 2001). In contrast, mice with targeted disruption of IGF-I in muscle demonstrate diminished muscle mass (Liu *et al.*, 1993). IGF-I administration increases skeletal muscle regeneration and ameliorates muscle wasting (Barton *et al.*, 2002; Lynch *et al.*, 2001). Collectively, the literature suggests that the growth, development, and regeneration of muscle fibers are controlled by both circulating and tissue concentrations of IGF-I (Frost and Lang, 2003).

The most critical regulators of plasma IGF-I levels are nutrient intake and growth hormone. The responsiveness of target tissues to GH is dependent on the cellular expression of the GHR, postreceptor-signaling events and the regulation of GH-mediated gene expression (Carter-Su *et al.*, 1996; Kopchick and Andry, 2000). The first step in activating GH-inducible gene expression involves the sequential binding of GH with two transmembrane receptors and the association of GH-$(GHR)_2$ with Janus kinase 2 (JAK2), an intracellular protein kinase that forms an activated multiprotein-signaling complex (Argetsinger *et al.*, 1993; Herrington and Carter-Su, 2001; Ihle

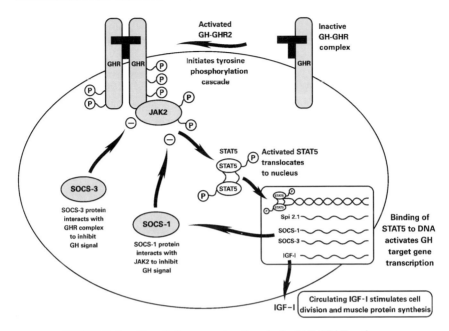

FIGURE 1.   Growth hormone signaling via the JAK/STAT pathway.

et al., 1995; Zhu *et al.*, 2001) (Fig. 1). The activated GHR/JAK2 complex forms high-affinity–binding sites for several signaling and regulatory proteins which propagate signaling via multiple pathways including the JAK/ signal transducer and activator of transcription (STAT), mitogen-activated protein kinase (MAPK), and PI-3 kinase pathways (Herrington and Carter-Su, 2001). The activation of transcription factors like c-Fos, c-Jun, and STAT by GH activates the transcription of multiple genes including IGF-I, IGF-binding protein-3 (IGFBP-3), serine protease inhibitor 2.1 (Spi 2.1), acid labile subunit (ALS), and the suppressors of cytokine signaling (SOCS) (Davey *et al.*, 1999, 2001; Woelfle and Rotwein, 2004). For example, GH stimulates the tyrosine phosphorylation of STAT5b by JAK2 and serine/ threonine phosphorylation of STAT5b by the MAPK pathway (Chow *et al.*, 1996). Phosphorylated STAT5b forms homodimers and heterodimers which translocate to the nucleus and bind specific DNA sequences in the promoter region of target genes to regulate transcriptional activity (Gebert *et al.*, 1999).

Studies performed using DNA microarray technology suggest that GH stimulates the expression of 8–30 genes in liver, depending on the dose and timing of GH administration (Ahluwalia *et al.*, 2004; Thompson *et al.*, 2000; Tollet-Egnell *et al.*, 2004). Because hepatocytes synthesize and secrete IGF-I into the bloodstream in response to GH or nutrient-intake, the regulation of IGF-I gene expression has been studied extensively in liver (Bichell *et al.*, 1992; Carter-Su *et al.*, 1996; Ribaux *et al.*, 2002). In mammals, the IGF-I gene consists of six exons with alternative promoters, transcription start sites, and splicing variants resulting in multiple mRNA species (Rotwein, 1999). Although the regulation of IGF-I gene expression remains incompletely understood, studies in STAT5b knockout mice suggest that STAT5b is required for both basal and GH-induced expression of hepatic IGF-I (Davey *et al.*, 2001). STAT5b dominant negative adenoviral transfection was shown to inhibit GH-mediated hepatic IGF-I gene transcription (Woelfle *et al.*, 2003a). The identification of tandem STAT5-binding sites in intron 2 of the IGF gene that mediate activation of IGF-I transcription by GH provides additional evidence for the JAK2/STAT5 pathway in regulating the induction of IGF-I by GH (Woelfle *et al.*, 2003b).

IX. CATABOLIC ILLNESS AND GH RESISTANCE

The development of GH resistance is one of the major metabolic derangements observed in patients with systemic infection, major trauma, or burn injury (Bistrian *et al.*, 1992; Dahn *et al.*, 1988; Wilmore, 1991). The clinical consequences of GH resistance include the loss of lean body mass, negative nitrogen balance, impaired wound healing, prolonged recovery, diminished mobility, prolonged recovery, and impaired survival. As previously mentioned, the inflammatory cytokines TNF and IL-1 have been implicated in the pathogenesis of both GH resistance and the loss of lean body mass. Incubation of IL-1 or TNF with muscle tissue *in vitro* shows no direct effect of either cytokine on muscle protein synthesis (Moldawer *et al.*, 1987). Consequently, the effects of TNF and IL-1 on the GH/IGF-I system have been implicated in the pathogenesis of GH resistance and indirectly in the loss of muscle mass.

The GH resistant state is characterized by elevations in plasma GH, decreased circulating and tissue levels of IGF-I, and reductions in the anabolic response to GH (Jenkins and Ross, 1996). In septic patients, increased levels of proinflammatory cytokines and GH resistance are commonly observed together (Dahn *et al.*, 1988; Guirao and Lowry, 1996). In animals, GH resistance is caused by the induction of abdominal sepsis, and the systemic administration of LPS, TNF, or IL-1β (Fan *et al.*, 1994, 1995a,b, 1996; Lang *et al.*, 1997, 1998a,b; Peisen *et al.*, 1995). Chronic GH administration is unable to reverse the endotoxin-induced reductions in serum IGF-I (Liao *et al.*, 1997). However, inhibition of cytokine activity by infusion of specific TNF or IL-1 antagonists attenuates both the sepsis-induced alterations in the GH/IGF-I system and prevents the catabolism of muscle protein (Cooney et al., 1999b; Fan et al., 1995a; Lang et al., 1996). The role of IGF-I as a mediator of muscle protein synthesis in septic rats was confirmed in isolated hind limb perfusions whereby increasing the concentration of IGF-I in the perfusate produced a dose-dependent increase in muscle protein synthesis (Jurasinski and Vary, 1995). Collectively, these results provide evidence that the inhibitory effects of cytokines on skeletal muscle protein synthesis during sepsis are mediated indirectly by changes in the GH/IGF-I system.

Although the role of inflammatory cytokines in the genesis of GH resistance seems relatively well established, the molecular mechanisms of GH resistance at the cellular level remain poorly defined. The development of sepsis- or cytokine-mediated GH resistance may be caused by alterations in the expression of cellular GHR levels, postreceptor defects in GH signaling, or inhibitory effects on GH-inducible gene expression. The next portion of this chapter will examine the potential mechanisms for sepsis- and cytokine-mediated GH resistance.

X. GHR EXPRESSION IN GH RESISTANCE

Studies examining the relative abundance of GH receptor in liver tissue from septic rats have yielded conflicting results. In LPS-treated rats, a 50% reduction in hepatic GH-binding sites was observed 5–10 h after LPS administration using a bovine GH binding assay (Defalque et al., 1999). In this study, GH administration failed to prevent the reductions in serum IGF-I levels and liver GHR, suggesting that GH resistance might be caused by the loss of liver GHR in endotoxemic rats. Although a 50% reduction in hepatic GHR and IGF-I mRNA was noted on day 5 of abdominal sepsis, the levels of hepatic GHR protein (by immunoblot analysis) were not different in control and septic rats (Yumet et al., 2002). When the effects of LPS were studied in Wistar and Lewis rats which differ in their adrenal response to inflammation, LPS decreased hepatic GHR and IGF-I mRNA only in Wistar rats, while serum concentrations of IGF-I were significantly decreased in both strains (Priego et al., 2002). These differing responses to LPS were attributed to activation of the adrenal axis rather than to the release of cytokines. Although reductions in hepatic GHR mRNA have been observed following LPS administration or sepsis (Hermansson et al., 1997; Ketelslegers et al., 1996), levels of GHR protein were not decreased (Mao et al., 1999; Yumet et al., 2002) suggesting that postreceptor defects in GH signaling were the most likely cause of GH resistance.

Cultured hepatocytes have also been utilized to investigate the mechanisms of hepatic GH resistance. In primary hepatocytes, the inhibitory effects of IL-1β on the induction of IGF-I by GH were attributed to reductions in

GHR mRNA expression (Thissen and Verniers, 1997; Wolf et al., 1996). However, reductions in GHR expression were not observed when cells were pretreated with TNF-α or IL-6 (Thissen and Verniers, 1997). In contrast, when studies were performed in an SV40 immortalized rat hepatocyte cell line (CWSV-1), IL-1β inhibited the induction of IGF-I by GH, but the relative abundance of GHR protein was unaltered (Shumate et al., 2005). These results suggest that postreceptor defects represent the most likely mechanism for IL-1 mediated GH resistance.

Suffice it to say that differences in experimental methods related to animal strain, cell type, catabolic insult (LPS, sepsis, cytokine administration), and measurement of GHR (binding curves versus immunoblot) appear to explain the inconsistencies in the literature regarding the effects of sepsis and inflammatory cytokines on hepatic GHR levels. Although several of these studies report reductions in hepatic GHR mRNA, the majority found no change in the levels of GHR protein (Mao et al., 1999; Yumet et al., 2002).

XI. HEPATIC GH SIGNALING VIA THE JAK2/STAT5 PATHWAY

Several studies have identified postreceptor defects in GH signaling via the JAK/STAT pathway as the potential etiology of hepatic GH resistance (Bergad et al., 2000; Mao et al., 1999). In LPS-treated rats stimulated with GH, an increase in total JAK2 protein was observed in conjunction with significant reductions in the ratio of tyrosine phosphorylated/total JAK2 and phosphorylated/total STAT5 (Bergad et al., 2000; Mao et al., 1999). The induction of abdominal sepsis also inhibits hepatic GH signaling via the JAK/STAT pathway as evidenced by: (1) decreased duration of STAT5 phosphorylation, (2) attenuated nuclear translocation of STAT5, and (3) reduced STAT5 DNA binding by electrophoretic mobility shift assay (Denson et al., 2001; Hong-Brown et al., 2003; Yumet et al., 2006). The reductions in STAT5 phosphorylation and activity observed in liver tissue from GH-treated septic rats were associated with decreased synthesis of both IGF-I and Spi 2.1 (Bergad et al., 2000; Defalque et al., 1999; Yumet et al., 2002). Since hepatic GHR protein levels were not altered by the septic insult, postreceptor defects in JAK/STAT signaling were hypothesized to explain the development of hepatic GH resistance.

The effects of inflammatory cytokines (TNF and IL-1) on GH signaling were studied in CWSV-1 hepatocytes (Shumate et al., 2005; Yumet et al., 2002). Incubation of hepatocytes with TNF prior to GH-stimulation attenuated the duration of STAT5 phosphorylation by GH, inhibited STAT5-DNA binding, and resulted in decreased IGF-I expression. Pretreatment with TNF did not influence the relative abundance of total GHR, JAK2, or STAT5 protein. Consequently, the decreased duration of STAT5 phosphorylation in

TNF-treated cells cannot be attributed to reductions in GHR or JAK/STAT-signaling proteins (Yumet *et al.*, 2002). The effects of IL-1β pretreatment on the time course of GH signaling via the JAK/STAT pathway were also evaluated in CWSV-1 hepatocytes (Shumate *et al.*, 2005). In contrast to TNF, only a transient reduction in STAT5b phosphorylation was noted in IL-1-treated cells and the magnitude of these changes did not correlate with the observed reductions in IGF-I or Spi 2.1 mRNA (Shumate *et al.*, 2005). IL-1 pretreatment did not alter the level of total GHR, JAK2, or STAT5 protein and no significant impairment of STAT5-DNA binding could be detected in IL-1-treated cells. Although collectively these results suggest that post-receptor defects are responsible for cytokine-mediated hepatic GH resistance, the relative importance of attenuated JAK/STAT signaling and its causal relationship with decreased GH-inducible gene expression remain unknown.

XII. GH SIGNALING BY P38/C-JUN/MAPK PATHWAYS

The "mitogen activated" or MAPK pathway is one of the major signaling pathways activated by GH in liver tissue (Carter-Su and Smit, 1998; Herrington and Carter-Su, 2001) and is involved in the regulation of transcriptional activity through serine phosphorylation of STAT5 (Gebert *et al.*, 1997; Horvath and Darnell, 1997; Park *et al.*, 2001; Ram *et al.*, 1996). GH activates MAP kinase kinase (MEK) resulting in the phosphorylation of the extracellular signal-regulated kinases (ERKs) 1 and 2. The ERKs then activate several transcription factors including STAT5a, STAT5b (Gebert *et al.*, 1997; Ram *et al.*, 1996), and Elk-1, which stimulates the transcription of c-Fos and c-Jun by GH (Hodge *et al.*, 1998). Ultimately, induction of this pathway influences inflammatory responses, cell division, and apoptosis in various cell types (Hodge *et al.*, 1998; Park *et al.*, 2001). A number of signaling proteins in mitogen- or stress-activated pathways undergo both serine/threonine and tyrosine phosphorylation resulting in "cross talk" between pathways. In fact, studies indicate that serine phosphorylation of STAT5b by ERK1 and ERK2 is necessary to achieve complete transcriptional activation by GH (Park *et al.*, 2001). Serine-phosphorylated STAT5b interaction may vary with different promoters and has been suggested as a potential regulatory mechanism for GH-inducible, STAT5 target genes (Park *et al.*, 2001). Consequently, inhibition of GH signaling or cross talk by inflammatory cytokines represents a potential mechanism for the inhibition of GH-inducible gene expression.

Studies in GH-stimulated primary hepatocytes have demonstrated a 24% inhibition in IGF-I mRNA with MAPK kinase inhibition (Shoba *et al.*, 2001). Treatment of CWSV-1 hepatocytes with the MAP kinase inhibitor PD98059 also resulted in a significant reduction in IGF-I in GH-stimulated cells (Shumate *et al.*, 2005), providing evidence for the involvement of the

MAP kinase pathway in the regulation of IGF-I expression by GH. To determine whether the inhibitory effects of cytokines on GH signaling involved the MAPK pathway, the effects of TNF and IL-1 on the activation of ERK1 and ERK2 by GH were examined in CWSV-1 hepatocytes. The induction of ERK1/2 phosphorylation/activation by GH was inhibited by TNF in CWSV-1 hepatocytes (unpublished results). However, IL-1 did not significantly alter either the magnitude or time course of ERK1 and ERK2 phosphorylation by GH (Shumate et al., 2005). Furthermore, pretreatment with IL-1 had no effect on GH signaling via the p38 MAPK and JNK pathways in CWSV-1 hepatocytes (unpublished results). Collectively, these results suggest that neither of these GH signaling pathways is responsible for IL-1-mediated GH resistance in CWSV-1 hepatocytes. Consequently, while the inhibitory effects of TNF on GH-inducible gene expression might involve the MAPK pathway, IL-1 appears to employ another mechanism to interfere with GH signaling.

XIII. SUPPRESSORS OF CYTOKINE SIGNALING: INHIBITORS OF JAK/STAT SIGNALING

The magnitude and duration of GH signaling in target cells, key to the extent of target gene expression, are controlled by several independent regulatory mechanisms. The SOCS are proteins induced by GH and other cytokines which inhibit JAK/STAT signaling by what appears to be a classic negative feedback loop (Cooney, 2002; Hansen et al., 1999; Ram and Waxman, 1999). The SOCS proteins, normally expressed at low levels, are rapidly induced by GH and cytokines (Adams et al., 1998; Alexander et al., 1999; Tollet-Egnell et al., 1999) (Fig. 1). Increased expression of SOCS proteins inhibits GH signaling through several different mechanisms including the indirect inhibition of JAK2 kinase activity by SOCS-1, interference with GHR-mediated JAK2 signaling by SOCS-3 (via tyrosines 333 and 338), and reductions in GH signaling by direct binding of CIS to the growth hormone receptor (Flores-Morales et al., 2005; Ram and Waxman, 1999). Furthermore, overexpression of individual SOCS proteins by cotransfection has been shown to influence GH-mediated gene expression in Chinese hamster ovary (CHO) cells. In these studies, coexpression of CIS with a GH-responsive Spi 2.1 promoter-CAT reporter construct had no effect on promoter activity, whereas overexpression of SOCS-3 blocked transactivation of the Spi 2.1 reporter and SOCS-2 enhanced the Spi 2.1 response to GH (Adams et al., 1998; Tollet-Egnell et al., 1999). Although these studies provide evidence that SOCS overexpression can influence GH-mediated gene expression, the role of SOCS in regulating GH activity and IGF-I expression under more physiologic conditions remains poorly understood (Hansen et al., 1999).

Several lines of evidence suggest that cytokine-induced SOCS expression during sepsis is an important factor in the development of hepatic GH resistance (Boisclair *et al.*, 2000; Hong-Brown *et al.*, 2003; Mao *et al.*, 1999; Yumet *et al.*, in press). First, the expression of SOCS in liver tissue is transiently increased during abdominal sepsis and endotoxemia (Alexander *et al.*, 1999; Mao *et al.*, 1999; Yumet *et al.*, in press). Second, hepatic GH signaling via the JAK/STAT pathway is attenuated either concomitantly or shortly after the period of maximal SOCS expression (Mao *et al.*, 1999; Yumet *et al.*, in press) and the induction of IGF-I by GH in septic rats is impaired when GH is administered during maximal SOCS expression (Yumet *et al.*, in press). Third, treatment of healthy animals or cells with inflammatory cytokines (TNF, IL-1, and IL-6) induces SOCS expression (Cooney, 2002; Shumate *et al.*, 2005; Yumet *et al.*, in press). Finally, the defects in GH signaling and gene expression induced by IL-1 pretreatment of H4IIE hepatocytes temporally correlates with increased SOCS-3 expression (Boisclair *et al.*, 2000). Collectively, these studies provide support for the hypothesis that cytokine-mediated SOCS expression is important in the pathogenesis of hepatic GH resistance during systemic infection.

Despite the temporal association of increased SOCS expression with the onset of hepatic GH resistance, the current studies in this area have been unable to prove "cause and effect." Although both IL-1 and GH stimulate SOCS-3 mRNA expression in CWSV-1 hepatocytes, IL-1 does not appear to significantly inhibit the time course of GH signaling via the JAK/STAT pathway in these cells (Shumate *et al.*, 2005). Based on this finding, a case could be made that the inhibitory effects of IL-1 are not due to increased SOCS expression. An alternative explanation for the inhibitory effects of inflammatory cytokines on GH-inducible gene expression is that they directly or indirectly influence GH-mediated gene expression.

XIV. INHIBITION OF GH-INDUCIBLE GENE EXPRESSION BY CYTOKINES (IL-1)

Cytokine-mediated inhibition of GH-inducible gene expression represents yet another potential mechanism for hepatic growth hormone resistance. The lack of GH receptor and IGF-I expression in many immortalized hepatocyte cell lines and the technical limitations of primary hepatocyte studies have been major obstacles to mechanistic studies of cytokines and GH-inducible gene expression. However, the promoters for the GH target genes Spi 2.1 and acid labile subunit (ALS) have been cloned, and the inhibitory effects of cytokines on their expression have been studied in various cell culture systems (Bergad *et al.*, 2000; Boisclair *et al.*, 2000; Simar-Blanchet *et al.*, 1998). The role of STAT5 in the regulation of GH-mediated hepatic gene expression is mediated by STAT5 binding to γ-interferon activated sequences (GAS) in the promoter region for both Spi 2.1 and ALS (Bergad *et al.*, 1995; Ooi *et al.*, 1998). Although the promoter elements responsible for basal IGF-I transcription are contained in the 5′ untranslated region (UTR), the exact mechanisms of IGF-I activation by GH remain poorly characterized (An and Lowe, 1995; Mittanck *et al.*, 1997; Wang *et al.*, 1998, 2000). The identification of a GH-regulated DNAse-I hypersensitive site (HS7) in intron 2 of the IGF-I gene suggests that alterations in chromatin structure are required for GH activation (Bichell *et al.*, 1992; Thomas *et al.*, 1995). Tandem STAT5-binding sites were identified in HS7 by chromatin immunoprecipitation assays which showed that GH-induced STAT5 binding to these GH response element (GHRE) sites was required for activation of IGF-I transcription (Woelfle *et al.*, 2003b). In contrast to IGF-I, the STAT5-binding sites for GH activation are located in 5′ UTR of the Spi 2.1 and ALS genes (Bergad *et al.*, 1995; Boisclair *et al.*, 2000; Le Cam *et al.*, 1998).

In primary rat hepatocytes, GH induces the expression of Spi 2.1 mRNA and the inflammatory cytokines (TNF, IL-1, and IL-6) have been shown to inhibit GH-induction of Spi 2.1 gene expression in this model (Bergad *et al.*, 2000; Le Cam *et al.*, 1998). Likewise, IL-1β has been shown to inhibit the induction of ALS mRNA by GH in primary rat hepatocytes and to inhibit ALS promoter activity in H4IIE rat hepatoma cells (Boisclair *et al.*, 2000). However, IL-1β did not inhibit GH-dependent binding of STAT5 to the ALS GAS1 element that mediates the transcriptional effects of GH on ALS gene expression. Our laboratory has shown that TNF pretreatment of CWSV-1 hepatocytes inhibits the induction of Spi 2.1-promoter luciferase activity by GH and by cotransfection of a constitutively active STAT5 vector (unpublished data). Collectively, these results suggest that the regulation of GH-inducible gene transcription by inflammatory cytokines represents a potentially important mechanism for hepatic GH resistance.

XV. CONCLUSIONS

In summary, the inflammatory cytokines are important mediators of systemic inflammation following injury and infection. Both TNF and IL-1 regulate the catabolism of muscle protein during sepsis through inflammation-induced changes in the GH/IGF-I system referred to as the GH resistant state. The onset of hepatic GH resistance is one of the major metabolic derangements observed in patients with catabolic illness. The development of cytokine-mediated GH resistance may be caused by reduced expression of cellular GHR levels, postreceptor defects in GH signaling, inhibitory effects of increased SOCS expression on JAK/STAT signaling, or by direct suppression of GH-inducible gene expression. Although reductions in hepatic GHR mRNA have been described, decreased levels of GHR protein do not appear to be the primary cause for GH resistance. Postreceptor defects in hepatic

GH signaling have been described with *in vivo* models of sepsis and in cultured hepatocytes. Although it is tempting to attribute the defects in GH-inducible gene expression to perturbations in GH signaling, there is some evidence that GH resistance may be caused by altered regulation of gene transcription. Despite the progress that has been made, additional studies will be required to determine the exact mechanisms by which IL-1 inhibits the induction of gene expression by GH.

REFERENCES

Adams, T. E., Hansen, J. A., Starr, R., Nicola, N. A., Hilton, D. J., and Billestrup, N. (1998). Growth hormone preferentially induces the rapid, transient expression of SOCS-3, a novel inhibitor of cytokine receptor signaling. *J. Biol. Chem.* **273**, 1285–1287.

Ahluwalia, A., Clodfelter, K. C., and Waxman, D. J. (2004). Sexual dimorphism of rat liver gene expression: Regulatory role of growth hormone revealed by deoxyribonucleic acid microarray analysis. *Mol. Endocrinol.* **18**, 747–760.

Akira, S., and Takeda, K. (2004). Toll-like receptor signalling. *Nat. Rev. Immunol.* **4**, 499–511.

Alexander, W. S., Starr, R., Metcalf, D., Nicholson, S. E., Farley, A., Elefanty, A. G., Brysha, M., Kile, B. T., Richardson, R., Baca, M., Zhang, J. G., Willson, T. A., *et al.* (1999). Suppressors of cytokine signaling (SOCS): Negative regulators of signal transduction. *J. Leukoc. Biol.* **66**, 588–592.

An, M. R., and Lowe, W. L. J. (1995). The major promoter of the rat insulin-like growth factor-I gene binds a protein complex that is required for basal expression. *Mol. Cell Endocrinol.* **114**, 77–89.

Arend, W. P., Welgus, H. G., Thompson, R. C., and Eisenberg, S. P. (1990). Biological properties of recombinant human monocyte-derived interleukin-1 receptor antagonist. *J. Clin. Invest.* **85**, 1694–1697.

Arend, W. P. (1991). Interleukin 1 receptor antagonist. A new member of the interleukin 1 family. *J. Clin. Invest.* **88**, 1445–1451.

Arend, W. P., Smith, M. F., Jr., Janson, R. W., and Joslin, F. G. (1991). IL-1 receptor antagonist and IL-1 beta production in human monocytes are regulated differently. *J. Immunol.* **147**, 1530–1536.

Argetsinger, L. S., Campbell, G. S., Yang, X., Witthuhn, B. A., Silvennoinen, O., Ihle, J. N., and Carter-Su, C. (1993). Identification of Jak2 as a growth hormone receptor-associated tyrosine kinase. *Cell* **74**, 237–244.

Auron, P. E., and Webb, A. C. (1994). Interleukin-1: A gene expression system regulated at multiple levels. *Eur. Cytokine Netw.* **5**, 573–592.

Bagby, G. C. (1989). Interleukin-1 and hematopoiesis. *Blood Rev.* **3**, 152–161.

Barton, E. R., Morris, L., Musaro, A., Rosenthal, N., and Sweeney, H. L. (2002). Muscle-specific expression of insulin-like growth factor I counters muscle decline in mdx mice. *J. Cell Biol.* **157**, 137–148.

Bergad, P. L., Shis, H. M., Towle, H. C., Schwarzenberg, S. J., and Berry, S. A. (1995). Growth hormone induction of hepatic serine protease inhibitor 2.1 transcription is mediated by a Stat5-related factor binding synergistically to two γ-activated sites. *J. Biol. Chem.* **270**, 24903–24910.

Bergad, P. L., Schwarzenberg, S. J., Humbert, J. T., Morrison, M., Amarasinghe, S., Towle, H. C., and Berry, S. A. (2000). Inhibition of growth hormone action in models of inflammation. *Am. J. Physiol. Cell Physiol.* **279**, C1906–C1917.

Bichell, D. P., Kikuchi, K., and Rotwein, P. (1992). Growth hormone rapidly activates insulin-like growth factor-I gene transcription *in vivo*. *Mol. Endocrinol.* **6,** 1899–1908.

Bistrian, B. R., Schwartz, J., and Istfan, N. W. (1992). Cytokines, muscle proteolysis, and the catabolic response to infection and inflammation. *Proc. Soc. Exp. Biol. Med.* **200,** 220–223.

Boisclair, Y. R., Wang, J., Shi, J., Hurst, K. R., and Ooi, G. T. (2000). Role of the suppressor of cytokine signaling-3 in mediating the inhibitory effects of interleukin-1β on the growth hormone-dependent transcription of the acid-labile subunit gene in liver cells. *J. Biol. Chem.* **275,** 3841–3847.

Cannon, J. G., Friedberg, J. S., Gelfand, J. A., Tompkins, R. G., Burke, J. F., and Dinarello, C. A. (1992). Circulating interleukin-1β and tumor necrosis factor-α concentrations after burn injury in humans. *Crit. Care Med.* **20,** 1414–1419.

Carter-Su, C., and Smit, L. S. (1998). Signaling via JAK tyrosine kinases: Growth hormone receptor as a model system. *Recent Prog. Horm. Res.* **53,** 61–83.

Carter-Su, C., Schwartz, J., and Smit, L. S. (1996). Molecular mechanism of growth hormone action. *Ann. Rev. Physiol.* **58,** 187–207.

Casey, L. C., Balk, R. A., and Bone, R. C. (1993). Plasma cytokine and endotoxin levels correlate with survival in patients with the sepsis syndrome. *Ann. Intern. Med.* **119,** 771–778.

Cerra, F. B., Siegal, J. H., Coleman, B., Border, J. R., and McNenamy, R. R. (1980). Septic autocannibalism: A failure of exogenous nutritional support. *Ann. Surg.* **192,** 570–580.

Cerretti, D. P., Kozlosky, C. J., Mosley, B., Nelson, N., van Ness, K., Greenstreet, T. A., March, C. J., Kronheim, S. R., Druck, T., Cannizaro, L. A., Huebner, K., and Black, R. A. (1992). Molecular cloning of the interleukin-1 beta converting enzyme. *Science* **256,** 97–100.

Chow, J. C., Ling, P. R., Qu, Z., Laviola, L., Ciccarone, A., Bistrian, B. R., and Smith, R. J. (1996). Growth hormone stimulates tyrosine phosphorylation of JAK2 and STAT5 but not insulin response substrate-1 or SHC proteins in liver and skeletal muscle of normal rats *in vivo*. *Endocrinology* **137,** 2880–2886.

Coculescu, M. (1999). Blood-brain barrier for human growth hormone and insulin-like growth factor-I. *J. Pediatr. Endocrinol. Metab.* **12,** 113–124.

Colotta, F., Re, F., Muzio, M., Bertini, R., Polentarutti, N., Sironi, M., Giri, J. G., Dower, S. K., Sims, J. E., and Mantovani, A. (1993). Interleukin-1 type II receptor: A decoy target for IL-1 that is regulated by IL-1. *Science* **261,** 472–474.

Cooney, R. N. (2002). Suppressors of cytokine signaling (SOCS): Inhibitors of the JAK/STAT pathway. *Shock* **17,** 83–90.

Cooney, R. N., Kimball, S. R., and Vary, T. C. (1997). Regulation of skeletal muscle protein turnover during sepsis: Mechanisms and mediators. *Shock* **7,** 1–16.

Cooney, R. N., Maish, G. O., III, Gilpin, T., Shumate, M. L., Lang, C. H., and Vary, T. C. (1999a). Mechanism of IL-1-induced inhibition of protein synthesis in skeletal muscle. *Shock* **11,** 235–241.

Cooney, R. N., Kimball, S. R., Eckman, R., Maish, G. O., 3rd, Shumate, M., and Vary, T. C. (1999b). TNF-binding protein ameliorates inhibition of skeletal muscle protein synthesis during sepsis. *Am. J. Physiol. Endocrinol. Metab.* **276**(39), E611–E619.

Dahn, M. S., Lange, P., and Jacobs, L. A. (1988). Insulin-like growth factor I production is inhibited in human sepsis. *Arch. Surg.* **123,** 1409–1414.

Davey, H. W., McLachlan, M. J., Wilkins, R. J., Hilton, D. J., and Adams, T. E. (1999). STAT5b mediates the GH-induced expression of SOCS-2 and SOCS-3 mRNA in the liver. *Mol. Cell Endocrinol.* **158,** 111–116.

Davey, H. W., Xie, T., McLachlan, M. J., Wilkins, R. J., Waxman, D. J., and Grattan, D. R. (2001). STAT5b is required for GH-induced liver IGF-I gene expression. *Endocrinology* **142,** 3836–3841.

Davidson, M. B. (1987). Effect of growth hormone on carbohydrate and lipid metabolism. *Endocr. Rev.* **8,** 115–131.

Defalque, D., Brandt, N., Ketelslegers, J. M., and Thissen, J. P. (1999). GH insensitivity induced by endotoxin injection is associated with decreased liver GH receptors. *Am. J. Physiol. Endocrinol. Metab.* **276**, E565–E572.

Denson, L. A., Menon, R. K., Shaufl, A., Bajwa, H. S., Williams, C. R., and Karpen, S. J. (2001). TNF-α downregulates murine hepatic growth hormone receptor expression by inhibiting Sp1 and Sp3 binding. *J. Clin. Invest.* **107**, 1451–1458.

Dinarello, C. A. (1991). Interleukin-1 and interleukin-1 antagonism. *Blood* **77**, 1627–1652.

Dinarello, C. A. (1996). Biological basis for interleukin-1 in disease. *Blood* **87**, 2095–2147.

Dinarello, C. A. (1997). Interleukin-1. *Cytok. Growth Factor Rev.* **8**(4), 253–265.

Dinarello, C. A. (2000). Proinflammatory cytokines. *Chest* **118**, 503–508.

Dinarello, C. A. (2005). Blocking IL-1 in systemic inflammation. *JEM* **201**, 1355–1359.

Dinarello, C. A., and Wolff, S. M. (1993). The role of interleukin-1 in disease. *N. Engl. J. Med.* **328**, 106–113.

Dinarello, C. A., Clowes, G. H., Gordon, A. H., Sapavis, A., and Wolff, S. M. (1984). Cleavage of human interleukin-1: Isolation of a peptide from the plasma of febrile humans and activated monocytes. *J. Immunol.* **133**, 1332–1338.

Dunne, A., and O'Neill, L. A. J. (2003). The interleukin-1 receptor/Toll-like receptor superfamily: Signal transduction during inflammation and host defense. *STKE* **171**, 1–17.

Eastgate, J. A., Symons, J. A., Wood, N. C., Grinlinton, F. M., di Giovine, F. S., and Duff, G. W. (1988). Correlation of plasma interleukin-1 levels with disease activity in rheumatoid arthritis. *Lancet* **2**, 706–709.

Fan, J., Molina, P. E., Gelato, M. C., and Lang, C. H. (1994). Differential tissue regulation of insulin-like growth factor-I content and binding proteins after endotoxin. *Endocrinology* **134**, 1685–1692.

Fan, J., Char, D., Bagby, G. J., Gelato, M. C., and Lang, C. H. (1995a). Regulation of insulin-like growth factor-I (IGF-I) and IGF-binding proteins by tumor necrosis factor. *Am. J. Physiol.* **269**, R1204–R1212.

Fan, J., Char, D., Kolasa, A. J., Pan, W., Maitra, S. R., Patlak, C. S., Spolarics, Z., Gelato, M. C., and Lang, C. H. (1995b). Alterations in hepatic production and peripheral clearance of IGF-I after endotoxin. *Am. J. Physiol. Endocrinol. Metab.* **269**, E33–E42.

Fan, J., Wojnar, M., Theodorakis, M., and Lang, C. H. (1996). Regulation of insulin-like growth factor (IGF-I) mRNA and peptide and IGF-binding proteins by interleukin-1. *Am. J. Physiol. Regul. Integr. Comp. Physiol.* **270**, R621–R629.

Fischer, E., Marano, M. A., Barber, A. E., Hudson, A., Lee, K., Rock, C. S., Hawes, A. S., Thompson, R. C., Hayes, T. J., Anderson, T. D., Benjamin, W. R., Lowry, S. R., *et al.* (1991). Comparison between effects of interleukin-1α administration and sublethal endotoxemia in primates. *Am. J. Physiol.* **261**, R442–R452.

Flores-Morales, A., Greenhalgh, C. J., Norstedt, G., and Rico-Bautista, E. (2006). Negative regulation of GH receptor signaling. *Mol. Endocrin.* **20**, 241–253.

Fong, Y., Moldawer, L. L., Marano, M., Wei, H., Barger, A., Manogue, K., Tracey, K. J., Kuo, G., Fischman, D. A., Cerami, A., and Lowry, S. F. (1989). Cachetin, TNF or IL-1 alpha induces cachexia with redistribution of body proteins. *Am. J. Physiol. Regul. Integr. Comp. Physiol.* **256**, R659–R665.

Freshney, N. W., Rawlinson, L., Guesdon, F., Jones, E., Cowley, S., Hsuan, J., and Saklatvala, J. (1994). Interleukin-1 activates a novel protein cascade that results in the phosphorylation of hsp27. *Cell* **78**, 1039–1049.

Frost, R. A., and Lang, C. H. (2003). Regulation of insulin-like growth factor-I in skeletal muscle and muscle cells. *Minerva Endocrinol.* **28**, 53–73.

Gebert, C. A., Park, S. H., and Waxman, D. J. (1997). Regulation of STAT5b activation by the temporal pattern of growth hormone stimulation. *Mol. Endocrinol.* **11**, 400–414.

Gebert, C. A., Park, S. H., and Waxman, D. J. (1999). Termination of growth hormone pulse-induced STAT5b signaling. *Mol. Endocrinol.* **13**, 38–56.

Granowitz, E. V., Mancilla, J., Clark, B. D., and Dinarello, C. A. (1991). The IL-1 receptor antagonist inhibits IL-1 binding to the type II IL-1 receptor. *J. Biol. Chem.* **266**, 14147–14150.

Greenfeder, S. A., Nunes, P., Kwee, L., Labow, M., Chizzonite, R. A., and Ju, G. (1995). Molecular cloning and characterization of a second subunit of the interleukin-1 receptor complex. *J. Biol. Chem.* **270**, 13757–13765.

Guirao, X., and Lowry, S. F. (1996). Biologic control of injury and inflammation: Much more than too little or too late. *World J. Surg.* **20**, 437–446.

Hansen, J. A., Lindberg, K., Hilton, D. J., Nielsen, J. H., and Billestrup, N. (1999). Mechanism of inhibition of growth hormone receptor signaling by suppressor of cytokine signaling proteins. *Mol. Endocrinol.* **13**, 1832–1843.

Hauser, C., Saurat, J. H., Schmitt, A., Jaunin, F., and Dayer, J. M. (1986). Interleukin-1 is present in normal human epidermis. *J. Immunol.* **136**, 3317–3323.

Hermansson, M., Wickelgren, R. B., Hammarqvist, F., Bjarnason, R., Wennstrom, I., Wernerman, J., Carlsson, B., and Carlsson, L. M. (1997). Measurement of human growth hormone receptor messenger ribonucleic acid by a quantitative polymerase chain reaction-based assay: Demonstration of reduced expression after elective surgery. *J. Clin. Endocrinol. Metab.* **82**, 421–428.

Herrington, J., and Carter-Su, C. (2001). Signaling pathways activated by the growth hormone receptor. *Trends Endocrinol. Metab.* **12**, 252–257.

Hodge, C., Liao, J., Stofega, M., Guan, K., Carter-Su, C., and Schwartz, J. (1998). Growth hormone stimulates phosphorylation and activation of Elk-1 and expression of c-fos, egr-1, and junB through activation of extracellular signal-related kinases 1 and 2. *J. Biol. Chem.* **273**, 31327–31336.

Hong-Brown, L. Q., Brown, C. R., Cooney, R. N., Frost, R. A., and Lang, C. H. (2003). Sepsis-induced muscle growth hormone resistance occurs independently of STAT5 phosphorylation. *Am. J. Physiol. Endocrinol. Metab.* **285**, E63–E72.

Horvath, C. M., and Darnell, J. E. (1997). The state of the STATs: Recent developments in the study of signal transduction to the nucleus. *Curr. Opin. Cell. Biol.* **9**, 233–239.

Ihle, J. N., Witthuhn, B. A., Quelle, F. W., Yamamoto, K., and Silvennoinen, O. (1995). Signaling through the hematopoietic cytokine receptors. *Annu. Rev. Immunol.* **13**, 369–398.

Jeay, S., Sonenshein, G. E., Postel-Vinay, M. C., Kelly, P. A., and Baixeras, E. (2002). Growth hormone can act as a cytokine controlling survival and proliferation of immune cells: New insights into signaling pathways. *Mol. Cell. Endocrinol.* **188**, 1–7.

Jenkins, R. C., and Ross, R. J. (1996). Acquired growth hormone resistance in catabolic states. *Baillieres Clin. Endocrinol. Metab.* **10**, 411–419.

Jurasinski, C. V., and Vary, T. C. (1995). Insulin-like growth factor-I accelerates protein synthesis in skeletal muscle during sepsis. *Am. J. Physiol.* **269**, E977–E981.

Ketelslegers, J. M., Maiter, D., Maes, M., Underwood, L. E., and Thissen, J. P. (1996). Nutritional regulation of the growth hormone and insulin-like growth factor-binding proteins. *Horm. Res.* **45**, 252–257.

Kopchick, J. J., and Andry, J. M. (2000). Growth hormone (GH), GH receptor, and signal transduction. *Mol. Genet. Metab.* **71**, 293–314.

Lang, C. H., Fan, J., Cooney, R. N., and Vary, T. C. (1996). IL-1ra attenuates sepsis-induced alterations in the IGF system and protein synthesis. *Am. J. Physiol.* **270**, E430–E437.

Lang, C. H., Pollard, V., Traber, L. D., Frost, R. A., Gelato, M. C., and Prough, D. S. (1997). Acute alterations in growth hormone-insulin-like growth factor axis in humans injected with endotoxin. *Am. J. Physiol. Regul. Integr. Comp. Physiol.* **273**, R371–R378.

Lang, C. H., Fan, J., Wojnar, M. M., Vary, T. C., and Cooney, R. (1998a). Role of central IL-1 in regulating peripheral IGF-I during endotoxemia and sepsis. *Am. J. Physiol. Regul. Integr. Comp. Physiol.* **274**, 956–962.

Lang, C. H., Frost, R. A., Ejiofor, J., Lacy, D. B., and McGuinness, O. P. (1998b). Hepatic production and intestinal uptake of IGF-I: Response to infection. *Am. J. Physiol. Gastrointest. Liver Physiol.* **275**(6), G1291–G1298.

Le Cam, A., Conception, P., and Thissen, J. P. (1998). Growth hormone-mediated transcriptional activation of the rat serine protease inhibitor 2. 1 gene involves both interleukin-1β-sensitive and -insensitive pathways. *Biochem. Biophys. Res. Commun.* **253**, 311–314.

Le Roith, D., Bondy, C., Yakar, S., Liu, J. L., and Butler, A. (2001). The somatomedin hypothesis: 2001. *Endocr. Rev.* **22**, 53–74.

Liao, W., Rudling, M., and Angelin, B. (1997). Contrasting effects of growth hormone and insulin-like growth factor I on the biological activities of endotoxin in the rat. *Endocrinology* **138**, 289–295.

Liu, J. P., Baker, J., Perkins, A. S., Robertson, E. J., and Efstratiadis, A. (1993). Mice carrying null mutations of the genes encoding insulin-like growth factor I (Igf-1) and type 1 IGF receptor (Igf1r). *Cell* **75**, 59–72.

Lombardi, G., Colao, A., Ferone, D., Marzullo, P., Orio, F., Longobardi, S., and Merola, B. (1997). Effect of growth hormone on cardiac function. *Horm. Res.* **48**, 38–42.

Lynch, G. S., Cuffe, S. A., Plant, D. R., and Gregorevic, P. (2001). IGF-I treatment improves the functional properties of fast- and slow-twitch skeletal muscles from dystrophic mice. *Neuromuscul. Disord.* **11**, 260–268.

Mao, Y., Ling, P. R., Fitzgibbons, T. P., McCowen, K. C., Frick, G. P., Bistrian, B. R., and Smith, R. J. (1999). Endotoxin-induced inhibition of growth hormone receptor signaling in rat liver *in vivo*. *Endocrinology* **140**, 5505–5515.

March, C. J., Moseley, B., Larsen, A., Cerretti, D. P., Braedt, G., Price, V., Gillis, S., Henney, C. S., Kronheim, S. R., Grabstein, K., Conlon, P. J., Hopp, T. P., *et al.* (1985). Cloning, sequence, and expression of two distinct human interleukin-1 complementary DNAs. *Nature* **315**, 641–647.

Marshall, J. C. (2000). SIRS and MODS: What is their relevance to the science and practice of intensive care? *Shock* **14**, 586–589.

Martin, M. U., and Wesche, H. (2002). Summary and comparison of the signaling mechanisms of the toll/interleukin-1 receptor family. *Biochim. Biophys. Acta* **1592**, 265–280.

Matthews, L. S., Enberg, B., and Norstedt, G. (1989). Regulation of rat growth hormone receptor gene expression. *J. Biol. Chem.* **264**, 9905–9919.

Mittanck, D. W., Kim, S. W., and Rotwein, P. (1997). Essential promoter elements are located within the 5″ untranslated region of human insulin-like growth factor-I exon I. *Mol. Cell Endocrinol.* **126**, 153–163.

Moldawer, L. L., Svaninger, G., Gelin, J., and Lundholm, K. G. (1987). Interleukin-1 and tumor necrosis factor do not regulate protein balance in skeletal muscle. *Am. J. Physiol.* **253**, C766–C773.

Ooi, G. T., Kelley, R. H., Poy, M. N., Rechler, M. M., and Boisclair, Y. R. (1998). Binding of STAT5a and STAT5b to a single element resembling a γ-interferon-activated sequence mediates the growth hormone induction of the mouse acid-labile subunit promoter in liver cells. *Mol. Endocrinol.* **12**, 675–687.

Okusawa, S., Gelfand, J. A., Ikejima, T., Connolly, R. J., and Dinarello, C. A. (1988). Interleukin 1 induces a shock-like state in rabbits: Synergism with tumor necrosis factor and the effect of cyclooxygenase inhibition. *J. Clin. Invest.* **81**, 1162–1172.

Park, S. H., Yamashita, H., Rui, H., and Waxman, D. J. (2001). Serine phosphorylation of GH-activated signal transducer and activator of transcription 5a (STAT5a) and STAT5b: Impact on STAT5 transcriptional activity. *Mol. Endocrinol.* **15**, 2157–2171.

Peisen, J. N., McDonnell, K. J., Mulroney, S. E., and Lumpkin, M. D. (1995). Endotoxin-induced suppression of the somatotropic axis is mediated by interleukin-1 beta and corticotropin-releasing factor in the juvenile rat. *Endocrinology* **136**, 3378–3390.

Priego, T., Ibanez de Caceres, I., Martin, A. I., Villanua, M. A., and Lopez-Calderon, A. (2002). Glucocorticoids are not necessary for the inhibitory effect of endotoxic shock on serum IGF-I and hepatic IGF-I mRNA. *J. Endocrinol.* **172**, 449–456.

Ram, P. A., and Waxman, D. J. (1999). SOCS/CIS protein inhibition of growth hormone-stimulated STAT5 signaling by multiple mechanisms. *J. Biol. Chem.* **274**, 35553–35561.

Ram, P. A., Park, S. H., Choi, H. K., and Waxman, D. J. (1996). Growth hormone activation of Stat 1, Stat 3, and Stat 5 in rat liver. Differential kinetics of hormone desensitization and growth hormone stimulation of both tyrosine phosphorylation and serine/threonine phosphorylation. *J. Biol. Chem.* **271**, 5929–5940.

Rennie, M. J. (1985). Muscle protein turnover and the wasting due to injury and disease. *Br. Med. Bull.* **41**, 257–264.

Ribaux, P., Gjinovci, A., Sadowski, H. B., and Iynedjian, P. B. (2002). Discrimination between signaling pathways in regulation of specific gene expression by insulin and growth hormone in hepatocytes. *Endocrinology* **143**, 3766–3773.

Rotwein, P. (1999). Part I. Molecular Biology of the IGF System. Molecular Biology of IGF-I and IGF-II. *In* "The IGF System, Molecular Biology, Physiology, and Clinical Applications" (R. Rosenfield and C. J. Roberts, Eds.), pp. 19–35. Humana, Totowa, NJ.

Roubenoff, R., Roubenoff, R. A., Ward, L. M., and Stevens, M. B. (1990). Catabolic effects of high-dose corticosteroids persist despite therapeutic benefit in rheumatoid arthritis. *Am. J. Clin. Nutr.* **52**, 1113–1117.

Roubenoff, R., Roubenoff, R. A., Cannon, J. G., Kehayias, J. J., Zhuang, H., Dawson-Hughes, B., Dinarello, C. A., and Rosenber, I. H. (1994). Rheumatoid cachexia: Cytokine-drive hypermetabolism accompanying reduced body cell mass in chronic inflammation. *J. Clin. Invest.* **93**, 2379–2386.

Roux-Lombard, P. (1998). The interleukin family. *Eur. Cytokine Netw.* **9**, 565–576.

Saxne, T., Pallodino, M. A., Jr., Heinegard, D., Talal, N., and Wollheim, F. A. (1988). Detection of tumor necrosis factor alpha but not tumor necrosis factor beta in rheumatoid arthritis synovial fluid and serum. *Arthritis Rheum.* **31**, 1041–1044.

Schindler, R., Clark, B. D., and Dinarello, C. A. (1990). Dissociation between interleukin-1b mRNA and protein synthesis in human peripheral mononuclear cells. *J. Biol. Chem.* **265**, 10232–10237.

Shoba, L. N., Newman, M., Liu, W., and Lowe, W. L., Jr. (2001). LY294002, an inhibitor of phosphatidylinositol 3-kinase, inhibits GH-mediated expression of the IGF-I gene in rat hepatocytes. *Endocrinology* **142**, 3980–3986.

Shumate, M. L., Yumet, G., Ahmed, T. A., and Cooney, R. N. (2005). Interleukin-1 inhibits the induction of insulin-like growth factor-I by growth hormone in CWSV-1 hepatocytes. *Am. J. Physiol. Gastrointes. Liver Physiol.* **289**, G227–G239.

Simar-Blanchet, A. E., Legraverend, C., Thissen, J. P., and Le Cam, A. (1998). Transcription of the rat serine protease inhibitor 2. 1 gene *in vivo*: Correlation with GAGA box promoter occupancy and mechanism of cytokine-mediated down-regulation. *Mol. Endocrinol.* **12**, 391–404.

Sims, J. E., Giri, J. G., and Dower, S. K. (1994). The two interleukin-1 receptors play different roles in IL-1 activities. *Clin. Immunol. Immunopathol.* **72**, 9–14.

Smith, J. W., 2nd, Urba, W. J., Curti, B. D., Elwood, L. J., Steis, R. G., Janik, R. E., Sharfman, W. H., Miller, L. L., Fenton, R. G., Conlon, K. C., Sznol, M., Greekmore, S. P., *et al.* (1992). The toxic and hematologic effects of interleukin-1 alpha administered in a phase I trial to patients with advanced malignancies. *J. Clin. Oncol.* **10**, 1141–1152.

Stevenson, F. T., Torrano, F., Locksley, R. M., and Lovett, D. H. (1992). Interleukin-1: The patterns of translation and intracellular distribution support alternative secretory mechanisms. *J. Cell. Physiol.* **152**, 223–231.

Symons, J. A., Eastgate, J. A., and Duff, G. W. (1991). Purification and characterization of a novel soluble receptor for interleukin 1. *J. Exp. Med.* **174**, 1251–1254.

Tatakis, D. N. (1993). Interleukin-1 and bone metabolism: A review. *J. Peridontol.* **64,** 416–431.

Tatar, M., Bartke, A., and Antebi, A. (2003). The endocrine regulation of aging by insulin-like signals. *Science* **299,** 1346–1351.

Thissen, J. P., and Verniers, J. (1997). Inhibition by interleukin-1 beta and tumor necrosis factor-alpha of the insulin-like growth factor I messenger ribonucleic acid response to growth hormone in rat hepatocyte primary culture. *Endocrinology* **138,** 1078–1084.

Thomas, M. J., Kikuchi, K., Bichell, D. P., and Rotwein, P. (1995). Characterization of deoxyribonucleic acid–protein interactions at a growth hormone-inducible nuclease hypersensitive site in the rat insulin-like growth factor-I gene. *Endocrinology* **136,** 562–569.

Thompson, B. J. L., Shang, C. A., and Waters, M. J. (2000). Identification of genes induced by growth hormone in rat liver using cDNA arrays. *Endocrinology* **141,** 4321–4324.

Tollet-Egnell, P., Flores-Morales, A., Stavreus-Evers, A., Sahlin, L., and Norstedt, G. (1999). Growth hormone regulation of SOCS-2, SOCS-3, and CIS messenger ribonucleic acid expression in the rat. *Endocrinology* **140,** 3693–3704.

Tollet-Egnell, P., Parini, P., Stahlberg, N., Lonnstedt, I., Lee, N. H., Rudling, M., Flores-Morales, A., and Norstedt, G. (2004). Growth hormone-mediated alteration of fuel metabolism in the aged rat as determined from transcript profiles. *Physiol. Genomics* **16,** 261–267.

Touw, I. P., De Koning, J. P., Ward, A. C., and Hermans, M. H. (2000). Signaling mechanisms of cytokine receptors and their perturbances in disease. *Mol. Cell. Endocrinol.* **160,** 1–9.

Van der Meer, J. W. M., Barza, M., Wolff, S. M., and Dinarello, C. A. (1988). A low dose of recombinant interleukin 1 protects granulocytopenic mice from lethal gram-negative infection. *Proc. Natl. Acad. Sci. USA* **85,** 1620–1623.

Vannier, E., Miller, L. C., and Dinarello, C. A. (1992). Coordinated anti-inflammatory effects of interleukin-4: Interleukin-4 suppresses IL-1 production, but up-regulates gene expression of IL1 receptor antagonist. *Proc. Natl. Acad. Sci. USA* **89,** 4076–4080.

Vary, T. C., and Kimball, S. R. (1992). Sepsis-induced changes in protein synthesis: Differential effects on fast- and slow-twitch muscles. *Am. J. Physiol.* **262,** C1513–C1519.

Wang, L., Wang, X., and Adamo, M. L. (2000). Two putative GATA motifs in the proximal exon 1 promoter of the rat insulin-like growth factor-I gene regulate basal promoter activity. *Endocrinology* **141,** 1118–1126.

Wang, X., Talamantez, J. L., and Adamo, M. L. (1998). A CACCC box in the proximal exon 2 promoter of the rat insulin-like growth factor I gene is required for basal promoter activity. *Endocrinology* **139,** 1054–1066.

Webb, A. C., Collins, K. L., Auron, P. E., Eddy, R. L., Nakai, H., Byers, M. G., Haley, W. M., and Shows, T. B. (1986). Interleukin-1 gene assigned to long arm or chromosome 2. *Lymphokine Res.* **5,** 77–85.

Wilmore, D. W. (1991). Catabolic illness: Strategies for enhancing recovery. *N. Engl. J. Med.* **325,** 695–702.

Wilmore, D. W. (2000). Metabolic response to severe surgical illness: Overview. *World J. Surg.* **6,** 705–711.

Woelfle, J., and Rotwein, P. (2004). *In vivo* regulation of growth hormone-stimulated gene transcription by STAT5b. *Am. J. Physiol. Endocrinol. Metab.* **286,** E393–E401.

Woelfle, J., Billiard, J., and Rotwein, P. (2003a). Acute control of IGF-I gene transcription by growth hormone through Stat5b. *J. Biol. Chem.* **278,** 22696–22702.

Woelfle, J., Chia, D. J., and Rotwein, P. (2003b). Mechanisms of growth hormone action: Identification of conserved STAT5 binding sites that mediate GH-induced insulin-like growth factor-I gene activation. *J. Biol. Chem.* **278,** 51261–51266.

Woelfle, J., Chia, D. J., Massart-Schlesinger, M. B., Moyano, P., and Rotwein, P. (2005). Molecular physiology, pathology, and regulation of the growth hormone/insulin-like growth factor-I system. *Pediatr. Nephrol.* **20,** 295–302.

Wolf, M., Bohm, S., Brand, M., and Kreymann, G. (1996). Proinflammatory cytokines interleukin 1 beta and tumor necrosis factor alpha inhibit growth hormone stimulation of insulin-like growth factor I synthesis and growth hormone receptor mRNA levels in cultured rat liver cells. *Eur. J. Endocrinol.* **135**, 729–737.

Yoshizato, H., Fujikawa, T., Soya, H., Tanaka, M., and Nakashima, K. (1998). The growth hormone (GH) gene is expressed in the lateral hypothalamus: Enhancement by GH-releasing hormone and repression by restraint stress. *Endocrinology* **139**, 2545–2551.

Yumet, G., Shumate, M. L., Bryant, D. P., Lin, C. M., Lang, C. H., and Cooney, R. N. (2002). Tumor necrosis factor mediates hepatic growth hormone resistance during sepsis. *Am. J. Physiol. Endocrinol. Metab.* **283**, E472–E481.

Yumet, G., Shumate, M. L., Bryant, D. P., Lang, C. H., and Cooney R. N. (2006). Hepatic growth hormone resistance during sepsis is associated with increased suppressors of cytokine signaling expression and impaired growth hormone signaling. *Crit. Care Med.* **34**, 1420–1427.

Zamir, O., Hasselgren, P. O., O'Brien, W. O., Thompson, R. C., and Fischer, E. J. (1992). Muscle protein breakdown during endotoxemia in rats and after treatment with IL-1ra. *Ann. Surg.* **216**, 381–387.

Zhu, T., Goh, E. L. K., Graichen, R., Ling, L., and Lobie, P. E. (2001). Signal transduction via the growth hormone receptor. *Cell Signal* **13**, 599–616.

14

THE ROLE OF THE INTERLEUKIN-6/GP130 SIGNALING PATHWAY IN BONE METABOLISM

XIN-HUA LIU,* ALEXANDER KIRSCHENBAUM,[†] SHEN YAO,* AND ALICE C. LEVINE*

*Department of Medicine, Division of Endocrinology, Diabetes and Bone Diseases
Mount Sinai School of Medicine, New York, New York 10029
[†]Department of Urology, Mount Sinai School of Medicine
New York, New York 10029

0083-6729/06 $35.00
DOI: 10.1016/S0083-6729(06)74014-6

I. INTRODUCTION

The interleukin-6 (IL-6) family of cytokines includes IL-6, IL-11, leukemia inhibitory factor (LIF), oncostain M (OSM), ciliary neurotrophic factor (CNTF), and cardiotrophin-1 (CT-1) (Kishimoto et al., 1995). Increasing evidence suggests that IL-6-type cytokines regulate immune and inflammatory responses, hepatic acute-phase protein synthesis, hematopoiesis, and bone metabolism (Kishimoto, 1989). All of the members of the IL-6 family have overlapping functions and utilize the same receptor subunit, glycoprotein 130 (gp130), a critical signal-transducing component previously identified as IL-6 receptor-β (IL-6Rβ) (Kishimoto et al., 1995). In target cells, IL-6 can simultaneously induce functionally distinct and even contradictory signals through its receptor complex, IL-6Rα (or soluble receptor, sIL-6R) and gp130. The binding of IL-6 to IL-6Rα induces dimerization of gp130 (Taga and Kishimoto, 1997), and initiates a cascade of intracellular signaling that leads to activation of signal transducers and activators of transcription (STAT)1/3 and/or SHP2/ras/MAPK, a process that culminates in modulation of gene transcription (Heymann and Rousselle, 2000; Kamimura et al., 2003; O'Brien et al., 2000).

There is ample evidence that IL-6-type cytokines play an important role in skeletal homeostasis (Manolagas and Jilka, 1995; Martin et al., 1998; Suda et al., 1999). IL-6 influences both osteoblast and osteoclast activities through a variety of complex mechanisms. For example, IL-6 has been shown to promote the differentiation of macrophages and bone marrow stromal cells into osteoclasts and osteoblasts, respectively (Erices et al., 2002; Manolagas, 1998; Sims et al., 2004). In addition, IL-6 interacts with other factors that are critically involved in bone remodeling, including the OPG/RANKL/RANK system, sex steroids (estrogens and androgens), prostaglandin E_2 (PGE_2), tumor necrosis factor (TNF)-α, parathyroid hormone (PTH), IL-11, and IL-1, to regulate bone turnover (Grey et al., 1999; Liu et al., 2005; Steeve et al., 2004). In this chapter, we will highlight the biological effects and clinical relevance of IL-6 and its associated receptors in bone development and remodeling. Recent data on the regulation of IL-6/gp130 signaling pathway in bone homeostasis will also be discussed with an emphasis on how one cytokine can initiate diverse effects in bone in a cell-specific fashion.

II. EFFECT OF IL-6 ON BONE RESORPTION

Bone tissue remodeling results from the coordinate activities of osteoblasts and osteoclasts. Osteoclasts are derived from hematopoietic precursors of the bone marrow (Roodman, 1996) and are highly specialized, multinucleated cells that are uniquely capable of lacunar bone resorption. Imbalances in the bone remodeling process result in metabolic bone diseases characterized by either enhanced osteoclast activity and increased bone resorption (i.e., osteoporosis and osteolytic bone lesions in cancer) or increased osteoblastic bone formation (i.e., osteopetrosis and prostate cancer-induced osteoblastic metastases) (Fohr *et al.*, 2003; Ohlsson *et al.*, 1998).

IL-6 increases osteoclast recruitment by acting on early hematopoietic cells from the granulocyte-macrophage lineage that contain the progenitors of the osteoclastic lineage (Otsuka *et al.*, 1991). IL-6 has also been shown to play a specific role in postmenopausal osteoporosis (Jilka *et al.*, 1992; Poli *et al.*, 1994; Tarura *et al.*, 1993). A possible mechanism for this effect was decreased osteoclast formation due to the lack of IL-6 (Tarura *et al.*, 1993). A cross-sectional study in humans compared bone turnover and bone mineral density (BMD) in healthy postmenopausal women with different G-C polymorph-isms at position –174 in the IL-6 promoter. Patients with either CG or GG genotypes were associated with higher bone resorption and lower BMD at the hip and forearm compared with those in patients with the CC genotype (Ferrari, 2001). The study suggests that allelic variations in the IL-6 promoter influence IL-6 production and contribute to increased bone resorption and decreased BMD. High IL-6 levels also correlate with high bone resorption indices in patients with rheumatoid arthritis. Clinical studies reveal a negative correlation between BMD and the combination of intracellular and cell-surface-bound levels of IL-6 in peripheral blood monocytes from rheumatoid arthritis patients (Verbruggen *et al.*, 1999). In multiple myeloma, IL-6 is one of the cytokines that promote bone destruction (Kuehl and Bergsagel, 2002). Multiple myeloma is a plasma cell dyscrasia characterized by proliferation of malignant B cells in the bone marrow and severe bone loss. Higher IL-6 serum levels in multiple myeloma are associated with more advanced stages of the disease (II and III). Furthermore, the serum level of IL-6 has been identified as a significant prognostic marker in multiple myeloma. Ludwig *et al.* (1991) found that survival times differed significantly between patients whose IL-6 levels at the time of diagnosis fell below 7 pg/ml and those with higher levels. The 50% of patients in the former category exhibited a medium survival of 53.7 months as compared with only 2.7 months in the latter category (Ludwig *et al.*, 1991). Although the mechanisms underlying these observed effects of IL-6 are not well understood, one report demonstrated that IL-6 modulates trabecular and endochondral bone turnover *in vivo* by stimulating osteoclast differentiation (Rozen *et al.*, 2000).

Bone remodeling is the result of the coordinate and interactive effects of both types of osteogenic cells (osteoblasts and osteoclasts). Although high levels of IL-6 stimulate bone resorption directely, IL-6, like many other regulatory factors (i.e., growth factors, hormones, cytokines), predominantly modulates osteoclast activity and bone resorption indirectly by influencing osteoblast differentiation and secretion. In bone cells, IL-6 production is limited to cells of the osteoblastic lineage (Holt *et al.*, 1996; Legrand-Poels *et al.*, 2000). Moreover, although both osteoblasts and osteoclasts express the

IL-6 receptor, functional studies demonstrate that IL-6-induced osteoclast differentiation is dependent upon IL-6 receptor expression by the osteoblast, but not the osteoclast (Udagawa *et al.*, 1995). In agreement with these observations, our *in vitro* studies demonstrate that IL-6 significantly stimulates osteoclast differentiation *only* when they are grown in coculture with osteoblasts (Liu *et al.*, 2005). However, a direct effect of IL-6 on inducing osteoclast formation has also been reported in several osteolytic bone disorders (Kudo *et al.*, 2003).

III. EFFECT OF IL-6 ON BONE FORMATION

Mature osteoblasts are derived from multipotent mesenchymal stem cells of the bone marrow that also give rise to the fibroblast cells of the marrow stroma, chondrocytes, adipocytes, and muscle cells (Aubin, 1998). Stromal cells of the bone marrow and osteoblasts exhibit an extensive overlap of phenotypic properties (Manolagas, 1998). The initial evidence that the IL-6 family of cytokines influences bone formation was provided by the observation that overexpression of either LIF or OSM gene (two IL-6 family members) in mice induces excessive bone formation (Lowe *et al.*, 1991; Malik *et al.*, 1995; Metcalf and Gearing, 1989). In addition, IL-6, LIF, and OSM have been reported to confer an antiapoptotic phenotype on osteoblastic cells via enhanced transcriptional activation of the *p21* gene (Bellido *et al.*, 1998; Jilka *et al.*, 1998; Steeve *et al.*, 2004). IL-6 also promotes osteogenic lineage commitment. IL-6 plus soluble IL-6 receptor or LIF stimulates the commitment of embryonic fibroblasts (12th–14th day of gestation) toward the osteoblast phenotype without any promotion of differentiation toward adipocytes, chondrocytes, or muscle cells (Tagochi *et al.*, 1998). It has also been reported that the differentiation of mesenchymal progenitors of osteoblasts in the murine bone marrow can be stimulated by IL-6 plus soluble IL-6 receptor or LIF (Tagochi *et al.*, 1998). IL-6 as well as LIF, IL-11, CNTF, and OSM promote the differentiation of committed osteoblast cells toward a more mature phenotype, and this action of the IL-6 family of cytokines is mediated by the activation of the Janus Kinase (JAK)/STAT pathway (Bellido *et al.*, 1997). However, Hughes and Howells (1993) have shown an inhibitory effect of IL-6 on bone formation *in vitro*. These apparently contradictory observations may be due to the differences in the experimental systems and methods utilized in the two studies. Both osteoblasts and osteoclasts express the IL-6 receptor subunits, that is, gp130 and soluble IL-6 receptor. However, the intracellular signaling cascades induced by IL-6 activation of gp130 are complex and may be cell specific. It is possible that the observed dual effect of IL-6 on bone is due to cell-specific activation of different intracellular signaling pathways in osteoblasts versus osteoclasts (Sims *et al.*, 2004).

IV. INTERACTIONS BETWEEN IL-6/GP130
SIGNALING AND THE
OPG/RANKL/RANK SYSTEM

Osteoblast function is intimately tied to osteoclast activity. The interactions between osteoblasts and osteoclasts can be established through cell–cell contact (Jimi *et al.*, 1996) and are mediated by receptor activator of nuclear factor-kappaB (NF-κB) ligand (RANKL) produced by osteoblasts and receptor activator of NF-κB (RANK) on the osteoclast surface (Nakagawa *et al.*, 1998; Yasuda *et al.*, 1998). Bone marrow stromal cells (osteoblast precursor cells) also produce a soluble glycoprotein called osteoprotegerin (OPG), a decoy receptor for RANKL that prevents osteoclast activation (Simonet and Luthy, 1997; Yasuda *et al.*, 1998). OPG and RANKL, synthesized by stromal cells/osteoblasts, have been identified as the two principal cytokines that regulate osteoclast differentiation and activation (Lacey *et al.*, 1998; Simonet and Luthy, 1997). Hormones, growth factors, cytokines, and prostaglandins regulate these processes (Brandstrom *et al.*, 2001; Ohlsson *et al.*, 1998) mainly via effects on osteoblasts. In general, the osteoblasts receive input directly from a variety of regulatory factors and then transmit these signals to the neighboring osteoclasts via the OPG/RANKL/RANK system. RANKL and IL-6 production by osteoblasts/stromal cells are coupled in the process of osteoclastogenesis and in diseases where there is excessive osteolysis (Steeve *et al.*, 2004). IL-6 modulates this vital communication network between the osteoblasts and osteoclasts. The first action of IL-6 is to stimulate osteoblastic production and secretion of factors that regulate osteoclastic activity, like RANKL (Steeve *et al.*, 2004). Although IL-6 was reported to increase RANKL secretion by osteoblasts in one study (Nakashima *et al.*, 2000), we observed only a minor effect of IL-6 on this parameter (Liu *et al.*, 2005). Our data are in agreement with that reported by Steeve *et al.* (2004) and O'Brien *et al.* (2000) that neither IL-6 nor soluble IL-6 receptor stimulates bone resorption when added separately. In contrast, significant stimulation of RANKL secretion and osteoclastogenesis was observed when IL-6 and sIL-6R were added in combination (O'Brien *et al.*, 2000; Steeve *et al.*, 2004). In addition, these studies showed that combination treatment with IL-6 and sIL-6R receptor stimulates OPG secretion by osteoblasts and inhibits RANK expression by osteoclasts (O'Brien *et al.*, 2000; Steeve *et al.*, 2004). However, we reported somewhat divergent effects of IL-6 on the OPG/RANKL/RANK system. Our *in vitro* studies demonstrate that IL-6 alone has no significant effect on RANKL secretion by osteoblasts. IL-6 addition, however, increases RANK expression by osteoclasts. Finally, although exogenous IL-6 had no detectable effect on osteoblastic OPG production, IL-6 neutralizing antibodies increased OPG secretion and reversed the observed suppression of OPG secretion by PGE$_2$, suggesting a role for endogenous IL-6 in mediating basal and inducible OPG production by osteoblasts (Liu *et al.*, 2005). The net

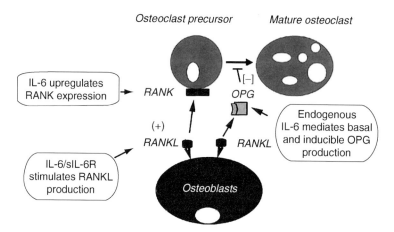

FIGURE 1.   Interaction between IL-6 and the OPG/RANKL/RANK system in osteoclas-togenesis. The binding of RANKL to RANK activates osteoclasts, whereas RANKL binding to OPG, a decoy receptor, suppresses osteoclast activation. IL-6 primarily modulates osteoclast functions via effects on osteoblasts and the OPG/RANKL/RANK system. Overall effect is inhibition of OPG, activation of RANKL/RANK, and promotion of osteoclast activation.

result of these effects of IL-6 (suppression of osteoblast OPG production and increased RANK expression in osteoclasts) is increased osteoclastic activity (Fig. 1). However, the precise mechanisms underlying the interaction between IL-6 and the OPG/RANKL/RANK system in the regulation of osteoclastogenesis are unclear. It has been proposed that the activation of STAT3 induced by IL-6/sIL-6R/gp130 signaling not only increases RANKL expression but also enhances the sensitivity of osteoclast precursors to RANKL stimulation (Steeve et al., 2004), presumably by increasing RANK expression on these cells (Liu et al., 2005). Moreover, both RANKL and IL-6 have been shown to activate protein kinase C (PKC) and the members of the MAPK signaling pathway (Sims et al., 2004; Steeve et al., 2004), such as ERK1/2, JNK, and p38, suggesting that IL-6/sIL-6/gp130 signaling and the OPG/RANKL/RANK system may share similar down-stream signaling pathways and have synergistic effects on osteoclastogenesis.

V. CROSS TALK BETWEEN IL-6 AND STEROID HORMONES, PTH, PGE$_2$, AND CYTOKINES

The process of bone remodeling is the result of an elaborate network composed of growth factors, sex steroids, cytokines, and prostaglandins. IL-6 has been shown to specifically interact with these other factors to promote osteoclastogenesis.

A. IL-6 AND SEX STEROIDS

Androgens and estrogens are key regulators of bone metabolism. Loss of gonadal function in either sex increases osteoclast precursor formation and inhibits osteoblast activity in the bone marrow, resulting in increased bone resorption and bone loss. Replacement of sex steroids in hypogonadal individuals of either sex prevents these changes (Bellido *et al.*, 1995; Jilka *et al.*, 1992). Estrogens specifically inhibit osteoclast activation with little or no direct effect on osteoblasts. This effect of estrogen is due, at least in part, to an interaction with IL-6 (Jilka *et al.*, 1992; Manolagas, 1998). It has been shown that loss of estrogens increases IL-6 production in response to 1,25-dihydroxyvitamin D3 (1,25(OH)2D3) or PTH by *in vitro* bone marrow cell cultures. IL-6-deficient mice do not exhibit an increase in osteoclastogenesis after ovariectomy and are protected from the bone loss caused by disrupted ovarian function (Poli *et al.*, 1994). Increased osteoclastogenic activity resulting from loss of ovarian function *in vivo* is accompanied by elevated levels of IL-6 in the microenvironment of the bone marrow (Jilka *et al.*, 1992). Notably, these changes were prevented by the administration of 17β-estradiol or neutralizing antibodies to IL-6 (Jilka *et al.*, 1992; Poli *et al.*, 1994). Taken together, these data indicate that estrogen signaling in osteoclasts is mediated by IL-6. This effect of estrogens is regulated by protein–protein interactions between the estrogen receptor and other transcriptional factors such as NF-κB or NF-IL-6 (Galien *et al.*, 1996; Hughes and Howells, 1993). Similarly, in a separate study, orchiectomy in male mice resulted in an increase in osteoclast progenitors in the bone marrow, and this effect was prevented by either androgen replacement or administration of IL-6 neutralizing antibodies (Bellido *et al.*, 1995). Bone histomorphometric analysis of trabecular bone reveals that IL-6-deficient mice exhibit no evidence of bone loss or elevated osteoclastic activity (Bellido *et al.*, 1995; Manolagas, 1998). These data indicate that sex steroids, both estrogens and androgens, inhibit IL-6 gene expression, and that IL-6 mediates their effects on bone metabolism.

B. IL-6 AND PTH

PTH stimulates bone resorption indirectly by promoting the release of paracrine agents produced by osteoblasts, which recruit and activate osteoclasts. Among those factors, IL-6 has been shown to be one of the critical cytokine mediators of PTH action. IL-6 is produced by osteoblasts in response to PTH (Lowik *et al.*, 1989). PTH-induced bone resorption by osteoclast-like cells is inhibited by neutralizing antibodies to the IL-6 receptor (Greenfield *et al.*, 1995). *In vivo* studies confirm that IL-6 levels are increased by PTH in experimental animals (Grey *et al.*, 1999). In addition, circulating levels of IL-6 are elevated in patients with primary hyper-parathyroidism and correlate with increased biochemical markers of bone resorption, suggesting that IL-6 plays a permissive role in PTH-induced bone effects (Grey et al., 1999).

C. IL-6 AND PGE$_2$

The roles of cyclooxygenase (COX)-2 and PGE$_2$, a major eicosanoid product of the COX-2-catalyzed reaction, in bone remodeling have been described in studies with mice that are genetically deficient in COX-2. Mice lacking COX-2 expression display reduced bone resorption in response to PTH or 1,25(OH)2D3 (Okada et al., 2000). In an in vitro study, COX-2 and PGE$_2$ have been shown to play important roles in osteoclast formation (Ono et al., 2002) and are required for debris-induced osteoclastogenesis and osteolysis in an in vivo mouse calvaria model (Zhang et al., 2001). COX-2/PGE$_2$ also participate in bone formation. Systemic or local injection of PGE$_2$ stimulates bone formation in response to mechanical strain (Supo-nitzky and Weinreb, 1998), and this effect is mediated by the COX-2-cata-lyzed pathway (Forwood, 1996). In addition, COX-2 has been demonstrated to be a critical regulator of mesenchymal cell differentiation into osteoblasts and an essential element in bone repair (Zhang et al., 2002). These data indicate that COX-2 and PGE$_2$ are involved in both cytokine-mediated osteoclast activation and osteoblastic bone formation. Moreover, it has been demonstrated that the actions of PGE$_2$ in bone homeostasis are mediated through the cAMP signaling pathway, activated by the binding of PGE$_2$ to subtypes of E-series of prostaglandin (EP) receptor, particularly the EP$_2$ and EP$_4$ receptor subtypes (Li et al., 2000; Miyaura et al., 2000).

Several lines of evidence support the notion that IL-6 interacts with PGE$_2$ in different systems. EP$_4$ receptor knockout mice have reduced circulating levels of IL-6 and significantly less IL-6 production by liver and macro-phages (McCoy et al., 2002). COX-2-promoted human oropharyngeal carci-noma growth is mediated by IL-6 (Hong et al., 2000). We observed that PGE$_2$ stimulation of human prostate intraepithelial neoplasia cell growth is through activation of the IL-6/gp130/STAT3 signaling pathway (Liu et al., 2002). Consistent with this data, it has been shown that stromal osteoblast cells support osteoclast differentiation by their ability to secrete IL-6 and RANKL in response to PTH, 1,25(OH)2D3, and PGE$_2$ (Gruber et al., 2000; Kozawa et al., 1998). These data provide mechanistic evidence of cross-talk between the COX-2/PGE$_2$ and IL-6 signaling systems. As previously men-tioned, we demonstrated that IL-6 stimulation of osteoclast differentiation in cocultures (with osteoblasts) was due to both an increase in RANK expres-sion by osteoclasts and reciprocal interactions with the COX-2/PGE$_2$ system (Liu et al., 2005). In that same report, neutralizing antibodies to IL-6 increased basal OPG secretion by osteoblasts and reversed the inhibitory effects of PGE_2 on this parameter, indicating that endogenous IL-6 mediates PGE_2 effects on osteoblastic OPG secretion. IL-6 also increased COX-2 expression and PGE_2 production in osteoblasts. Finally, there is evidence that IL-6 interacts with the EP receptor system in inflammatory carcinogenesis and rheumatoid arthritis (Hong et al., 2000; Sugiyama, 2001) through activation of the gp130/STAT3 signaling pathway (Gruber et al., 2000; Ni et al., 2000). Our data indicate that IL-6 increases the expression of the EP_4 receptor subtype in both osteoblasts and osteoclast precursors. IL-6 also induces the EP_2 receptor subtype expression in osteoblasts (Liu et al., 2005). The induction of EP_4 and EP_2 by IL-6 in osteoblasts, in turn, amplifies the effects of PGE_2 on the inhibition of OPG production and stimulation of membrane-bound RANKL expression and soluble RANKL release. All of these events, coordinately, tip the balance of the OPG/RANKL/RANK system in favor of increased osteoclastogenesis and enhanced bone resorption. These results demonstrate significant cross talk between the IL-6/gp130 and COX-2/PGE_2 signaling systems in the regulation of osteoclastogenesis and indicate that these effects are mediated by the OPG/RANKL/RANK system.

D. IL-6 AND OTHER INFLAMMATORY CYTOKINES

TNF-α and IL-1 are important cytokines that are involved in the regulation of bone metabolism. Experimental data indicate that TNF-α, IL-1, and IL-6 stimulate osteoclast differentiation in a synergistic fashion (Ragab et al., 2002), primarily via effects on the OPG/RANKL/RANK system (Steeve et al., 2004). These factors increase the production of both OPG and RANKL, but tip the balance in favor of increased RANKL/OPG production. TNF-α has also been shown to stimulate both the proliferation and differentiation of cells in the osteoclast lineage (Kobayashi et al., 2000; Kudo et al., 2002). TNF-α can act in combination with RANKL produced in the marrow microenvironment to enhance the actions of macrophage colony-stimulating factor (MCSF) on osteoclast formation (Kudo et al., 2002), and this effect can be significantly increased by combination treatment with TNF-α and IL-6 (Gorny et al., 2004). In addition, TNF-α stimulates a significant increase in IL-6 production by osteoblasts. However, it is not clear whether the effect of TNF-α is directly mediated by its effect on IL-6 secretion in bone cells. IL-1 increases RANKL expression by osteoblasts and this effect is significantly enhanced by IL-6 (Gorny et al., 2004; Kudo et al., 2002). The interactive effects of IL-6, TNF-α, and IL-1 have been proposed to involve activation/inactivation of a cascade of intracellular signaling events including the activation of two members of the MAPK family (i.e., ERK and p38) and JNK (Steeve et al., 2004). The ERK pathway negatively regulates osteoclastogenesis whereas the p38 pathway promotes this process (Steeve et al., 2004).

VI. GP130 SIGNALING AND BONE
REMODELING

IL-6-type cytokines regulate bone remodeling by activating the gp130 receptor subunit, which, in turn, stimulates the intracellular cascade of signal transduction and induces target gene expression. The expression levels of gp130 in bone marrow stromal cells have been shown to determine the magnitude of the cascade signals generated by IL-6-type cytokines (O'Brien, *et al.*, 2000). Recent studies demonstrate that gp130 signaling proceeds via at least two intracellular pathways, that is, the STAT1/3 (Stahl *et al.*, 1995) and SHP2/ras/MAPK (Fukuta, 1996) pathways. The activation of these pathways is ligand- and tissue-specific and leads to induction of distinct sets of target genes and, thus, distinct biological consequences (Kamimura *et al.*, 2003; Sims *et al.*, 2004). The effects of the activation of these two gp130-associated pathways on bone remodeling have been investigated. Sims *et al.* (2004) analyzed mice in which gp130 signaling via either the STAT1/3 or MAPK pathway was attenuated by conditional mutation and demonstrated a dual role for gp130 in osteoclastogenesis based on its simultaneous expression in osteoblast and osteoclast precursors (Gao *et al.*, 1998; Sims *et al.*, 2004). These studies also revealed that there are three key pathways by which gp130 signaling contributes to bone cell interactions. First, the activation of STAT1/3 pathway induced by gp130 cytokines plays an essential role in stimulating chondrocyte proliferation and disruption of this pathway results in premature growth plate closure and reduced bone size. Second, the SHP2/ras/MAPK pathway of the gp130 signaling plays an equally key role in the inhibition of osteoclastogenesis. In the absence of this latter pathway, a high level of osteoclastogenesis is observed that leads to trabecular and cortical bone loss. Finally, IL-6 stimulates osteoblasts, and this effect is mediated by the gp130-STAT1/3 pathway. The IL-6/gp130-STAT1/3 activation of osteoblast function is exaggerated in the absence of the gp130-SHP2/ras/MAPK pathway, producing increased osteoblastic bone formation (Sims *et al.*, 2004). The exact pathway whereby IL-6 type cytokines stimulate osteoclastic activity has not been elucidated. These available data indicate that IL-6-type cytokines have diverse effects on bone metabolism depending upon cell-specific intracellular signaling cascades (either STAT1/3 or SHP2/ras/MAPK pathway, or both) in response to gp130 activation.

VII. SUMMARY

There is increasing evidence that the IL-6 family of cytokines and signaling pathways downstream of the common gp130 receptor subunit play critical roles in the processes of bone homeostasis and remodeling. The binding of IL-6 to sIL-6R is a prerequisite step for the activation of gp130/STAT3 signaling. Once gp130 is activated, there are at least two intracellular signaling cascades that can transmit divergent signals to bone cells. Although there is some conflicting data regarding the effects of IL-6 on bone, it is generally accepted that the primary effect of this cytokine group is the stimulation of osteoclastic bone resorption. In addition, IL-6 effects on osteoclasts appear to be predominantly indirect via modulation of osteo-blasts and the OPG/RANKL/RANK system that coordinates the functions and activities of osteoblasts and osteoclasts. IL-6 alone has minimal effects on osteoclast differentiation and activation. However, IL-6 acts synergisti-cally with growth factors, steroid hormones, inflammatory cytokines, and prostaglandins in bone cells. Reciprocal interactions between IL-6 and PGE_2 are particularly relevant to bone metabolism. IL-6 enhances the expression of two subtypes of EP receptor and mediates PGE_2-induced suppression of OPG secretion. A better understanding of the complex, cell-specific, interactive effects of IL-6 and various bone modulators may uncover new paradigms for the treatment of bone diseases.

REFERENCES

Aubin, J. E. (1998). Advances in the osteoblast lineage. *Biochem. Cell Biol.* **76**, 899–910.

Bellido, T., Jilka, R. J., Boyce, B. F., Girasole, G., Broxmeyer, H., Dalrymple, S. A., Murray, R., and Manolagas, S. C. (1995). Regulation of interleukin-6, osteo-clastogenesis and bone mass by androgens: The role of the androgen receptor. *J. Clin. Invest.* **95**, 2886–2895.

Bellido, T., Borba, V. Z., Roberson, P., and Monolagas, S. C. (1997). Activation of the Janus kinase/STAT signal transduction pathway by interleukin-6-type cytokines promotes osteoblast differentiation. *Endocrinology* **138**, 3666–3676.

Bellido, T., O'Brien, C. A., Roberson, P. K., and Manolagas, S. C. (1998). Transcriptional activation of the p21^{waf-1} gene by interleukin-6 type cytokines. A prerequisite for their pro-differentiating and anti-apoptotic effect on human osteoblastic cells. *J. Biol. Chem.* **273**, 21137–21144.

Brandstrom, H., Bjorkman, T., and Ljunggren, O. (2001). Regulation of osteopro-tegerin secretion from primary cultures of human bone marrow stromal cells. *Biochem. Biophys. Res. Commun.* **280**, 831–835.

Erices, A., Conget, P., Rojas, C., and Minguell, J. (2002). gp130 activation by soluble interleukin 6 receptor/interleukin 6 enhances osteoblastic differentiation of human bone marrow-derived from mesenchymal stem cells. *Exp. Cell Res.* **180**, 24–32.

Ferrari, S. L., Garnero, P., Emond, S., Montgomery, H., Humphries, S. E., and Greenspan, S. L. (2001). A functional polymorphic variant in the interleukin-6 gene promoter associated with low bone resorption in postmenopausal women. *Arthritis Rheum.* **44**, 196–201.

Fohr, B., Dunstan, C. R., and Seibel, M. J. (2003). Markers of bone remodeling in metastatic bone disease. *J. Clin. Endo & Meta* **88**, 5059–5075.

Forwood, M. R. (1996). Inducible COX-2 mediates the induction of bone formation by mechanical loading *in vivo. J. Bone Miner. Res.* **11**, 1688–1693.

Fukuta, T. (1996). Two signals are necessary for cell proliferation induced by a cytokine receptor gp130: Involvement of STAT3 in anti-apoptosis. *Immunity* **5**, 449–460.

Galien, R., Evans, H., and Garcia, T. (1996). Involvment of CCAAT/enhancer-binding protein and NF-κB binding sites in IL-6 promoter inhibition by estrogens. *Mol. Endocrinol.* **10**, 713–722.

Gao, Y., Morita, I., Maruo, N., Kubota, T., Murota, S., and Aso, T. (1998). Expression of IL-6 receptor and gp130 in mouse bone marrow cells during osteoclast differentiation. *Bone* **22,** 487–493.

Gorny, G., Shaw, A., and Oursler, M. J. (2004). IL-6, LIF, and TNFα regulation of GM-CSF inhibition of osteoclastogenesis *in vitro*. *Exp. Cell Res.* **294,** 149–158.

Greenfield, E. M., Shaw, S. M., Gornik, S. A., and Banks, M. A. (1995). Adenyl cyclase and IL-6 are downstream effectors of parathyroid hormone regulating in stimulation of bone resorption. *J. Clin. Invest.* **96,** 1238–1244.

Grey, A., Mitnick, M.-A., Masiukiewicz, U., Sun, B. H., Rudikoff, S., Jilka, R. L., Manolagas, S. C., and Insogna, K. (1999). A role for IL-6 in parathyroid hormone-induced bone resorption *in vivo*. *Endocrinology* **140,** 4683–4690.

Gruber, R., Nothegger, G., Ho, G. M., Willheim, M., and Peterlik, M. (2000). Differential stimulation by prostaglandin E_2 and calcemic hormones of interleukin-6 in stromal/osteoblastic cells. *Biochem. Biophys. Res. Commun.* **270,** 1080–1085.

Heymann, D., and Rousselle, A.-V. (2000). gp130 cytokine family and bone cells. *Cytokine* **12,** 1455–1468.

Holt, I., Davie, M. W. J., and Marshall, M. J. (1996). Osteoclast are not the major source of interleukin-6 in mouse parietal bone. *Bone* **18,** 221–226.

Hong, S. H., Ondrey, F. C., Avis, I. M., Chen, Z., Loukinova, E., Cavanaugh, P. F., Jr., Waes, C. V., and Mulshine, J. L. (2000). Cyclooxygenase regulates human oropharyngeal carcinomas via the proinflammatory cytokine interleukin-6: A general role for inflammation? *FASEB J.* **14,** 1499–1507.

Hughes, F. J., and Howells, G. L. (1993). Interleukin-6 inhibits bone formation *in vitro*. *Bone Miner.* **21,** 21–28.

Jilka, R. L., Hangoc, G., Girasole, G., Passeri, G., Williams, D. C., Abrams, J. S., Boyce, B., Broxmeyer, H., and Manolagas, S. C. (1992). Increased osteoclast development after estrogen loss: Mediation by interleukin-6. *Science* **257,** 88–91.

Jilka, R. L., Weinstein, R. S., Bellido, T., Parfitt, A. M., and Manolagas, S. C. (1998). Osteoblast programmed cell death (apoptosis): Modulation by growth factor and cytokines. *J. Bone Miner. Res.* **13,** 793–802.

Jimi, E., Nakamura, I., Amano, H., Taguchi, Y., Tsurakai, T., Tamura, M., Takahashi, N., and Suda, T. (1996). Osteoclst function is activated by osteoblastic cells through mechanism involving cell-to-cell contact. *Endocrinology* **137,** 2187–2190.

Kamimura, D., Ishihara, K., and Hirano, T. (2003). IL-6 signal transduction and its physiological roles: The signal orchestration model. *Rev. Physiol. Biochem. Pharmacol.* **149,** 1–38.

Kishimoto, T. (1989). The biology of interleukin-6. *Blood* **74,** 1–10.

Kishimoto, T., Akira, S., Narazaki, M., and Taga, T. (1995). Interleukin-6 family of cytokines and gp130. *Blood* **86,** 1243–1254.

Kozawa, O., Suzuki, A., Tokuda, H., Kaida, T., and Uematsu, T. (1998). IL-6 synthesis induced by prostaglandin E_2: Cross-talk regulation by protein kinase C. *Bone* **22,** 355–360.

Kudo, O., Fujikawa, Y., Itonaga, I., Sabokbar, A., Torisu, T., and Athanasou, N. A. (2002). Proinflammatory cytokines (TNFα/IL-1α) induction of human osteoclast formation. *J. Pathol.* **198,** 220–227.

Kudo, O., Sabokbar, A., Pocock, A., Itonaga, I., Fujikawa, Y., and Athanasou, N. A. (2003). Interleukin-6 and interleukin-11 support human osteoclast formation by a RANKL-independent mechanism. *Bone* **32,** 1–7.

Kuehl, W. M., and Bergsagel, P. L. (2002). Multiple myeloma: Evolving genetic events and host interactions. *Nature Rev. Cancer* **1,** 175–187.

Kobayashi, K., Takahashi, N., Jimi, E., Udagawa, N., Takami, M., and Kotake, S. (2000). Tumor necrosis factor alpha stimulates osteoclast differentiation by a mechanism independent of the OPG/RANKL/RANK interaction. *J. Exp. Med.* **191,** 275–286.

Lacey, D. L., Timms, E., Tan, H. L., Keller, M., Dunstan, C. R., and Burgess, T. (1998). Osteoprotegerin ligand is a cytokine that regulates osteoclast differentiation and activation. *Cell* **93**, 165–176.

Legrand-Poels, S., Schoonbroodt, S., and Piette, J. (2000). Regulation of interleukin-6 gene expression by pro-inflammatory cytokines in a colon cancer cell line. *Biochem. J.* **349**, 765–773.

Li, X. D., Okada, Y., Pilbeam, C. C., Lorenzo, J. A., Kennedy, C. R. J., Breyer, R. M., and Raisz, L. G. (2000). Knockout of the murine prostaglandin EP_2 receptor impairs osteoclastogenesis *in vitro. Endocrinology* **141**, 2054–2061.

Liu, X. H., Kirschenbaum, A., Lu, M., Yao, S., Klausner, A., Preston, C., Holland, J. F., and Levine, A. C. (2002). Prostaglandin E_2 stimulates prostatic intraepithelial neoplasia cell growth through activation of the interleukin-6/gp130/STAT-3 signaling pathway. *Biochem. Biophys. Res. Commun.* **290**, 249–255.

Liu, X. H., Kirshenbaum, A., Yao, S., and Levine, A. C. (2005). Cross-talk between the interleukin-6 and prostaglandin E_2 signaling system results in enhancement of osteo-clastogenesis through effects on the OPG/RANKL/RANK system. *Endocrinology* **146**, 1991–1998.

Lowe, C., Cornish, J., Callon, K., Martin, T. J., and Reid, L. R. (1991). Regulation of osteoblast proliferation by leukemia inhibitory factor. *J. Bone Miner. Res.* **6**, 1277–1283.

Lowik, C. W., van der Pluijm, G., Bloys, H., Hoekman, K., Bijvoet, O. L. M., Aarden, L. A., and Papapoulos, S. A. (1989). Parathyroid hormone (PTH) and PTH- like protein (PLP) stimulate interleukin-6 production by osteogenic cells: A possible role of interleukin-6 in osteoclastogenesis. *Biochem. Biophys. Res. Commun.* **162**, 1546–1552.

Ludwig, H., Nachbaur, D. M., Fritz, E., Krainer, M., and Huber, H. (1991). Interleukin-6 is a prognostic factor in multiple myeloma. *Blood* **77**, 2794–2795.

Malik, N., Haugen, H. S., Modrell, B., Shoyab, M., and Clegg, C. (1995). Development abnormalities in mice. *Mol. Cell Biol.* **15**, 2349–2358.

Manolagas, S. C. (1998). The role of IL-6 type cytokines and their receptors in bone. *Ann. N. Y. Acad. Sci.* **840**, 194–204.

Manolagas, S. C., and Jilka, R. L. (1995). Bone marrow, cytokines, and bone remodeling: Emerging insights into the pathophysiology of osteoprosis. *N. Engl. J. Med.* **332**, 305.

Martin, T. J., Romas, E., and Gillespie, M. T. (1998). Interleukins in the control of osteoclast differentiation. *Crit. Rev. Eukary. Gene Expression* **8**, 107.

McCoy, J. M., Wicks, J. R., and Audoly, L. P. (2002). The role of prostaglandin E_2 receptors in the pathogenesis of rheumatoid arthritis. *J. Clin. Invest.* **110**, 651–658.

Metcalf, D., and Gearing, G. P. (1989). Fatal syndrome in mice engrafted with cells producing high levels of the leukemia inhibitory factor. *Proc. Natl. Acad. Sci. USA* **86**, 5948–5952.

Miyaura, C., Inada, M., Suzawa, T., Sugimoto, Y., Ushikubi, F., Ichikawa, A., Narumiya, S., and Suda, T. (2000). Impaired bone resorption to PGE_2 in prosta-glandin E receptor EP_4-knockout mice. *J. Biol. Chem.* **275**, 19819–19823.

Nakagawa, N., Kinosaki, M., Yamaguchi, K., Shima, N., Yasuda, H., Yano, K., Morinaga, T., and Higashio, K. (1998). RANK is the essential signaling receptor for osteoclast differention factor in osteoclastogenesis. *Biochem. Biophys. Res. Commun.* **253**, 395–400.

Nakashima, T., Kobayashi, Y., Yamasaki, S., Kawakami, A., Eguchi, K., Sasaki, H., and Sakai, H. (2000). Protein expression and functional difference of membrane-bound and soluble receptor activator of NF-κB ligand: Modulation of the expression by osteotropic factors and cytokines. *Biochem. Biophys. Res. Commun.* **275**, 768–775.

Ni, Z., Lou, W., Leman, E. S., and Gao, A. C. (2000). Inhibition of constitutively activated Stat-3 signaling pathway suppresses growth of prostate cancer cells. *Cancer Res.* **60**, 1225–1228.

O'Brien, C. A., Lin, S. C., Bellido, T., and Manolagas, S. C. (2000). Expression levels of gp130 in bone marrow stromal cells determine the magnitude of osteo-clastogenic signals generated by IL-6-type cytokines. *J. Cell. Biochem.* **79**, 532–549.

Ohlsson, C., Bengtsson, B. A., Isakasson, O. G., Andreassen, T. T., and Slootweg, M. C. (1998). Growth hormone and bone. *Endocr. Rev.* **19**, 55–79.

Okada, Y., Lorenzo, J. A., Freeman, A. M., Tomita, M., Morham, S. G., Raisz, L.G, and Pilbeam, C. C. (2000). COX-2 is required for maximal formation of osteoclast-like cells in culture. *J. Clin. Invest.* **105**, 823–832.

Ono, K., Akatsu, T., Murakami, T., Kitamura, R., Yamamoto, M., Rokutanda, M., Nagata, N., and Kugai, N. (2002). Involvement of cyclooxygenase-2 in osteoclast formation and bone destruction in bone metastasis of mammary carcinoma cell lines. *J. Bone Miner. Res.* **17**, 774–781.

Otsuka, T., Thacker, J. D., and Hogge, D. E. (1991). The effects of interleukin-6 and interleukin-3 on early hemotopoietic events in long-term cultures of human bone marrow. *Exp. Hematol.* **19**, 1042–1048.

Poli, V., Balena, R., Fattori, E., Markatos, A., Yamamoto, M., Tanake, H., Ciliberto, G., Rodan, G. A., and Costantini, F. (1994). IL-6 deficient mice are protected from bone loss caused by estrogen depletion. *EMBO J.* **13**, 1189–1196.

Ragab, A. A., Nalepka, J. L., Bi, Y., and Greenfield, E. M. (2002). Cytokines synergistically induce osteoclast differentiation: Support by immortalized or normal calvarial cells. *Am. J. Physiol. Cell Physiol.* **283**, C679–C687.

Roodman, G. D. (1996). Advances in bone biology: The osteoclast. *Endocr. Rev.* **17**, 308–332.

Rozen, N., Ish-Shalom, S., Rachmiel, A., Stein, H., and Lewinson, D. (2000). IL-6 modulates trabecular and endochondral bone turnover in the nude mouse by stimulating osteoclast differentiation. *Bone* **26**, 469–474.

Simonet, W. S., and Luthy, R. (1997). OPG: A novel secreted protein involved in the regulation of bone density. *Cell* **89**, 309–319.

Sims, N. A., Jenkins, B. J., Quinn, J. M., Nakamura, A., Glatt, M., Gillespie, M. T., Ernst, M., and Martin, T. J. (2004). Glycoprotein 130 regulates bone turnover and bone size by distinct downstream signaling pathways. *J. Clin. Invest.* **113**, 379–389.

Stahl, N., Farruggella, T. J., Boulton, T. G., Zhong, Z., Darnell, J. E., Jr., and Yancopoulos, G. D. (1995). Choice of STATs and other substrates specified by modular tyrosin-based motifs in cytokine receptors. *Science* **267**, 1349–1353.

Steeve, K. T., Marc, P., Sandrine, T., Heymann, D., and Yannick, F. (2004). IL-6, RANKL, TNFα/IL-1: Interactions in bone resorption pathophysiology. *Cytokines Growth Factor Rev.* **15**, 49–60.

Suda, T., Takahashi, N., Udagawa, E., Jimi, M. T., and Martin, T. J. (1999). Modulation of osteoclast differentiation and function by the new members of the TNF receptor and ligand families. *Endocr. Rev.* **20**, 345–357.

Sugiyama, T. (2001). Involvement of interleukin-6 and prostaglandin E_2 in periarticular osteoporosis of postmenopausal woman with rheumatoid arthritis. *J. Bone Miner. Metab.* **19**, 89–96.

Suponitzky, I., and Weinreb, M. (1998). Differential effects of systemic PGE_2 on bone mass in rat long bones and calvariae. *J. Endocrinol.* **156**, 51–57.

Taga, T., and Kishimoto, T. (1997). gp130 and the interleukin 6 family of cytokines. *Annu. Rev. Immunol.* **15**, 797–819.

Tagochi, Y., Yamamoto, M., Yamate, T., Lin, S. C., Mocharla, H., DeTogni, P., Nakayama, N., Boyce, B. F., Abe, E., and Manolagas, S. C. (1998). Interleukin-6-type cytokines stimulate meshenchymal progenitor differentiation toward the osteoblastic lineage. *Proc. Assoc. Am. Physicians.* **110**, 559–574.

Tarura, T., Udagawa, N., Takahashi, N., Miyaura, C., Tanaka, S., and Yamada, Y. (1993). Soluble IL-6 receptor triggers osteoclast formation by IL-6. *Proc. Natl. Acad. Sci. USA* **90**, 11924–11928.

Udagawa, N., Takahashi, N., Katagiri, T., Tamura, T., Wada, S., Findlay, D. M., Martin, T. J., Hirota, H., Taga, T., Kishimoto, T., and Suda, T. (1995). IL-6 induction of osteoclast differentiation depends on IL-6 receptors expressed on osteoblastic cells but not on osteoclast progenitors. *J. Exp. Med.* **182,** 1461–1468.

Verbruggen, A., De Clerck, L. S., Bridts, C. H., van Offel, J. F., and Stevens, W. J. (1999). Flow cytometric determination of interleukin-1β, interleukin-6 and tumor necrosis factor-α in monocytes of rheumatoid arthritis patients: Relation with parameters of osteoporosis. *Cytokines* **11,** 869–874.

Yasuda, H., Shima, N., Nakagawa, N., Yamaguchi, K., Kinosaki, M., Mochizuki, S., Tomoyasu, A., Yano, K., Goto, M., Murakami, A., Tsuda, E., Morinaga, T., *et al.* (1998). Osteoclast differentiation factor is a ligand for OPG/osteoclastogenesis-inhibitory factor and is identical to TRANCE/RANKL. *Proc. Natl. Acad. Sci. USA* **95,** 3597–3602.

Zhang, X., Morham, S. G., Langenbach, R., Young, D. A., Xing, L., Boyce, B. F., Puzas, E. J., Rosier, R. N., O'Keefe, R. J., and Schwarz, E. M. (2001). Evidence for a direct role of cyclooxygenase-2 in implant wear debris induced osteolysis. *J. Bone Miner. Res.* **16,** 660–669.

Zhang, X., Schwarz, E. M., Young, D. A., Puzas, J., Rosier, R. N., and O'Keefe, R. J. (2002). Cyclooxygenase-2 regulates mesenchymal cell differentiation into the osteoblast lineage and is critically involved in bone repair. *J. Clin. Invest.* **109,** 1405–1415.

15

REGULATION OF OSTEOCLAST DIFFERENTIATION AND FUNCTION BY INTERLEUKIN-1

ICHIRO NAKAMURA* AND EIJIRO JIMI[†]

*Department of Rheumatology, Yugawara Kosei-Nenkin Hospital
Ashigara-shimo, Kanagawa 259-0314, Japan
[†]Department of Bioscience, Division of Molecular Biochemistry
Kyushu Dental College, Kita-Kyushu, Fukuoka 803-8580, Japan

Interleukin-1 (IL-1) is a multifunctional cytokine that regulates various cellular and tissue functions. Among tissues, bone is the most sensitive to IL-1. IL-1 is a potent cytokine for bone resorption and participates in the multiple steps of osteoclast recruitment, such as differentiation,

multinucleation, activation, and survival. On the other hand, considerable evidence has been accumulated over the past 10 years to indicate
that this cytokine plays key roles in pathological bone destruction in a
variety of human diseases, including rheumatoid arthritis, osteoporosis,
and periodontal disease. In this chapter, we review the history of "IL-1
in bone" and the locus of this cytokine "from laboratory bench to
bedside." A better understanding of the role of IL-1 in osteoclastic bone
resorption would provide opportunities for developing new therapeutics
to treat diseases of the bone. © 2006 Elsevier Inc.

I. INTRODUCTION

Osteoclasts are terminally differentiated multinucleated cells that are
responsible for bone resorption (Nakamura et al., 2003; Suda et al., 1999;
Teitelbaum, 2000). They are the principal, if not exclusive, resorptive cell of
bone, playing a central role in the formation of the skeleton and regulation
of its mass. Osteoclastic bone resorption consists of multiple steps: the proliferation of osteoclast progenitors, differentiation of progenitors into mononuclear prefusion osteoclasts (pOCs), fusion of pOCs into multinucleated
osteoclasts, clear zone (actin ring) and ruffled border formation (activation),
and apoptosis. Findings indicate that several cytokines and hormones including macrophage colony-stimulating factor (M-CSF, also called CSF-1)
(Fuller et al., 1993; Yoshida et al., 1990), interleukin-1 (IL-1) (Jimi et al., 1995,
1999a), receptor activator of NF-κB ligand (RANKL) (Jimi et al., 1999b;
Lacey et al., 1998; Yasuda et al., 1998), and tumor necrosis factor-α (TNF-α)
(Kim et al., 2005; Kobayashi et al., 2000) regulate differentiation, activation,
and survival of osteoclasts.

IL-1 is a multifunctional cytokine that regulates various cellular and tissue
functions (Dinarello, 1994). This cytokine refers to two polypeptides, IL-1α
and IL-1β. Although IL-1α and IL-1β are independent gene products, they
recognize the same cell-surface receptors (type I and type II) and elicit similar
biological responses through the type I receptor (Dinarello, 1994). A natural
inhibitor to IL-1 has been identified (Arend et al., 1990; Dinarello, 1994).
This peptide, IL-1 receptor antagonist (IL-1Ra) is a naturally occurring
structure variant of IL-1 that binds to, but does not activate, IL-1 receptors.
Among the tissues, bone is most sensitive to IL-1. Historically, activated
monocytes/macrophages were shown to produce a potent bone-resorbing
factor initially termed "osteoclast-activating factor (OAF)" (Gowen et al.,
1983), and this factor was later identified as IL-1β (Dewhirst et al., 1985).
In the 1980s, several lines of evidence demonstrated that IL-1 exhibits
potent bone-resorbing activity in in vitro organ cultures (Gowen et al., 1984;

Lorenzo *et al.*, 1987). In the opposite way, IL-1Ra blocks the ability of IL-1 to stimulate bone resorption in organ cultures (Seckinger *et al.*, 1990). IL-1 also stimulates bone resorption when infused *in vivo* and causes a substantial increase in plasma calcium levels (Boyce *et al.*, 1989; Sabatini *et al.*, 1988). At the cellular level, IL-1 participates in the multiple steps of osteoclastic bone resorption, such as differentiation, multinucleation, activation, and survival. IL-1 also plays critical roles in the pathological bone destruction associated with multiple myeloma, rheumatoid arthritis, and osteoporosis (Dinarello, 1994). Here, we discuss the involvement of IL-1 in osteoclast differentiation and function, mainly from the viewpoint of osteoclast cell biology.

II. INTERLEUKIN-1 AND OSTEOCLAST DIFFERENTIATION

The molecular events involved in the differentiation and activation of osteoclasts had not been clarified until recently due to the lack of suitable *in vitro* models to investigate osteoclast biology. However, the development of reliable methods to isolate and culture large number of primary osteoclasts or to generate osteoclasts in *in vitro* culture systems allowed remarkable progress in the field of osteoclast research over the course of the last decade. Takahashi *et al.* (1988) developed an excellent *in vitro* culture system of osteoclast differentiation, so-called "Takahashi's coculture system," in which mouse osteoblastic cells and spleen cells were cocultured in presence of osteotropic factors, such as $1\alpha,25$-dihydroxyvitamin D_3 [$1\alpha,25(OH)_2D_3$] and prostaglandin E_2 (PGE_2). This murine coculture system has made it possible to investigate the molecular mechanism of osteoclast differentiation, finally leading to the historic discovery of RANKL, the master molecule for osteoclast differentiation (Lacey *et al.*, 1998; Yasuda *et al.*, 1998). It is now a well-established concept that various osteotropic factors, such as $1\alpha,25(OH)_2D_3$, PGE_2, parathyroid hormone (PTH), and IL-11 induce RANKL expression on the surface of osteoblasts/stromal cells, leading to the differentiation of hematopoietic cells into osteoclasts (Suda *et al.*, 1999).

The involvement of IL-1 in osteoclast differentiation was analyzed using this murine coculture system. Akatsu *et al.* (1991) clearly demonstrated that IL-1 stimulated osteoclast formation not directly but indirectly via PGE_2 synthesis in cocultures of murine osteoblastic cells and spleen cells. However, in terms of the multinucleation of osteoclasts, IL-1 plays a direct role. Using the culture system of purified pOCs established by Wesolowski *et al.* (1995), we reported that IL-1 induces the fusion of mononuclear prefusion osteoclasts (Jimi *et al.*, 1999a). In this sense, IL-1 is indirectly involved in osteoclast differentiation and directly involved in osteoclast multinucleation (Fig. 1). On the other hand, M-CSF, RANKL, and TNF-α among

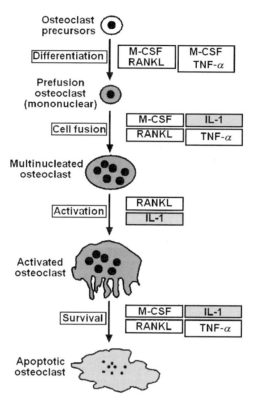

FIGURE 1. The differentiation and activation pathway of osteoclast progenitors into functionally active osteoclasts and the cytokines required for each step.

other related cytokines, have been demonstrated to play essential roles in osteoclast differentiation (Kobayashi *et al.*, 2000; Kong *et al.*, 1999; Yoshida *et al.*, 1990) and induce cell fusion of osteoclasts (Amano *et al.*, 1998; Jimi *et al.*, 1999a,b) (Fig. 1).

III. INTERLEUKIN-1 AND OSTEOCLAST ACTIVATION

A. MECHANISM OF ACTION OF IL-1 IN OSTEOCLAST ACTIVATION AT THE CELLULAR LEVEL

The most important involvement of IL-1 in osteoclasts is the activation of the bone-resorbing activity of these cells. Thomson *et al.* (1986) first reported that IL-1 stimulated the pit-forming activity of isolated rat osteoclasts. They showed that this effect of IL-1 was not due to a direct action of the cytokine,

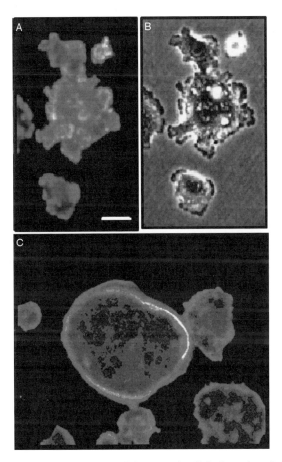

FIGURE 2. Effects of IL-1 on cytoskeleton and cell fusion of prefusion osteoclasts. Prefusion osteoclasts were plated on vitronectin (20 μg/ml)-coated dishes in the absence of serum. After culture for 60 min, cells were treated with IL-1 (10 ng/ml) for 0 (A, B) and 30 (C) min. Cells were fixed and stained for tartrate-resistant acid phosphatase (B) or F-actin (A, C). Note that IL-1 induces actin ring formation and the multinucleation of osteoclasts. Bar = 10 μm (See Color Insert.)

but was mediated by soluble factor(s) secreted by osteoblasts. Nowadays, however, several lines of evidence have clearly demonstrated the expression of IL-1 receptors in mature osteoclasts *in vivo* and *in vitro*, suggesting the direct action of IL-1 on osteoclasts (Jimi *et al.*, 1998; Xu *et al.*, 1996). Activated osteoclasts resorbing bone have a specific ringed organization of F-actin, known as the actin ring, which is now recognized as a marker for osteoclast activation (Lakkakorpi and Väänänen, 1991; Nakamura *et al.*, 1996; Turksen *et al.*, 1988). Using the purified pOC culture system, we have demonstrated that IL-1 directly induces actin ring formation (Fig. 2) and the activation of osteoclasts at the cellular level (Jimi *et al.*, 1999a; Kobayashi *et al.*, 2000, Nakamura *et al.*, 2002).

B. MECHANISM OF ACTION OF IL-1 IN OSTEOCLAST ACTIVATION AT THE MOLECULAR LEVEL

Then, how is IL-1-initiated signaling transduced in osteoclasts, resulting in actin ring formation and bone resorption? The first molecule to be discussed is TRAF6 (Fig. 3). TRAF, TNF receptor-associated factor family proteins, are adaptor molecules that mediate the intracellular signaling of various cytokine receptors, including the TNF receptor superfamily and the Toll/IL-1 receptor family (Inoue *et al.*, 2000). To date, six members of the TRAF family have been identified. TRAF6 is the only TRAF that is involved in the signal from the Toll/IL-1 receptor family by interacting with the IL-1 receptor-associated kinase (IRAK). The essential role of TRAF6 in physiological bone development has now been clarified by the results from TRAF6-deficient mice, in which the osteopetrotic phenotype was observed. According to the report by Lomaga *et al.* (1999), in these mice, abundant dysfunctional osteoclasts were found in their skeletal tissues, which is compatible with the direct involvement of IL-1 in osteoclast activation, but not in osteoclast differentiation. Armstrong *et al.* (2002) confirmed the involvement of TRAF6 in osteoclast activation in *in vitro* cultures. Kim *et al.* (2005) also showed that TRAF6 is essential for osteoclast function, but not for osteoclast differentiation, using cell cultures from TRAF6 null mice.

Another question to be answered is: What is the next molecule for osteoclast activation? Generally, IL-1 enhances various intracellular signal transduction pathways, including NF-κB activation, ERK activation, and so forth. The interesting aspect was the similar phenotype of TRAF6-deficient

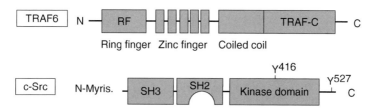

FIGURE 3. Structural features of c-Src and TRAF6. Src kinase contains a unique N-terminal region, an SH3 (Src-homology-3) domain that binds to proline-rich motifs, an SH2 domain that binds to phosphotyrosine-containing motifs, a kinase domain, and a C-regulatory sequence that is phosphorylated by the Csk protein-tyrosine kinase. Domains within TRAF6 include ring finger (RF), zinc finger, coiled coil, and TRAF-C domains. The direct interaction of TRAF6 and c-Src is mediated by the RPTIPRNPK motif (aa 469–477) in TRAF6 and the SH3 domain in c-Src.

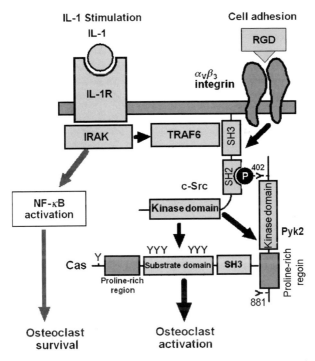

FIGURE 4. Our proposed model of IL-1-induced signaling pathways in osteoclasts. Osteoclast adhesion via $\alpha_V\beta_3$ integrin induces c-Src-dependent tyrosine phosphorylation of Pyk2 and p130^{Cas}, leading to the cytoskeletal organization of osteoclasts. IL-1 signaling cross talks with this tyrosine phosphorylation pathway via the association of TRAF6 with c-Src, leading to the formation of a huge molecular complex including TRAF6, c-Src, Pyk2, and p130^{Cas}, and results in osteoclast activation. On the other hand, IL-1-induced NF-κB activation plays an important role in osteoclast survival.

mice to that of c-Src-deficient mice. c-*src* was first identified as the normal cellular counterpart of the oncogene encoded by Rous sarcoma virus, v-*src* (Thomas and Brugge, 1997). The protooncogene product c-Src is a 60-kDa protein and belongs to the nonreceptor-type tyrosine kinase family, the structural feature of which is shown in Fig. 3. Soriano *et al.* (1991) reported that the targeted disruption of c-*src* in mice induced osteopetrosis. The absence of c-Src is sufficient to abolish bone resorption *in vivo,* without reducing the osteoclast number (Boyce *et al.*, 1992), suggesting that c-Src plays an essential role in osteoclast activation. The similarity of these two knockout mice suggests that both c-Src and TRAF6 have some mutual relationship in osteoclast function. In fact, we found that IL-1 stimulation induced the activation of c-Src kinase, tyrosine phosphorylation of Pyk2 and p130^{Cas}, the substrates of c-Src (Duong *et al.*, 1998; Nakamura *et al.*, 1998), and the formation of a huge molecular complex, including TRAF6, c-Src, Pyk2, and p130^{Cas}, resulting in the actin ring formation and osteoclast activation (Nakamura *et al.*, 2002). In Src$^{-/-}$ osteoclasts, IL-1 did not induce the tyrosine phosphorylation of Pyk2 and p130^{Cas} and did not rescue the bone-resorbing activity of Src$^{-/-}$ osteoclasts, suggesting the functional interaction of TRAF6 and c-Src (Nakamura *et al.*, 2002). Wong *et al.* (1999) also reported the association of TRAF6 and c-Src in the signal transduction pathway of RANKL, which led to the activation of Akt/PKB and osteoclast survival. According to their report, the direct interaction of TRAF6 and c-Src is mediated by the RPTIPRNPK motif (aa 469–477) in TRAF6 and the SH3 domain in c-Src. The molecular mechanism of action of IL-1 in osteoclast activation is proposed in Fig. 4.

Several findings retorting against the concept mentioned earlier were also reported. Naito *et al.* (1999) reported that TRAF6 was an essential transducer for osteoclast differentiation, since their TRAF6$^{-/-}$ mice were defective in osteoclast formation and exhibited severe osteopetrosis. Miyazaki *et al.* (2000) reported that NF-κB activation plays a key role in IL-1-induced osteoclast function, using adenovirus vectors carrying dominant negative IκB kinase 2 (IKK2) and constitutively active IKK2. Further studies will be required to explain this discrepancy. On the other hand, among the other related cytokines, RANKL is also involved in osteoclast function (Burgess *et al.*, 1999; Jimi *et al.*, 1999b), although neither M-CSF nor TNF-α can induce actin ring formation and osteoclast activation (Jimi *et al.*, 1999a; Kim *et al.*, 2005) (Fig. 1).

IV. INTERLEUKIN-1 AND OSTEOCLAST SURVIVAL

Another important involvement of IL-1 in bone resorption is the survival of osteoclasts. When osteoclasts were purified by removing osteoblasts from cocultures, osteoclasts rapidly died within 48 h due to spontaneously occurring apoptosis. The addition of IL-1 to the purified osteoclasts prolonged the survival of these cells (Jimi *et al.*, 1995). Thus, IL-1 is involved in prolonging the lifespan of osteoclasts as well as in the activation of osteoclasts. Besides IL-1, M-CSF (Fuller *et al.*, 1993), RANKL (Jimi *et al.*, 1999b), and TNF-α (unpublished observation) also induce osteoclast survival (Fig. 1).

Although the involvement of IL-1 in osteoclast survival at the cellular level is now well accepted, its molecular mechanism still remains to be discussed. We have shown that IL-1 activated NF-κB in osteoclasts and that the activation of NF-κB is involved in the survival of osteoclasts, using antisense oligodeoxynucleotides to NF-κB (Rel A/p65 and p50) and proteasome inhibitors (Jimi *et al.*, 1996, 1998). On the other hand, M-CSF, another survival factor of osteoclasts, does not activate NF-κB in osteoclasts (Jimi *et al.*, 1996), indicating that some signals other than NF-κB should be involved in the survival of osteoclasts due to M-CSF. As pointed out by Miyazaki *et al.* (2000), ERK is a candidate molecule for M-CSF-induced osteoclast survival. Akiyama *et al.* (2003) also reported that the proapoptotic BH3-only Bcl-2 family member Bim is critical for controlling osteoclast survival and apoptosis. In spite of distinct pathways for IL-1- and M-CSF-induced cell survival, there must be a common downstream pathway in these signals. In this sense, Okahashi *et al.* (1998) reported that both IL-1 and M-CSF reduce caspase activity, which is known to induce apoptosis in osteoclasts.

There are several reports retorting against our findings. Lee *et al.* (2002) showed the IL-1α-stimulated osteoclast survival through the PI 3-kinase/Akt and ERK pathways. Miyazaki *et al.* (2000) also demonstrated that ERK activation plays a key role in IL-1-induced osteoclast survival, using adenovirus vectors carrying dominant negative Ras and constitutively active MEK1. Further studies are necessary to elucidate the precise role of NF-κB-mediated signals in osteoclast activation and survival.

V. INTERLEUKIN-1 AND RHEUMATOID ARTHRITIS

Considerable evidence has accumulated over the past 10 years to indicate that IL-1 mediates inflammation and pathological bone destruction in a variety of human diseases associated with multiple myeloma, rheumatoid arthritis (RA), osteoporosis, and periodontal disease. Pacifici's group reported that IL-1 is implicated as a potential mediator of bone resorption and increased bone turnover in postmenopausal osteoporosis (Pacifici *et al.*, 1989) and that the *in vivo* administration of IL-1Ra inhibited the bone loss that occurs in ovariectomized rats (Kimble *et al.*, 1994).

On the other hand, one of the most-studied diseases is RA. Eastgate *et al.* (1988) first demonstrated the correlation of plasma IL-1 levels with disease activity in RA. The important involvement of IL-1 in RA has been further confirmed by the results of studies on mice that are genetically engineered to overproduce IL-1Ra (transgenic mice) or those that lack the capacity to make any isoforms of IL-1Ra (knockout mice). Collagen-induced arthritis in mice was reduced in incidence and severity in IL-1Ra transgenic mice, whereas the opposite pattern was observed in IL-1Ra-deficient mice (Ma *et al.*, 1998). Another report showed that IL-1Ra-deficietnt mice, when crossed into the BALB/cA background, spontaneously developed an inflammatory arthritis that exhibited many features of RA (Horai *et al.*, 2000). Moreover, there is the increasing evidence that the ratio of IL-1Ra and IL-1 may be under genetic control and may influence the development or severity of certain disease. Actually, a possible association between polymorphisms in the IL-1Ra gene and various rheumatic diseases has been studied

(Barrera *et al.*, 2001; Cantagrel *et al.*, 1999; Cvetkovic *et al.*, 2002; Genevay *et al.*, 2002; Perrier *et al.*, 1998).

These numerous studies at the genetic, molecular, cellular, and *in vivo* (animal model) levels have indicated that the exogenous administration of IL-1Ra might be therapeutically beneficial for RA. Clinical trials in RA examining the administration of recombinant human IL-1Ra by subcutaneous injection have yielded positive results. A total of 472 patients with active and severe RA were studied in a 24-week, double-blind, randomized, placebo-controlled, multicentered clinical trial (Bresnihan *et al.*, 1998). In patients treated with the highest dose of IL-1Ra (a single daily subcutaneous injection of IL-1Ra at 150 mg), 43% achieved an American College of Rheumatology (ACR) 20 response, compared with 27% in the placebo group. In addition, the IL-1Ra-treated group overall demonstrated a lower rate of radiological progression over 48 weeks (Jiang *et al.*, 2000). Histological studies on serial synovial biopsies revealed a reduction in mononuclear cell infiltration in four patients with a favorable clinical response (Cunnane *et al.*, 2001). This therapy with IL-1Ra has now been approved by the regulatory agencies in the United States and Europe.

VI. PROSPECTS

In the near future, studies of "IL-1 in bone" should be focused on the precise molecular mechanism of action of this cytokine in osteoclast activation. Especially, in terms of the role of NF-κB in osteoclast function, molecular biology studies and the analysis of other knockout mice would allow us to achieve a more precise understanding of the intracellular function of this molecule. In the long term, these continuous trials for the better understanding of osteoclast biology would lead to the availability of new therapeutic agents to treat diseases of bone.

REFERENCES

Akatsu, T., Takahashi, N., Udagawa, N., Imamura, K., Yamaguchi, A., Sato, K., Nagata, N., and Suda, T. (1991). Role of prostaglandins in interleukin-1-induced bone resorption in mice *in vitro*. *J. Bone Miner. Res.* **6**, 183–190.

Akiyama, T., Bouillet, P., Miyazaki, T., Kadono, Y., Chikuda, H., Chung, U. I., Fukuda, A., Hikita, A., Seto, H., Okada, T., Inaba, T., Sanjay, A., *et al.* (2003). Regulation of osteoclast apoptosis by ubiquitylation of proapoptotic BH3-only Bcl-2 family member Bim. *EMBO J.* **22**, 6653–6664.

Amano, H., Yamada, S., and Felix, R. (1998). Colony-stimulating factor-1 stimulates the fusion process in osteoclasts. *J. Bone Miner. Res.* **13**, 846–853.

Arend, W. P., Welgus, H. G., Thompson, R. C., and Eisenberg, S. P. (1990). Biological properties of recombinant human monocyte-derived interleukin 1 receptor antagonist. *J. Clin. Invest.* **85**, 1694–1697.

Armstrong, A. P., Tometsko, M. E., Glaccum, M., Sutherland, C. L., Cosman, D., and Dougall, W. C. (2002). A RANK/TRAF6-dependent signal transduction pathway is essential for osteoclast cytoskeletal organization and resorptive function. *J. Biol. Chem.* **277**, 44347–44356.

Barrera, P., Faure, S., Prud'homme, J. F., Balsa, A., Migliorini, P., Chimenti, D., Radstake, T. R., van de Putte, L. B., Pascual-Salcedo, D., Westhovens, R., Maenaut, K., Alves, H., *et al.*, European Consortium on Rheumatoid Arthritis Families (ECRAF) (2001). European genetic study on rheumatoid arthritis: Is there a linkage of the interleukin-1 (IL-1), IL-10 or IL-4 genes to RA? *Clin. Exp. Rheumatol.* **19**, 709–714.

Boyce, B. F., Aufdemorte, T. B., Garrett, I. R., Yates, A. J. P., and Mundy, G. R. (1989). Effects of interleukin-1 on bone turnover in normal mice. *Endocrinology* **125**, 1142–1150.

Boyce, B. F., Yoneda, T., Lowe, C., Soriano, P., and Mundy, G. R. (1992). Requirement of pp60$^{c\text{-}src}$ expression for osteoclasts to form ruffled border and resorb bone in mice. *J. Clin. Invest.* **90**, 1622–1627.

Bresnihan, B., Alvaro-Gracia, J. M., Cobby, M., Doherty, M., Domljan, Z., Emery, P., Nuki, G., Pavelka, K., Rau, R., Rozman, B., Watt, I., Williams, B., *et al.* (1998). Treatment of rheumatoid arthritis with recombinant human interleukin-1 receptor antagonist. *Arthritis Rheum.* **41**, 2196–2204.

Burgess, T. L., Qian, Y., Kaufman, S., Ring, B. D., Van, G., Capparelli, C., Kelley, M., Hsu, H., Boyle, W. J., Dunstan, C. R., Hu, S., and Lacey, D. L. (1999). The ligand for osteoprotegerin (OPGL) directly activates mature osteoclasts. *J. Cell Biol.* **145**, 527–538.

Cantagrel, A., Navaux, F., Loubet-Lescoulie, P., Nourhashemi, F., Enault, G., Abbal, M., Constantin, A., Laroche, M., and Mazieres, B. (1999). Interleukin-1 beta, interleukin-1 receptor antagonist, interleukin-4, and interleukin-10 gene polymorphisms: Relationship to occurrence and severity of rheumatoid arthritis. *Arthritis Rheum.* **42**, 1093–1100.

Cunnane, G., Madigan, A., Murphy, E., FitzGerald, O., and Bresnihan, B. (2001). The effects of treatment with interleukin-1 receptor antagonist on the inflamed synovial membrane in rheumatoid arthritis. *Rheumatology (Oxford)* **40**, 62–69.

Cvetkovic, J. T., Wallberg-Jonsson, S., Stegmayr, B., Rantapaa-Dahlqvist, S., and Lefvert, A. K. (2002). Susceptibility for and clinical manifestations of rheumatoid arthritis are associated with polymorphisms of the TNF-alpha, IL-1beta, and IL-1Ra genes. *J. Rheumatol.* **29**, 212–219.

Dewhirst, F. E., Stashenko, P. P., Mole, J. E., and Tsurumachi, T. (1985). Purification and partial sequence of human osteoclast-activating factor: Identity with interleukin 1β. *J. Immunol.* **135**, 2562–2568.

Dinarello, C. A. (1994). The interleukin-1 family: 10 years of discovery. *FASEB J.* **8**, 1314–1325.

Duong, L. T., Lakkakorpi, P. T., Nakamura, I., Machwate, M., Nagy, R. M., and Rodan, G. A. (1998). PYK2 in osteoclasts is an adhesion kinase, localized in the sealing zone, activated by $\alpha v \beta 3$ integrin, and associated with SRC kinase. *J. Clin. Invest.* **102**, 881–892.

Eastgate, J. A., Symons, J. A., Wood, N. C., Grinlinton, F. M., di Giovine, F. S., and Duff, G. W. (1988). Correlation of plasma interleukin 1 levels with disease activity in rheumatoid arthritis. *Lancet* **8613**, 706–709.

Fuller, K., Owens, J. M., Jagger, C. J., Wilson, A., Moss, R., and Chambers, T. J. (1993). Macrophage colony-stimulating factor stimulates survival and chemotactic behavior in isolated osteoclasts. *J. Exp. Med.* **178**, 1733–1744.

Genevay, S., Di Giovine, F. S., Perneger, T. V., Silvestri, T., Stingelin, S., Duff, G., and Guerne, P. A. (2002). Association of interleukin-4 and interleukin-1B gene variants with Larsen score progression in rheumatoid arthritis. *Arthritis Rheum.* **47**, 303–309.

Gowen, M., Wood, D. D., Ihrie, E. J., Mcguire, M. K. B., and Russell, R. G. G. (1983). An interleukin 1 like factor stimulates bone resorption *in vitro*. *Nature* **306**, 378–380.

Gowen, M., Wood, D. D., Ihrie, E. J., Meats, J. E., and Russell, R. G. (1984). Stimulation by human interleukin 1 of cartilage breakdown and production of collagenase and proteoglycanase by human chondrocytes but not by human osteoblasts *in vitro. Biochim. Biophys. Acta* **797**, 186–193.

Horai, R., Saijo, S., Tanioka, H., Nakae, S., Sudo, K., Okahara, A., Ikuse, T., Asano, M., and Iwakura, Y. (2000). Development of chronic inflammatory arthropathy resembling rheumatoid arthritis in interleukin 1 receptor antagonist-deficient mice. *J. Exp. Med.* **191**, 313–320.

Inoue, J., Ishida, T., Tsukamoto, N., Kobayashi, N., Naito, A., Azuma, S., and Yamamoto, T. (2000). Tumor necrosis factor receptor-associated factor (TRAF) family: Adaptor proteins that mediate cytokine signaling. *Exp. Cell Res.* **254**, 14–24.

Jiang, Y., Genant, H. K., Watt, I., Cobby, M., Bresnihan, B., Aitchison, R., and McCabe, D. (2000). A multicenter, double-blind, dose-ranging, randomized, placebo-controlled study of recombinant human interleukin-1 receptor antagonist in patients with rheumatoid arthritis: Radiologic progression and correlation of Genant and Larsen scores. *Arthritis Rheum.* **43**, 1001–1009.

Jimi, E., Shuto, T., and Koga, T. (1995). Macrophage colony-stimulating factor and interleukin-1α maintain the survival of osteoclast-like cells. *Endocrinology* **136**, 808–811.

Jimi, E., Ikebe, T., Takahashi, N., Hirata, M., Suda, T., and Koga, T. (1996). Interleukin-1 activates an NF-κB-like factor in osteoclast-like cells. *J. Biol. Chem.* **271**, 4605–4608.

Jimi, E., Nakamura, I., Ikebe, T., Akiyama, S., Takahashi, N., and Suda, T. (1998). Activation of NF-κB is involved in the survival of osteoclasts promoted by interleukin-1. *J. Biol. Chem.* **273**, 8799–8805.

Jimi, E., Nakamura, I., Duong, L. T., Ikebe, T., Takahashi, N., Rodan, G. A., and Suda, T. (1999a). Interleukin 1 induces multinucleation and bone-resorbing activity of osteoclasts in the absence of osteoblasts/stromal cells. *Exp. Cell Res.* **247**, 84–93.

Jimi, E., Akiyama, S., Tsurukai, T., Okahashi, N., Kobayashi, K., Udagawa, N., Nishihara, T., Takahashi, N., and Suda, T. (1999b). Osteoclast differentiation factor acts as a multifunctional regulator in murine osteoclast differentiation and function. *J. Immunol.* **163**, 434–442.

Kim, N., Kadono, Y., Takami, M., Lee, J., Lee, S. H., Okada, F., Kim, J. H., Kobayashi, T., Odgren, P. R., Nakano, H., Yeh, W. C., Lee, S. K., *et al.* (2005). Osteoclast differentiation independent of the TRANCE-RANK-TRAF6 axis. *J. Exp. Med.* **202**, 589–595.

Kimble, R. B., Vannice, J. L., Bloedow, D. C., Thompson, R. C., Hopfer, W., Kung, V. T., Brownfield, C., and Pacifici, R. (1994). Interleukin-1 receptor antagonist decreases bone loss and bone resorption in ovariectomized rats. *J. Clin. Invest.* **93**, 1959–1967.

Kobayashi, K., Takahashi, N., Jimi, E., Udagawa, N., Takami, M., Kotake, S., Nakagawa, N., Kinosaki, M., Yamaguchi, K., Shima, N., Yasuda, H., Morinaga, T., *et al.* (2000). Tumor necrosis factor alpha stimulates osteoclast differentiation by a mechanism independent of the ODF/RANKL-RANK interaction. *J. Exp. Med.* **191**, 275–286.

Kong, Y. Y., Yoshida, H., Sarosi, I., Tan, H. L., Timms, E., Capparelli, C., Morony, S., Oliveira-dos-Santos, A. J., Van, G., Itie, A., Khoo, W., Wakeham, A., *et al.* (1999). OPGL is a key regulator of osteoclastogenesis, lymphocyte development and lymph-node organogenesis. *Nature* **397**, 315–323.

Lacey, D. L., Timms, E., Tan, H. L., Kelley, M., Dunstan, C. R., Burgess, T., Elliott, R., Colombero, A., Elliott, G., Scully, S., Hsu, H., Sullivan, J., *et al.* (1998). Osteoprotegerin ligand is a cytokine that regulates osteoclast differentiation and activation. *Cell* **93**, 165–176.

Lakkakorpi, P. T., and Väänänen, H. K. (1991). Kinetics of the osteoclast cytoskeleton during the resorption cycle *in vitro. J. Bone Miner. Res.* **6**, 817–826.

Lee, Z. H., Lee, S. E., Kim, C. W., Lee, S. H., Kim, S. W., Kwack, K., Walsh, K., and Kim, H. H. (2002). IL-1alpha stimulation of osteoclast survival through the PI 3-kinase/Akt and ERK pathways. *J. Biochem. (Tokyo)* **131**, 161–166.

Lomaga, M. A., Yeh, W.-C., Sarosi, I., Duncan, G. S., Furlonger, C., Ho, A., Morony, S., Capparelli, C., Van, G., Kaufman, S., van der Heiden, A., Itie, A., et al. (1999). TRAF6 deficiency results in osteopetrosis and defective interlerkin-1, CD40, and LPS signaling. Genes Dev. 13, 1015–1024.

Lorenzo, J. A., Sousa, S. L., Alender, C., Raisz, L. G., and Dinarello, A. (1987). Comparison of the bone-resorbing activity in the supernatants from phytohemagglutinin-stimulated human peripheral blood mononuclear cells with that of cytokines through the use of an antiserum to interleukin 1. Endocrinology 121, 1164–1170.

Ma, Y., Thornton, S., Boivin, G. P., Hirsh, D., Hirsch, R., and Hirsch, E. (1998). Altered susceptibility to collagen-induced arthritis in transgenic mice with aberrant expression of interleukin-1 receptor antagonist. Arthritis Rheum. 41, 1798–1805.

Miyazaki, T., Katagiri, H., Kanegase, Y., Takayanagi, H., Sawada, Y., Yamamoto, A., Pando, M. P., Asano, T., Verma, I. M., Oda, H., Nakamura, K., and Tanaka, S. (2000). Reciprocal role of ERK and NF-kappaB pathways in survival and activation of osteoclasts. J. Cell. Biol 148, 333–342.

Naito, A., Azuma, S., Tanaka, S., Miyazaki, T., Takaki, S., Takatsu, K., Nakao, K., Nakamura, K., Katsuki, M., Yamamoto, T., and Inoue, J. (1999). Severe osteopetrosis, defective interleukin-1 siganalling and lymph node organogenesis in TRAF6-deficient mice. Genes Cells 4, 353–362.

Nakamura, I., Takahashi, N., Sasaki, T., Jimi, E., Kurokawa, T., and Suda, T. (1996). Chemical and physical properties of the extracellular matrix are required for the actin ring formation in osteoclasts. J. Bone. Miner. Res. 12, 1873–1879.

Nakamura, I., Jimi, E., Duong, L. T., Sasaki, T., Takahashi, N., Rodan, G. A., and Suda, T. (1998). Tyrosine phosphorylation of p130^{Cas} is involved in actin organization in osteoclasts. J. Biol. Chem. 273, 11144–11149.

Nakamura, I., Kadono, Y., Takayanagi, H., Jimi, E., Miyazaki, T., Oda, H., Nakamura, K., Tanaka, S., Rodan, G. A., and Duong, L. T. (2002). IL-1 regulates cytoskeletal organization in osteoclasts via TNF receptor-associated factor 6/c-Src complex. J. Immunol. 168, 5103–5109.

Nakamura, I., Rodan, G. A., and Duong, L. T. (2003). Regulatory mechanism of osteoclast activation. J. Electron Microsc. 52, 527–533.

Okahashi, N., Koide, M., Jimi, E., Suda, T., and Nishihara, T. (1998). Caspases (interleukin-1β converting enzyme family proteases) are involved in the regulation of the survival of osteoclasts. Bone 23, 33–41.

Pacifici, R., Rifas, L., McCracken, R., Vered, I., McMurtry, C., Avioli, L. V., and Peck, W. A. (1989). Ovarian steroid treatment blocks a postmenopausal increase in blood monocyte interleukin 1 release. Proc. Natl. Acad. Sci. USA 86, 2398–2402.

Perrier, S., Coussediere, C., Dubost, J. J., Albuisson, E., and Sauvezie, B. (1998). IL-1 receptor antagonist (IL-1RA) gene polymorphism in Sjogren's syndrome and rheumatoid arthritis. Clin. Immunol. Immunopathol. 87, 309–313.

Sabatini, M., Boyce, B., Aufdemorte, T., Bonewald, L., and Mundy, G. R. (1988). Infusions of recombinant human interleukins 1 alpha and 1 beta cause hypercalcemia in normal mice. Proc. Natl. Acad. Sci. USA 85, 5235–5239.

Seckinger, P., Klein-Nulend, J., Alender, C., Thompson, R. C., Dayer, J.-M., and Raisz, L. G. (1990). Natural and recombinant human IL-1 receptor antagonists block the effects of IL-1 on bone resorption and prostaglandin production. J. Immunol. 145, 4181–4184.

Soriano, P., Montgomery, C., Geske, R., and Bradley, A. (1991). Targeted disruption of the c-src proto-oncogene leads to osteopetrosis in mice. Cell 64, 693–702.

Suda, T., Takahashi, N., Udagawa, N., Jimi, E., Gillespie, M. T., and Martin, T. J. (1999). Modulation of osteoclast differentiation and function by the new members of the tumor necrosis factor receptor and ligand families. Endocr. Rev. 20, 345–357.

Takahashi, N., Akatsu, T., Sasaki, T., Nicholson, G. C., Moseley, J. M., Martin, T. J., and Suda, T. (1988). Induction of calcitonin receptors by $1\alpha,25$-dihydroxyvitamin D_3 in osteoclast-like multinucleated cells formed from mouse bone marrow cells. *Endocrinology* **123**, 1504–1510.

Teitelbaum, S. L. (2000). Bone resorption by osteoclasts. *Science* **289**, 1504–1508.

Thomas, S. M., and Brugge, J. S. (1997). Cellular functions regulated by Src family kinases. *Annu. Rev. Cell Dev. Biol.* **13**, 513–609.

Thomson, B. M., Saklatvala, J., and Chambers, T. J. (1986). Osteoblasts mediate interleukin 1 stimulation of bone resorption by rat osteoclasts. *J. Exp. Med.* **164**, 104–112.

Turksen, K., Kanehisa, J., Opas, M., Heersche, J. N., and Aubin, J. E. (1988). Adhesion patterns and cytoskeleton of rabbit osteoclasts on bone slices and glass. *J. Bone Miner. Res.* **3**, 389–400.

Wesolowski, G., Duong, L. T., Lakkakorpi, P. T., Nagy, R. M., Tezuka, K., Tanaka, H., Rodan, G. A., and Rodan, S. B. (1995). Isolation and characterization of highly enriched, prefusion mouse osteoclastic cells. *Exp. Cell Res.* **219**, 679–686.

Wong, B. R., Besser, D., Kim, N., Arron, J. R., Vologodskaia, M., Hanafusa, H., and Choi, Y. (1999). TRANCE, a TNF family member, activates Akt/PKB through a signaling complex involving TRAF6 and c-Src. *Mol. Cell* **4**, 1041–1049.

Xu, L. X., Kukita, T., Nakano, Y., Yu, H., Hotokebuchi, T., Kuratani, T., Iijima, T., and Koga, T. (1996). Osteoclasts in normal and adjuvant arthritis bone tissues express the mRNA for both type I and II interleukin-1 receptors. *Lab. Invest.* **75**, 677–687.

Yasuda, H., Shima, N., Nakagawa, N., Yamaguchi, K., Kinosaki, M., Mochizuki, S., Tomoyasu, A., Yano, K., Goto, M., Murakami, A., Tsuda, E., Morinaga, T., *et al.* (1998). Osteoclast differentiation factor is a ligand for steoprotegerin/osteoclastogenesis-inhibitory factor and is identical to TRANCE/RANKL. *Proc. Natl. Acad. Sci. USA* **95**, 3597–3602.

Yoshida, H., Hayashi, S., Kunisada, T., Ogawa, M., Nishikawa, S., Okumuram, H., Sudo, T., Shultz, L. D., and Nishikawa, S. (1990). The murine mutation osteopetrosis is in the coding region of the macrophage colony stimulating factor gene. *Nature* **345**, 442–444.

16

THE ROLE OF IL-1 AND IL-1RA IN JOINT INFLAMMATION AND CARTILAGE DEGRADATION

CLAIRE JACQUES,* MARJOLAINE GOSSET,* FRANCIS BERENBAUM,*,† AND CEM GABAY‡

*UMR 7079 CNRS, Physiology and Physiopathology Laboratory, University Paris 6 Paris, 75252 Cedex 5, France
†Department of Rheumatology, APHP Saint-Antoine Hospital, 75012 Paris, France
‡Division of Rheumatology, University Hospital of Geneva, Geneva 14, Switzerland

Vitamins and Hormones, Volume 74
0083-6729/06 $35.00
DOI: 10.1016/S0083-6729(06)74016-X

Copyright 2006, Elsevier Inc. All rights reserved.

Interleukin (IL)-1 is a cytokine that plays a major role in inflammatory responses in the context of infections and immune-mediated diseases. IL-1 refers to two different cytokines, termed IL-1α and IL-1β, produced from two genes. IL-1α and IL-1β are produced by different cell types following stimulation by bacterial products, cytokines, and immune complexes. Monocytes/macrophages are the primary source of IL-1β. Both cytokines do not possess leader peptide sequences and do not follow a classical secretory pathway. IL-1α is mainly cell associated, whereas IL-1β can be released from activated cells after cleavage of its amino-terminal region by caspase-1. IL-1 is present in the synovial tissue and fluids of patients with rheumatoid arthritis. Several *in vitro* studies have shown that IL-1 stimulates the production of mediators such as prostaglandin E_2, nitric oxide, cytokines, chemokines, and adhesion molecules that are involved in articular inflammation. Furthermore, IL-1 stimulates the synthesis and activity of matrix metalloproteinases and other enzymes involved in cartilage destruction in rheumatoid arthritis and osteoarthritis. The effects of IL-1 are inhibited *in vitro* and *in vivo* by natural inhibitors such as IL-1 receptor antagonist and soluble receptors. IL-1 receptor antagonist belongs to the IL-1 family of cytokines and binds to IL-1 receptors but does not induce any intracellular response. IL-1 receptor antagonist inhibits the effect of IL-1 by blocking its interaction with cell surface receptors. The use of IL-1 inhibitors in experimental models of inflammatory arthritis and osteoarthritis has provided a strong support for the role of IL-1 in the pathogeny of these diseases. Most importantly, these findings have been confirmed in clinical trials in patients with rheumatic diseases. Additional strategies aimed to block the effect of IL-1 are tested in clinical trials.

I. INTRODUCTION

Many joint diseases are associated with matrix cartilage degradation such as rheumatoid arthritis (RA) and osteoarthritis (OA). RA is an immune-mediated chronic inflammatory disease of unknown etiology characterized by synovial cell proliferation and inflammation with destruction of cartilage and subchondral bone. OA is the most frequent cause of musculoskeletal disability associated with a loss of articular cartilage macromolecules that are involved in its biomechanical and functional properties. In both diseases, cartilage degradation is the result of overexpression and increased activity of multiple enzymes that largely belong to the matrix metalloproteinase (MMP) family. Pro- and anti-inflammatory cytokines are key mediators in this process as demonstrated by the success of anticytokine therapies in blunting the destructive process in RA. Some of these cytokines are directly involved in the regulation of MMPs expression by acting at the transcriptional, translational, or posttranslational level. Among these cytokines, it is widely accepted that interleukin (IL)-1 and its natural inhibitor, IL-1 receptor antagonist (IL-1Ra) are critical in this regulation. Moreover, IL-1 is involved in the synthesis of other mediators that have themselves deleterious effects on cartilage, such as prostaglandins (PG) or nitric oxide (NO). Finally, IL-1 can trigger a vicious loop in facilitating the synthesis of proinflammatory cytokines that eventually enhance cartilage degradation.

This chapter will highlight the role of IL-1 family members, their receptors, and IL-1-induced pathways. Based on this description, present and future therapies aimed to target IL-1 will be discussed.

II. IL-1 AND IL-1 RECEPTORS

A. IL-1 FAMILY OF CYTOKINES

The IL-1 family of cytokines includes eleven individual members but only four, namely IL-1α, IL-1β, IL-18, and IL-1Ra, have been thoroughly described and implicated in pathological process (Dinarello, 2002). There is a strong homology between IL-1α, IL-1β, and IL-1Ra. The amino acid identities between these human proteins are: IL-1α and IL-1β 22%, IL-1α and IL-1Ra 18%, and IL-1β and IL-1Ra 26%. Moreover, human IL-1α is approximately 55% identical to the murine and rat forms of this molecule, with IL-1β being approximately 78% identical and IL-1Ra approximately 76% identical. The genes for IL-1α, IL-1β, and IL-1Ra are located close to each other in the human chromosome 2q14 region (Patterson et al., 1993; Steinkasserer et al., 1992). The genes for these three members of the IL-1 family are quite similar, indicating an origin by gene duplication. Further analysis of the protein structures suggest that IL-1Ra separated from a primordial IL-1 molecule about 360 million years ago, whereas the separation between IL-1α and IL-1β is a more recent event occurring about 285 million years ago (Eisenberg et al., 1991).

Both IL-1α and IL-1β are synthesized as 31-kDa precursor peptides (pre-IL-1α and pre-IL-1β) that are cleaved to generate 17-kDa mature IL-1α and IL-1β. IL-1β is primarily produced by macrophages and is secreted after cleavage of its proform by the cysteine protease caspase-1 (also termed IL-1β

converting enzyme or ICE) (Black *et al.*, 1988). Pre-IL-1α is cleaved by calpain proteases to release mature carboxy-terminal IL-1α. Most IL-1α is placed on the plasma membrane and can exert its function by stimulating cells by direct cell–cell interaction (Niki *et al.*, 2004). In addition, pre-IL-1α contains a nuclear localization sequence in its amino-terminal domain allowing the nuclear translocation of pre-IL-1α and its amino-terminal 16-kDa propiece (Wessendorf *et al.*, 1993) where they exert different effects on cell growth, tumor transformation, apoptosis, procollagen-I and cytokine production, and NF-κB activation (Hu *et al.*, 2003; Pollock *et al.*, 2003; Stevenson *et al.*, 1997; Werman *et al.*, 2004).

IL-1Ra is a naturally occurring IL-1 inhibitor. The purification and cDNA cloning have been described in a previous review article (Arend *et al.*, 1998). IL-1Ra is produced as four different isoforms derived from the same gene by alternative mRNA splicing and alternative translation initiation. A 17-kDa secreted isoform is expressed as variably glycosylated species of 22–25 kDa (Carter *et al.*, 1990; Eisenberg *et al.*, 1990), now termed sIL-1Ra. An 18-kDa intracellular isoform, created by alternate transcriptional splice of an upstream exon, termed icIL-1Ra1, is a major protein in keratinocytes and other epithelial cells, monocytes, macrophages, fibroblasts, and endothelial cells (Dewberry *et al.*, 2000; Haskill *et al.*, 1991; Maret *et al.*, 2004). icIL-1Ra2 is produced by alternate transcriptional splice from an exon located between icIL-1Ra1 and sIL-1Ra first exons (Muzio *et al.*, 1995). A third 16-kDa intracellular isoform of IL-1Ra, termed icIL-1Ra3, was found in human monocytes, neutrophils, and hepatocytes (Gabay *et al.*, 1997; Malyak *et al.*, 1998). This low-molecular-weight species of IL-1Ra may be formed by alternative translational initiation (Malyak *et al.*, 1998) or by an alternative transcriptional splice mechanism (Weissbach *et al.*, 1998). Both sIL-1Ra and icIL-1Ra1 bind avidly to IL-1 receptor type 1 and inhibit IL-1 effects. Some icIL-1Ra1 may be released from keratinocytes and endothelial cells, and inhibit receptor binding of IL-1. In addition, findings indicate that icIL-1Ra1 carries out additional and unique functions inside cells (Banda *et al.*, 2005; Garat and Arend, 2003; Merhi-Soussi *et al.*, 2005).

B. IL-1 RECEPTORS

The IL-1 receptor family includes three members, IL-1 receptor type I, IL-1RI (80 kDa), IL-1RII (68 kDa), and IL-1 receptor accessory protein, IL-1RAcP that are able to bind the three members of the IL-1 family (IL-1α, IL-1β, IL-1Ra) and are expressed either as membrane-bound or soluble proteins (Fig. 1). IL-1RI, IL-1RII, and IL-1RAcP belong to the immunoglobulin (Ig) gene superfamily with their extracellular segment containing three Ig-like domains. IL-1RI and IL-1RAcP, but not IL-1RII, have cytoplasmic domains that are related to the Toll-like receptor (TLR) superfamily,

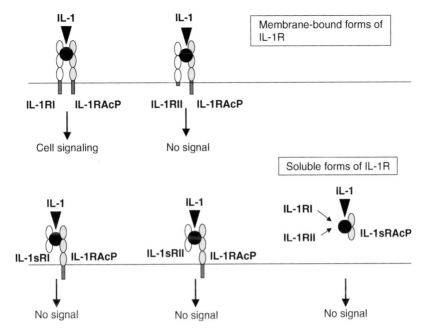

FIGURE 1.   The family of IL-1 receptors (membrane-bound and soluble forms) and their role in IL-1 signal transduction regulation. Interleukin-1 signals into the cell on binding to IL-1 receptor type I (IL-1RI), which subsequently recruits IL-1 receptor accessory protein (IL-1RAcP). IL-1 signaling is regulated by different combinations between membrane-bound and soluble IL-1 receptor type II (IL-1RII) and soluble forms of IL-1RI and sIL-1RAcP. IL-1RII lacks a long cytoplasmic domain and does not exert any signaling activity on IL-1 binding (decoy receptor). Proteolytic cleavage of the extracellular domain of IL-1RII plays an additional role in the control of IL-1 activities, by preventing the interaction between IL-1 and cell surface receptors. Additionally, sIL-1RAcP competes with membrane-bound IL-1RAcP for interacting with IL-1RI, and therefore neutralizes the effect of IL-1.

the Toll-like IL-1R (TIR) domains. The most striking structural difference between IL-1RI and IL-1RII is the short cytoplasmic domain of IL-1RII (29 amino acids), whereas IL-1RI possesses a cytoplasmic tail of 213 residues (Sims *et al.*, 1994). After IL-1 binding, intracellular signaling occurs only through IL-1RI, whereas IL-1RII may exist only as a decoy receptor either on the cell surface or in the cell microenvironment as a soluble form after enzymatic cleavage of the extracellular portion (Colotta *et al.*, 1994).

Of the three members of the IL-1 family (IL-1α, IL-1β, IL-1 Ra), IL-1β has the lowest affinity for the cell-bound form of IL-1RI. The binding of IL-1α to the soluble form of IL-1RI is lower than to the membrane-bound receptor. IL-1Ra has the greatest binding affinity for IL-1RI. The off-rate is slow and binding IL-1Ra to the cell surface IL-1RI is nearly irreversible. In contrast, IL-1β binds to IL-1RII with a greatest affinity than does IL-1α and

IL-1Ra. Moreover, the binding of IL-1β to soluble IL-1RII is nearly irreversible due to a long dissociation rate (2 h). Thus, both membrane-bound
and soluble IL-1RII function as natural inhibitors of IL-1β signaling.

1. Signal Transduction

When IL-1 binds to IL-1RI, a high-affinity trimeric complex is formed
with the IL-1RAcP (Lang *et al.*, 1998). The intracellular domains of
each receptor form a heterodimer that activates IL-1 transduction (Fig. 2).
The TIR domain of adaptor molecule MyD88 interacts with TIR domain
of IL-1RAcP and recruits IRAK-4 and IRAK-1 through death domain

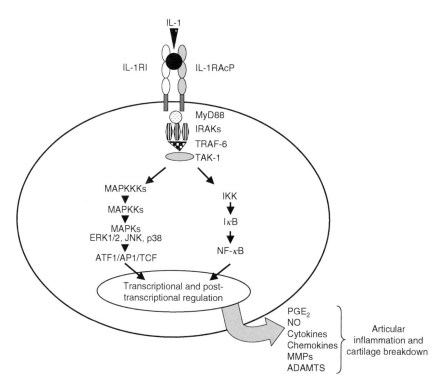

FIGURE 2.   Intracellular-signaling pathways activated by IL-1 in articular chondrocytes.
IL-1 forms a ternary complex with membrane-bound IL-1RI and IL-1RAcP resulting in the
recruitment of MyD88, IL-1 receptor activating kinases (IRAK), and TNF receptor activating
factor-6 (TRAF-6). Following phosphorylation of IRAK and TRAF-6, TGFβ activated
protein kinase 1 (TAK-1) is then phosphorylated. Two major signaling pathways are activated:
(1) the mitogen activated protein kinase (MAPK) pathway, leading to the activation of the
transcription factors ATF1/AP1/TCF, and (2) the NF-κB pathway. These signals activate gene
transcription and posttranscriptional modifications. IL-1 induces the synthesis of PGE$_2$, NO,
cytokines, chemokines, MMPs, and ADAMTS, which are responsible of articular inflammation
and cartilage breakdown.

interactions and TNF receptor associated factor (TRAF)-6 resulting in the formation of a receptor complex (Cao *et al.*, 1996; Lye *et al.*, 2004, Suzuki *et al.*, 2002; Wesche *et al.*, 1997). Phosphorylation of IRAK leads to the formation of a larger complex that is released from the IL-1 receptor and interacts with membrane-bound preassociated transforming growth factor-*β* activated kinase (TAK)-1-transforming growth factor-*β* activated protein kinase 1 binding protein (TAB)1-TAB2 (Jiang *et al.*, 2002). Activation of TAK-1 in the cytosol leads to the activation of IKK (Zandi *et al.*, 1997), phosphorylation and degradation of IκB proteins, and NF-κB activation. Activated TAK-1 is also thought to participate to activation of p38 MAP kinase, JNK, and ERK1/2 pathways (Ninomiya-Tsuji *et al.*, 1999). In addition to TAK-1, mitogen-activated extracellular signal-regulated kinase-activating kinase (MEKK)3 has also been implicated in NF-κB activation through interaction with TRAF-6 (Huang *et al.*, 2004). The use of gene knockout mice has demonstrated the essential role of MyD88, IRAK family members, and TRAF-6 in IL-1 signal transduction (Kawai *et al.*, 1999; Naito *et al.*, 1999; Thomas *et al.*, 1999).

2. IL-1R Distribution in Cartilage

By using gene-array analysis, Attur *et al.* (2000) have demonstrated the presence of IL-1RI, but not IL-1RII, in human normal and OA-affected cartilage, suggesting that human articular chondrocytes may lack a naturally occurring defense mechanism against IL-1 (Attur *et al.*, 2000). However, others have shown that constitutive mRNA and protein expression of all IL-1 receptors exists in human healthy and OA cartilage, but IL-1RII appears to be slightly more expressed than IL-1RI. In order to explain the absence of IL-1RII mRNA on isolated OA chondrocytes precedently found by Attur *et al.* (2000), these authors suggested that an inhibition or an absence of stimulation at IL-1RII gene level exists, implicating a lack of anti-inflammatory signal (Silvestri *et al.*, 2005). Actually, two main pathways of regulation of IL-1RII release have been described. Anti-inflammatory cytokines increase receptor gene expression and therefore its surface level (Colotta *et al.*, 1996), whereas proinflammatory mediators induce shedding of receptors from the cell surface via MMP involvement (Colotta *et al.*, 1995).

Expression of IL-1 receptors varies with physiopathological conditions. IL-1RI expression was decreased in pathological chondrocytes, whereas IL-1-RII did not. IL-1RI was expressed at high level in cartilage from OA than in inflammatory arthritis, whereas IL-1RII showed a similar level of expression in cartilage from OA and inflammatory arthritis (Silvestri *et al.*, 2005).

3. Regulation of the IL-1 Activity by IL-1 Receptor

The function of IL-1RII as a decoy receptor is based on the binding of IL-1*β* to the cell surface form of this receptor. IL-1RII may recruit the coreceptor IL-1RAcP to form the trimeric complex IL-1β, IL-1RAcP, and IL-1RII, thus subtracting the coreceptor from IL-1RI signaling (Lang *et al.*, 1998; Malinowsky *et al.*, 1998). Injections of soluble IL-1RII in rabbits result in dose-dependent decrease of parameters of inflammation in antigen-induced arthritis (Dawson *et al.*, 1999). Moreover, transfection of IL-1RII in cells expressing only IL-1R1 triggers an inhibition of IL-1 responsiveness (Sirum and Brinckerhoff, 1989).

Regulation of IL-1 activity in cell exists via IL-1RI. Binding IL-1Ra to IL-1RI does not recruit IL-1RAcP, thus preventing formation of the signaling complex. In addition, IL-1 soluble receptors (sIL-1R) are able to bind IL-1, thus diminishing the concentration of soluble free cytokines. *In vitro* studies have suggested that the simultaneous presence of both IL-1Ra and sIL-1RII are able to abolish most of the IL-1 inflammatory response (Burger *et al.*, 1995).

Finally, an alternative splice transcript of the membrane IL-1RAcP encoding a smaller soluble protein sIL-1RAcP has been described (Jensen and Whitehead, 2003, Jensen *et al.*, 2000). sIL-1RAcP is constitutively present in normal human serum at a concentration greater than 300 ng/ml (Smith *et al.*, 2003) but it seems that its expression could be tissue specific (Jensen and Whitehead, 2004). sIL-1RAcP adds another layer of complexity to the regulation of IL-1 action. Smith *et al.* (2003) reported that soluble form of IL-1RAcP increases the binding affinity of human IL-1α and IL-1β to the soluble form of IL-1RII. Overexpression of sIL-1RAcP ameliorates joint and systemic manifestations of collagen-induced arthritis in mice (Smeets *et al.*, 2005).

III. ROLE OF IL-1 AND IL-1RA IN ARTICULAR INFLAMMATION

Strong evidence favors a central role for proinflammatory cytokines such as IL-1β in cartilage degradation both in inflammatory arthritis and OA (Goldring, 2000). Chondrocytes in OA cartilage, especially those in clonal clusters, are positive for IL-1 immunostaining (Moos *et al.*, 1999; Tetlow *et al.*, 2001; Towle *et al.*, 1997) and produce caspase-1 and IL-1RI (Martel-Pelletier *et al.*, 1992). Therefore, chondrocytes in OA cartilage may be exposed continuously to the autocrine and paracrine effects of IL-1 and other catabolic factors at high local concentrations.

A. PROSTAGLANDIN E$_2$ SYNTHESIS

IL-1 stimulates the synthesis of prostaglandin E$_2$ (PGE$_2$) and nitric oxide (NO), which regulates type II collagen gene transcription (Goldring *et al.*, 1990, 1996) and modulates aggrecan synthesis in chondrocytes (Hauselmann *et al.*, 1994), respectively. Moreover, it has been evidenced that mice deficient for EP4, a membrane receptor for PGE$_2$, results in the absence of cartilage degradation in collagen-induced arthritis (McCoy *et al.*, 2002).

The synthesis of PGE$_2$ is the endpoint of a sequence of enzymatic reactions, including the release of arachidonic acid from membrane phospholipids by soluble phospholipase A2 (sPLA2) and conversion of this substrate to prostaglandin H2 (PGH2) by cyclooxygenase (COX)-1 and COX-2, also known as PGH1 and PGH2. PGH2 is subsequently metabolized by PGE synthase to form PGE$_2$ (Fig. 3). The COX-1 isoform is expressed constitutively by many types of cells, whereas COX-2 requires specific induction by inflammatory mediators such as lipopolysaccharide (LPS) and cytokines (Crofford *et al.*, 1994, 2000). In articular chondrocytes, IL-1β and TNF-α synergistically induce COX-2, whereas COX-1 expression remains unchanged (Berenbaum *et al.*, 1996). The prostaglandin E synthase (PGES) catalyzes the conversion of PGH2 to PGE$_2$. Three forms of PGES have been cloned and

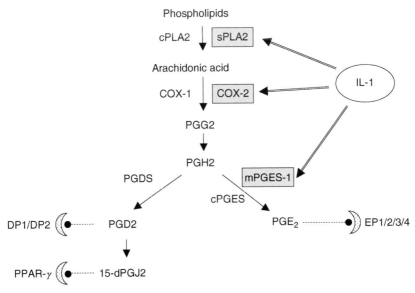

FIGURE 3. The arachidonic acid cascade and the targets of IL-1. The release of arachidonic acid from membrane phospholipids and its conversion to prostaglandin (PG) E2 occurs by a sequence of enzymatic reactions involving isoforms of phospholipase (PL) A2, cyclooxygenase (COX), and PGE synthase (PGES). Cytosolic PLA2, COX-1, and cytosolic PGES are constitutive isoforms, whereas secreted PLA2, COX-2, and microsomal PGES-1 isoforms are IL-1 inducible. Prostaglandin H2 may also be converted to PGD2 by prostaglandin D synthase (PGDS). Then PGD2 can be dehydrated in 15-dPGJ2 that may act as anti-inflammatory mediator. After release from cells, PGE$_2$, PGD2, and 15-dPGJ2 interact with specific EP, DP, and PPAR-γ receptors, respectively.

characterized (Jakobsson *et al.*, 1999; Tanioka *et al.*, 2000) including cytosolic PGE synthase (cPGES) and two microsomal forms: glutathione-specific mPGES-1 and glutathione nonspecific mPGES-2. Although cPGES is constitutively expressed and unresponsive to inflammatory stimuli, mPGES-1 is inducible by LPS and inflammatory cytokines (Jakobsson *et al.*, 1999; Murakami *et al.*, 2000; Tanioka *et al.*, 2000). The coordinate regulation and functional coupling of mPGES-1 and COX-2 have been reported (Murakami *et al.*, 2000). In mice lacking mPGES-1, decreased cartilage destruction accompanies impaired inflammatory response in collagen-induced arthritis (Trebino *et al.*, 2003). Therefore, mPGES-1 may be a novel target for selective inhibition of PGE_2 synthesis without affecting other COX-2 products in joint tissues.

The observation that IL-1β induces the expression of mPGES-1 in rheumatoid synovial cells (Stichtenoth *et al.*, 2001) prompted examination of this response in chondrocytes, where mPGES-1 expression is regulated by p38 MAPK and ERK1/2 pathways (Masuko-Hongo *et al.*, 2004). Although the IL-1-induced COX-2 response is dependant on the differentiated phenotype of the chondrocyte (Thomas *et al.*, 2002), PGE_2 paradoxically opposes the effects of IL-1 on cartilage matrix synthesis by inhibiting type I collagen synthesis and by stimulating type II collagen production in dedifferenciated chondrocytes (Goldring *et al.*, 1994; Riquet *et al.*, 2000). If, as suggested by Melchiorri *et al.* (1998), the superficial zone chondrocytes express IL-1β and IL-1 receptors at higher levels than deep zone chondrocytes in OA cartilage, then a gradient of PGE_2 may be produced in order to counteract IL-1-induced dedifferenciation (Melchiorri *et al.*, 1998).

B. NO PRODUCTION

Proinflammatory cytokines increase the synthesis of NO through the inducible enzyme, iNO synthase (iNOS). IL-1 induces NO release by chondrocytes *in vitro* (Palmer *et al.*, 1993, Stadler *et al.*, 1991). The various effects of NO as a mediator of IL-1-induced responses, including inhibition of aggrecan and type II collagen synthesis (Cao *et al.*, 1997; Hauselmann *et al.*, 1994; Taskiran *et al.*, 1994), enhancement of MMP activity, chondrocyte apoptosis (Blanco *et al.*, 1995; Clancy *et al.*, 1998; Sasaki *et al.*, 1998), and inhibition of IL-1Ra production (Maneiro *et al.*, 2001, Pelletier *et al.*, 1996) have been reported. Nitric oxide may also increase chondrocyte susceptibility to injury by other oxidants such as H_2O_2 and contributes to resistance against the anabolic effects of insulin-like growth factor-I (Clancy *et al.*, 1997; Loeser *et al.*, 2002; Studer *et al.*, 2000; van de Loo *et al.*, 1998).

Nitric oxide also has been implicated as an important mediator of chondrocyte apoptosis (Blanco *et al.*, 1995; Hashimoto *et al.*, 1998). The failure to induce arthritis in iNOS-deficient mice (van de Loo *et al.*, 1998) and the cartilage protection provided by NO inhibitors in animal models of arthritis

(Ohtsuka et al., 2002; Pelletier et al., 2000; Presle et al., 1999) further argue for a role of NO in cartilage damage. In contrast, other studies showed that NO may inhibit cytokine production or activity in chondrocytes (Henrotin et al., 1998) and that selective inhibition of iNOS may exacerbate erosive arthritis (Clements et al., 2003; McCartney-Francis et al., 2001). Furthermore, IL-1 seems to protect chondrocytes from apoptosis by a mechanism that is independent of IL-1-induced NO (Kuhn et al., 2000, 2003). Therefore, the balance of mediators determining normal homeostasis is complex, and modulation of their activities may produce positive or negative effects on chondrocyte function depending on the extracellular medium.

C. PEROXISOME PROLIFERATOR-ACTIVATED RECEPTOR-γ

15-deoxy-delta12,14-prostaglandin J2 (15d-PGJ2), a dehydration product of PGD2, arises from the conversion of PGH2 by PGD synthase. Prostaglandin J2 acts as the natural ligand of the peroxisome proliferator-activated receptor-γ (PPAR-γ) which is a transcription factor belonging to the nuclear receptor superfamily (Issemann and Green, 1990). In addition to driving PPAR-γ-dependent adipogenesis, 15d-PGJ2 promotes apoptosis and inhibits inflammation (Hortelano et al., 2000; Rossi et al., 2000; Shibata et al., 2002). Similar to 15d-PGJ2, leukiotriene B4 can ligate PPAR-γ (Devchand et al., 1996), and the localization of COX-1 and COX-2 to the nuclear envelope suggests that other eicosanoids may engage nuclear receptors (Spencer et al., 1998). However, 15d-PGJ2 is not formed in mammalian cells in sufficient amounts to drive PPAR-γ-dependent adipogenesis (Bell-Parikh et al., 2003; Ide et al., 2003). Nevertheless, the use of exogenous 15d-PGJ2 and synthetic PPAR-γ ligands to evoke biologic responses has permitted examination of their efficacy as pharmacological mediators. Studies in human chondrocytes and synovial cells show that PPAR-γ ligands are capable of opposing many of the actions of IL-1. 15d-PGJ2 inhibits IL-1-induced NO, MMP-13, and COX-2 production in human chondrocytes (Boyault et al., 2001; Fahmi et al., 2001), and MMP-1 production in human synovial fibroblasts (Fahmi et al., 2002). Conversely, IL-1 decreases PPAR-γ expression in rat and human chondrocytes (Bordji et al., 2000; Boyault et al., 2001) suggesting that PPAR-γ and IL-1 pathways regulate their actions.

D. ANIMAL MODELS

Several experimental models of chronic arthritis have confirmed the pivotal role of IL-1 in joint damage. Elevated levels of IL-1 have been reported in the early phase of experimental arthritis (Eastgate et al., 1988; van de Loo et al., 1995; Van Lent et al., 1995). Intra-articular injection of

IL-1 into rabbit knee joints induces the accumulation of polymorphonuclear and mononuclear leukocytes in the joint space and the loss of proteoglycan from the articular cartilage (Henderson and Pettipher, 1989). Expression of human IL-1β using an *ex vivo* gene transfer method of delivery into the knee joints of rabbits resulted in a severe, highly aggressive form of arthritis reproducing some of the features of RA in humans (Ghivizzani *et al.*, 1997a,b). A role of IL-1 in joint destruction is also evident in IL-1β-deficient mice. When streptococcal cell wall (SCW) arthritis was induced in IL-1β-deficient mice, cartilage damage and sustained cellular infiltration in the synovium were greatly reduced as compared to arthritis in wild-type controls (van den Berg *et al.*, 1999). Joint swelling, however, was not reduced in IL-1β-deficient mice. Repeated administration of small amounts of streptococcal cell walls at sites of ongoing arthritis produces arthritis episodes. When this chronic relapsing model of arthritis was evaluated in IL-1-deficient mice, cartilage erosion was essentially abolished and the synovial infiltrate was significantly reduced. These results suggest that IL-1 may produce joint damage in the SCW arthritis model, whereas inflammation is caused by additional mechanisms.

IL-1 is present in the synovial lining layer and in focal areas of the inflamed synovium of mice with antigen-induced arthritis (van de Loo *et al.*, 1995). Furthermore, a single injection of rabbit anti-IL-1α and anti-IL-1β antibodies resulted in reduced joint swelling by 30–40% and proteoglycan breakdown (Van Lent *et al.*, 1995). In a study comparing the effect of IL-1β and tumor necrosis factor (TNF)-α, the authors showed distinct time-dependent patterns of acute arthritis in the rat knee. They demonstrate that IL-1β impels joint lesions to a substantially greater degree and for a longer time than does an equivalent dose of TNF-α (Bolon *et al.*, 2004).

To further examine the role of IL-1 in pathophysiologic events of articular inflammation, administration of recombinant IL-1Ra was used in several models of inflammatory arthritis. The chronic phase of SCW arthritis in rats was markedly reduced by intraperitoneal (IP) injections of IL-1Ra at the time of reactivation of the disease (Schwab *et al.*, 1991). Although IL-1Ra was found not to reduce inflammation in murine SCW arthritis, continuous IP infusion of IL-1Ra led to a marked reversal of the inhibition of proteoglycan synthesis as well as to decreased inflammatory cell influx and proteoglycan depletion in articular cartilage (Kuiper *et al.*, 1998). The greater effect of IL-1Ra on reducing cartilage and bone destruction were described in immune complex-induced arthritis in mice (Van Lent *et al.*, 1995), antigen-induced arthritis in rabbits (Arner *et al.*, 1995), and collagen-induced arthritis in mice (Joosten *et al.*, 1996, 1999). These successful therapeutic approaches have been complemented by the use of gene therapy techniques to deliver IL-1Ra to the joint. *Ex vivo* gene therapy has been carried out by transfection of the IL-1Ra cDNA into cultured rabbit synovial fibroblasts. The cells secrete IL-1Ra into the synovial fluid preventing IL-1-induced migration of neutrophils (Bandara *et al.*, 1993; Hung *et al.*, 1994) and proteoglycan degradation in the articular cartilage (Hung *et al.*, 1994, Roessler *et al.*, 1995). *Ex vivo* gene therapy with IL-1Ra also suppressed antigen-induced arthritis in rabbits (Otani *et al.*, 1996), bacterial cell wall–induced arthritis in rats (Makarov *et al.*, 1996), and both ipsilateral and contralateral arthritis in collagen-induced arthritis in mice (Bakker *et al.*, 1997). Gene transfer carried out by injection of viral vectors containing the IL-1Ra cDNA directly in the joint was successful in adjuvant arthritis in rats (Nguyen *et al.*, 1998), antigen-induced arthritis in rabbits (Ghivizzani *et al.*, 1998), IL-1-induced arthritis in rabbits (Oligino *et al.*, 1996), and LPS-induced arthritis in rats (Pan *et al.*, 2000). Transgenic mice overexpressing sIL-1Ra or icIL-1Ra1 were protected from the occurrence of collagen-induced arthritis (Palmer *et al.*, 2003). Thus, all of the above-mentioned studies indicate that experimental animal models of inflammatory arthritis are significantly prevented or ameliorated by blocking IL-1.

IV. ROLE OF IL-1 IN CARTILAGE BREAKDOWN

Articular cartilage consists of a highly structured extracellular matrix composed primarily of type II collagen and proteoglycans that account for the tensile strength and load-bearing capacity of the joint. Chondrocytes are embedded within this matrix and participate in the degradation of the extracellular matrix as well as the synthesis of new matrix proteins (Dijkgraaf *et al.*, 1995). Under normal conditions, these processes are maintained in balance by various cytokines and growth factors. In RA and OA, however, this balance is tipped in favor of matrix destruction. Although the clinical features of arthritic diseases differ, IL-1 is believed to play a central role in the cartilage destruction inherent to both RA and OA (Martel-Pelletier *et al.*, 1999). The degradation of cartilage is mediated by a number of different proteases, including neutral endopeptidases of the metalloproteinase superfamily of enzymes. Members of two metalloproteinase families, MMP and ADAMTS (a disintegrin and metalloproteinase with thrombospondin motifs), have been implicated in cartilage matrix destruction (Koshy *et al.*, 2002).

A. MATRIX METALLOPROTEINASES

Matrix metalloproteinases are synthesized as latent proenzymes that require activation in order to degrade cartilage extracellular matrix proteins (Malemud *et al.*, 2003). Three types of enzymes including collagenases, stromelysin, and gelatinases are believed to regulate the turnover of extracellular matrix proteins.

Collagenases (MMP-1 and -13) are responsible for degradation of native collagen fibers. MMP-1 breaks down the helical region of the fibrillar collagens, with greatest degradative activity toward collagen type III, followed by type I, and then type II (Goupille *et al.*, 1998; Shingleton *et al.*, 2000). MMP-13, called collagenase-3, is more effective than other collagenases at cleaving triple helices, particularly those of type II collagen (Goupille *et al.*, 1998), which is the most abundant collagen in the articular cartilage (Malemud *et al.*, 2003). It has also been shown to cleave gelatin with greater efficiency than other collagenases and hence, acts to further degrade the initial cleavage products of the collagenases (Goupille *et al.*, 1998). IL-1β markedly stimulated MMP-1 gene expression in cultured chondrocytes as compared to unstimulated chondrocytes at days 21 and 28. In contrast, the expression of MMP-13 was markedly higher in IL-1β-stimulated chondrocytes than that of unstimulated cells on day 1, but a reverse pattern was observed after day 7 of culture. Therefore, these results suggest that IL-1β may induce MMP-13 gene expression in the initial stage of arthritis leading to rapid type II collagen degradation in articular cartilage. IL-1β may subsequently induce late MMP-1 gene expression which further cleaves other collagens.

Stromelysin (MMP-3) degrades proteoglycans and type IX collagen (Flannery *et al.*, 1992; Wu *et al.*, 1991) and appears to be involved in the pathogenesis of osteoarthritis (Hembry *et al.*, 1995; Sirum and Brinckerhoff, 1989). Human chondrocytes isolated from femoral head osteoarthritis cartilage express MMP-3 constitutively *in vitro* (Ganu *et al.*, 1994). Gelatinases (MMP-2) degrades denatured collagen, proteoglycans, fibronectin, and type IX collagen. IL-1β stimulated the production of MMP-2 and -3 in cultured chondrocytes (Aida *et al.*, 2005). These results suggest that the denatured collagen present after cleavage by MMP-13 and -1 may be hydrolyzed by MMP-2, whereas other components of articular cartilage such as proteoglycans, fibronectin, link protein, and type IX collagen may be hydrolyzed by MMP-3.

Tissue inhibitors of matrix metalloproteinases (TIMPs) inhibit the enzymatic activities of MMPs (Smith *et al.*, 1999). TIMPs are known endogenous protease inhibitors that bind to active MMPs in a 1:1 molar ratio (Cawston, 1996). TIMP-1 binds activated forms of MMP-1, -3, and -13 and both latent and active MMP-9. In contrast, TIMP-2 is mainly associated with MMP-2 (Martin *et al.*, 2004). It has been shown that the expression of TIMP-1 was increased in the presence of IL-1β compared with that of unstimulated chondrocytes on days 21 and 28 of culture. In contrast, the expression of TIMP-2 is significantly decreased on day 1, whereas its expression is increased after 3 days of culture. These findings suggest that MMP-1, -2, and -3 may be inhibited by TIMP-1 or -2 at later stage of joint inflammation, whereas MMP-13 enzymatic activities during early stage of arthritis may be unaffected by these inhibitors.

B. AGGRECANASES

Aggrecan, a large aggregating proteoglycan, forms a macromolecular complex with hyaluronan and link protein. It swells within the interstices of the collagen framework and provides compressibility to cartilage (Koshy *et al.*, 2002; Nagase and Kashiwagi, 2003). The loss of aggrecan is considered to be a critical early event in cartilage destruction, occurring initially at the joint surface and progressing to the deeper zones. This step is followed by degradation of collagen fibrils and mechanical failure of the tissue (Nagase and Kashiwagi, 2003). Aggrecan is degraded by one or more "aggrecanases" from the ADAMTS family of proteases. The ADAMTS family contains 19 individual gene products (Apte, 2004). Certain members of the ADAMTS family (ADAMTS-1, -4, -5, -8, -9, and -15), called aggrecanases, can proteolytically process aggrecan within the interglobular domain separating its globular G1 and G2 domains at a specific Glu373–Ala374 bond (Apte, 2004, Tortorella *et al.*, 2002) or at one or more sites within the more C-terminal glycosaminoglycan (GAG)-bearing region (Kuno *et al.*, 2000). Proteolytic liberation of the GAG-bearing regions reduces the load-bearing properties of articular cartilage and may accompany or initiate a series of cellular responses that culminate in loss of joint cartilage. These proteases are believed to be active in both inflammatory arthritis and osteoarthritis. Aggrecanase activity was first detected in bovine articular cartilage treated with IL-1β, but it is also enhanced by TNF-α or retinoic acid (Flannery *et al.*, 1999; Sandy *et al.*, 1991). These data support the hypothesis that aggrecanases are active early in the disease process of arthritis or during acute inflammatory episodes. However, the exact enzyme(s) responsible for cartilage aggrecan degradation, both during active inflammation and as arthritis progresses, are still unknown (Kevorkian *et al.*, 2004). ADAMTS-4 (aggrecanase 1), ADAMTS-5 (aggrecanase 2), and subsequently, ADAMTS-1 were the first proteases to which significant aggrecanase activity was attributed (Kuno *et al.*, 2000; Sandy *et al.*, 1991; Tortorella *et al.*, 2002), although their specific importance in the context of arthritis is not yet fully established. Like ADAMTS-4 and ADAMTS-1, ADAMTS-9, ADAMTS-8, and ADAMTS-15 were shown to be aggrecanases (Cal *et al.*, 2002; Collins-Racie *et al.*, 2004; Porter *et al.*, 2005). In gene profiling studies, ADAMTS-9 was expressed in the setting of osteoarthritis (Kevorkian *et al.*, 2004; Somerville *et al.*, 2003). The effects of two major proinflammatory cytokines, IL-1β and TNF-α, were investigated to determine how and which aggrecanase may play a role in arthritis. *ADAMTS-9* was the most highly induced of the aggrecanase family gene in IL-1β-stimulated chondrosarcoma-derived cells and isolated chondrocytes (Demircan *et al.*, 2005). Previous studies demonstrated the synergistic induction of *ADAMTS-4* and *ADAMTS-5* genes expression by a combination of IL-1β and oncostatin M (Koshy *et al.*, 2002). It appears that expression of aggrecanase genes is synergistically induced by cytokines/growth factors, which is relevant to the complex extracellular milieu in arthritis. A study demonstrates that ADAMTS-5 is the major aggrecanase in mouse cartilage, both *in vitro* and in a mouse model of OA and of inflammatory arthritis (Glasson *et al.*, 2005; Stanton *et al.*, 2005). Data suggest that ADAMTS-5 may be a suitable target for the development of new drugs designed to inhibit cartilage destruction in arthritis, although further work will be required to determine whether ADAMTS-5 is also the major aggrecanase in human arthritis. A study shows that ADAMTS-1 is the first matrix-degrading enzyme downregulated by IL-1β *in vitro* (Wachsmuth *et al.*, 2004).

The role of IL-1 in articular cartilage degradation was also examined in experimental models of osteoarthritis. Transplantation of IL-1Ra-transduced chondrocytes onto the articular surface of osteoarthritic cartilage organ cultures protected against IL-1-induced proteoglycan degradation (Baragi *et al.*, 1995). The progression of experimental OA in dogs was prevented by IL-1Ra administered by intraarticular injections of recombinant protein (Caron *et al.*, 1996), *ex vivo* gene therapy (Pelletier *et al.*, 1997), or *in vivo* gene therapy (Fernandes *et al.*, 1999).

V. THE ROLE OF THE BALANCE BETWEEN ENDOGENOUS IL-1 AND IL-1RA

An important anti-inflammatory role for endogenous IL-1Ra in arthritis was suggested by a study that compared the clinical course of knee arthritis in patients with Lyme disease. Patients with high concentrations of synovial fluid IL-1Ra and low concentrations of IL-1β had rapid resolution of acute attacks of arthritis, whereas patients with the reverse pattern of cytokine concentrations had a more protracted course (Miller *et al.*, 1993). In addition, several studies demonstrated that the IL-1Ra/IL-1β ratio was low in RA, thus leading to the perpetuation of articular inflammation and subsequent tissue destruction (Deleuran *et al.*, 1992). The IL-1β/IL-1Ra ratio is elevated in the synovium of mice with collagen-induced arthritis and correlated to the severity of joint score. In contrast, the IL-1β/IL-1Ra ratio decreases at later time points. These changes are associated with a progressive reduction in the levels of inflammatory activity in the joints, thus further emphasizing the role of the balance between IL-1 and IL-1Ra in the modulation of the inflammatory response (Gabay *et al.*, 2001).

The physiologic function of endogenous IL-1 and IL-1Ra has been further demonstrated in several studies by blocking endogenous production of IL-1 and IL-1Ra by using gene deletion. IL-1β- and IL-1RI-deficient mice are protected from the development of collagen-induced arthritis. IL-1Ra knockout mice had a significantly earlier onset of collagen-induced arthritis and more severe synovitis, often accompanied by bony erosions (Ma *et al.*,

1998). The absence of IL-1Ra by gene deletion in BALB/cA mice was associated with the spontaneous development of chronic polyarthritis with the presence of autoantibodies, thus reproducing some of the clinical and biological features of RA (Horai *et al.*, 2000). Taken together, these findings indicate that an imbalance between IL-1 and IL-1Ra may predispose to inflammatory diseases and that endogenous IL-1Ra may serve an important role in preventing or limiting organ damage in IL-1-mediated diseases.

VI. TARGETING IL-1 IN THE TREATMENT OF RHEUMATIC DISEASES

As depicted in Fig. 4, different approaches have been designed and tested in clinical trials to inhibit IL-1 activities (Table I), including inhibition of IL-1 production, the use of specific antibodies targeting IL-1 or its receptors, and a recombinant receptor antagonist.

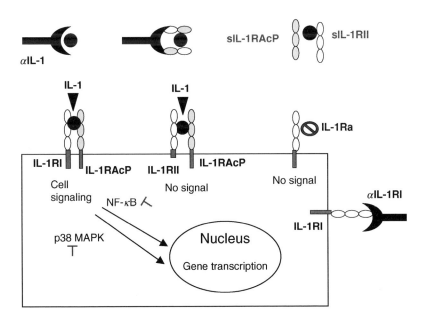

FIGURE 4.   Potential strategies to block the effect of IL-1. The maturation and release of IL-1β can be inhibited by caspase-1 (not depicted in this figure). Extracellular free IL-1 can be blocked by specific antibodies (αIL-1), fusion molecules containing binding motifs of IL-1 receptors (IL-1 trap), and soluble receptors (sIL-1RII, sIL-1RAcP). Binding to cell surface receptors can be inhibited by IL-1Ra and antibodies directed against IL-1RI (αIL-1RI). Postreceptor-signaling inhibitors targeting p38 MAPK and NF-κB pathways can block the biological effect of IL-1 and of other cytokines.

TABLE I. Targeting IL-1 in Rheumatic Diseases[a]

Rheumatic disease	Treatment	Efficacy	Studies
Rheumatoid arthritis (RA)	Anakinra	+ + +	Bresnihan et al., 1998
	Anakinra + MTX	+ + +	Cohen et al., 2003
	sIL-1RI	−	Drevlow et al., 1996
	IL-1 trap	+/−	Guler et al., 2001
	Pralnacasan	−	Pavelka et al., 2002
Osteoarthritis (OA)	Anakinra	+/−	Chevalier et al., 2005
Adult Still's disease	Anakinra	+ + ++	Fitzgerald et al., 2005
Systemic-onset JIA	Anakinra	+ + ++	Pascual et al., 2005
Lupus arthritis	Anakinra	+ +	Ostendorf et al., 2005
Ankylosing spondylitis	Anakinra	+	Tan et al., 2004
			Haibel et al., 2005

[a]MTX, methotrexate; JIA, juvenile idiopathic arthritis.

A. ANAKINRA (IL-1RA)

Anakinra is approved for the treatment of RA and is now commercially available as Kineret®. A randomized double-blind, placebo-controlled multicenter trial including 472 patients with RA demonstrated that after 24 weeks, the American College of Rheumatology 20% (ACR20) response was achieved by 43% of the patients receiving the largest dose (150 mg per injection) of anakinra in monotherapy in comparison with 27% of those in the placebo group (Bresnihan et al., 1998). A 24-week extension of this study confirmed these results with sustained efficacy of anakinra without additional adverse events (Nuki et al., 2002). The radiological evaluation, performed using the Genant score that distinguishes the joint space narrowing and the presence of bony erosions, showed greater reduction in joint space narrowing (58% compared with placebo) than in erosion (38% versus placebo), raising the possibility that IL-1 inhibition provides a greater protection for cartilage than for subchondral bone (Jiang et al., 2000). Serial synovial biopsies were performed in 12 patients from the 24-week randomized trial and the extension study. The results showed a reduction in intimal macrophages and subintimal macrophages and lymphocytes, and a downregulation of E-selectin and vascular cell adhesion molecule-1 in patients receiving 150 mg/day anakinra. The absence of progression in radiological signs of joint damage seen in some patients correlated with the decrease in intimal macrophages (Cunnane et al., 2001).

The effect of anakinra in combination with methotrexate has been studied in a randomized, double-blind, placebo-controlled, multicenter trial including 419 patients with active RA despite being treated with methotrex-ate for six consecutive months. ACR20 rates were significantly higher in patients who received the combination of methotrexate and 1 mg/kg ana-kinra than those who received methotrexate and the placebo only (42% versus 23%). The percentage of patients who achieved more stringent re-sponse criteria such as ACR50 and ACR70 was also significantly higher among those treated with 1 mg/kg and 2 mg/kg anakinra than those who received placebo (Cohen *et al.*, 2003). Most withdrawal in the IL-1Ra 1 and 2 mg/kg groups were due to injection site reactions (6.8% and 9.7%, respec-tively). Five patients withdrew of the study because of leukopenia. White blood cell count returned to normal values after discontinuation of IL-1Ra treatment. Leukopenia was not associated with episodes of infection. Results of larger population indicate that anakinra in combination with methotrexate as well as other disease modifying antirheumatic drugs (DMARDs) is safe with a rate of serious infections slightly higher in the anakinra than in the placebo group (2.1% versus 0.4%). Opportunistic infection and tuberculosis have not been reported to date.

The efficacy and safety of anakinra and etanercept combination was examined in RA patients. The results did not show any advantage of the combination over etanercept alone. However, the percentage of infectious adverse events was significantly higher in patients treated with the combina-tion of biological agents indicating that blockade of two cytokines involved in innate immune responses to microorganisms may result in increased susceptibility to infections (Genovese *et al.*, 2004). The use of anakinra in patients who had a previous incomplete response to TNF-α inhibitors did not show any advantage in a study (Buch *et al.*, 2004).

The efficacy and safety of anakinra were also investigated in other rheu-matic diseases. Anakinra is dramatically successful in systemic-onset juvenile idiopathic arthritis and in adult Still's disease (Fitzgerald *et al.*, 2005; Pascual *et al.*, 2005). Anakinra led to interesting results in a few patients with lupus arthritis (Ostendorf *et al.*, 2005) and in patients with osteoarthri-tis, the latter after intra-articular injection (Chevalier *et al.*, 2005). The results of a randomized, double-blind, placebo-controlled study failed to show a positive effect of a single intraarticular injection of anakinra in knee OA at the 12-week evaluation (Chevalier *et al.*, 2005). Anakinra treatment was only modestly successful in a subset of patients with ankylosing spondylitis (Haibel *et al.*, 2005; Tan *et al.*, 2004).

B. SOLUBLE RECEPTORS

The administration of human soluble IL-1RI exhibited some beneficial effects in antigen-induced arthritis in mice (Dower *et al.*, 1994). In contrast, treatment with soluble IL-1RI administered either by intra-articular or subcutaneous injection was devoid of significant effect in patients with RA

(Drevlow *et al.*, 1996). The administration of soluble IL-1RI may have inhibited binding of IL-1Ra to cell surface IL-1 receptors, thus further enhancing the inflammatory effects of IL-1 on target cells (Arend *et al.*, 1994). Soluble IL-1RII binds to IL-1β with higher affinity than IL-1Ra. The administration of soluble IL-1RII in experimental models resulted in a marked inhibition of joint swelling and joint damage and exerts a chondroprotective effect *in vitro* (Attur *et al.*, 2002; Bessis *et al.*, 2000; Dawson *et al.*, 1999).

IL-1 trap is a fusion protein containing some of the extracellular-binding motifs of IL-1RI and IL-1RAcP coupled to the Fc fraction of the human immunoglobulin IgG. IL-1 trap binds IL-1β and IL-1α with high affinity (K_d = 1.5 and 3 pM, respectively). Most importantly, IL-1 trap binds IL-1β with a much stronger affinity than IL-1Ra. Thus, administration of IL-1 trap should not affect the anti-inflammatory effect of endogenous IL-1Ra. Administration of a murine form of IL-1 trap almost completely blocked the development of collagen-induced arthritis (Economides *et al.*, 2003).

The safety and efficacy of IL-1 trap was assessed in a phase Ib randomized, dose-escalating, double-blind, placebo-controlled trial including four groups of 15–20 patients with active RA. After 6 weeks, an average ACR20 was achieved by 74% of patients receiving the highest dose of IL-1 trap as compared with 36% of placebo-treated patients (Guler *et al.*, 2001). The results of a multicenter, randomized, placebo-controlled, double-blind phase II trial including 200 RA patients failed to show a significant effect even in patients receiving the highest dose of IL-1 trap (100 mg weekly). Approximately two-third of the patients were on DMARDs during the trial. After 12 weeks, the ACR20 response rates were 30.9, 34.8, 20.8, and 46% in patients treated with placebo and in those receiving weekly subcutaneous injections of 25, 50, and 100 mg IL-1 trap, respectively. The response rate was slightly better in patients treated with DMARDs, reaching statistical significance for the ACR50 response rate (11.1% versus 29.4% in placebo and 100 mg IL-1 trap, respectively). The safety profile of IL-1 trap during the trial was good (unpublished data). IL-1 trap was used with success in a few patients with periodic fever syndromes (Canna *et al.*, 2005).

C. INHIBITOR OF IL-1β PRODUCTION

IL-1β is synthesized in the cytoplasm as an inactive precursor 31-kDa pro-IL-1β that is cleaved by caspase-1 to generate mature and biologically active 17-kDa IL-1β. In addition, caspase-1 cleaves pro-IL-18 to generate mature and active IL-18, a cytokine that has been shown to play an important role in experimental models of arthritis (Plater-Zyberk *et al.*, 2001). Finally, caspase-1 cleaves IL-33, the recently described member of the IL-1 family of cytokines (Schmitz *et al.*, 2005). Taken together, these findings suggest that caspase-1 is a potential target in the treatment of arthritis. Consistent with this hypothesis, the administration of caspase-1 inhibitors blocked the progression of collagen-induced arthritis in mice (Ku *et al.*, 1996). The efficacy and safety of pralnacasan, a caspase-1 inhibitor, was examined in a 12-week phase II placebo-controlled multicenter study in RA patients receiving concurrent DMARDs. ACR20 response rate was not significantly higher in patients treated with pralnacasan than in those in the placebo group (Pavelka *et al.*, 2002). This disappointing result can be partly explained by the fact that other enzymes are also able to cleave pro-IL-1β. In addition, caspase-1 does not influence the biological effects of IL-1α.

VII. CONCLUSIONS

The results of *in vitro* and *in vivo* studies have demonstrated that IL-1 plays a major role in articular inflammation and subsequent tissue damage. The biological effects of this cytokine are tightly controlled by a complex system at the level of production and maturation, its concentration as a free cytokine, and its interaction with cell surface receptors. Several examples obtained in mouse models indicate that an imbalance between IL-1 and IL-1Ra, its natural inhibitor, results in excessive inflammation and organ damage. In contrast, administration of IL-1Ra is successful in the treat-ment of experimental models of inflammatory arthritis and OA. The results of clinical trials using therapies aimed to inhibit the effect of IL-1 in patients with inflammatory rheumatic diseases provided encouraging results. Furthermore, these treatments have proven to be well tolerated and safe. Future approaches including neutralizing antibodies against IL-1, IL-1RI, and locally delivered gene therapy may provide additional options for the clinicians.

REFERENCES

Aida, Y., Maeno, M., Suzuki, N., Shiratsuchi, H., Motohashi, M., and Matsumura, H. (2005). The effect of IL-1beta on the expression of matrix metalloproteinases and tissue inhibitors of matrix metalloproteinases in human chondrocytes. *Life Sci.* **77,** 3210–3221.

Apte, S. S. (2004). A disintegrin-like and metalloprotease (reprolysin type) with thrombos-pondin type 1 motifs: The ADAMTS family. *Int. J. Biochem. Cell Biol.* **36,** 981–985.

Arend, W. P., Malyak, M., Smith, M. F., Jr., Whisenand, T. D., Slack, J. L., Sims, J. E., Giri, J. G., and Dower, S. K. (1994). Binding of IL-1 alpha, IL-1 beta, and IL-1 receptor antagonist by soluble IL-1 receptors and levels of soluble IL-1 receptors in synovial fluids. *J. Immunol.* **153,** 4766–4774.

Arend, W. P., Malyak, M., Guthridge, C. J., and Gabay, C. (1998). Interleukin-1 receptor antagonist: Role in biology. *Annu. Rev. Immunol.* **16,** 27–55.

Arner, E. C., Harris, R. R., DiMeo, T. M., Collins, R. C., and Galbraith, W. (1995). Interleukin-1 receptor antagonist inhibits proteoglycan breakdown in antigen induced but not polycation induced arthritis in the rabbit. *J. Rheumatol.* **22,** 1338–1346.

Attur, M. G., Dave, M., Cipolletta, C., Kang, P., Goldring, M. B., Patel, I. R., Abramson, S. B., and Amin, A. R. (2000). Reversal of autocrine and paracrine effects of interleukin 1 (IL-1) in human arthritis by type II IL-1 decoy receptor. Potential for pharmacological intervention. *J. Biol. Chem.* **275**, 40307–40315.

Attur, M. G., Dave, M. N., Leung, M. Y., Cipolletta, C., Meseck, M., Woo, S. L., and Amin, A. R. (2002). Functional genomic analysis of type II IL-1beta decoy receptor: Potential for gene therapy in human arthritis and inflammation. *J. Immunol.* **168**, 2001–2010.

Bakker, A. C., Joosten, L. A., Arntz, O. J., Helsen, M. M., Bendele, A. M., van de Loo, F. A., and van den Berg, W. B. (1997). Prevention of murine collagen-induced arthritis in the knee and ipsilateral paw by local expression of human interleukin-1 receptor antagonist protein in the knee. *Arthritis Rheum.* **40**, 893–900.

Banda, N. K., Guthridge, C., Sheppard, D., Cairns, K. S., Muggli, M., Bech-Otschir, D., Dubiel, W., and Arend, W. P. (2005). Intracellular IL-1 receptor antagonist type 1 inhibits IL-1-induced cytokine production in keratinocytes through binding to the third component of the COP9 signalosome. *J. Immunol.* **174**, 3608–3616.

Bandara, G., Mueller, G. M., Galea-Lauri, J., Tindal, M. H., Georgescu, H. I., Suchanek, M. K., Hung, G. L., Glorioso, J. C., Robbins, P. D., and Evans, C. H. (1993). Intraarticular expression of biologically active interleukin 1-receptor-antagonist protein by *ex vivo* gene transfer. *Proc. Natl. Acad. Sci. USA* **90**, 10764–10768.

Baragi, V. M., Renkiewicz, R. R., Jordan, H., Bonadio, J., Hartman, J. W., and Roessler, B. J. (1995). Transplantation of transduced chondrocytes protects articular cartilage from interleukin 1-induced extracellular matrix degradation. *J. Clin. Invest.* **96**, 2454–2460.

Bell-Parikh, L. C., Ide, T., Lawson, J. A., McNamara, P., Reilly, M., and FitzGerald, G. A. (2003). Biosynthesis of 15-deoxy-delta12,14-PGJ2 and the ligation of PPARgamma. *J. Clin. Invest.* **112**, 945–955.

Berenbaum, F., Jacques, C., Thomas, G., Corvol, M. T., Bereziat, G., and Masliah, J. (1996). Synergistic effect of interleukin-1 beta and tumor necrosis factor alpha on PGE2 production by articular chondrocytes does not involve PLA2 stimulation. *Exp. Cell Res.* **222**, 379–384.

Bessis, N., Guery, L., Mantovani, A., Vecchi, A., Sims, J. E., Fradelizi, D., and Boissier, M. C. (2000). The type II decoy receptor of IL-1 inhibits murine collagen-induced arthritis. *Eur. J. Immunol.* **30**, 867–875.

Black, R. A., Kronheim, S. R., Cantrell, M., Deeley, M. C., March, C. J., Prickett, K. S., Wignall, J., Conlon, P. J., Cosman, D., Hopp, T. P., and Mochizuki, D. Y. (1988). Generation of biologically active interleukin-1 beta by proteolytic cleavage of the inactive precursor. *J. Biol. Chem.* **263**, 9437–9442.

Blanco, F. J., Ochs, R. L., Schwarz, H., and Lotz, M. (1995). Chondrocyte apoptosis induced by nitric oxide. *Am. J. Pathol.* **146**, 75–85.

Bolon, B., Campagnuolo, G., Zhu, L., Duryea, D., Zack, D., and Feige, U. (2004). Interleukin-1beta and tumor necrosis factor-alpha produce distinct, time-dependent patterns of acute arthritis in the rat knee. *Vet. Pathol.* **41**, 235–243.

Bordji, K., Grillasca, J. P., Gouze, J. N., Magdalou, J., Schohn, H., Keller, J. M., Bianchi, A., Dauca, M., Netter, P., and Terlain, B. (2000). Evidence for the presence of peroxisome proliferator-activated receptor (PPAR) alpha and gamma and retinoid Z receptor in cartilage. PPARgamma activation modulates the effects of interleukin-1beta on rat chondrocytes. *J. Biol. Chem.* **275**, 12243–12250.

Boyault, S., Simonin, M. A., Bianchi, A., Compe, E., Liagre, B., Mainard, D., Becuwe, P., Dauca, M., Netter, P., Terlain, B., and Bordji, K. (2001). 15-Deoxy-delta12,14-PGJ2, but not troglitazone, modulates IL-1beta effects in human chondrocytes by inhibiting NF-kappaB and AP-1 activation pathways. *FEBS Lett.* **501**, 24–30.

Bresnihan, B., Alvaro-Gracia, J. M., Cobby, M., Doherty, M., Domljan, Z., Emery, P., Nuki, G., Pavelka, K., Rau, R., Rozman, B., Watt, I., Williams, B., *et al.* (1998). Treatment of rheumatoid arthritis with recombinant human interleukin-1 receptor antagonist. *Arthritis Rheum.* **41**, 2196–2204.

Buch, M. H., Bingham, S. J., Seto, Y., McGonagle, D., Bejarano, V., White, J., and Emery, P. (2004). Lack of response to anakinra in rheumatoid arthritis following failure of tumor necrosis factor alpha blockade. *Arthritis Rheum.* **50**, 725–728.

Burger, D., Chicheportiche, R., Giri, J. G., and Dayer, J. M. (1995). The inhibitory activity of human interleukin-1 receptor antagonist is enhanced by type II interleukin-1 soluble receptor and hindered by type I interleukin-1 soluble receptor. *J. Clin. Invest.* **96**, 38–41.

Cal, S., Obaya, A. J., Llamazares, M., Garabaya, C., Quesada, V., and Lopez-Otin, C. (2002). Cloning, expression analysis, and structural characterization of seven novel human ADAMTSs, a family of metalloproteinases with disintegrin and thrombospondin-1 domains. *Gene* **283**, 49–62.

Canna, S., Gelabert, A., Aksentijevich, I., Mellis, S., Radin, A., Papadopoulos, J., Barham, B., Wilson, M., Hawkins, P. N., Kastner, D. L., and Goldbach-Mansky, R. (2005). Treatment of 4 patients with cryopyrin-associated periodic syndromes with the long-acting Il-1 inhibitor Il-1 trap. *Arthritis Rheum.* **52**, S274.

Cao, M., Westerhausen-Larson, A., Niyibizi, C., Kavalkovich, K., Georgescu, H. I., Rizzo, C. F., Hebda, P. A., Stefanovic-Racic, M., and Evans, C. H. (1997). Nitric oxide inhibits the synthesis of type-II collagen without altering Col2A1 mRNA abundance: Prolyl hydroxylase as a possible target. *Biochem. J.* **324**(Pt. 1), 305–310.

Cao, Z., Xiong, J., Takeuchi, M., Kurama, T., and Goeddel, D. V. (1996). TRAF6 is a signal transducer for interleukin-1. *Nature* **383**, 443–446.

Caron, J. P., Fernandes, J. C., Martel-Pelletier, J., Tardif, G., Mineau, F., Geng, C., and Pelletier, J. P. (1996). Chondroprotective effect of intraarticular injections of interleukin-1 receptor antagonist in experimental osteoarthritis. Suppression of collagenase-1 expression. *Arthritis Rheum.* **39**, 1535–1544.

Carter, D. B., Deibel, M. R., Jr., Dunn, C. J., Tomich, C. S., Laborde, A. L., Slightom, J. L., Berger, A. E., Bienkowski, M. J., Sun, F. F., McEwan, R. N., Harris, P. K. W., and Yem, A. W. (1990). Purification, cloning, expression and biological characterization of an interleukin-1 receptor antagonist protein. *Nature* **344**, 633–638.

Cawston, T. E. (1996). Metalloproteinase inhibitors and the prevention of connective tissue breakdown. *Pharmacol. Ther.* **70**, 163–182.

Chevalier, X., Giraudeau, B., Conrozier, T., Marliere, J., Kiefer, P., and Goupille, P. (2005). Safety study of intraarticular injection of interleukin 1 receptor antagonist in patients with painful knee osteoarthritis: A multicenter study. *J. Rheumatol.* **32**, 1317–1323.

Clancy, R. M., Abramson, S. B., Kohne, C., and Rediske, J. (1997). Nitric oxide attenuates cellular hexose monophosphate shunt response to oxidants in articular chondrocytes and acts to promote oxidant injury. *J. Cell Physiol.* **172**, 183–191.

Clancy, R. M., Amin, A. R., and Abramson, S. B. (1998). The role of nitric oxide in inflammation and immunity. *Arthritis Rheum.* **41**, 1141–1151.

Clements, K. M., Price, J. S., Chambers, M. G., Visco, D. M., Poole, A. R., and Mason, R. M. (2003). Gene deletion of either interleukin-1beta, interleukin-1beta-converting enzyme, inducible nitric oxide synthase, or stromelysin 1 accelerates the development of knee osteoarthritis in mice after surgical transection of the medial collateral ligament and partial medial meniscectomy. *Arthritis Rheum.* **48**, 3452–3463.

Cohen, S. B., Woolley, J. M., and Chan, W. (2003). Interleukin 1 receptor antagonist anakinra improves functional status in patients with rheumatoid arthritis. *J. Rheumatol.* **30**, 225–231.

Collins-Racie, L. A., Flannery, C. R., Zeng, W., Corcoran, C., Annis-Freeman, B., Agostino, M. J., Arai, M., DiBlasio-Smith, E., Dorner, A. J., Georgiadis, K. E., Jin, M., Tan, X. Y., *et al.* (2004). ADAMTS-8 exhibits aggrecanase activity and is expressed in human articular cartilage. *Matrix Biol.* **23**, 219–230.

Colotta, F., Dower, S. K., Sims, J. E., and Mantovani, A. (1994). The type II 'decoy' receptor: A novel regulatory pathway for interleukin 1. *Immunol. Today* **15**, 562–566.

Colotta, F., Orlando, S., Fadlon, E. J., Sozzani, S., Matteucci, C., and Mantovani, A. (1995). Chemoattractants induce rapid release of the interleukin 1 type II decoy receptor in human polymorphonuclear cells. *J. Exp. Med.* **181**, 2181–2186.

Colotta, F., Saccani, S., Giri, J. G., Dower, S. K., Sims, J. E., Introna, M., and Mantovani, A. (1996). Regulated expression and release of the IL-1 decoy receptor in human mononuclear phagocytes. *J. Immunol.* **156**, 2534–2541.

Crofford, L. J., Wilder, R. L., Ristimaki, A. P., Sano, H., Remmers, E. F., Epps, H. R., and Hla, T. (1994). Cyclooxygenase-1 and -2 expression in rheumatoid synovial tissues. Effects of interleukin-1 beta, phorbol ester, and corticosteroids. *J. Clin. Invest.* **93**, 1095–1101.

Crofford, L. J., Lipsky, P. E., Brooks, P., Abramson, S. B., Simon, L. S., and van de Putte, L. B. (2000). Basic biology and clinical application of specific cyclooxygenase-2 inhibitors. *Arthritis Rheum.* **43**, 4–13.

Cunnane, G., Madigan, A., Murphy, E., FitzGerald, O., and Bresnihan, B. (2001). The effects of treatment with interleukin-1 receptor antagonist on the inflamed synovial membrane in rheumatoid arthritis. *Rheumatology (Oxford)* **40**, 62–69.

Dawson, J., Engelhardt, P., Kastelic, T., Cheneval, D., MacKenzie, A., and Ramage, P. (1999). Effects of soluble interleukin-1 type II receptor on rabbit antigen-induced arthritis: Clinical, biochemical and histological assessment. *Rheumatology (Oxford)* **38**, 401–406.

Deleuran, B. W., Chu, C. Q., Field, M., Brennan, F. M., Katsikis, P., Feldmann, M., and Maini, R. N. (1992). Localization of interleukin-1 alpha, type 1 interleukin-1 receptor and interleukin-1 receptor antagonist in the synovial membrane and cartilage/pannus junction in rheumatoid arthritis. *Br. J. Rheumatol.* **31**, 801–809.

Demircan, K., Hirohata, S., Nishida, K., Hatipoglu, O. F., Oohashi, T., Yonezawa, T., Apte, S. S., and Ninomiya, Y. (2005). ADAMTS-9 is synergistically induced by interleukin-1beta and tumor necrosis factor alpha in OUMS-27 chondrosarcoma cells and in human chondrocytes. *Arthritis Rheum.* **52**, 1451–1460.

Devchand, P. R., Keller, H., Peters, J. M., Vazquez, M., Gonzalez, F. J., and Wahli, W. (1996). The PPARalpha-leukotriene B4 pathway to inflammation control. *Nature* **384**, 39–43.

Dewberry, R., Holden, H., Crossman, D., and Francis, S. (2000). Interleukin-1 receptor antagonist expression in human endothelial cells and atherosclerosis. *Arterioscler. Thromb. Vasc. Biol.* **20**, 2394–2400.

Dijkgraaf, L. C., de Bont, L. G., Boering, G., and Liem, R. S. (1995). Normal cartilage structure, biochemistry, and metabolism: A review of the literature. *J. Oral Maxillofac. Surg.* **53**, 924–929.

Dinarello, C. A. (2002). The IL-1 family and inflammatory diseases. *Clin. Exp. Rheumatol.* **20**, S1–S13.

Dower, S. K., Fanslow, W., Jacobs, C., Waugh, S., Sims, J. E., and Widmer, M. B. (1994). Interleukin-1 antagonists. *Therapeutic Immunol.* **1**, 113–122.

Drevlow, B. E., Lovis, R., Haag, M. A., Sinacore, J. M., Jacobs, C., Blosche, C., Landay, A., Moreland, L. W., and Pope, R. M. (1996). Recombinant human interleukin-1 receptor type I in the treatment of patients with active rheumatoid arthritis. *Arthritis Rheum.* **39**, 257–265.

Eastgate, J. A., Symons, J. A., Wood, N. C., Grinlinton, F. M., di Giovine, F. S., and Duff, G. W. (1988). Correlation of plasma interleukin 1 levels with disease activity in rheumatoid arthritis. *Lancet* **2**, 706–709.

Economides, A. N., Carpenter, L. R., Rudge, J. S., Wong, V., Koehler-Stec, E. M., Hartnett, C., Pyles, E. A., Xu, X., Daly, T. J., Young, M. R., Fandl, J. P., Lee, F., *et al.* (2003). Cytokine traps: Multi-component, high-affinity blockers of cytokine action. *Nat. Med.* **9**, 47–52.

Eisenberg, S. P., Evans, R. J., Arend, W. P., Verderber, E., Brewer, M. T., Hannum, C. H., and Thompson, R. C. (1990). Primary structure and functional expression from complementary DNA of a human interleukin-1 receptor antagonist. *Nature* **343**, 341–346.

Eisenberg, S. P., Brewer, M. T., Verderber, E., Heimdal, P., Brandhuber, B. J., and Thompson, R. C. (1991). Interleukin 1 receptor antagonist is a member of the interleukin 1 gene family: Evolution of a cytokine control mechanism. *Proc. Natl. Acad. Sci. USA* **88,** 5232–5236.

Fahmi, H., Di Battista, J. A., Pelletier, J. P., Mineau, F., Ranger, P., and Martel-Pelletier, J. (2001). Peroxisome proliferator-activated receptor gamma activators inhibit interleukin-1beta-induced nitric oxide and matrix metalloproteinase 13 production in human chondrocytes. *Arthritis Rheum.* **44,** 595–607.

Fahmi, H., Pelletier, J. P., Di Battista, J. A., Cheung, H. S., Fernandes, J. C., and Martel-Pelletier, J. (2002). Peroxisome proliferator-activated receptor gamma activators inhibit MMP-1 production in human synovial fibroblasts likely by reducing the binding of the activator protein 1. *Osteoarthritis Cartilage* **10,** 100–108.

Fernandes, J., Tardif, G., Martel-Pelletier, J., Lascau-Coman, V., Dupuis, M., Moldovan, F., Sheppard, M., Krishnan, B. R., and Pelletier, J. P. (1999). *In vivo* transfer of interleukin-1 receptor antagonist gene in osteoarthritic rabbit knee joints: Prevention of osteoarthritis progression. *Am. J. Pathol.* **154,** 1159–1169.

Fitzgerald, A. A., Leclercq, S. A., Yan, A., Homik, J. E., and Dinarello, C. A. (2005). Rapid responses to anakinra in patients with refractory adult-onset Still's disease. *Arthritis Rheum.* **52,** 1794–1803.

Flannery, C. R., Lark, M. W., and Sandy, J. D. (1992). Identification of a stromelysin cleavage site within the interglobular RT domain of human aggrecan. Evidence for proteolysis at this site *in vivo* in human articular cartilage. *J. Biol. Chem.* **267,** 1008–1014.

Flannery, C. R., Little, C. B., Hughes, C. E., and Caterson, B. (1999). Expression of ADAMTS homologues in articular cartilage. *Biochem. Biophys. Res. Commun.* **260,** 318–322.

Gabay, C., Smith, M. F., Eidlen, D., and Arend, W. P. (1997). Interleukin 1 receptor antagonist (IL-1Ra) is an acute-phase protein. *J. Clin. Invest.* **99,** 2930–2940.

Gabay, C., Marinova-Mutafchieva, L., Williams, R. O., Gigley, J. P., Butler, D. M., Feldmann, M., and Arend, W. P. (2001). Increased production of intracellular interleukin-1 receptor antagonist type I in the synovium of mice with collagen-induced arthritis: A possible role in the resolution of arthritis. *Arthritis Rheum.* **44,** 451–462.

Ganu, V. S., Hu, S. I., Melton, R., Winter, C., Goldberg, V. M., Haqqi, T. M., and Malemud, C. J. (1994). Biochemical and molecular characterization of stromelysin synthesized by human osteoarthritic chondrocytes stimulated with recombinant human interleukin-1. *Clin. Exp. Rheumatol.* **12,** 489–496.

Garat, C., and Arend, W. P. (2003). Intracellular IL-1Ra type 1 inhibits IL-1-induced IL-6 and IL-8 production in Caco-2 intestinal epithelial cells through inhibition of p38 mitogen-activated protein kinase and NF-kappaB pathways. *Cytokine* **23,** 31–40.

Genovese, M. C., Cohen, S., Moreland, L., Lium, D., Robbins, S., Newmark, R., and Bekker, P. (2004). Combination therapy with etanercept and anakinra in the treatment of patients with rheumatoid arthritis who have been treated unsuccessfully with methotrexate. *Arthritis Rheum.* **50,** 1412–1419.

Ghivizzani, S. C., Kang, R., Georgescu, H. I., Lechman, E. R., Jaffurs, D., Engle, J. M., Watkins, S. C., Tindal, M. H., Suchanek, M. K., McKenzie, L. R., Evans, C. H., and Robbins, P. D. (1997a). Constitutive intra-articular expression of human IL-1 beta following gene transfer to rabbit synovium produces all major pathologies of human rheumatoid arthritis. *J. Immunol.* **159,** 3604–3612.

Ghivizzani, S. C., Lechman, E. R., Tio, C., Mule, K. M., Chada, S., McCormack, J. E., Evans, C. H., and Robbins, P. D. (1997b). Direct retrovirus-mediated gene transfer to the synovium of the rabbit knee: Implications for arthritis gene therapy. *Gene Ther.* **4,** 977–982.

Ghivizzani, S. C., Lechman, E. R., Kang, R., Tio, C., Kolls, J., Evans, C. H., and Robbins, P. D. (1998). Direct adenovirus-mediated gene transfer of interleukin 1 and tumor necrosis factor alpha soluble receptors to rabbit knees with experimental arthritis has local and distal anti-arthritic effects. *Proc. Natl. Acad. Sci. USA* **95,** 4613–4618.

Glasson, S. S., Askew, R., Sheppard, B., Carito, B., Blanchet, T., Ma, H. L., Flannery, C. R., Peluso, D., Kanki, K., Yang, Z., Majumdar, M. K., and Morris, E. A. (2005). Deletion of active ADAMTS5 prevents cartilage degradation in a murine model of osteoarthritis. *Nature* **434,** 644–648.

Goldring, M. B. (2000). Osteoarthritis and cartilage: The role of cytokines. *Curr. Rheumatol. Rep.* **2,** 459–465.

Goldring, M. B., Sohbat, E., Elwell, J. M., and Chang, J. Y. (1990). Etodolac preserves cartilage-specific phenotype in human chondrocytes: Effects on type II collagen synthesis and associated mRNA levels. *Eur. J. Rheumatol. Inflamm.* **10,** 10–21.

Goldring, M. B., Fukuo, K., Birkhead, J. R., Dudek, E., and Sandell, L. J. (1994). Transcriptional suppression by interleukin-1 and interferon-gamma of type II collagen gene expression in human chondrocytes. *J. Cell Biochem.* **54,** 85–99.

Goldring, M. B., Suen, L. F., Yamin, R., and Lai, W. F. (1996). Regulation of collagen gene expression by prostaglandins and interleukin-1beta in cultured chondrocytes and fibroblasts. *Am. J. Ther.* **3,** 9–16.

Goupille, P., Jayson, M. I., Valat, J. P., and Freemont, A. J. (1998). Matrix metalloproteinases: The clue to intervertebral disc degeneration? *Spine* **23,** 1612–1626.

Guler, H. P., Caldwell, J., Littlejohn, T., McIlwain, H., Offenberg, H., and Stahl, N. (2001). A phase 1, single dose escalation study of IL-1 Trap in patients with rheumatoid arthritis. *Arthritis Rheum.* **44,** S370.

Haibel, H., Rudwaleit, M., Listing, J., and Sieper, J. (2005). Open label trial of anakinra in active ankylosing spondylitis over 24 weeks. *Ann. Rheum. Dis.* **64,** 296–298.

Hashimoto, S., Takahashi, K., Amiel, D., Coutts, R. D., and Lotz, M. (1998). Chondrocyte apoptosis and nitric oxide production during experimentally induced osteoarthritis. *Arthritis Rheum.* **41,** 1266–1274.

Haskill, S., Martin, G., Van Le, L., Morris, J., Peace, A., Bigler, C. F., Jaffe, G. J., Hammerberg, C., Sporn, S. A., Fong, S., Arend, W. P., and Ralph, P. (1991). cDNA cloning of an intracellular form of the human interleukin 1 receptor antagonist associated with epithelium. *Proc. Natl. Acad. Sci. USA* **88,** 3681–3685.

Hauselmann, H. J., Oppliger, L., Michel, B. A., Stefanovic-Racic, M., and Evans, C. H. (1994). Nitric oxide and proteoglycan biosynthesis by human articular chondrocytes in alginate culture. *FEBS Lett.* **352,** 361–364.

Hembry, R. M., Bagga, M. R., Reynolds, J. J., and Hamblen, D. L. (1995). Immunolocalisation studies on six matrix metalloproteinases and their inhibitors, TIMP-1 and TIMP-2, in synovia from patients with osteo and rheumatoid arthritis. *Ann. Rheum. Dis.* **54,** 25–32.

Henderson, B., and Pettipher, E. R. (1989). Arthritogenic actions of recombinant IL-1 and tumour necrosis factor alpha in the rabbit: Evidence for synergistic interactions between cytokines *in vivo. Clin. Exp. Immunol.* **75,** 306–310.

Henrotin, Y. E., Zheng, S. X., Deby, G. P., Labasse, A. H., Crielaard, J. M., and Reginster, J. Y. (1998). Nitric oxide downregulates interleukin 1beta (IL-1beta) stimulated IL-6, IL-8, and prostaglandin E2 production by human chondrocytes. *J. Rheumatol.* **25,** 1595–1601.

Horai, R., Saijo, S., Tanioka, H., Nakae, S., Sudo, K., Okahara, A., Ikuse, T., Asano, M., and Iwakura, Y. (2000). Development of chronic inflammatory arthropathy resembling rheumatoid arthritis in interleukin 1 receptor antagonist-deficient mice. *J. Exp. Med.* **191,** 313–320.

Hortelano, S., Castrillo, A., Alvarez, A. M., and Bosca, L. (2000). Contribution of cyclopentenone prostaglandins to the resolution of inflammation through the potentiation of apoptosis in activated macrophages. *J. Immunol.* **165,** 6525–6531.

Hu, B., Wang, S., Zhang, Y., Feghali, C. A., Dingman, J. R., and Wright, T. M. (2003). A nuclear target for interleukin-1alpha: Interaction with the growth suppressor necdin modulates proliferation and collagen expression. *Proc. Natl. Acad. Sci. USA* **100,** 10008–10013.

Huang, Q., Yang, J., Lin, Y., Walker, C., Cheng, J., Liu, Z. G., and Su, B. (2004). Differential regulation of interleukin 1 receptor and Toll-like receptor signaling by MEKK3. *Nat. Immunol.* **5**, 98–103.

Hung, G. L., Galea-Lauri, J., Mueller, G. M., Georgescu, H. I., Larkin, L. A., Suchanek, M. K., Tindal, M. H., Robbins, P. D., and Evans, C. H. (1994). Suppression of intra-articular responses to interleukin-1 by transfer of the interleukin-1 receptor antagonist gene to synovium. *Gene Ther.* **1**, 64–69.

Ide, T., Egan, K., Bell-Parikh, L. C., and FitzGerald, G. A. (2003). Activation of nuclear receptors by prostaglandins. *Thromb. Res.* **110**, 311–315.

Issemann, I., and Green, S. (1990). Activation of a member of the steroid hormone receptor superfamily by peroxisome proliferators. *Nature* **347**, 645–650.

Jakobsson, P. J., Thoren, S., Morgenstern, R., and Samuelsson, B. (1999). Identification of human prostaglandin E synthase: A microsomal, glutathione-dependent, inducible enzyme, constituting a potential novel drug target. *Proc. Natl. Acad. Sci. USA* **96**, 7220–7225.

Jensen, L. E., and Whitehead, A. S. (2003). Expression of alternatively spliced interleukin-1 receptor accessory protein mRNAs is differentially regulated during inflammation and apoptosis. *Cell Signal* **15**, 793–802.

Jensen, L. E., and Whitehead, A. S. (2004). The 3′ untranslated region of the membrane-bound IL-1R accessory protein mRNA confers tissue-specific destabilization. *J. Immunol.* **173**, 6248–6258.

Jensen, L. E., Muzio, M., Mantovani, A., and Whitehead, A. S. (2000). IL-1 signaling cascade in liver cells and the involvement of a soluble form of the IL-1 receptor accessory protein. *J. Immunol.* **164**, 5277–5286.

Jiang, Y., Genant, H. K., Watt, I., Cobby, M., Bresnihan, B., Aitchison, R., and McCabe, D. (2000). A multicenter, double-blind, dose-ranging, randomized, placebo-controlled study of recombinant human interleukin-1 receptor antagonist in patients with rheumatoid arthritis: Radiologic progression and correlation of Genant and Larsen scores. *Arthritis Rheum.* **43**, 1001–1009.

Jiang, Z., Ninomiya-Tsuji, J., Qian, Y., Matsumoto, K., and Li, X. (2002). Interleukin-1 (IL-1) receptor-associated kinase-dependent IL-1-induced signaling complexes phosphorylate TAK1 and TAB2 at the plasma membrane and activate TAK1 in the cytosol. *Mol. Cell. Biol.* **22**, 7158–7167.

Joosten, L. A., Helsen, M. M., van de Loo, F. A., and van den Berg, W. B. (1996). Anticytokine treatment of established type II collagen-induced arthritis in DBA/1 mice. A comparative study using anti-TNF alpha, anti-IL-1 alpha/beta, and IL-1Ra. *Arthritis Rheum.* **39**, 797–809.

Joosten, L. A., Helsen, M. M., Saxne, T., van De Loo, F. A., Heinegard, D., and van Den Berg, W. B. (1999). IL-1 alpha beta blockade prevents cartilage and bone destruction in murine type II collagen-induced arthritis, whereas TNF-alpha blockade only ameliorates joint inflammation. *J. Immunol.* **163**, 5049–5055.

Kawai, T., Adachi, O., Ogawa, T., Takeda, K., and Akira, S. (1999). Unresponsiveness of MyD88-deficient mice to endotoxin. *Immunity* **11**, 115–122.

Kevorkian, L., Young, D. A., Darrah, C., Donell, S. T., Shepstone, L., Porter, S., Brockbank, S. M., Edwards, D. R., Parker, A. E., and Clark, I. M. (2004). Expression profiling of metalloproteinases and their inhibitors in cartilage. *Arthritis Rheum.* **50**, 131–141.

Koshy, P. J., Lundy, C. J., Rowan, A. D., Porter, S., Edwards, D. R., Hogan, A., Clark, I. M., and Cawston, T. E. (2002). The modulation of matrix metalloproteinase and ADAM gene expression in human chondrocytes by interleukin-1 and oncostatin M: A time-course study using real-time quantitative reverse transcription-polymerase chain reaction. *Arthritis Rheum.* **46**, 961–967.

Ku, G., Faust, T., Lauffer, L. L., Livingston, D. J., and Harding, M. W. (1996). Interleukin-1 beta converting enzyme inhibition blocks progression of type II collagen-induced arthritis in mice. *Cytokine* **8**, 377–386.

Kuhn, K., Hashimoto, S., and Lotz, M. (2000). IL-1 beta protects human chondrocytes from CD95-induced apoptosis. *J. Immunol.* **164,** 2233–2239.

Kuhn, K., Shikhman, A. R., and Lotz, M. (2003). Role of nitric oxide, reactive oxygen species, and p38 MAP kinase in the regulation of human chondrocyte apoptosis. *J. Cell. Physiol.* **197,** 379–387.

Kuiper, S., Joosten, L. A., Bendele, A. M., Edwards, C. K., III, Arntz, O. J., Helsen, M. M., Van de Loo, F. A., and Van den Berg, W. B. (1998). Different roles of tumour necrosis factor alpha and interleukin 1 in murine streptococcal cell wall arthritis. *Cytokine* **10,** 690–702.

Kuno, K., Okada, Y., Kawashima, H., Nakamura, H., Miyasaka, M., Ohno, H., and Matsushima, K. (2000). ADAMTS-1 cleaves a cartilage proteoglycan, aggrecan. *FEBS Lett.* **478,** 241–245.

Lang, D., Knop, J., Wesche, H., Raffetseder, U., Kurrle, R., Boraschi, D., and Martin, M. U. (1998). The type II IL-1 receptor interacts with the IL-1 receptor accessory protein: A novel mechanism of regulation of IL-1 responsiveness. *J. Immunol.* **161,** 6871–6877.

Loeser, R. F., Carlson, C. S., Del Carlo, M., and Cole, A. (2002). Detection of nitrotyrosine in aging and osteoarthritic cartilage: Correlation of oxidative damage with the presence of interleukin-1beta and with chondrocyte resistance to insulin-like growth factor 1. *Arthritis Rheum.* **46,** 2349–2357.

Lye, E., Mirtsos, C., Suzuki, N., Suzuki, S., and Yeh, W. C. (2004). The role of interleukin 1 receptor-associated kinase-4 (IRAK-4) kinase activity in IRAK-4-mediated signaling. *J. Biol. Chem.* **279,** 40653–40658.

Ma, Y., Thornton, S., Boivin, G. P., Hirsh, D., Hirsch, R., and Hirsch, E. (1998). Altered susceptibility to collagen-induced arthritis in transgenic mice with aberrant expression of interleukin-1 receptor antagonist. *Arthritis Rheum.* **41,** 1798–1805.

Makarov, S. S., Olsen, J. C., Johnston, W. N., Anderle, S. K., Brown, R. R., Baldwin, A. S., Jr., Haskill, J. S., and Schwab, J. H. (1996). Suppression of experimental arthritis by gene transfer of interleukin 1 receptor antagonist cDNA. *Proc. Natl. Acad. Sci. USA* **93,** 402–406.

Malemud, C. J., Islam, N., and Haqqi, T. M. (2003). Pathophysiological mechanisms in osteoarthritis lead to novel therapeutic strategies. *Cells Tissues Organs* **174,** 34–48.

Malinowsky, D., Lundkvist, J., Laye, S., and Bartfai, T. (1998). Interleukin-1 receptor accessory protein interacts with the type II interleukin-1 receptor. *FEBS Lett.* **429,** 299–302.

Malyak, M., Smith, M. F., Jr., Abel, A. A., Hance, K. R., and Arend, W. P. (1998). The differential production of three forms of IL-1 receptor antagonist by human neutrophils and monocytes. *J. Immunol.* **161,** 2004–2010.

Maneiro, E., Lopez-Armada, M. J., Fernandez-Sueiro, J. L., Lema, B., Galdo, F., and Blanco, F. J. (2001). Aceclofenac increases the synthesis of interleukin 1 receptor antagonist and decreases the production of nitric oxide in human articular chondrocytes. *J. Rheumatol.* **28,** 2692–2699.

Maret, M., Chicheportiche, R., Dayer, J. M., and Gabay, C. (2004). Production of intracellular IL-1alpha, IL-1beta, and IL-1Ra isoforms by activated human dermal and synovial fibroblasts: Phenotypic differences between human dermal and synovial fibroblasts. *Cytokine* **25,** 193–203.

Martel-Pelletier, J., McCollum, R., DiBattista, J., Faure, M. P., Chin, J. A., Fournier, S., Sarfati, M., and Pelletier, J. P. (1992). The interleukin-1 receptor in normal and osteoarthritic human articular chondrocytes. Identification as the type I receptor and analysis of binding kinetics and biologic function. *Arthritis Rheum.* **35,** 530–540.

Martin, G., Andriamanalijaona, R., Grassel, S., Dreier, R., Mathy-Hartert, M., Bogdanowicz, P., Boumediene, K., Henrotin, Y., Bruckner, P., and Pujol, J. P. (2004). Effect of hypoxia and reoxygenation on gene expression and response to interleukin-1 in cultured articular chondrocytes. *Arthritis Rheum.* **50,** 3549–3560.

Masuko-Hongo, K., Berenbaum, F., Humbert, L., Salvat, C., Goldring, M. B., and Thirion, S. (2004). Up-regulation of microsomal prostaglandin E synthase 1 in osteoarthritic human cartilage: Critical roles of the ERK-1/2 and p38 signaling pathways. *Arthritis Rheum.* **50**, 2829–2838.

McCartney-Francis, N. L., Song, X., Mizel, D. E., and Wahl, S. M. (2001). Selective inhibition of inducible nitric oxide synthase exacerbates erosive joint disease. *J. Immunol.* **166**, 2734–2740.

McCoy, J. M., Wicks, J. R., and Audoly, L. P. (2002). The role of prostaglandin E2 receptors in the pathogenesis of rheumatoid arthritis. *J. Clin. Invest.* **110**, 651–658.

Melchiorri, C., Meliconi, R., Frizziero, L., Silvestri, T., Pulsatelli, L., Mazzetti, I., Borzi, R. M., Uguccioni, M., and Facchini, A. (1998). Enhanced and coordinated *in vivo* expression of inflammatory cytokines and nitric oxide synthase by chondrocytes from patients with osteoarthritis. *Arthritis Rheum.* **41**, 2165–2174.

Merhi-Soussi, F., Berti, M., Wehrle-Haller, B., and Gabay, C. (2005). Intracellular interleukin-1 receptor antagonist type 1 antagonizes the stimulatory effect of interleukin-1alpha precursor on cell motility. *Cytokine* **32**, 163–170.

Miller, L. C., Lynch, E. A., Isa, S., Logan, J. W., Dinarello, C. A., and Steere, A. C. (1993). Balance of synovial fluid IL-1 beta and IL-1 receptor antagonist and recovery from Lyme arthritis. *Lancet* **341**, 146–148.

Moos, V., Fickert, S., Muller, B., Weber, U., and Sieper, J. (1999). Immunohistological analysis of cytokine expression in human osteoarthritic and healthy cartilage. *J. Rheumatol.* **26**, 870–879.

Murakami, M., Naraba, H., Tanioka, T., Semmyo, N., Nakatani, Y., Kojima, F., Ikeda, T., Fueki, M., Ueno, A., Oh, S., and Kudo, I. (2000). Regulation of prostaglandin E2 biosynthesis by inducible membrane-associated prostaglandin E2 synthase that acts in concert with cyclooxygenase-2. *J. Biol. Chem.* **275**, 32783–32792.

Muzio, M., Polentarutti, N., Sironi, M., Poli, G., De Gioia, L., Introna, M., Mantovani, A., and Colotta, F. (1995). Cloning and characterization of a new isoform of the interleukin 1 receptor antagonist. *J. Exp. Med.* **182**, 623–628.

Nagase, H., and Kashiwagi, M. (2003). Aggrecanases and cartilage matrix degradation. *Arthritis Res. Ther.* **5**, 94–103.

Naito, A., Azuma, S., Tanaka, S., Miyazaki, T., Takaki, S., Takatsu, K., Nakao, K., Nakamura, K., Katsuki, M., Yamamoto, T., and Inoue, J. (1999). Severe osteopetrosis, defective interleukin-1 signalling and lymph node organogenesis in TRAF6-deficient mice. *Genes Cells* **4**, 353–362.

Nguyen, K. H., Boyle, D. L., McCormack, J. E., Chada, S., Jolly, D. J., and Firestein, G. S. (1998). Direct synovial gene transfer with retroviral vectors in rat adjuvant arthritis. *J. Rheumatol.* **25**, 1118–1125.

Niki, Y., Yamada, H., Kikuchi, T., Toyama, Y., Matsumoto, H., Fujikawa, K., and Tada, N. (2004). Membrane-associated IL-1 contributes to chronic synovitis and cartilage destruction in human IL-1 alpha transgenic mice. *J. Immunol.* **172**, 577–584.

Ninomiya-Tsuji, J., Kishimoto, K., Hiyama, A., Inoue, J., Cao, Z., and Matsumoto, K. (1999). The kinase TAK1 can activate the NIK-I kappaB as well as the MAP kinase cascade in the IL-1 signalling pathway. *Nature* **398**, 252–256.

Nuki, G., Bresnihan, B., Bear, M. B., and McCabe, D. (2002). Long-term safety and maintenance of clinical improvement following treatment with anakinra (recombinant human interleukin-1 receptor antagonist) in patients with rheumatoid arthritis: Extension phase of a randomized, double-blind, placebo-controlled trial. *Arthritis Rheum.* **46**, 2838–2846.

Ohtsuka, M., Konno, F., Honda, H., Oikawa, T., Ishikawa, M., Iwase, N., Isomae, K., Ishii, F., Hemmi, H., and Sato, S. (2002). PPA250 [3-(2,4-difluorophenyl)-6-[2-[4-(1H-imidazol-1-ylmethyl) phenoxy]ethoxy]-2-phenylpyridine], a novel orally effective inhibitor of the dimerization of inducible nitric-oxide synthase, exhibits an anti-inflammatory effect in animal models of chronic arthritis. *J. Pharmacol. Exp. Ther.* **303**, 52–57.

Oligino, T. J., Ghivizzani, S., and Wolfe, D. (1996). Intra-articular delivery of a herpes simplex virus IL-1Ra gene vector reduces inflammation in a rabbit model of arthritis. *Gene Ther.* **6**, 1713–1720.

Ostendorf, B., Iking-Konert, C., Kurz, K., Jung, G., Sander, O., and Schneider, M. (2005). Preliminary results of safety and efficacy of the interleukin 1 receptor antagonist anakinra in patients with severe lupus arthritis. *Ann. Rheum. Dis.* **64,** 630–633.

Otani, K., Nita, I., Macaulay, W., Georgescu, H. I., Robbins, P. D., and Evans, C. H. (1996). Suppression of antigen-induced arthritis in rabbits by *ex vivo* gene therapy. *J. Immunol.* **156,** 3558–3562.

Palmer, G., Talabot-Ayer, D., Szalay-Quinodoz, I., Maret, M., Arend, W. P., and Gabay, C. (2003). Mice transgenic for intracellular interleukin-1 receptor antagonist type 1 are protected from collagen-induced arthritis. *Eur. J. Immunol.* **33,** 434–440.

Palmer, R. M., Hickery, M. S., Charles, I. G., Moncada, S., and Bayliss, M. T. (1993). Induction of nitric oxide synthase in human chondrocytes. *Biochem. Biophys. Res. Commun.* **193,** 398–405.

Pan, R. Y., Chen, S. L., Xiao, X., Liu, D. W., Peng, H. J., and Tsao, Y. P. (2000). Therapy and prevention of arthritis by recombinant adeno-associated virus vector with delivery of interleukin-1 receptor antagonist. *Arthritis Rheum.* **43,** 289–297.

Pascual, V., Allantaz, F., Arce, E., Punaro, M., and Banchereau, J. (2005). Role of interleukin-1 (IL-1) in the pathogenesis of systemic onset juvenile idiopathic arthritis and clinical response to IL-1 blockade. *J. Exp. Med.* **201,** 1479–1486.

Patterson, D., Jones, C., Hart, I., Bleskan, J., Berger, R., Geyer, D., Eisenberg, S. P., Smith, M. F., Jr., and Arend, W. P. (1993). The human interleukin-1 receptor antagonist (IL1RN) gene is located in the chromosome 2q14 region. *Genomics* **15,** 173–176.

Pavelka, K., Rasmussen, M. J., Mikkelsen, K., Tamasi, L., Vitek, P., and Rozman, B. (2002). Clinical effects of pralnacasan (PRAL), an orally-active interleukin-1 beta converting enzyme (ICE) inhibitor, in a 285 patient Phase II trial in rheumatoid arthritis. *Arthritis Rheum.* **46,** LB02.

Pelletier, J. P., Mineau, F., Ranger, P., Tardif, G., and Martel-Pelletier, J. (1996). The increased synthesis of inducible nitric oxide inhibits IL-1ra synthesis by human articular chondrocytes: Possible role in osteoarthritic cartilage degradation. *Osteoarthritis Cartilage* **4,** 77–84.

Pelletier, J. P., Caron, J. P., Evans, C., Robbins, P. D., Georgescu, H. I., Jovanovic, D., Fernandes, J. C., and Martel-Pelletier, J. (1997). *In vivo* suppression of early experimental osteoarthritis by interleukin-1 receptor antagonist using gene therapy. *Arthritis Rheum.* **40,** 1012–1019.

Pelletier, J. P., Jovanovic, D. V., Lascau-Coman, V., Fernandes, J. C., Manning, P. T., Connor, J. R., Currie, M. G., and Martel-Pelletier, J. (2000). Selective inhibition of inducible nitric oxide synthase reduces progression of experimental osteoarthritis *in vivo*: Possible link with the reduction in chondrocyte apoptosis and caspase 3 level. *Arthritis Rheum.* **43,** 1290–1299.

Plater-Zyberk, C., Joosten, L. A., Helsen, M. M., Sattonnet-Roche, P., Siegfried, C., Alouani, S., van De Loo, F. A., Graber, P., Aloni, S., Cirillo, R., Lubberts, E., Dinarello, C. A., *et al.* (2001). Therapeutic effect of neutralizing endogenous IL-18 activity in the collagen-induced model of arthritis. *J. Clin. Invest.* **108,** 1825–1832.

Pollock, A. S., Turck, J., and Lovett, D. H. (2003). The prodomain of interleukin 1alpha interacts with elements of the RNA processing apparatus and induces apoptosis in malignant cells. *FASEB J.* **17,** 203–213.

Porter, S., Clark, I. M., Kevorkian, L., and Edwards, D. R. (2005). The ADAMTS metalloproteinases. *Biochem. J.* **386,** 15–27.

Presle, N., Cipolletta, C., Jouzeau, J. Y., Abid, A., Netter, P., and Terlain, B. (1999). Cartilage protection by nitric oxide synthase inhibitors after intraarticular injection of interleukin-1beta in rats. *Arthritis Rheum.* **42,** 2094–2102.

Riquet, F. B., Lai, W. F., Birkhead, J. R., Suen, L. F., Karsenty, G., and Goldring, M. B. (2000). Suppression of type I collagen gene expression by prostaglandins in fibroblasts is mediated at the transcriptional level. *Mol. Med.* **6,** 705–719.

Roessler, B. J., Hartman, J. W., Vallance, D. K., Latta, J. M., Janich, S. L., and Davidson, B. L. (1995). Inhibition of interleukin-1-induced effects in synoviocytes transduced with the human IL-1 receptor antagonist cDNA using an adenoviral vector. *Hum. Gene Ther.* **6,** 307–316.

Rossi, A., Kapahi, P., Natoli, G., Takahashi, T., Chen, Y., Karin, M., and Santoro, M. G. (2000). Anti-inflammatory cyclopentenone prostaglandins are direct inhibitors of IkappaB kinase. *Nature* **403,** 103–108.

Sandy, J. D., Neame, P. J., Boynton, R. E., and Flannery, C. R. (1991). Catabolism of aggrecan in cartilage explants. Identification of a major cleavage site within the interglobular domain. *J. Biol. Chem.* **266,** 8683–8685.

Sasaki, K., Hattori, T., Fujisawa, T., Takahashi, K., Inoue, H., and Takigawa, M. (1998). Nitric oxide mediates interleukin-1-induced gene expression of matrix metalloproteinases and basic fibroblast growth factor in cultured rabbit articular chondrocytes. *J. Biochem. (Tokyo)* **123,** 431–439.

Schmitz, J., Owyang, A., Oldham, E., Song, Y., Murphy, E., McClanahan, T. K., Zurawski, G., Moshrefi, M., Qin, J., Li, X., Gorman, D. M., Bazan, J. F., *et al.* (2005). IL-33, an interleukin-1-like cytokine that signals via the IL-1 receptor-related protein ST2 and induces T helper type 2-associated cytokines. *Immunity* **23,** 479–490.

Schwab, J. H., Anderle, S. K., Brown, R. R., Dalldorf, F. G., and Thompson, R. C. (1991). Pro- and anti-inflammatory roles of interleukin-1 in recurrence of bacterial cell wall-induced arthritis in rats. *Infect. Immun.* **59,** 4436–4442.

Shibata, T., Kondo, M., Osawa, T., Shibata, N., Kobayashi, M., and Uchida, K. (2002). 15-deoxy-delta 12,14-prostaglandin J2. A prostaglandin D2 metabolite generated during inflammatory processes. *J. Biol. Chem.* **277,** 10459–10466.

Shingleton, W. D., Ellis, A. J., Rowan, A. D., and Cawston, T. E. (2000). Retinoic acid combines with interleukin-1 to promote the degradation of collagen from bovine nasal cartilage: Matrix metalloproteinases-1 and -13 are involved in cartilage collagen breakdown. *J. Cell Biochem.* **79,** 519–531.

Silvestri, T., Pulsatelli, L., Dolzani, P., Frizziero, L., Facchini, A., and Meliconi, R. (2006). *In vivo* expression of inflammatory cytokine receptors in the joint compartments of patients with arthritis. *Rheumatol. Int.* **26,** 360–368.

Sims, J. E., Giri, J. G., and Dower, S. K. (1994). The two interleukin-1 receptors play different roles in IL-1 actions. *Clin. Immunol. Immunopathol.* **72,** 9–14.

Sirum, K. L., and Brinckerhoff, C. E. (1989). Cloning of the genes for human stromelysin and stromelysin 2: Differential expression in rheumatoid synovial fibroblasts. *Biochemistry* **28,** 8691–8698.

Smeets, R. L., Joosten, L. A., Arntz, O. J., Bennink, M. B., Takahashi, N., Carlsen, H., Martin, M. U., van den Berg, W. B., and van de Loo, F. A. (2005). Soluble interleukin-1 receptor accessory protein ameliorates collagen-induced arthritis by a different mode of action from that of interleukin-1 receptor antagonist. *Arthritis Rheum.* **52,** 2202–2211.

Smith, D. E., Hanna, R., Della, F., Moore, H., Chen, H., Farese, A. M., MacVittie, T. J., Virca, G. D., and Sims, J. E. (2003). The soluble form of IL-1 receptor accessory protein enhances the ability of soluble type II IL-1 receptor to inhibit IL-1 action. *Immunity* **18,** 87–96.

Somerville, R. P., Longpre, J. M., Jungers, K. A., Engle, J. M., Ross, M., Evanko, S., Wight, T. N., Leduc, R., and Apte, S. S. (2003). Characterization of ADAMTS-9 and ADAMTS-20 as a distinct ADAMTS subfamily related to Caenorhabditis elegans GON-1. *J. Biol. Chem.* **278,** 9503–9513.

Spencer, A. G., Woods, J. W., Arakawa, T., Singer, I. I., and Smith, W. L. (1998). Subcellular localization of prostaglandin endoperoxide H synthases-1 and -2 by immunoelectron microscopy. *J. Biol. Chem.* **273,** 9886–9893.

Stadler, J., Stefanovic-Racic, M., Billiar, T. R., Curran, R. D., McIntyre, L. A., Georgescu, H. I., Simmons, R. L., and Evans, C. H. (1991). Articular chondrocytes synthesize nitric oxide in response to cytokines and lipopolysaccharide. *J. Immunol.* **147,** 3915–3920.

Stanton, H., Rogerson, F. M., East, C. J., Golub, S. B., Lawlor, K. E., Meeker, C. T., Little, C. B., Last, K., Farmer, P. J., Campbell, I. K., Fourie, A. M., and Fosang, A. J. (2005). ADAMTS5 is the major aggrecanase in mouse cartilage *in vivo* and *in vitro*. *Nature* **434**, 648–652.

Steinkasserer, A., Spurr, N. K., Cox, S., Jeggo, P., and Sim, R. B. (1992). The human IL-1 receptor antagonist gene (IL1RN) maps to chromosome 2q14-q21, in the region of the IL-1 alpha and IL-1 beta loci. *Genomics* **13**, 654–657.

Stevenson, F. T., Turck, J., Locksley, R. M., and Lovett, D. H. (1997). The N-terminal propiece of interleukin 1 alpha is a transforming nuclear oncoprotein. *Proc. Natl. Acad. Sci. USA* **94**, 508–513.

Stichtenoth, D. O., Thoren, S., Bian, H., Peters-Golden, M., Jakobsson, P. J., and Crofford, L. J. (2001). Microsomal prostaglandin E synthase is regulated by proinflammatory cytokines and glucocorticoids in primary rheumatoid synovial cells. *J. Immunol.* **167**, 469–474.

Studer, R. K., Levicoff, E., Georgescu, H., Miller, L., Jaffurs, D., and Evans, C. H. (2000). Nitric oxide inhibits chondrocyte response to IGF-I: Inhibition of IGF-IRbeta tyrosine phosphorylation. *Am. J. Physiol. Cell Physiol.* **279**, C961–C969.

Suzuki, N., Suzuki, S., Duncan, G. S., Millar, D. G., Wada, T., Mirtsos, C., Takada, H., Wakeham, A., Itie, A., Li, S., Penninger, J. M., Wesche, H., *et al.* (2002). Severe impairment of interleukin-1 and Toll-like receptor signalling in mice lacking IRAK-4. *Nature* **416**, 750–756.

Tan, A. L., Marzo-Ortega, H., O'Connor, P., Fraser, A., Emery, P., and McGonagle, D. (2004). Efficacy of anakinra in active ankylosing spondylitis: A clinical and magnetic resonance imaging study. *Ann. Rheum. Dis.* **63**, 1041–1045.

Tanioka, T., Nakatani, Y., Semmyo, N., Murakami, M., and Kudo, I. (2000). Molecular identification of cytosolic prostaglandin E2 synthase that is functionally coupled with cyclooxygenase-1 in immediate prostaglandin E2 biosynthesis. *J. Biol. Chem.* **275**, 32775–32782.

Taskiran, D., Stefanovic-Racic, M., Georgescu, H., and Evans, C. (1994). Nitric oxide mediates suppression of cartilage proteoglycan synthesis by interleukin-1. *Biochem. Biophys. Res. Commun.* **200**, 142–148.

Tetlow, L. C., Adlam, D. J., and Woolley, D. E. (2001). Matrix metalloproteinase and proinflammatory cytokine production by chondrocytes of human osteoarthritic cartilage: Associations with degenerative changes. *Arthritis Rheum.* **44**, 585–594.

Thomas, B., Thirion, S., Humbert, L., Tan, L., Goldring, M. B., Bereziat, G., and Berenbaum, F. (2002). Differentiation regulates interleukin-1beta-induced cyclo-oxygenase-2 in human articular chondrocytes: Role of p38 mitogen-activated protein kinase. *Biochem. J.* **362**, 367–373.

Thomas, J. A., Allen, J. L., Tsen, M., Dubnicoff, T., Danao, J., Liao, X. C., Cao, Z., and Wasserman, S. A. (1999). Impaired cytokine signaling in mice lacking the IL-1 receptor-associated kinase. *J. Immunol.* **163**, 978–984.

Tortorella, M. D., Liu, R. Q., Burn, T., Newton, R. C., and Arner, E. (2002). Characterization of human aggrecanase 2 (ADAM-TS5): Substrate specificity studies and comparison with aggrecanase 1 (ADAM-TS4). *Matrix Biol.* **21**, 499–511.

Towle, C. A., Hung, H. H., Bonassar, L. J., Treadwell, B. V., and Mangham, D. C. (1997). Detection of interleukin-1 in the cartilage of patients with osteoarthritis: A possible autocrine/paracrine role in pathogenesis. *Osteoarthritis Cartilage* **5**, 293–300.

Trebino, C. E., Stock, J. L., Gibbons, C. P., Naiman, B. M., Wachtmann, T. S., Umland, J. P., Pandher, K., Lapointe, J. M., Saha, S., Roach, M. L., Carter, D., Thomas, N. A., *et al.* (2003). Impaired inflammatory and pain responses in mice lacking an inducible prostaglandin E synthase. *Proc. Natl. Acad. Sci. USA* **100**, 9044–9049.

van de Loo, A. A., Arntz, O. J., Bakker, A. C., van Lent, P. L., Jacobs, M. J., and van den Berg, W. B. (1995). Role of interleukin 1 in antigen-induced exacerbations of murine arthritis. *Am. J. Pathol.* **146**, 239–249.

van de Loo, F. A., Arntz, O. J., van Enckevort, F. H., van Lent, P. L., and van den Berg, W. B. (1998). Reduced cartilage proteoglycan loss during zymosan-induced gonarthritis in NOS2-deficient mice and in anti-interleukin-1-treated wild-type mice with unabated joint inflammation. *Arthritis Rheum.* **41**, 634–646.

van den Berg, W. B., Joosten, L. A., Kollias, G., and van De Loo, F. A. (1999). Role of tumour necrosis factor alpha in experimental arthritis: Separate activity of interleukin 1beta in chronicity and cartilage destruction. *Ann. Rheum. Dis.* **58**(Suppl. 1), I40–I48.

Van Lent, P. L., Van De Loo, F. A., Holthuysen, A. E., Van Den Bersselaar, L. A., Vermeer, H., and Van Den Berg, W. B. (1995). Major role for interleukin 1 but not for tumor necrosis factor in early cartilage damage in immune complex arthritis in mice. *J. Rheumatol.* **22**, 2250–2258.

Wachsmuth, L., Bau, B., Fan, Z., Pecht, A., Gerwin, N., and Aigner, T. (2004). ADAMTS-1, a gene product of articular chondrocytes *in vivo* and *in vitro*, is downregulated by interleukin 1beta. *J. Rheumatol.* **31**, 315–320.

Weissbach, L., Tran, K., Colquhoun, S. A., Champliaud, M. F., and Towle, C. A. (1998). Detection of an interleukin-1 intracellular receptor antagonist mRNA variant. *Biochem. Biophys. Res. Commun.* **244**, 91–95.

Werman, A., Werman-Venkert, R., White, R., Lee, J. K., Werman, B., Krelin, Y., Voronov, E., Dinarello, C. A., and Apte, R. N. (2004). The precursor form of IL-1alpha is an intracrine proinflammatory activator of transcription. *Proc. Natl. Acad. Sci. USA* **101**, 2434–2439.

Wesche, H., Henzel, W. J., Shillinglaw, W., Li, S., and Cao, Z. (1997). MyD88: An adapter that recruits IRAK to the IL-1 receptor complex. *Immunity* **7**, 837–847.

Wessendorf, J. H., Garfinkel, S., Zhan, X., Brown, S., and Maciag, T. (1993). Identification of a nuclear localization sequence within the structure of the human interleukin-1 alpha precursor. *J. Biol. Chem.* **268**, 22100–22104.

Wu, J. J., Lark, M. W., Chun, L. E., and Eyre, D. R. (1991). Sites of stromelysin cleavage in collagen types II, IX, X and XI of cartilage. *J. Biol. Chem.* **266**, 5625–5628.

Zandi, E., Rothwarf, D. M., Delhase, M., Hayakawa, M., and Karin, M. (1997). The IkappaB kinase complex (IKK) contains two kinase subunits, IKKalpha and IKKbeta, necessary for IkappaB phosphorylation and NF-kappaB activation. *Cell* **91**, 243–252.

17

CYTOKINES IN TYPE 2 DIABETES

DANIEL R. JOHNSON,*,† JASON C. O'CONNOR,‡
ANSUMAN SATPATHY,† AND GREGORY G. FREUND*,†

*Department of Animal Sciences, University of Illinois
Urbana, Illinois 61801
†Department of Pathology, University of Illinois
Urbana, Illinois 61801
‡Division of Nutritional Sciences, University of Illinois
Urbana, Illinois 61801

I. INTRODUCTION

The Center for Disease Control and Prevention defines diabetes mellitus as "a group of diseases characterized by high levels of blood glucose resulting from defects in insulin production, insulin action, or both" (National Diabetes Fact Sheet, 2003). Of the more than 18 million Americans with diabetes, 90–95% of those are type 2, costing an estimated 132 billion dollars annually (National Diabetes Fact Sheet, 2003). Type 2 diabetes is distinguished by the development of insulin resistance, a condition where normal physiological levels of insulin are insufficient in maintaining glucose homeostasis. As hyperglycemia develops the pancreas increases insulin production in an effort to achieve normal glucose levels, creating a state of hyperinsulinemia. Eventually uncontrolled hyperglycemia results in overcompensation by and ultimately destruction of the pancreatic β-cells (Hennige et al., 2003).

A. INSULIN AND ITS RECEPTOR

The pathogenesis of insulin resistance has been intensely studied (Aguirre et al., 2002; Arkan et al., 2005; Bandyopadhyay et al., 2005; Cai et al., 2005; Kido et al., 2000; Ueki et al., 2004a,b; Werner et al., 2004; Zisman et al., 2000), but is not fully understood. Since its first identification as a pancreatic factor with a hypoglycemic function by Banting and Best in 1921, insulin has proven to be the key hormone involved in the maintenance of whole body glucose homeostasis (Park and Johnson, 1955). Insulin facilitates glucose uptake in muscle and adipose tissue while inhibiting gluconeogenesis and stimulating glycogen storage in the liver (Best, 1972; Bogardus et al., 1984; Nadkarni and Chitnis, 1963; Renold et al., 1950). Insulin is also involved in gene regulation, cellular differentiation, mitogenesis, protein and fatty acid synthesis, and increasing the permeability of certain cells to potassium, magnesium, and phosphate ions. Insulin can regulate enzymes such as hexokinase and glucose-6-phosphatase (Gagnon and Sorisky, 1998; Ish-Shalom et al., 1997; Jones and Dohm, 1997; Krahl, 1962; Monaco and Lippman, 1977; Prager et al., 1990; Ronnett et al., 1982; Rosic et al., 1985; Suzuki et al., 1984; Taub et al., 1987; Vileisis and Oh, 1983; Wang and Scott, 1991; Wool and Krahl, 1959). This multifunctional hormone is continually discharged into the blood, but its secretion by pancreatic beta cells is increased in response to elevated blood glucose (Barrnett et al., 1955; Humbel, 1963; Rickert and Fischer, 1975).

In the "classic" insulin sensitive tissues, muscle and adipose, the insulin/ insulin receptor interaction brings about a well-studied series of intracellular signals. The insulin receptor is transmembrane consisting of 2 alpha and 2 beta subunits linked by disulfide bonds. It is in a family of receptors that exhibit receptor tyrosine kinase (RTK)[1] activity. RTKs are essential components of the signal transduction pathways that affect cell proliferation, differentiation, migration, and metabolism and are subdivided into four classes. Class I receptors include epidermal growth factor (EGF) receptor, while the receptors for insulin and insulin-like growth factor-1 (IGF-1) are class II. The class III and IV receptors include the platelet-derived growth factor (PDGF) family, colony-stimulating factor-1 (CSF-1), and fibroblast growth factor. Receptor activation occurs upon ligand binding, facilitating interreceptor interactions and subsequent autophosphorylation of specific tyrosine residues in the cytoplasmic domain (Heffetz and Zick, 1986; Kahn et al., 1978). In the basal state, the receptor is phosphorylated on Ser and Thr residues, which is increased by phorbol esters, cAMP, and certain cytokines. These serine phosphorylations appear to reduce insulin receptor signaling (Haring et al., 1986; Lewis et al., 1990a,b; Stadtmauer and Rosen, 1986; Takayama et al., 1984, 1988). Activation of the insulin receptor by insulin binding to the receptor alpha subunit triggers a conformation change that releases the intrinsic tyrosine kinase activity of the beta subunit. Receptor autophosphorylation then occurs at multiple sites including Tyr 1158/62/63, 1328/34, and ultimately Tyr 972, which is the major docking site for interacting proteins (Kido et al., 2001; Tornqvist et al., 1987; Ullrich and Schlessinger, 1990; White et al., 1988). The tyrosine kinase protein targets interacting with Tyr 972 include the insulin receptor substrates (IRSs) 1, 2, 3, 4, 5, 6; Grb-2-associated binding protein-1 (Gab-1); and Shc (Cai et al., 2003; Holgado-Madruga et al., 1996; Lavan et al., 1997a,b; Myers and White, 1996; Ricketts et al., 1996; Sasaoka et al., 1994; Sun et al., 1995; White, 1997).

B. INSULIN RECEPTOR SUBSTRATES AND THEIR DOWNSTREAM TARGETS

Of the potential insulin receptor targets, IRSs are the most important (Sun et al., 1991, 1992) coordinating the phosphoinositide-3 kinase (PI-3K) pathway (Saltiel and Kahn, 2001) that is necessary to insulin-induced glucose transport (Sanchez-Margalet et al., 1994; Standaert et al., 1995; Tsakiridis et al., 1995). PI-3K binding to phosphorylated tyrosines on IRSs leads to activation of PI-3K and generation of phosphatidyl-inositol-3, 4-biphosphate (PIP2), and phosphatidyl-inositol-3,4,5-triphosphate (PIP3) (Alessi and Cohen, 1998). PIP3 recruits the serine kinases pyruvate

---

[1]Abbreviations: CVD, cardiovascular disease; GLUT4, glucose transporter 4; IGF-1, insulin-like growth factor-1; IL-1RA, IL-1 receptor antagonist; IL-1R2, type-2 IL-1 receptor; IRS, insulin receptor substrates; JAK, Janus kinase; LPS, lipopolysaccharide; MAPK, mitogen-activated protein kinase; mTOR, mammalian target of rapamycin; PI-3K, phosphatidylinositol-3 kinase; PKB, protein kinase B; PKC, protein kinase C; RTK, receptor tyrosine kinase; SOCS, suppressor of cytokine signaling; TNF, tumor necrosis factor.

dehydrogenase kinase-1 (PDK-1), protein kinase B (PKB), and protein kinase C (PKCs) ζ/λ at the plasma membrane and PDK-1 is simultaneously activated by PIP3 where it phosphorylates PKB and PKCs (Brazil and Hemmings, 2001; Vanhaesebroeck and Alessi, 2000). This activation results in plasma membrane glucose transporter 4 (GLUT4) translocation (Khan and Pessin, 2002), glycogen synthesis (Cross *et al.*, 1995), and lipogenesis (Girard *et al.*, 1994). In addition, activated PKB descaffolds from the plasma membrane to affect metabolic processes in the cytoplasm and/or tranlocates to the nucleus to influence gene expression (Andjelkovic *et al.*, 1997; Meier *et al.*, 1997; Vanhaesebroeck and Alessi, 2000). Substrates for PKB include PKCs, protein phosphatase 2A (PP2A), glycogen synthase kinase-3 (GSK-3), Forkhead (*Drosophila*) homolog-(rhabdomyosarcoma)-like 1 (FKHR-L1), BCL2-antagonist of cell death (BAD), mammalian target of rapamycin (mTOR), and phosphofruco-kinase 2 (Bevan, 2001).

Finally, other signal transduction proteins that interact with IRS molecules include SH2-containing protein tyrosine phosphatase 2 (SHP2), a protein-tyrosine phosphatase (PTP). In addition, growth factor receptor bound protein 2 (Grb-2) associates with IRSs and is constitutively associated with murine son of sevenless (mSOS), a guanine nucleotide exchange factor and a component of the cascade from Ras to Raf to mitogen activated kinase kinase (MEK) that leads to the activation of mitogen-activated protein kinases (MAPK) and expression of transcription factors Fos and Elk1.

II. PROINFLAMMATORY CYTOKINES IN TYPE 2 DIABETES

The role of proinflammatory cytokines in the pathogenesis of insulin resistance and augmenting the complications associated with type 2 diabetes is becoming clearer. In general, cytokines are low molecular weight proteins produced by nearly all cells of the immune system as well as many cells not normally considered immune cells, that is, epithelial cells and adipocytes. Cytokines are chemical messengers and coordinate the myriad host responses during immunological challenge. They initiate the innate immune response and coordinate the adaptive immune response by directing the Th1/Th2 course. Discovered in the late 1960s the diverse action of cytokines is continuously being expanded. Many cell types have been shown to have cytokine receptors and the action of cytokines on neurons, adipocytes, fibroblasts, epithelial cells, and so on has been intensely studied. Over the past decade, a link between metabolic processes and immunity has emerged. It is now well established that obesity is associated with low-grade chronic inflammation and that this inflammation, orchestrated by the classic proinflammatory cytokines tumor necrosis factor-α (TNF-α), interleukin-6 (IL-6), and IL-1β, may be a causative factor in the development of diabetes and/or its complications.

A. TNF-α

In the late nineteenth century an observation of tumor regression in cancer patients who recovered from bacterial infections (Old, 1988) sparked the search for a "tumor necrosis factor." Carswell *et al.* identified the factor, TNF in 1975 while investigating the antitumor activity of normal sera (Carswell *et al.*, 1975). Until 1985 when Beutler *et al.* identified TNF as a critical mediator of lethal endotoxin shock, produced by macrophages, little was known about the function of TNF in immunity (Beutler *et al.*, 1985). Since this landmark discovery two decades ago, it is now known that TNF-α is a proinflammatory cytokine that has many biological actions including induction of acute phase protein production, dendritic cell migration to lymph nodes and mediating specific components of the brain-based sickness response to lipopolysaccharide (LPS), such as reduced social exploration (Bluthe *et al.*, 1994; Cumberbatch and Kimber, 1995; Gresser *et al.*, 1987; Warren *et al.*, 1987). The first evidence pointing to diabetes as a disease of immunological origin was the discovery by Lang *et al.* in 1992 showing that TNF-α reduced peripheral glucose disposal and hepatic glucose output (Lang *et al.*, 1992). Although immunological dysfunction was inherently obvious in patients suffering from diabetes, this finding gave the first inclination that the link between immunity and diabetes may not be unidirectional. Hotamisligil *et al.* and others advanced this hypothesis by showing that adipocytes express TNF-α mRNA and that neutralization of TNF-α improves insulin sensitivity (Hotamisligil *et al.*, 1993, 1994, 1995). Persons with type 2 diabetes appear to have elevated levels of plasma TNF-α, which is adipocyte derived (Esposito *et al.*, 2002a), although this finding is somewhat controversial.

1. TNF-α and Insulin Resistance

When bound by its ligand, the TNF receptor initiates a signaling cascade that results in activation of, c-Jun NH$_2$-terminal kinase (JNK) 1/2/3, mitogen-activated protein kinase (MAPK) 1/2, p38 MAPK, and NF-κB. JNK phosphorylates a number of proteins, including IRS1/2, Shc, and Gab-1 (Aguirre *et al.*, 2000).

The major JNK phosphorylation site in rat IRS1 is located at Ser307 (Ser312 in human IRS1), which is located on the C-terminal side of the phosphotyrosine-binding (PTB) domain (Aguirre *et al.*, 2000). Rui *et al.* and others showed that TNF-α induced Ser 307 phosphorylation of IRS1 requires MEK1 activation and others have demonstrated that TNF-α induced serine phosphorylation of IRS1 was achieved through activation of p38 MAPK and IκB kinase (IKK) (Ricketts *et al.*, 1996; Saltiel *et al.*, 2001; Sanchez-Margalet *et al.*, 1994). Insulin also induces Ser 307 phosphorylation; however this is

PI-3K dependent. Thus, in the prediabetic condition of hyperinsulinemia and elevated TNF-α, insulin resistance through serine phosphorylation of IRS1 is exacerbated by both insulin and TNF-α, through independent pathways (Rui et al., 2001). Ser 307 of IRS-1 is located in the phosphotyrosine-binding (PTB) domain and phosphorylation impairs docking of IRS-1 to the insulin receptor, thereby preventing insulin from eliciting its biological effects although binding its receptor (Aguirre et al., 2002). IRS-1 associates with the insulin receptor entirely through the association of the phosphorylated insulin receptor to the PTB domain in IRS-1 (Aguirre et al., 2000; Craparo et al., 1995; Gustafson et al., 1995; O'Neill et al., 1994). Although of uncertain biologic significance, the ability of PI-3K to dock to the tyrosine phosphorylated insulin receptor is decreased by TNF-α, in turn, preventing tyrosine phosphorylation of PI-3K by the insulin receptor (Miura et al., 1999). Additionally, TNF-α activates the protein tyrosine phosphatase SH-PTPase, which is critical to the negative regulation of insulin signaling by dephosphorylating tyrosine residues on the insulin receptor (Engelman et al., 2000; Maegawa et al., 1994). These studies exhibit the expansive influence TNF-α has on insulin signaling. By preventing multiple protein–protein interactions from fully eliciting the appropriate biological effects of insulin, TNF-α initiates and/or exacerbates insulin resistance.

The overproduction of TNF-α in adipose tissue from diabetic animal models is still controversial. It appears as though mRNA production of TNF-α is elevated in adipose from diabetic subjects, protein measurements however, show attenuated TNF-α protein levels in these same tissues (Hotamisligil et al., 1993, 1995; Kern et al., 2001). When circulating levels of TNF-α are elevated, as in cachexia, insulin resistance is often observed. However, it has been reported that individuals suffering from obesity and/or type 2 diabetes have decreased levels of circulating TNF-α as compared to healthy individual (Kern et al., 2001; Koistinen et al., 2000). Borst et al. showed that blocking TNF-α in insulin resistant rats reversed insulin resistance and reduced TNF-α in muscle, but not fat (Borst and Bagby, 2002). Experiments involving TNF-α knockout mice show that they have improved glucose tolerance and were protected against insulin resistance resulting from gold-thioglucose-induced hyperphagia. While ob/ob mice with the p75 TNF-α receptor knocked out, also, exhibit improved glucose tolerance (Hotamisligil, 1999a,b; Voros et al., 2004). To date, anti-TNF-α therapies have proved unsuccessful in improving insulin sensitivity in humans, but have decreased insulin resistance in Zucker fatty rats (Hotamisligil et al., 1993; Paquot et al., 2000). Therefore, while TNF-α can significantly impact insulin signaling, its role as the causative agent of diabetes-associated insulin resistance is unlikely.

2. TNF-α and Diabetic Complications

Finally, the impact of TNF-α in cardiovascular complications is of importance since cardiovascular disease (CVD) is the principal killer of those with type 2 diabetes (National Diabetes Fact Sheet, 2003). Persons with type 2 diabetes suffer from cardiovascular disease at a rate 2 to 4 times higher than their healthy counterparts (National Diabetes Fact Sheet, 2003), and when stricken they exhibit increased severity of symptoms and mortality (National Diabetes Fact Sheet, 2003). Evidence indicates that atherogenesis is driven by an inflammatory process, linking diabetes-associated chronic inflammation to CVD (Danesh et al., 2000; Ferencik et al., 2005; Koenig et al., 2005; Rattazzi et al., 2005; Schwartz et al., 1985; Xanthoulea et al., 2005). TNF-α has been shown to increase the expression of endothelin-1 (Klemm et al., 1995; Lees et al., 2000; Marsden and Brenner, 1992) and angiotensinogen (Brasier et al., 1996; Wang et al., 2005) both of which have been shown to accelerate the atherosclerotic process (Ishigami et al., 1995; Keavney and McKenzie, 1995; Lerman et al., 1991; Sugiyama et al., 1997; Winkles et al., 1993; Zeiher et al., 1994). In addition, a spontaneous hypertensive rat model produces elevated levels of TNF-α in response to LPS as compared to control rats (Brasier et al., 1996; Kahaleh and Fan, 1997; Nyui et al., 1997), and blood monocytes from hypertensive patients produce elevated amounts of TNF-α (Dorffel et al., 1999; Zinman et al., 1999). The ratio of soluble TNF receptors, sTNFR2/sTNFR1, an indicator of TNF-α system activation, is positively correlated with systolic and diastolic blood pressure, and the ratio is greater in persons with type 2 diabetes as compared to those without (Fernandez-Real et al., 2002). Shedding of TNF receptors is associated with insulin resistance and vascular dysfunction in type 2 diabetes by, decreasing TNFR1 shedding, thus decreasing the TNFR2/TNFR1 ratio (Fernandez-Real et al., 2002). Compounding the prohypertensive aspect of TNF is its tie to dyslipidemia. TNF-α has been shown to increase serum triglyceride levels through increased very low density lipoprotein (VLDL) and decreased high density lipoprotein (HDL) production (Feingold et al., 1990; Krauss et al., 1990; McDonagh et al., 1992), and a positive correlation exists between sTNFR2 concentration and plasma triglyceride levels (Fernandez-Real et al., 1999, 2002). VLDL levels in both healthy and post-infarction patients is positively correlated to plasma TNF-α concentrations and it has been demonstrated that plasma TNF-α is elevated in low density lipoprotein (LDL) receptor knockout animals (Ettinger et al., 1990; Jovinge et al., 1998; Skoog et al., 2002). In addition, TNF-α administration has been shown to increase plasma LDL. In addition, hypercholesterolemic animals produce elevated levels of TNF-α in response to infection (Brito et al., 1995; Fleet et al., 1992; Lopes-Virella and Virella, 1996; Mehta et al., 1998). Taken together, these finding provide a link between plasma TNF-α and/or its receptors and the lipid profile in both healthy and diabetic subjects. Pausova et al., using the haplotype relative-risk test, demonstrated a significant association between the TNF-α gene locus, obesity, and obesity-associated hypertension in persons of French-Canadian origin (Pausova et al., 2000). Therefore, the positive interaction between TNF-α and dyslipidemia/

hypertension may not just be a phenomenological association resulting from cytokine and/or lipid unbalance, but may also have a significant genetic component.

B. IL-6

IL-6 is a multifunctional cytokine most often grouped with TNF-α and IL-1β as proinflammatory. Produced principally by macrophages in the liver as an acute phase protein, it can also be elaborated by adipose (Kern et al., 2001), muscle (Bartoccioni et al., 1994; Loppnow and Libby, 1989, 1990), endothelial (Jirik et al., 1989; Loppnow and Libby, 1989; May et al., 1989; Podor et al., 1989), T and B cells (Hodgkin et al., 1988; Van Damme et al., 1988) and cancer cells (Baffet et al., 1991; Siegall et al., 1990). Elevated plasma IL-6 is linked with obesity; however, conflicting data exists on whether plasma IL-6 alters glucose metabolism. Febbraio and colleagues reported IL-6 as a mediator of glucose homeostasis during muscle contraction, while others have reported no affect on glucose uptake or production in healthy subjects at rest (Febbraio et al., 2004; Rotter Sopasakis et al., 2004). These findings indicate IL-6 may participate in improved glucose tolerance observed in exercised diabetic individuals (Bruunsgaard, 2005; Monzillo et al., 2003; Shephard, 2002). Carey et al. (2004) reported no increase in plasma IL-6 or TNF-α concentrations in diabetic subjects, but did find a correlation between elevated IL-6 and body mass index (BMI). Others have negatively correlated increased adipose IL-6 mRNA to insulin-stimulated glucose disposal (Rotter et al., 2003). Insulin resistant individuals receiving recombinant human IL-6 (rhIL-6) exhibit decreased plasma insulin, increased growth hormone, cortisol, fatty acid turnover, and lipid oxidation (Rotter Sopasakis et al., 2004).

1. IL-6 and Insulin Resistance

Although the mechanisms involved in IL-6 mediated disruption of glucose homeostasis is unclear, it is evident that IL-6 is critical in the development and/ or pathology of insulin resistance. Experiments utilizing IL-6 knockout mice show that they have impaired glucose tolerance and develop mature-onset diabetes and obesity. Treating these animals with IL-6 resulted in reduced body fat mass in knockout, but not control mice (Di Gregorio et al., 2004; Faldt et al., 2004). Neutralizing IL-6 in ob/ob mice improves insulin sensitivity, decreased signal transducers and activators of transcription 3 (STAT3) phosphorylation and increased insulin receptor autophosphorylation and PKB activation by 50%, demonstrating the significant impact IL-6 has on elements of the insulin-signaling cascade (Di Gregorio et al., 2004; Klover et al., 2005). Additionally, IL-6 has been shown to reduce GLUT4 and IRS1 mRNA expression in adipocytes, as well as reduce tyrosine phosphorylation of IRS1, further exacerbating the negative impact IL-6 has on insulin-induced glucose uptake (Rotter *et al.*, 2003). No suppression of insulin receptor signaling has been observed in skeletal muscle in rats treated with IL-6, but a significant reduction in insulin signaling is seen in hepatic tissue (Klover *et al.*, 2003). Since hepatic regulation of glucose storage and release is integral to maintaining euglycemia, these findings point to IL-6 as a mediator of glucose intolerance via multiple methods, including disruption of the insulin-signaling cascade in muscle, fat, and liver, and downregulation of proteins necessary for normal glucose uptake in fat and muscle. Cai *et al.* (2005) found that hepatic NF-κB activation results in systemic insulin resistance and using antibodies to NF-κB and IL-6 they reversed the effect. These finding suggests IL-6 exerts its influence on plasma glucose via multiple pathways. It is generally accepted that IL-6 induces insulin resistance in hepatocytes. In response to IL-6 these cells exhibit reduced glycogen synthase activity, decreased suppression of glycogen phosphorylase and decreased synthesis and increased breakdown of glycogen, as well as inhibition of insulin-induced activation of glucokinase (Kanemaki *et al.*, 1998). This alteration of hepatic enzyme activity results in impaired glucose storage and subsequent elevation of plasma glucose. Finally, IL-6 impairs insulin sensitivity through multiple physiological processes and it appears that the IL-6/ diabetes association may also have a genetic component. A polymorphism in the IL-6 gene promoter linking IL-6 and type 2 diabetes has been discovered (Fernandez-Real *et al.*, 2000a,b), although not all persons with type 2 diabetics possess this polymorphism.

2. SOCS and Insulin Resistance

An attractive mechanistic model of how IL-6 antagonizes insulin action is via the upregulation of the suppressor of cytokine-signaling (SOCS) proteins. SOCS are a family of proteins that include eight members, cytokine-inducible SH2 protein (CIS) and SOCS1–7 (Alexander and Hilton, 2004; Kubo *et al.*, 2003; Yoshimura *et al.*, 2005). Each SOCS member contains a central SH2 domain, an N-terminal variable length sequence and a C-terminal, 40 amino acid SOCS box (Kubo *et al.*, 2003). The best-characterized SOCS proteins are CIS and SOCS-1/2/3, which were initially identified as negative regulators of JAK-STAT signal transduction. IL-6 signals through the JAK1/STAT3 pathway and subsequent upregulation of SOCS-3 serves as a negative feedback loop. SOCS-3 binds to Tyr 759 of the gp130 phosphopeptide (Lehmann *et al.*, 2003). The consensus SOCS-3-binding motif has been identified by De Souza *et al.* (2002) as Ptyr-(Ser/Ala/ Val/Tyr/Phe)-hydrophobic-hydrophobic, which is highly homologous to Tyr 759 of gp130. The prediction that SOCS3-binding sites were likely to exist on other tyrosine phosphorylated receptors has also turned out to be correct, as SOCS-3 has now been shown to associate with several receptors, including the insulin receptor (Ueki *et al.*, 2004).

Mooney and colleagues first identified the ability of SOCS to block insulin signaling by disrupting the formation of signaling complexes at the insulin receptor (Mooney et al., 2001). Their studies suggested that SOCS-1 and SOCS-6 block insulin signaling by associating with the insulin receptor and inhibiting insulin receptor catalytic activity. This association resulted in a decrease of p85 association with IRS1, decreased PI-3K activation and reduced activation of downstream proteins PKB, MAPK, and STAT5. Further studies supported this conclusion, demonstrating that SOCS-3 binds directly to the insulin receptor at Tyr 960 through its SH2 domain (Ueki et al., 2004). SOCS-3 binding of the insulin receptor does not alter the phosphorylation state of the receptor or its kinase activity. Rather, this association prevents downstream signaling through IRS1 and IRS2 (Ueki et al., 2004). Tyr 960 is an essential binding target of the phosphotyrosine binding domains of IRS1/2. Thus, SOCS-3 exerts its inhibitory function by preventing downstream substrates from being phosphorylated by the activated insulin receptor (Ueki et al., 2004). White and colleagues later proposed an additional mechanism of SOCS involvement in insulin signaling and demonstrated that SOCS proteins associated with IRS1 and IRS2 in response to insulin stimulation, and not only inhibited tyrosine phosphorylation as previous studies had shown, but that expression of SOCS-1 and SOCS-3 correlate with the ubiquitination and degradation of IRS1 and IRS2 (Kawazoe et al., 2001; Rui et al., 2002). Ueki et al. (2004a,b) went on to show that overexpression of SOCS-1 and SOCS-3 in liver causes insulin resistance and conversely, inhibition of SOCS-1 and -3 in obese diabetic mice improves insulin sensitivity. Importantly, Fasshauer et al. (2004) found that TNF-alpha and IL-6 induced the expression of SOCS-1 and -3 mRNA and concluded that SOCS proteins could be an important intracellular mediator of insulin resistance in states of inflammation.

3. IL-6 and Diabetic Complications

In terms of diabetic complications, the role of IL-6 in cardiovascular disease is developing. Plasma levels of IL-6 correlated with fat percentage, diastolic blood pressure, and the risk of myocardial infarction (Bennet et al., 2003; Haider et al., 2004; Heliovaara et al., 2005). High IL-6 levels have been shown to predict CVD in men (Ridker et al., 2000b), women (Ridker et al., 2000a; Volpato et al., 2001) and the elderly (Harris et al., 1999; Jenny et al., 2002), and it has been demonstrated that plasma IL-6 is elevated in diabetic women with CVD (Tuttle et al., 2004). Although plasma IL-6 and CVD are closely related and it is apparent each sustains the other in the process, the mechanism is poorly understood. One of the hallmarks of CVD is hypertension, and IL-6 has been shown to be a potent stimulator of the central and sympathetic nervous system, both of which are involved in the onset of hypertension (Gordon et al., 1979; Nelson and Boulant, 1981; Smithwick, 1951; Uhari et al., 1979). IL-6 administration results in increased heart rate and angiotensinogen expression (Gonzalez *et al.*, 2000; Greenwel *et al.*, 1995; Lowe *et al.*, 1999; Takano *et al.*, 1993). Furthermore, CVD is characterized by the development of atherosclerotic plaques and IL-6 is involved plaque development. Intercellular adhesion molecule-1 (ICAM-1), an adhesion molecule on endothelial cells, is increased by exposure to IL-6 (Ikeda *et al.*, 1996). Also, IL-6 has been shown to stimulate coagulation in humans, which can contribute to arterial blockage and clot formation. High blood pressure and atherosclerosis, both significant risk factors in the development and mortality of CVD, are potentially worsened by increased IL-6, providing a mechanism for the increased incidence and poor prognosis of CVD in type 2 diabetes. CVD development is associated with dyslipidemia, and increased blood concentrations of IL-6 are associated with free fatty acid and triglyceride levels as well as increase hepatic triglyceride production (Fernandez-Real *et al.*, 2000b; Greenberg *et al.*, 1992; Nonogaki *et al.*, 1995; Stouthard *et al.*, 1995).

C. IL-1β

IL-1β is synthesized in an inactive, precursor form that is cleaved by interleukin-1β-converting enzyme to its 17.3-kDa biologically active form (Brazel *et al.*, 1991; Schmidt, 1984). Two receptors isoforms for IL-1β have been identified, these are the 80-kDa type 1 IL-1 receptor (IL-1R1) (Horuk *et al.*, 1987; Resch *et al.*, 1986; Spriggs *et al.*, 1992) and 68-kDa IL-1R2 (Re *et al.*, 1994). Both receptors bind IL-1β with similar affinity (Labriola-Tompkins *et al.*, 1991), but only the IL-1R1 receptor is physiologically functional, as the IL-1R2 receptor acts as a negative regulator of IL-1β signaling by binding IL-1β and not initiating an intracellular signaling cascade (Mantovani *et al.*, 1996; Re *et al.*, 1994). IL-1β induces many physiological responses, including induction of other cytokines, activation of the hypothalamic-pituitary-adrenal (HPA) axis, induction of fever, sickness behavior and anorexia (Bluthe *et al.*, 2000; Mrosovsky *et al.*, 1989; Stenzel-Poore *et al.*, 1993). IL-1β is released mainly from macrophages, but is produced by many other cells including neurons, microglial cells, and endothelial cells (Fontana *et al.*, 1984; Libby *et al.*, 1986; MacPherson *et al.*, 2005; Nawroth *et al.*, 1986; Wagner *et al.*, 1985; Xing *et al.*, 1994). Receptors for IL-1β have also been identified on many cell types throughout the periphery and the brain. In the brain, IL-1R1 is expressed in neurons of the hippocampus, the basolateral nucleus of the amygdala, and the basomedian nuclei of the hypothalamus (Ban *et al.*, 1991; Takao *et al.*, 1990), as well as microglial cells and astrocytes (Ban *et al.*, 1993; Gottschall *et al.*, 1991). IL-1R2 expression has been identified in the neuronal cells of the median preoptic area, dorsomedial, and paraventricular hypothalamic nuclei and various thalamic nuclei (Ban *et al.*, 1991; Takao *et al.*, 1990), as well as on the surface of microglial cells (Pinteaux *et al.*, 2002). In the periphery IL-1 receptors have been identified on macrophages (Granowitz *et al.*, 1992;

Spriggs *et al.*, 1992), endothelial cells (Boraschi *et al.*, 1991), adipose (Burysek *et al.*, 1993), and muscle cells (Lederer and Czuprynski, 1994; Mugridge *et al.*, 1991). The IL-1 receptors belong to subgroup 1, the immunoglobulin (Ig) subgroup, which contain extracellular Ig domains and include the IL-1 receptor accessory protein (IL-1RAcP). Binding of IL-1β, to IL-1R1 results in IL-1 receptor accessory protein (IL-1RAcP) forming a complex with the receptor, causing myeloid differentiation primary response gene 88 (MyD88) association, IL-1 receptor-associated kinase (IRAK) 1/2 activation, and ultimately leading to activation of NF-κB (Dunne and O'Neill, 2003).

1. Impaired Negative Regulation of IL-1β in Diabetes

Negative regulation of IL-1β through IL-1 receptor antagonist (IL-1RA) and type 2 IL-1 receptor (IL-1R2) is an essential element in returning the body and brain to a state of immunologic homeostasis when an infection is cleared and in maintaining equilibrium in a basal state. Evidence shows that persons with diabetes suffer from both increased basal inflammation and increased incidence severity and prolonged recovery from infection (Esposito *et al.*, 2002a; Fourrier *et al.*, 1975; Pickup *et al.*, 2000). Impaired negative regulation of cytokines such as IL-1β could potentially play a role in the pathogenesis of diabetes and its associated complications. We have shown that the *db/db* mouse fails to upregulate brain IL-1RA and IL-1R2 mRNA following LPS administration, contributing to delayed recovery from LPS and IL-1β-induced sickness behavior (O'Connor *et al.*, 2005). We have also shown that the dietary supplement vanadyl sulfate when administered intraperitoneally upregulates basal brain IL-1RA and IL-1R2 and improves recovery from LPS and IL-1β induced sickness behavior in both control and *db/db* mice (Johnson *et al.*, 2005). These findings implicate impaired central negative regulation of IL-1β as a contributor to the increased rate of infection, mortality and prolonged recovery observed in individuals with diabetes.

2. IL-1β in Diabetes

Elevated levels of IL-1β have been reported in sera of persons with type 2 diabetes, and these individuals produce more IL-1β in response to immune challenge (Dandona *et al.*, 2004; Pickup, 2004). We have shown that macrophages isolated from *db/db* mice are hyper-responsive to LPS, and when challenged with IL-1β or LPS, *db/db* mice exhibit impaired recovery from the effects of the sickness inducing effects of IL-1β (O'Connor *et al.*, 2005). Little evidence exists that IL-1β induces insulin resistance, although IRAK 1 has been shown to serine phosphorylate IRS1 (Kim *et al.*, 2005). The largest body of work on IL-1-β and diabetes focuses on IL-1β toxicity to pancreatic beta cells in type 1 diabetes, which has been thoroughly reviewed elsewhere (Helqvist, 1994; Hohmeier *et al.*, 2003; Maedler and Donath, 2004; Mandrup-Poulsen *et al.*, 1993). IL-1β-dependent pancreatic β-cell toxicity can also be seen in type 2 diabetes. One of the earliest features of insulitis are changes in endothelial cell changes along with the appearance of macrophages and dendritic cells within the islets of Langerhans. This is followed by infiltration with CD4+ and later CD8+ T lymphocytes (Kolb-Bachofen and Kolb, 1989). Additionally, IL-1β has been shown to inhibit glucose-stimulated insulin secretion from islets (Mandrup-Poulsen et al., 1985, 1986), as well as induce DNA damage (Delaney et al., 1993), reduce DNA content (Sandler et al., 1987), and induce cell death (Bolaffi et al., 1994) in rodent and human islets, as well as in beta cell lines (Hamaguchi and Leiter, 1990; Janjic and Asfari, 1992; Sandler et al., 1989). This action of IL-1 apparently involves increases in inducible nitric oxide synthase (iNOS) and production of nitric oxide (NO) (Corbett et al., 1991; Southern et al., 1990; Welsh et al., 1991). Unlike rat islets, human and mouse islets are relatively more resistant to the effects of IL-1β and require a signal from interferon-γ (IFN-γ) and/or TNF-α for β-cell destruction to occur (Campbell et al., 1988; Kawahara and Kenney, 1991; Rabinovitch et al., 1990; Soldevila et al., 1991). Thus, in type 2 diabetes, suffering from chronic low-grade inflammation, elevated IL-β, TNF-α, and IFN-γ could potentially mediate β-cell destruction as the diabetic condition progresses.

3. IL-1β and Diabetic Complications

The involvement of IL-1β in the progression of complications associated with diabetes is significant. IL-1β appears to affect cells associated with vasculature, including endothelium and smooth muscle. In endothelial cells, IL-1β has been shown to increase expression of vascular adherence molecules, such as endothelial adhesion molecule-1 (ELAM-1) and the CD11/CD18 complex (Luscinskas et al., 1989). Additionally, Bevilacqua et al. demonstrated that IL-1 induces the expression of a tissue factor-like procoagulant activity and increases the adhesiveness of the endothelial cell surface for human peripheral blood polymorphonuclear leukocytes and monocytes (Bevilacqua et al., 1984, 1985). Others have shown IL-1β promotes platelet activating factor secretion from endothelial cells (Breviario et al., 1988) and vascular permeability (Martin et al., 1988). These findings indicate that elevated IL-1β potentially exacerbates the development of atherosclerosis through the induction of a phenotype in endothelial cells conducive to plaque formation. It is known that cardiovascular tissue mounts an inflammatory response to infection, and this response is exacerbated in diabetes (Lu et al., 2004). In addition to CVD, IL-1β has been linked to diabetic neuropathy. Macrophage infiltration and neuronal death, potentially mediated by IL-1β, has been observed in early experimental diabetic neuropathy (Conti et al., 2002). Also, prior to and during the early stages of diabetic neuropathy, the IL-1β–signaling pathway in schwann cells is activated (Skundric et al., 2002). Schwann cells make up the myelin sheath, aid in the clean up of debris, and guide the regrowth of neurons (Ernyei and Young, 1966; Gonatas et al., 1964).

III. IL-18 AND DIABETES

Finally, a more recently discovered proinflammatory cytokine emerging as a potential inducer of insulin resistance is IL-18. Synthesized as a 24-kDa inactive precursor that is cleaved by IL-1β converting enzyme to the biologically active 18-kDa form, this cytokine is predominately produced by the liver and is structurally related to IL-1β (Okamura et al., 1995). The IL-18 receptor is a member of the IL-1 receptor family and is expressed on multiple cell types including macrophages, endothelial, and smooth muscle cells (Gerdes et al., 2002). The biological functions of IL-18 include guiding the adaptive immune response to Th1 or Th2, depending on the immunological context (Nakanishi et al., 2001). Elevated plasma IL-18 is associated with insulin resistance and type 2 diabetes (Aso et al., 2003; Esposito et al., 2004; Fischer et al., 2005; Kawashima et al., 2001; Kretowski et al., 2002), however IL-18 administration results in delayed diabetic onset in diabetes-susceptible mice (Rothe et al., 1999). In Streptozocin-induced diabetic rats, however, blocking endogenous IL-18 reduces hyperglycemia (Nicoletti et al., 2003), and its role in type 1 diabetes seems greater than in type 2. The understanding of IL-18 in diabetes complications is emerging but it has been shown to be a predictor of cardiovascular mortality, obesity and polycystic ovary disease Escobar-Morreale et al., 2004; Esposito et al., 2002b; Hung et al., 2005).

IV. ANTI-INFLAMMATORY CYTOKINES IN DIABETES

Unlike the proinflammatory cytokines, much less is known about anti-inflammatory cytokines and type 2 diabetes. The anti-inflammatory cytokines are typically described as IL-4, IL-10, IL-13, IL-16, IGF-1, and IL-1RA. A subgroup of these cytokines, including IL-4, IL-10, and IGF-1, share common intracellular-signaling components with the insulin receptor. As noted earlier, the insulin-signaling cascade is required for GLUT4-dependent glucose transport (Lienhard et al., 1982; Park and Johnson, 1955) and induction of cellular responses ranging from glycogen (Renold et al., 1950) and protein synthesis (Krahl, 1962) to cell survival (Conejo and Lorenzo, 2001) and proliferation (Conejo and Lorenzo, 2001). Critical to the initiation of these cascades is the ability of the insulin receptor to autophosphorylate its own intracellular tyrosine residues and its subsequent tyrosine phosphorylation of IRSs (Sun et al., 1991, 1992). This IRS phosphorylation causes IRS/PI-3K association (Backer et al., 1992), enhanced PI-3K activation

(Okamoto *et al.*, 1993) as well as localization of PI-3K to membrane surfaces (Kelly *et al.*, 1992). Cytokine receptors that utilize the tyrosine-dependent IRS/PI-3K association as a means of conveying intracellular signals are potentially susceptible to the same impaired signaling that is seen during insulin resistance. Therefore, in the obese and/or type 2 diabetic individual "cytokine resistance" may exist side-by-side with insulin resistance.

A. CYTOKINE RESISTANCE

We have characterized this "cytokine resistance" in the diabetic state showing that hyperinsulinemia induces serine phosphorylation of IRSs, which blocks the ability of IRSs to serve as JAK substrates and associate with PI-3K (Cengel and Freund, 1999; Hartman *et al.*, 2001, 2004). In general, serine phosphorylation of IRSs can induce chronic inhibition of IRS-dependent signaling (Le Marchand-Brustel, 1999; White, 1998). Activators of IRS serine phosphorylation such as okadaic acid, phorbol esters, angiotensin II, endothelin-1, platelet-derived growth factor (PDGF), and TNF-α reduce the ability of IRSs to serve as receptor/kinase substrates (De Fea and Roth, 1997a,b; Folli *et al.*, 1997; Hotamisligil *et al.*, 1996; Kanety *et al.*, 1995; Li *et al.*, 1999; Ricort *et al.*, 1997; Tanti *et al.*, 1994). This loss of IRS tyrosine (Jullien *et al.*, 1993; Paz *et al.*, 1997; Tanti *et al.*, 1991) phosphorylation prevents IRSs from recruiting/activating PI-3K, an essential inducer of growth, differentiation and survival signals for a variety of cytokine receptors including IFN-γ (Tengku-Muhammad *et al.*, 1999), IL-13 (Wang *et al.*, 1995), IFN-α (Cengel and Freund, 1999; Hartman *et al.*, 2001), IL-10 (Zhou *et al.*, 2001), and IL-4 (Minshall *et al.*, 1996, 1997). This inhibitory type serine phosphorylation of IRSs is blocked by rapamycin (Li *et al.*, 1999). Since mTOR phosphorylates serines in motifs similar to those identified in IRS1, mTOR is likely a physiologic IRS serine kinase as we (Cengel and Freund, 1999) and others (Brown and Schreiber, 1996; Li *et al.*, 1999; Ozes *et al.*, 2001) have shown.

B. mTOR AND INSULIN RECEPTOR SUBSTRATES

In the PIK-related kinase family that includes such members as ataxia telangiectasia mutated (ATM), ATM and Rad3-related protein (ATR), DNA-dependent protein kinase (DNA-PK), and TOR1/2 (Brown and Schreiber, 1996; Dennis *et al.*, 1999; Kuruvilla and Schreiber, 1999; Schmelzle and Hall, 2000), mTOR is 289 kDa serine kinase. The inhibitory complex of FK506-binding protein (FKBP12) and rapamycin binds to mTOR and rapamycin is considered a highly specific inhibitor of mTOR, especially at nanomolar concentrations (Brown *et al.*, 1994; Sabers *et al.*, 1995). mTOR-dependent proteasomal degradation has been shown to be an important regulator of IRS1/2 signaling (Haruta *et al.*, 2000; Pederson *et al.*, 2001;

Rice *et al.*, 1993; Sun *et al.*, 1999). The proteasome comprises approximately 1% of cellular protein, and is present in both the cytoplasm and nucleus of eukaryotic cells. Targeting of proteins for degradation by the 26S proteasome depends on ubiquitination (Lee and Goldberg, 1998). Serine phosphorylation and proline rich motifs are mechanisms that target proteins for ubiquitination by ubiquitin ligases (Laney and Hochstrasser, 1999). With regard to hyper-insulinemia, a precursor to type 2 diabetes, the proteasome was first shown to be critical to chronic insulin dependent loss of IRS1 in 3T3-L1 adipocytes reducing the half-life of IRS1 from 25 to 2.5 h (Rice *et al.*, 1993). Inhibition of the 26S proteasome with the peptide aldehyde transition state analog MG-132 blocked the effects of chronic insulin exposure on IRS1 expression (Sun *et al.*, 1999). Furthermore, the mTOR inhibitor, rapamycin, also blocked chronic insulin-induced IRS1 degradation (Dennis *et al.*, 1999) suggesting that serine phosphorylation of IRS1 by mTOR targets IRS1 for degradation (Pederson *et al.*, 2001). In addition, mTOR was shown to phosphorylate IRS1 on serines 636/639 contained within SPXS motifs (Ozes *et al.*, 2001) homologous to ubiquitin-protein ligase-binding regions in other proteins (Laney and Hochstrasser, 1999).

1. Hyperglycemia Impairs IL-4 Activation of PI-3K via mTOR-Dependent Pathway

In our initial work, we found that okadaic acid [a potent PP1 and PP2A phosphatase inhibitor (Bialojan and Takai, 1988)], as well as, insulin induces IRS1 serine phosphorylation that blocks JAK1-dependent tyrosine phosphorylation of IRS-1 and its subsequent ability to bind to PI-3K (Cengel and Freund, 1999). We also found that this inhibitory serine phosphorylation can be induced by mTOR and that these inhibitory serines lie between residues 511 and 772 of rat IRS1 (Hartman *et al.*, 2001). We reported that chronic insulin and high glucose synergistically inhibited IL-4-dependent activation of PI-3K via the mTOR pathway (Hartman *et al.*, 2004). We found that resident peritoneal macrophages from *db/db* mice had a near 50% reduction in IL-4-stimulated IRS2-associated PI-3K activity when compared to macrophages from similarly treated control (*db/+*) mice. Importantly, IRS2 from *db/db* mouse macrophages had increased Ser/Thr-Pro motif phosphorylation without a loss in IRS2 mass (Hartman *et al.*, 2004). The relevance of IL-4 resistance to type 2 diabetes is that IL-4 leads to an "alternative activation phenotype" in macrophages. This IL-4-dependent macrophage activation results in an absence of NO production, suppressive activity directed toward T cells, and generation of IL-10 and IL-1RA (Mosser, 2003). Failure to express IL-1RA and appropriately upregulate it in response to LPS appears responsible for LPS hypersensitivity and prolonged LPS-induced sickness in type 2-like diabetic mice, as we have shown (Johnson *et al.*, 2005; O'Connor *et al.*, 2005).

V. LEPTIN

Leptin is a 16-kDa adipokine, that has proven to be a major mediator of metabolic, neuroendocrine, and immune function, produced mainly by white adipose tissue (Ahima and Flier, 2000; Zhang *et al.*, 1994). A member of the type I cytokine superfamily, it is encoded by the *obese (ob)* gene and is structurally related to growth hormone, prolactin, and IL-3 (Ahima and Flier, 2000; Zhang *et al.*, 1994). The leptin receptor (Ob-R), encoded by the *diabetes (db)* gene, is a member of the class I cytokine receptor superfamily, which also includes the receptors for IL-6, G-CSF, and others (Tartaglia, 1995, 1997). There are six known isoforms of the receptor, including Ob-Ra, Ob-Rb, Ob-Rc, Ob-Rd, Ob-Re, and Ob-Rf, with Ob-Rb, the long receptor isoform, seemingly of the most biological significance. (Fei *et al.*, 1997; Lee *et al.*, 1996). Binding of leptin to the Ob-Rb receptor activates JAK2 and the STATs (Bjorbaek *et al.*, 1997; Ghilardi *et al.*, 1996). The biological functions of leptin are diverse, ranging from an indicator of energy stores to an immunomodulator that is produced in response to inflammatory stimuli and has been shown to induce the production of IL-1RA in pancreatic β-cells (Ahima *et al.*, 1996; Faggioni *et al.*, 2001; Maedler *et al.*, 2004). The relationship between leptin and diabetes is solid, but due to the complexity of both the biological activities of leptin and the pathology of diabetes, the mechanistic link is poorly understood.

A. LEPTIN IN THE STUDY OF DIABETES

Two widely used mouse models employed in the study of diabetes are products of mutation of leptin or its Ob-Rb receptor, the *ob/ob* and *db/db* mice, respectively. The *ob/ob* mouse model possesses a mutation of the *ob* gene and does not express functional leptin (Zhang *et al.*, 1994). Mutant mice exhibit a rapid increase in body weight and may weigh three times that of wild type animals. Obesity in *ob/ob* mice is marked by an increase in size and number of adipose cells (Kaplan *et al.*, 1976). In addition to obesity, mutant mice exhibit hyperphagia, glucose intolerance, elevated plasma insulin, impaired wound healing, hypothermia, and an increase in hormone production from the pituitary and adrenal glands (Boozer and Mayer, 1976; Coleman, 1982; Edwardson and Hough, 1975; Flatt and Bailey, 1981; Ring *et al.*, 2000; Trayhurn *et al.*, 1977). Development of obesity occurs prior to the increase in plasma insulin, and it is the likely cause of hyperinsulinemia in *ob/ob* mice (Thenen and Mayer, 1976). The *db/db* mouse model possesses a mutation of the *db* gene, resulting in a truncated Ob-Rb receptor with no intracellular signaling domain (Lee *et al.*, 1996). These mice become obese at 3 to 4 weeks of age, hyperinsulinemic at 10 to 14 days, and hyperglycemia at 4 to 8 weeks (Coleman and Hummel, 1974). Mutant mice are polyphagic, polydipsic, polyuric, and exhibit delayed wound healing and increased metabolic efficiency (Coleman, 1985; Greenhalgh *et al.*, 1990; Hosokawa *et al.*, 1985).

B. LEPTIN, DIABETES, AND COMPLICATIONS

Intracellular leptin signaling via Ob-Rb has been shown to tyrosine phosphorylate IRS1, activate PI-3K and MAPK 1/2 (Banks *et al.*, 2000; Bjorbak *et al.*, 2000), and share other docking proteins with the insulin signaling cascade including p38 MAPK and Grb-2 (Gualillo *et al.*, 2002; van den Brink *et al.*, 2000). Hyperleptinemia and leptin resistance is commonly associated with obesity and/or type 2 diabetes and has been coupled to increased cardiovascular risk (Dagogo-Jack *et al.*, 1996; Leyva *et al.*, 1998; Sivitz *et al.*, 1998). Additionally, leptin appears to control total body sensitivity to insulin and triglycerides levels (Oral *et al.*, 2002), potentially through metabolic status signaling to the brain and tissues in the periphery such as adipose and pancreatic β-cells (Kieffer and Habener, 2000; Kieffer *et al.*, 1996). Hepatocytes exposed to leptin at physiological levels observed in obesity exhibit decreased insulin-responsive tyrosine phosphorylation of IRS1 and decreased IRS1/Grb2 association as well as upregulated phosphoenolpyruvate carboxykinase (PEPCK), resulting in increased gluconeogensis (Cohen *et al.*, 1996). In the leptin resistance and hyperleptinemia, it is apparent that leptin impairs the ability of insulin to properly transduce its intracellular-signaling cascade.

VI. CONCLUSIONS

Type 2 diabetes mellitus (DM) is a disease associated with subclinical systemic inflammation and this chronic inflammation provides a pathogenic tie between diabetes and its complications including "newly recognized" sequela such as depression, cognitive impairment, and dementia. While much work has been done to understand the underlying mechanisms how inflammation effects insulin resistance, the role of cytokines in the pathogenesis of diabetes and its associated complications remains poorly understood.

ACKNOWLEDGMENTS

This research was supported by grants from the National Institutes of Health (DK064862 to G. G. F. and Postdoctoral Fellowship PHS5 T32 DK59802–01 to J. C. O.), American Heart Association Predoctoral Fellowship to J. C. O. and University of Illinois Agricultural Experiment Station (to G. G. F.).

REFERENCES

Aguirre, V., Uchida, T., Yenush, L., Davis, R., and White, M. F. (2000). The c-Jun NH (2)-terminal kinase promotes insulin resistance during association with insulin receptor substrate-1 and phosphorylation of Ser (307). *J. Biol. Chem.* **275**, 9047–9054.

Aguirre, V., Werner, E. D., Giraud, J., Lee, Y. H., Shoelson, S. E., and White, M. F. (2002). Phosphorylation of Ser307 in insulin receptor substrate-1 blocks interactions with the insulin receptor and inhibits insulin action. *J. Biol. Chem.* **277**, 1531–1537. Epub 2001 Oct 1517.

Ahima, R. S., and Flier, J. S. (2000). Leptin. *Annu. Rev. Physiol.* **62**, 413–437.

Ahima, R. S., Prabakaran, D., Mantzoros, C., Qu, D., Lowell, B., Maratos-Flier, E., and Flier, J. S. (1996). Role of leptin in the neuroendocrine response to fasting. *Nature* **382**, 250–252.

Alessi, D. R., and Cohen, P. (1998). Mechanism of activation and function of protein kinase B. *Curr. Opin. Genet. Dev.* **8**, 55–62.

Alexander, W. S., and Hilton, D. J. (2004). The role of suppressors of cytokine signaling (SOCS) proteins in regulation of the immune response. *Annu. Rev. Immunol.* **22**, 503–529.

Andjelkovic, M., Alessi, D. R., Meier, R., Fernandez, A., Lamb, N. J., Frech, M., Cron, P., Cohen, P., Lucocq, J. M., and Hemmings, B. A. (1997). Role of translocation in the activation and function of protein kinase B. *J. Biol. Chem.* **272**, 31515–31524.

Arkan, M. C., Hevener, A. L., Greten, F. R., Maeda, S., Li, Z. W., Long, J. M., Wynshaw-Boris, A., Poli, G., Olefsky, J., and Karin, M. (2005). IKK-beta links inflammation to obesity-induced insulin resistance. *Nat. Med.* **11**, 191–198. Epub 2005 Jan 2030.

Aso, Y., Okumura, K., Takebayashi, K., Wakabayashi, S., and Inukai, T. (2003). Relationships of plasma interleukin-18 concentrations to hyperhomocysteinemia and carotid intimal-media wall thickness in patients with type 2 diabetes. *Diabetes Care* **26**, 2622–2627.

Backer, J. M., Myers, M. G., Jr., Shoelson, S. E., Chin, D. J., Sun, X. J., Miralpeix, M., Hu, P., Margolis, B., Skolnik, E. Y., Schlessinger, J., and White, M. F. (1992). Phosphatidylinositol 3'-kinase is activated by association with IRS-1 during insulin stimulation. *EMBO J.* **11**, 3469–3479.

Baffet, G., Braciak, T. A., Fletcher, R. G., Gauldie, J., Fey, G. H., and Northemann, W. (1991). Autocrine activity of interleukin 6 secreted by hepatocarcinoma cell lines. *Mol. Biol. Med.* **8**, 141–156.

Ban, E., Milon, G., Prudhomme, N., Fillion, G., and Haour, F. (1991). Receptors for interleukin-1 (alpha and beta) in mouse brain: Mapping and neuronal localization in hippocampus. *Neuroscience* **43**, 21–30.

Ban, E. M., Sarlieve, L. L., and Haour, F. G. (1993). Interleukin-1 binding sites on astrocytes. *Neuroscience* **52**, 725–733.

Bandyopadhyay, G. K., Yu, J. G., Ofrecio, J., and Olefsky, J. M. (2005). Increased p85/55/50 expression and decreased phosphotidylinositol 3-kinase activity in insulin-resistant human skeletal muscle. *Diabetes* **54**, 2351–2359.

Banks, A. S., Davis, S. M., Bates, S. H., and Myers, M. G., Jr. (2000). Activation of downstream signals by the long form of the leptin receptor. *J. Biol. Chem.* **275**, 14563–14572.

Barrnett, R. J., Marshall, R. B., and Seligman, A. M. (1955). Histochemical demonstration of insulin in the islets of Langerhans. *Endocrinology* **57**, 419–438.

Bartoccioni, E., Michaelis, D., and Hohlfeld, R. (1994). Constitutive and cytokine-induced production of interleukin-6 by human myoblasts. *Immunol. Lett.* **42**, 135–138.

Bennet, A. M., Prince, J. A., Fei, G. Z., Lyrenas, L., Huang, Y., Wiman, B., Frostegard, J., and Faire, U. (2003). Interleukin-6 serum levels and genotypes influence the risk for myocardial infarction. *Atherosclerosis* **171**, 359–367.

Best, C. H. (1972). Nineteen hundred twenty-one in Toronto. *Diabetes* **21**(2), 385–395.

Beutler, B., Milsark, I. W., and Cerami, A. C. (1985). Passive immunization against cachectin/tumor necrosis factor protects mice from lethal effect of endotoxin. *Science* **229**, 869–871.

Bevan, P. (2001). Insulin signalling. *J. Cell Sci.* **114,** 1429–1430.

Bevilacqua, M. P., Pober, J. S., Majeau, G. R., Cotran, R. S., and Gimbrone, M. A., Jr. (1984). Interleukin 1 (IL-1) induces biosynthesis and cell surface expression of procoagulant activity in human vascular endothelial cells. *J. Exp. Med.* **160,** 618–623.

Bevilacqua, M. P., Pober, J. S., Wheeler, M. E., Cotran, R. S., and Gimbrone, M. A., Jr. (1985). Interleukin-1 activation of vascular endothelium. Effects on procoagulant activity and leukocyte adhesion. *Am. J. Pathol.* **121,** 394–403.

Bialojan, C., and Takai, A. (1988). Inhibitory effect of a marine-sponge toxin, okadaic acid, on protein phosphatases. Specificity and kinetics. *Biochem. J.* **256,** 283–290.

Bjorbaek, C., Uotani, S., da Silva, B., and Flier, J. S. (1997). Divergent signaling capacities of the long and short isoforms of the leptin receptor. *J. Biol. Chem.* **272,** 32686–32695.

Bjorbak, C., Lavery, H. J., Bates, S. H., Olson, R. K., Davis, S. M., Flier, J. S., and Myers, M. G., Jr. (2000). SOCS3 mediates feedback inhibition of the leptin receptor via Tyr985. *J. Biol. Chem.* **275,** 40649–40657.

Bluthe, R. M., Pawlowski, M., Suarez, S., Parnet, P., Pittman, Q., Kelley, K. W., and Dantzer, R. (1994). Synergy between tumor necrosis factor alpha and interleukin-1 in the induction of sickness behavior in mice. *Psychoneuroendocrinology* **19,** 197–207.

Bluthe, R. M., Laye, S., Michaud, B., Combe, C., Dantzer, R., and Parnet, P. (2000). Role of interleukin-1beta and tumour necrosis factor-alpha in lipopolysaccharide-induced sickness behaviour: A study with interleukin-1 type I receptor-deficient mice. *Eur. J. Neurosci.* **12,** 4447–4456.

Bogardus, C., Lillioja, S., Howard, B. V., Reaven, G., and Mott, D. (1984). Relationships between insulin secretion, insulin action, and fasting plasma glucose concentration in nondiabetic and noninsulin-dependent diabetic subjects. *J. Clin. Invest.* **74,** 1238–1246.

Bolaffi, J. L., Rodd, G. G., Wang, J., and Grodsky, G. M. (1994). Interrelationship of changes in islet nicotine adeninedinucleotide, insulin secretion, and cell viability induced by interleukin-1 beta. *Endocrinology* **134,** 537–542.

Boozer, C. N., and Mayer, J. (1976). Effects of long-term restricted insulin production in obese-hyperglycemic (genotype ob/ob) mice. *Diabetologia* **12,** 181–187.

Boraschi, D., Rambaldi, A., Sica, A., Ghiara, P., Colotta, F., Wang, J. M., de Rossi, M., Zoia, C., Remuzzi, G., Bussolino, F., Scapigliati, G., Stoppacciaro, A., *et al.* (1991). Endothelial cells express the interleukin-1 receptor type I. *Blood* **78,** 1262–1267.

Borst, S. E., and Bagby, G. J. (2002). Neutralization of tumor necrosis factor reverses age-induced impairment of insulin responsiveness in skeletal muscle of Sprague-Dawley rats. *Metabolism* **51,** 1061–1064.

Brasier, A. R., Li, J., and Wimbish, K. A. (1996). Tumor necrosis factor activates angiotensinogen gene expression by the Rel A transactivator. *Hypertension* **27,** 1009–1017.

Brazel, D., Nakanishi, S., and Oster, W. (1991). Interleukin-1, characterization of the molecule, functional activity, and clinical implications. *Biotechnol. Ther.* **2,** 241–267.

Brazil, D. P., and Hemmings, B. A. (2001). Ten years of protein kinase B signalling: A hard Akt to follow. *Trends Biochem. Sci.* **26,** 657–664.

Breviario, F., Bertocchi, F., Dejana, E., and Bussolino, F. (1988). IL-1-induced adhesion of polymorphonuclear leukocytes to cultured human endothelial cells. Role of platelet-activating factor. *J. Immunol.* **141,** 3391–3397.

Brito, B. E., Romano, E. L., and Grunfeld, C. (1995). Increased lipopolysaccharide-induced tumour necrosis factor levels and death in hypercholesterolaemic rabbits. *Clin. Exp. Immunol.* **101,** 357–361.

Brown, E. J., and Schreiber, S. L. (1996). A signaling pathway to translational control. *Cell* **86,** 517–520.

Brown, E. J., Albers, M. W., Shin, T. B., Ichikawa, K., Keith, C. T., Lane, W. S., and Schreiber, S. L. (1994). A mammalian protein targeted by G1-arresting rapamycin-receptor complex. *Nature* **369,** 756–758.

425

Bruunsgaard, H. (2005). Physical activity and modulation of systemic low-level inflammation. *J. Leukoc. Biol.* **78,** 819–835. Epub 2005 Jul 2020.

Burysek, L., Tvrdik, P., and Houstek, J. (1993). Expression of interleukin-1 alpha and interleukin-1 receptor type I genes in murine brown adipose tissue. *FEBS Lett.* **334,** 229–232.

Cai, D., Dhe-Paganon, S., Melendez, P. A., Lee, J., and Shoelson, S. E. (2003). Two new substrates in insulin signaling, IRS5/DOK4 and IRS6/DOK5. *J. Biol. Chem.* **278,** 25323–25330. Epub 2003 May 25321.

Cai, D., Yuan, M., Frantz, D. F., Melendez, P. A., Hansen, L., Lee, J., and Shoelson, S. E. (2005). Local and systemic insulin resistance resulting from hepatic activation of IKK-beta and NF-kappaB. *Nat. Med.* **11,** 183–190. Epub 2005 Jan 2030.

Campbell, I. L., Iscaro, A., and Harrison, L. C. (1988). IFN-gamma and tumor necrosis factor-alpha. Cytotoxicity to murine islets of Langerhans. *J. Immunol.* **141,** 2325–2329.

Carey, A. L., Bruce, C. R., Sacchetti, M., Anderson, M. J., Olsen, D. B., Saltin, B., Hawley, J. A., and Febbraio, M. A. (2004). Interleukin-6 and tumor necrosis factor-alpha are not increased in patients with Type 2 diabetes: Evidence that plasma interleukin-6 is related to fat mass and not insulin responsiveness. *Diabetologia* **47,** 1029–1037. Epub 2004 May 1028.

Carswell, E. A., Old, L. J., Kassel, R. L., Green, S., Fiore, N., and Williamson, B. (1975). An endotoxin-induced serum factor that causes necrosis of tumors. *Proc. Natl. Acad. Sci. USA* **72,** 3666–3670.

Cengel, K. A., and Freund, G. G. (1999). JAK1-dependent phosphorylation of insulin receptor substrate-1 (IRS-1) is inhibited by IRS-1 serine phosphorylation. *J. Biol. Chem.* **274,** 27969–27974.

Cohen, B., Novick, D., and Rubinstein, M. (1996). Modulation of insulin activities by leptin. *Science* **274,** 1185–1188.

Coleman, D. L. (1982). Thermogenesis in diabetes-obesity syndromes in mutant mice. *Diabetologia* **22,** 205–211.

Coleman, D. L. (1985). Increased metabolic efficiency in obese mutant mice. *Int. J. Obes.* **9,** 69–73.

Coleman, D. L., and Hummel, K. P. (1974). Hyperinsulinemia in pre-weaning diabetes (db) mice. *Diabetologia* **10**(Suppl.), 607–610.

Conejo, R., and Lorenzo, M. (2001). Insulin signaling leading to proliferation, survival, and membrane ruffling in C2C12 myoblasts. *J. Cell Physiol.* **187,** 96–108.

Conti, G., Scarpini, E., Baron, P., Livraghi, S., Tiriticco, M., Bianchi, R., Vedeler, C., and Scarlato, G. (2002). Macrophage infiltration and death in the nerve during the early phases of experimental diabetic neuropathy: A process concomitant with endoneurial induction of IL-1beta and p75NTR. *J. Neurol. Sci.* **195,** 35–40.

Corbett, J. A., Lancaster, J. R., Jr., Sweetland, M. A., and McDaniel, M. L. (1991). Interleukin-1 beta-induced formation of EPR-detectable iron-nitrosyl complexes in islets of Langerhans. Role of nitric oxide in interleukin-1 beta-induced inhibition of insulin secretion. *J. Biol. Chem.* **266,** 21351–21354.

Craparo, A., O'Neill, T. J., and Gustafson, T. A. (1995). Non-SH2 domains within insulin receptor substrate-1 and SHC mediate their phosphotyrosine-dependent interaction with the NPEY motif of the insulin-like growth factor I receptor. *J. Biol. Chem.* **270,** 15639–15643.

Cross, D. A., Alessi, D. R., Cohen, P., Andjelkovich, M., and Hemmings, B. A. (1995). Inhibition of glycogen synthase kinase-3 by insulin mediated by protein kinase B. *Nature* **378,** 785–789.

Cumberbatch, M., and Kimber, I. (1995). Tumour necrosis factor-alpha is required for accumulation of dendritic cells in draining lymph nodes and for optimal contact sensitization. *Immunology* **84,** 31–35.

Dagogo-Jack, S., Fanelli, C., Paramore, D., Brothers, J., and Landt, M. (1996). Plasma leptin and insulin relationships in obese and nonobese humans. *Diabetes* **45,** 695–698.

Dandona, P., Aljada, A., and Bandyopadhyay, A. (2004). Inflammation: The link between insulin resistance, obesity and diabetes. *Trends Immunol.* **25**, 4–7.

Danesh, J., Whincup, P., Walker, M., Lennon, L., Thomson, A., Appleby, P., Gallimore, J. R., and Pepys, M. B. (2000). Low grade inflammation and coronary heart disease: Prospective study and updated meta-analyses. *BMJ* **321**, 199–204.

De Fea, K., and Roth, R. A. (1997a). Modulation of insulin receptor substrate-1 tyrosine phosphorylation and function by mitogen-activated protein kinase. *J. Biol. Chem.* **272**, 31400–31406.

De Fea, K., and Roth, R. A. (1997b). Protein kinase C modulation of insulin receptor substrate-1 tyrosine phosphorylation requires serine 612. *Biochemistry* **36**, 12939–12947.

De Souza, D., Fabri, L. J., Nash, A., Hilton, D. J., Nicola, N. A., and Baca, M. (2002). SH2 domains from suppressor of cytokine signaling-3 and protein tyrosine phosphatase SHP-2 have similar binding specificities. *Biochemistry* **41**, 9229–9236.

Delaney, C. A., Green, M. H., Lowe, J. E., and Green, I. C. (1993). Endogenous nitric oxide induced by interleukin-1 beta in rat islets of Langerhans and HIT-T15 cells causes significant DNA damage as measured by the 'comet' assay. *FEBS Lett.* **333**, 291–295.

Dennis, P. B., Fumagalli, S., and Thomas, G. (1999). Target of rapamycin (TOR): Balancing the opposing forces of protein synthesis and degradation. *Curr. Opin. Genet. Dev.* **9**, 49–54.

Di Gregorio, G. B., Hensley, L., Lu, T., Ranganathan, G., and Kern, P. A. (2004). Lipid and carbohydrate metabolism in mice with a targeted mutation in the IL-6 gene: Absence of development of age-related obesity. *Am. J. Physiol. Endocrinol. Metab.* **287**, E182–E187.

Dorffel, Y., Latsch, C., Stuhlmuller, B., Schreiber, S., Scholze, S., Burmester, G. R., and Scholze, J. (1999). Preactivated peripheral blood monocytes in patients with essential hypertension. *Hypertension* **34**, 113–117.

Dunne, A., and O'Neill, L. A. (2003). The interleukin-1 receptor/Toll-like receptor superfamily: Signal transduction during inflammation and host defense. *Sci. STKE* **2003**(171), re3.

Edwardson, J. A., and Hough, C. A. (1975). The pituitary-adrenal system of the genetically obese (ob/ob) mouse. *J. Endocrinol.* **65**, 99–107.

Engelman, J. A., Berg, A. H., Lewis, R. Y., Lisanti, M. P., and Scherer, P. E. (2000). Tumor necrosis factor alpha-mediated insulin resistance, but not dedifferentiation, is abrogated by MEK1/2 inhibitors in 3T3-L1 adipocytes. *Mol. Endocrinol.* **14**, 1557–1569.

Ernyei, S., and Young, M. R. (1966). Pulsatile and myelin-forming activities of Schwann cells *in vitro*. *J. Physiol.* **183**, 469–480.

Escobar-Morreale, H. F., Botella-Carretero, J. I., Villuendas, G., Sancho, J., and San Millan, J. L. (2004). Serum interleukin-18 concentrations are increased in the polycystic ovary syndrome: Relationship to insulin resistance and to obesity. *J. Clin. Endocrinol. Metab.* **89**, 806–811.

Esposito, K., Marfella, R., and Giugliano, D. (2004). Plasma interleukin-18 concentrations are elevated in type 2 diabetes. *Diabetes Care* **27**, 272.

Esposito, K., Nappo, F., Marfella, R., Giugliano, G., Giugliano, F., Ciotola, M., Quagliaro, L., Ceriello, A., and Giugliano, D. (2002a). Inflammatory cytokine concentrations are acutely increased by hyperglycemia in humans: Role of oxidative stress. *Circulation* **106**, 2067–2072.

Esposito, K., Pontillo, A., Ciotola, M., Di Palo, C., Grella, E., Nicoletti, G., and Giugliano, D. (2002b). Weight loss reduces interleukin-18 levels in obese women. *J. Clin. Endocrinol. Metab.* **87**, 3864–3866.

Ettinger, W. H., Miller, L. D., Albers, J. J., Smith, T. K., and Parks, J. S. (1990). Lipopolysaccharide and tumor necrosis factor cause a fall in plasma concentration of lecithin: Cholesterol acyltransferase in cynomolgus monkeys. *J. Lipid Res.* **31**, 1099–1107.

Faggioni, R., Feingold, K. R., and Grunfeld, C. (2001). Leptin regulation of the immune response and the immunodeficiency of malnutrition. *FASEB J.* **15**, 2565–2571.

Faldt, J., Wernstedt, I., Fitzgerald, S. M., Wallenius, K., Bergstrom, G., and Jansson, J. O. (2004). Reduced exercise endurance in interleukin-6-deficient mice. *Endocrinology* **145**, 2680–2686. Epub 2004 Feb 2626.

Fasshauer, M., Kralisch, S., Klier, M., Lossner, U., Bluher, M., Klein, J., and Paschke, R. (2004). Insulin resistance inducing cytokines differentially regulate SOCS mRNA expression via growth factor- and Jak/Stat-signaling pathways in 3T3-L1 adipocytes. *J. Endocrinol.* **181**, 129–138.

Febbraio, M. A., Hiscock, N., Sacchetti, M., Fischer, C. P., and Pedersen, B. K. (2004). Interleukin-6 is a novel factor mediating glucose homeostasis during skeletal muscle contraction. *Diabetes* **53**, 1643–1648.

Fei, H., Okano, H. J., Li, C., Lee, G. H., Zhao, C., Darnell, R., and Friedman, J. M. (1997). Anatomic localization of alternatively spliced leptin receptors (Ob-R) in mouse brain and other tissues. *Proc. Natl. Acad. Sci. USA* **94**, 7001–7005.

Feingold, K. R., Soued, M., Adi, S., Staprans, I., Shigenaga, J., Doerrler, W., Moser, A., and Grunfeld, C. (1990). Tumor necrosis factor-increased hepatic very-low-density lipoprotein production and increased serum triglyceride levels in diabetic rats. *Diabetes* **39**, 1569–1574.

Ferencik, M., Stvrtinova, V., and Hulin, I. (2005). Defects in regulation of local immune responses resulting in atherosclerosis. *Clin. Dev. Immunol.* **12**, 225–234.

Fernandez-Real, J. M., Gutierrez, C., Ricart, W., Castineira, M. J., Vendrell, J., and Richart, C. (1999). Plasma levels of the soluble fraction of tumor necrosis factor receptors 1 and 2 are independent determinants of plasma cholesterol and LDL-cholesterol concentrations in healthy subjects. *Atherosclerosis* **146**, 321–327.

Fernandez-Real, J. M., Broch, M., Vendrell, J., Gutierrez, C., Casamitjana, R., Pugeat, M., Richart, C., and Ricart, W. (2000a). Interleukin-6 gene polymorphism and insulin sensitivity. *Diabetes* **49**, 517–520.

Fernandez-Real, J. M., Broch, M., Vendrell, J., Richart, C., and Ricart, W. (2000b). Interleukin-6 gene polymorphism and lipid abnormalities in healthy subjects. *J. Clin. Endocrinol. Metab.* **85**, 1334–1339.

Fernandez-Real, J. M., Lainez, B., Vendrell, J., Rigla, M., Castro, A., Penarroja, G., Broch, M., Perez, A., Richart, C., Engel, P., and Ricart, W. (2002). Shedding of TNF-alpha receptors, blood pressure, and insulin sensitivity in type 2 diabetes mellitus. *Am. J. Physiol. Endocrinol. Metab.* **282**, E952–E959.

Fischer, C. P., Perstrup, L. B., Berntsen, A., Eskildsen, P., and Pedersen, B. K. (2005). Elevated plasma interleukin-18 is a marker of insulin-resistance in type 2 diabetic and non-diabetic humans. *Clin. Immunol.* **117**, 152–160. Epub 2005 Aug 2019.

Flatt, P. R., and Bailey, C. J. (1981). Development of glucose intolerance and impaired plasma insulin response to glucose in obese hyperglycaemic (ob/ob) mice. *Horm. Metab. Res.* **13**, 556–560.

Fleet, J. C., Clinton, S. K., Salomon, R. N., Loppnow, H., and Libby, P. (1992). Atherogenic diets enhance endotoxin-stimulated interleukin-1 and tumor necrosis factor gene expression in rabbit aortae. *J. Nutr.* **122**, 294–305.

Folli, F., Kahn, C. R., Hansen, H., Bouchie, J. L., and Feener, E. P. (1997). Angiotensin II inhibits insulin signaling in aortic smooth muscle cells at multiple levels. A potential role for serine phosphorylation in insulin/angiotensin II crosstalk. *J. Clin. Invest.* **100**, 2158–2169.

Fontana, A., Hengartner, H., de Tribolet, N., and Weber, E. (1984). Glioblastoma cells release interleukin 1 and factors inhibiting interleukin 2-mediated effects. *J. Immunol.* **132**, 1837–1844.

Fourrier, A., Montois, R., Socolovsky, C., Maisonneuve, B., and Mouton, Y. (1975). Incidence and severity of infection in diabetes. Comparative study of 142 patients. *Lille Med.* **20**, 653–656.

Gagnon, A., and Sorisky, A. (1998). The effect of glucose concentration on insulin-induced 3T3-L1 adipose cell differentiation. *Obes. Res.* **6,** 157–163.

Gerdes, N., Sukhova, G. K., Libby, P., Reynolds, R. S., Young, J. L., and Schonbeck, U. (2002). Expression of interleukin (IL)-18 and functional IL-18 receptor on human vascular endothelial cells, smooth muscle cells, and macrophages: Implications for atherogenesis. *J. Exp. Med.* **195,** 245–257.

Ghilardi, N., Ziegler, S., Wiestner, A., Stoffel, R., Heim, M. H., and Skoda, R. C. (1996). Defective STAT signaling by the leptin receptor in diabetic mice. *Proc. Natl. Acad. Sci. USA* **93,** 6231–6235.

Girard, J., Perdereau, D., Foufelle, F., Prip-Buus, C., and Ferre, P. (1994). Regulation of lipogenic enzyme gene expression by nutrients and hormones. *FASEB J.* **8,** 36–42.

Gonatas, N. K., Levine, S., and Shoulson, R. (1964). Phagocytosis and regeneration of myelin in an experimental leukoencephalopathy. *Am. J. Pathol.* **44,** 565–583.

Gonzalez, W., Fontaine, V., Pueyo, M. E., Laquay, N., Messika-Zeitoun, D., Philippe, M., Arnal, J. F., Jacob, M. P., and Michel, J. B. (2000). Molecular plasticity of vascular wall during N(G)-nitro-L-arginine methyl ester-induced hypertension: Modulation of proinflammatory signals. *Hypertension* **36,** 103–109.

Gordon, F. J., Brody, M. J., Fink, G. D., Buggy, J., and Johnson, A. K. (1979). Role of central catecholamines in the control of blood pressure and drinking behavior. *Brain Res.* **178,** 161–173.

Gottschall, P. E., Koves, K., Mizuno, K., Tatsuno, I., and Arimura, A. (1991). Glucocorticoid upregulation of interleukin 1 receptor expression in a glioblastoma cell line. *Am. J. Physiol.* **261,** E362–E368.

Granowitz, E. V., Clark, B. D., Vannier, E., Callahan, M. V., and Dinarello, C. A. (1992). Effect of interleukin-1 (IL-1) blockade on cytokine synthesis: I. IL-1 receptor antagonist inhibits IL-1-induced cytokine synthesis and blocks the binding of IL-1 to its type II receptor on human monocytes. *Blood* **79,** 2356–2363.

Greenberg, A. S., Nordan, R. P., McIntosh, J., Calvo, J. C., Scow, R. O., and Jablons, D. (1992). Interleukin 6 reduces lipoprotein lipase activity in adipose tissue of mice *in vivo* and in 3T3-L1 adipocytes: A possible role for interleukin 6 in cancer cachexia. *Cancer Res.* **52,** 4113–4116.

Greenhalgh, D. G., Sprugel, K. H., Murray, M. J., and Ross, R. (1990). PDGF and FGF stimulate wound healing in the genetically diabetic mouse. *Am. J. Pathol.* **136,** 1235–1246.

Greenwel, P., Iraburu, M. J., Reyes-Romero, M., Meraz-Cruz, N., Casado, E., Solis-Herruzo, J. A., and Rojkind, M. (1995). Induction of an acute phase response in rats stimulates the expression of alpha 1(I) procollagen messenger ribonucleic acid in their livers. Possible role of interleukin-6. *Lab. Invest.* **72,** 83–91.

Gresser, I., Delers, F., Tran Quangs, N., Marion, S., Engler, R., Maury, C., Soria, C., Soria, J., Fiers, W., and Tavernier, J. (1987). Tumor necrosis factor induces acute phase proteins in rats. *J. Biol. Regul. Homeost. Agents* **1,** 173–176.

Gualillo, O., Eiras, S., White, D. W., Dieguez, C., and Casanueva, F. F. (2002). Leptin promotes the tyrosine phosphorylation of SHC proteins and SHC association with GRB2. *Mol. Cell Endocrinol.* **190,** 83–89.

Gustafson, T. A., He, W., Craparo, A., Schaub, C. D., and O'Neill, T. J. (1995). Phosphotyrosine-dependent interaction of SHC and insulin receptor substrate 1 with the NPEY motif of the insulin receptor via a novel non-SH2 domain. *Mol. Cell. Biol.* **15,** 2500–2508.

Haider, A. W., Roubenoff, R., Wilson, P. W., Levy, D., D'Agostino, R., Silbershatz, H., and O'Donnell, C. J. (2004). Monocyte cytokine production, systemic inflammation and cardiovascular disease in very elderly men and women: The Framingham Heart Study. *Eur. J. Cardiovasc. Prev. Rehabil.* **11,** 214–215.

Hamaguchi, K., and Leiter, E. H. (1990). Comparison of cytokine effects on mouse pancreatic alpha-cell and beta-cell lines. Viability, secretory function, and MHC antigen expression. *Diabetes* **39**, 415–425.

Haring, H., Kirsch, D., Obermaier, B., Ermel, B., and Machicao, F. (1986). Tumor-promoting phorbol esters increase the Km of the ATP-binding site of the insulin receptor kinase from rat adipocytes. *J. Biol. Chem.* **261**, 3869–3875.

Harris, T. B., Ferrucci, L., Tracy, R. P., Corti, M. C., Wacholder, S., Ettinger, W. H., Jr., Heimovitz, H., Cohen, H. J., and Wallace, R. (1999). Associations of elevated interleukin-6 and C-reactive protein levels with mortality in the elderly. *Am. J. Med.* **106**, 506–512.

Hartman, M. E., Villela-Bach, M., Chen, J., and Freund, G. G. (2001). Frap-dependent serine phosphorylation of IRS-1 inhibits IRS-1 tyrosine phosphorylation. *Biochem. Biophys. Res. Commun.* **280**, 776–781.

Hartman, M. E., O'Connor, J. C., Godbout, J. P., Minor, K. D., Mazzocco, V. R., and Freund, G. G. (2004). Insulin receptor substrate-2-dependent interleukin-4 signaling in macrophages is impaired in two models of type 2 diabetes mellitus. *J. Biol. Chem.* **279**, 28045–28050. Epub 22004 Apr 28027.

Haruta, T., Uno, T., Kawahara, J., Takano, A., Egawa, K., Sharma, P. M., Olefsky, J. M., and Kobayashi, M. (2000). A rapamycin-sensitive pathway down-regulates insulin signaling via phosphorylation and proteasomal degradation of insulin receptor substrate-1. *Mol. Endocrinol.* **14**, 783–794.

Heffetz, D., and Zick, Y. (1986). Receptor aggregation is necessary for activation of the soluble insulin receptor kinase. *J. Biol. Chem.* **261**, 889–894.

Heliovaara, M. K., Teppo, A. M., Karonen, S. L., Tuominen, J. A., and Ebeling, P. (2005). Plasma IL-6 concentration is inversely related to insulin sensitivity, and acute-phase proteins associate with glucose and lipid metabolism in healthy subjects. *Diabetes Obes. Metab.* **7**, 729–736.

Helqvist, S. (1994). Interleukin 1 beta-mediated destruction of pancreatic beta-cells *in vitro*. A model of beta-cell destruction in insulin-dependent diabetes mellitus? *Dan. Med. Bull.* **41**, 151–166.

Hennige, A. M., Burks, D. J., Ozcan, U., Kulkarni, R. N., Ye, J., Park, S., Schubert, M., Fisher, T. L., Dow, M. A., Leshan, R., Zakaria, M., Mossa-Basha, M., *et al.* (2003). Upregulation of insulin receptor substrate-2 in pancreatic beta cells prevents diabetes. *J. Clin. Invest.* **112**, 1521–1532.

Hodgkin, P. D., Bond, M. W., O'Garra, A., Frank, G., Lee, F., Coffman, R. L., Zlotnik, A., and Howard, M. (1988). Identification of IL-6 as a T cell-derived factor that enhances the proliferative response of thymocytes to IL-4 and phorbol myristate acetate. *J. Immunol.* **141**, 151–157.

Hohmeier, H. E., Tran, V. V., Chen, G., Gasa, R., and Newgard, C. B. (2003). Inflammatory mechanisms in diabetes: Lessons from the beta-cell. *Int. J. Obes. Relat. Metab. Disord.* **27** (Suppl. 3), S12–S16.

Holgado-Madruga, M., Emlet, D. R., Moscatello, D. K., Godwin, A. K., and Wong, A. J. (1996). A Grb2-associated docking protein in EGF- and insulin-receptor signalling. *Nature* **379**, 560–564.

Horuk, R., Huang, J. J., Covington, M., and Newton, R. C. (1987). A biochemical and kinetic analysis of the interleukin-1 receptor. Evidence for differences in molecular properties of IL-1 receptors. *J. Biol. Chem.* **262**, 16275–16278.

Hosokawa, T., Ando, K., and Tamura, G. (1985). An ascochlorin derivative, AS-6, reduces insulin resistance in the genetically obese diabetic mouse, db/db. *Diabetes* **34**, 267–274.

Hotamisligil, G. S. (1999a). Mechanisms of TNF-alpha-induced insulin resistance. *Exp. Clin. Endocrinol. Diabetes* **107**, 119–125.

Hotamisligil, G. S. (1999b). The role of TNFalpha and TNF receptors in obesity and insulin resistance. *J. Intern. Med.* **245**, 621–625.

Hotamisligil, G. S., Shargill, N. S., and Spiegelman, B. M. (1993). Adipose expression of tumor necrosis factor-alpha: Direct role in obesity-linked insulin resistance. *Science* **259**, 87–91.

Hotamisligil, G. S., Murray, D. L., Choy, L. N., and Spiegelman, B. M. (1994). Tumor necrosis factor alpha inhibits signaling from the insulin receptor. *Proc. Natl. Acad. Sci. USA* **91**, 4854–4858.

Hotamisligil, G. S., Arner, P., Caro, J. F., Atkinson, R. L., and Spiegelman, B. M. (1995). Increased adipose tissue expression of tumor necrosis factor-alpha in human obesity and insulin resistance. *J. Clin. Invest.* **95**, 2409–2415.

Hotamisligil, G. S., Peraldi, P., Budavari, A., Ellis, R., White, M. F., and Spiegelman, B. M. (1996). IRS-1-mediated inhibition of insulin receptor tyrosine kinase activity in TNF-alpha- and obesity-induced insulin resistance. *Science* **271**, 665–668.

Humbel, R. E. (1963). Studies on isolated islets of Langerhans (Brockmann bodies) of teleost fishes. II. Evidence for insulin biosynthesis *in vitro*. *Biochim. Biophys. Acta.* **74**, 96–104.

Hung, J., McQuillan, B. M., Chapman, C. M., Thompson, P. L., and Beilby, J. P. (2005). Elevated interleukin-18 levels are associated with the metabolic syndrome independent of obesity and insulin resistance. *Arterioscler. Thromb. Vasc. Biol.* **25**, 1268–1273. Epub 2005 Mar 1224.

Ikeda, M., Ikeda, U., Shimada, K., Minota, S., and Kano, S. (1996). Regulation of ICAM-1 expression by inflammatory cytokines in rat mesangial cells. *Cytokine* **8**, 109–114.

Ishigami, T., Umemura, S., Iwamoto, T., Tamura, K., Hibi, K., Yamaguchi, S., Nyuui, N., Kimura, K., Miyazaki, N., and Ishii, M. (1995). Molecular variant of angiotensinogen gene is associated with coronary atherosclerosis. *Circulation* **91**, 951–954.

Ish-Shalom, D., Christoffersen, C. T., Vorwerk, P., Sacerdoti-Sierra, N., Shymko, R. M., Naor, D., and De Meyts, P. (1997). Mitogenic properties of insulin and insulin analogues mediated by the insulin receptor. *Diabetologia* **40**(Suppl. 2), S25–S31.

Janjic, D., and Asfari, M. (1992). Effects of cytokines on rat insulinoma INS-1 cells. *J. Endocrinol.* **132**, 67–76.

Jenny, N. S., Tracy, R. P., Ogg, M. S., Luong le, A., Kuller, L. H., Arnold, A. M., Sharrett, A. R., and Humphries, S. E. (2002). In the elderly, interleukin-6 plasma levels and the −174G > C polymorphism are associated with the development of cardiovascular disease. *Arterioscler. Thromb. Vasc. Biol.* **22**, 2066–2071.

Jirik, F. R., Podor, T. J., Hirano, T., Kishimoto, T., Loskutoff, D. J., Carson, D. A., and Lotz, M. (1989). Bacterial lipopolysaccharide and inflammatory mediators augment IL-6 secretion by human endothelial cells. *J. Immunol.* **142**, 144–147.

Johnson, D. R., O'Connor, J. C., Dantzer, R., and Freund, G. G. (2005). Inhibition of vagally mediated immune-to-brain signaling by vanadyl sulfate speeds recovery from sickness. *Proc. Natl. Acad. Sci. USA* **102**, 15184–15189. Epub 12005 Oct 15110.

Jones, J. P., and Dohm, G. L. (1997). Regulation of glucose transporter GLUT-4 and hexokinase II gene transcription by insulin and epinephrine. *Am. J. Physiol.* **273**, E682–E687.

Jovinge, S., Hamsten, A., Tornvall, P., Proudler, A., Bavenholm, P., Ericsson, C. G., Godsland, I., de Faire, U., and Nilsson, J. (1998). Evidence for a role of tumor necrosis factor alpha in disturbances of triglyceride and glucose metabolism predisposing to coronary heart disease. *Metabolism* **47**, 113–118.

Jullien, D., Tanti, J. F., Heydrick, S. J., Gautier, N., Gremeaux, T., Van Obberghen, E., and Le Marchand-Brustel, E. (1993). Differential effects of okadaic acid on insulin-stimulated glucose and amino acid uptake and phosphatidylinositol 3-kinase activity. *J. Biol. Chem.* **268**, 15246–15251.

Kahaleh, M. B., and Fan, P. S. (1997). Effect of cytokines on the production of endothelin by endothelial cells. *Clin. Exp. Rheumatol.* **15**, 163–167.

Kahn, C. R., Baird, K. L., Jarrett, D. B., and Flier, J. S. (1978). Direct demonstration that receptor crosslinking or aggregation is important in insulin action. *Proc. Natl. Acad. Sci. USA* **75,** 4209–4213.

Kanemaki, T., Kitade, H., Kaibori, M., Sakitani, K., Hiramatsu, Y., Kamiyama, Y., Ito, S., and Okumura, T. (1998). Interleukin 1beta and interleukin 6, but not tumor necrosis factor alpha, inhibit insulin-stimulated glycogen synthesis in rat hepatocytes. *Hepatology* **27,** 1296–1303.

Kanety, H., Feinstein, R., Papa, M. Z., Hemi, R., and Karasik, A. (1995). Tumor necrosis factor alpha-induced phosphorylation of insulin receptor substrate-1 (IRS-1). Possible mechanism for suppression of insulin-stimulated tyrosine phosphorylation of IRS-1. *J. Biol. Chem.* **270,** 23780–23784.

Kaplan, M. L., Trout, J. R., and Leveille, G. A. (1976). Adipocyte size distribution in ob/ob mice during preobese and obese phases of development. *Proc. Soc. Exp. Biol. Med.* **153,** 476–482.

Kawahara, D. J., and Kenney, J. S. (1991). Species differences in human and rat islet sensitivity to human cytokines. Monoclonal anti-interleukin-1 (IL-1) influences on direct and indirect IL-1-mediated islet effects. *Cytokine* **3,** 117–124.

Kawashima, M., Yamamura, M., Taniai, M., Yamauchi, H., Tanimoto, T., Kurimoto, M., Miyawaki, S., Amano, T., Takeuchi, T., and Makino, H. (2001). Levels of interleukin-18 and its binding inhibitors in the blood circulation of patients with adult-onset Still's disease. *Arthritis Rheum.* **44,** 550–560.

Kawazoe, Y., Naka, T., Fujimoto, M., Kohzaki, H., Morita, Y., Narazaki, M., Okumura, K., Saitoh, H., Nakagawa, R., Uchiyama, Y., Akira, S., and Kishimoto, T. (2001). Signal transducer and activator of transcription (STAT)-induced STAT inhibitor 1 (SSI-1)/ suppressor of cytokine signaling 1 (SOCS1) inhibits insulin signal transduction pathway through modulating insulin receptor substrate 1 (IRS-1) phosphorylation. *J. Exp Med.* **193,** 263–269.

Keavney, B., and McKenzie, C. (1995). Coronary atherosclerosis and the angiotensinogen gene. *Circulation* **92,** 2356–2357.

Kelly, K. L., Ruderman, N. B., and Chen, K. S. (1992). Phosphatidylinositol-3-kinase in isolated rat adipocytes. Activation by insulin and subcellular distribution. *J. Biol. Chem.* **267,** 3423–3428.

Kern, P. A., Ranganathan, S., Li, C., Wood, L., and Ranganathan, G. (2001). Adipose tissue tumor necrosis factor and interleukin-6 expression in human obesity and insulin resistance. *Am. J. Physiol. Endocrinol. Metab.* **280,** E745–E751.

Khan, A. H., and Pessin, J. E. (2002). Insulin regulation of glucose uptake: A complex interplay of intracellular signalling pathways. *Diabetologia* **45,** 1475–1483. Epub 2002 Oct 1418.

Kido, Y., Burks, D. J., Withers, D., Bruning, J. C., Kahn, C. R., White, M. F., and Accili, D. (2000). Tissue-specific insulin resistance in mice with mutations in the insulin receptor, IRS-1, and IRS-2. *J. Clin. Invest.* **105,** 199–205.

Kido, Y., Nakae, J., and Accili, D. (2001). Clinical review 125: The insulin receptor and its cellular targets. *J. Clin. Endocrinol. Metab.* **86,** 972–979.

Kieffer, T. J., and Habener, J. F. (2000). The adipoinsular axis: Effects of leptin on pancreatic beta-cells. *Am. J. Physiol. Endocrinol. Metab.* **278,** E1–E14.

Kieffer, T. J., Heller, R. S., and Habener, J. F. (1996). Leptin receptors expressed on pancreatic beta-cells. *Biochem. Biophys. Res. Commun.* **224,** 522–527.

Kim, J. A., Yeh, D. C., Ver, M., Li, Y., Carranza, A., Conrads, T. P., Veenstra, T. D., Harrington, M. A., and Quon, M. J. (2005). Phosphorylation of Ser24 in the pleckstrin homology domain of insulin receptor substrate-1 by Mouse Pelle-like kinase/interleukin-1 receptor-associated kinase: Cross talk between inflammatory signaling and insulin signaling that may contribute to insulin resistance. *J. Biol. Chem.* **280,** 23173–23183. Epub 22005 Apr 23122.

Klemm, P., Warner, T. D., Hohlfeld, T., Corder, R., and Vane, J. R. (1995). Endothelin 1 mediates *ex vivo* coronary vasoconstriction caused by exogenous and endogenous cytokines. *Proc. Natl. Acad. Sci. USA* **92**, 2691–2695.

Klover, P. J., Zimmers, T. A., Koniaris, L. G., and Mooney, R. A. (2003). Chronic exposure to interleukin-6 causes hepatic insulin resistance in mice. *Diabetes* **52**, 2784–2789.

Klover, P. J., Clementi, A. H., and Mooney, R. A. (2005). Interleukin-6 depletion selectively improves hepatic insulin action in obesity. *Endocrinology* **146**, 3417–3427. Epub 2005 Apr 3421.

Koenig, W., Meisinger, C., Baumert, J., Khuseyinova, N., and Lowel, H. (2005). Systemic low-grade inflammation and risk of coronary heart disease: Results from the MONICA/KORA Augsburg cohort studies. *Gesundheitswesen* **67**(Suppl. 1), S62–S67.

Koistinen, H. A., Bastard, J. P., Dusserre, E., Ebeling, P., Zegari, N., Andreelli, F., Jardel, C., Donner, M., Meyer, L., Moulin, P., Hainque, B., Riou, J. P., *et al.* (2000). Subcutaneous adipose tissue expression of tumour necrosis factor-alpha is not associated with whole body insulin resistance in obese nondiabetic or in type-2 diabetic subjects. *Eur. J. Clin. Invest.* **30**, 302–310.

Kolb-Bachofen, V., and Kolb, H. (1989). A role for macrophages in the pathogenesis of type 1 diabetes. *Autoimmunity* **3**, 145–154.

Krahl, M. E. (1962). Insulin and protein synthesis in isolated tissues. *Diabetes* **11**, 144–146.

Krauss, R. M., Grunfeld, C., Doerrler, W. T., and Feingold, K. R. (1990). Tumor necrosis factor acutely increases plasma levels of very low density lipoproteins of normal size and composition. *Endocrinology* **127**, 1016–1021.

Kretowski, A., Mironczuk, K., Karpinska, A., Bojaryn, U., Kinalski, M., Puchalski, Z., and Kinalska, I. (2002). Interleukin-18 promoter polymorphisms in type 1 diabetes. *Diabetes* **51**, 3347–3349.

Kubo, M., Hanada, T., and Yoshimura, A. (2003). Suppressors of cytokine signaling and immunity. *Nat. Immunol.* **4**, 1169–1176.

Kuruvilla, F. G., and Schreiber, S. L. (1999). The PIK-related kinases intercept conventional signaling pathways. *Chem. Biol.* **6**, R129–R136.

Labriola-Tompkins, E., Chandran, C., Kaffka, K. L., Biondi, D., Graves, B. J., Hatada, M., Madison, V. S., Karas, J., Kilian, P. L., and Ju, G. (1991). Identification of the discontinuous binding site in human interleukin 1 beta for the type I interleukin 1 receptor. *Proc. Natl. Acad. Sci. USA* **88**, 11182–11186.

Laney, J. D., and Hochstrasser, M. (1999). Substrate targeting in the ubiquitin system. *Cell* **97**, 427–430.

Lang, C. H., Dobrescu, C., and Bagby, G. J. (1992). Tumor necrosis factor impairs insulin action on peripheral glucose disposal and hepatic glucose output. *Endocrinology* **130**, 43–52.

Lavan, B. E., Fantin, V. R., Chang, E. T., Lane, W. S., Keller, S. R., and Lienhard, G. E. (1997a). A novel 160-kDa phosphotyrosine protein in insulin-treated embryonic kidney cells is a new member of the insulin receptor substrate family. *J. Biol. Chem.* **272**, 21403–21407.

Lavan, B. E., Lane, W. S., and Lienhard, G. E. (1997b). The 60-kDa phosphotyrosine protein in insulin-treated adipocytes is a new member of the insulin receptor substrate family. *J. Biol. Chem.* **272**, 11439–11443.

Le Marchand-Brustel, G. E. (1999). Molecular mechanisms of insulin action in normal and insulin-resistant states. *Exp. Clin. Endocrinol. Diabetes* **107**, 126–132.

Lederer, J. A., and Czuprynski, C. J. (1994). Species-specific binding of IL-1, but not the IL-1 receptor antagonist, by fibroblasts. *Cytokine* **6**, 154–161.

Lee, D. H., and Goldberg, A. L. (1998). Proteasome inhibitors: Valuable new tools for cell biologists. *Trends Cell Biol.* **8**, 397–403.

Lee, G. H., Proenca, R., Montez, J. M., Carroll, K. M., Darvishzadeh, J. G., Lee, J. I., and Friedman, J. M. (1996). Abnormal splicing of the leptin receptor in diabetic mice. *Nature* **379**, 632–635.

Lees, D. M., Pallikaros, Z., and Corder, R. (2000). The p55 tumor necrosis factor receptor (CD120a) induces endothelin-1 synthesis in endothelial and epithelial cells. *Eur. J. Pharmacol.* **390**, 89–94.

Lehmann, U., Schmitz, J., Weissenbach, M., Sobota, R. M., Hortner, M., Friederichs, K., Behrmann, I., Tsiaris, W., Sasaki, A., Schneider-Mergener, J., Yoshimura, A., Neel, B. G., et al. (2003). SHP2 and SOCS3 contribute to Tyr-759-dependent attenuation of interleukin-6 signaling through gp130. *J. Biol. Chem.* **278**, 661–671. Epub 2002 Oct 2027.

Lerman, A., Edwards, B. S., Hallett, J. W., Heublein, D. M., Sandberg, S. M., and Burnett, J. C., Jr. (1991). Circulating and tissue endothelin immunoreactivity in advanced atherosclerosis. *N. Engl. J. Med.* **325**, 997–1001.

Lewis, R. E., Cao, L., Perregaux, D., and Czech, M. P. (1990a). Threonine 1336 of the human insulin receptor is a major target for phosphorylation by protein kinase C. *Biochemistry* **29**, 1807–1813.

Lewis, R. E., Wu, G. P., MacDonald, R. G., and Czech, M. P. (1990b). Insulin-sensitive phosphorylation of serine 1293/1294 on the human insulin receptor by a tightly associated serine kinase. *J. Biol. Chem.* **265**, 947–954.

Leyva, F., Godsland, I. F., Ghatei, M., Proudler, A. J., Aldis, S., Walton, C., Bloom, S., and Stevenson, J. C. (1998). Hyperleptinemia as a component of a metabolic syndrome of cardiovascular risk. *Arterioscler. Thromb. Vasc. Biol.* **18**, 928–933.

Li, J., DeFea, K., and Roth, R. A. (1999). Modulation of insulin receptor substrate-1 tyrosine phosphorylation by an Akt/phosphatidylinositol 3-kinase pathway. *J. Biol. Chem.* **274**, 9351–9356.

Libby, P., Ordovas, J. M., Auger, K. R., Robbins, A. H., Birinyi, L. K., and Dinarello, C. A. (1986). Endotoxin and tumor necrosis factor induce interleukin-1 gene expression in adult human vascular endothelial cells. *Am. J. Pathol.* **124**, 179–185.

Lienhard, G. E., Kim, H. H., Ransome, K. J., and Gorga, J. C. (1982). Immunological identification of an insulin-responsive glucose transporter. *Biochem. Biophys. Res. Commun.* **105**, 1150–1156.

Lopes-Virella, M. F., and Virella, G. (1996). Cytokines, modified lipoproteins, and arteriosclerosis in diabetes. *Diabetes* **45**(Suppl. 3), S40–S44.

Loppnow, H., and Libby, P. (1989). Comparative analysis of cytokine induction in human vascular endothelial and smooth muscle cells. *Lymphokine Res.* **8**, 293–299.

Loppnow, H., and Libby, P. (1990). Proliferating or interleukin 1-activated human vascular smooth muscle cells secrete copious interleukin 6. *J. Clin. Invest.* **85**, 731–738.

Lowe, G. D., Rumley, A., Woodward, M., Reid, E., and Rumley, J. (1999). Activated protein C resistance and the FV:R506Q mutation in a random population sample: Associations with cardiovascular risk factors and coagulation variables. *Thromb. Haemost.* **81**, 918–924.

Lu, H., Raptis, M., Black, E., Stan, M., Amar, S., and Graves, D. T. (2004). Influence of diabetes on the exacerbation of an inflammatory response in cardiovascular tissue. *Endocrinology* **145**, 4934–4939. Epub 2004 Jul 4929.

Luscinskas, F. W., Brock, A. F., Arnaout, M. A., and Gimbrone, M. A., Jr. (1989). Endothelial-leukocyte adhesion molecule-1-dependent and leukocyte (CD11/CD18)-dependent mechanisms contribute to polymorphonuclear leukocyte adhesion to cytokine-activated human vascular endothelium. *J. Immunol.* **142**, 2257–2263.

MacPherson, A., Dinkel, K., and Sapolsky, R. (2005). Glucocorticoids worsen excitotoxin-induced expression of pro-inflammatory cytokines in hippocampal cultures. *Exp. Neurol.* **194**, 376–383.

Maedler, K., and Donath, M. Y. (2004). Beta-cells in type 2 diabetes: A loss of function and mass. *Horm. Res.* **62**, 67–73.

Maedler, K., Sergeev, P., Ehses, J. A., Mathe, Z., Bosco, D., Berney, T., Dayer, J. M., Reinecke, M., Halban, P. A., and Donath, M. Y. (2004). Leptin modulates beta cell expression of IL-1 receptor antagonist and release of IL-1beta in human islets. *Proc. Natl. Acad. Sci. USA* **101**, 8138–8143. Epub 2004 May 8112.

Maegawa, H., Ugi, S., Adachi, M., Hinoda, Y., Kikkawa, R., Yachi, A., Shigeta, Y., and Kashiwagi, A. (1994). Insulin receptor kinase phosphorylates protein tyrosine phosphatase containing Src homology 2 regions and modulates its PTPase activity *in vitro. Biochem. Biophys. Res. Commun.* **199**, 780–785.

Mandrup-Poulsen, T., Bendtzen, K., Nielsen, J. H., Bendixen, G., and Nerup, J. (1985). Cytokines cause functional and structural damage to isolated islets of Langerhans. *Allergy* **40**, 424–429.

Mandrup-Poulsen, T., Bendtzen, K., Nerup, J., Dinarello, C. A., Svenson, M., and Nielsen, J. H. (1986). Affinity-purified human interleukin I is cytotoxic to isolated islets of Langerhans. *Diabetologia* **29**, 63–67.

Mandrup-Poulsen, T., Zumsteg, U., Reimers, J., Pociot, F., Morch, L., Helqvist, S., Dinarello, C. A., and Nerup, J. (1993). Involvement of interleukin 1 and interleukin 1 antagonist in pancreatic beta-cell destruction in insulin-dependent diabetes mellitus. *Cytokine* **5**, 185–191.

Mantovani, A., Muzio, M., Ghezzi, P., Colotta, F., and Introna, M. (1996). Negative regulators of the interleukin-1 system: Receptor antagonists and a decoy receptor. *Int. J. Clin. Lab. Res.* **26**, 7–14.

Marsden, P. A., and Brenner, B. M. (1992). Transcriptional regulation of the endothelin-1 gene by TNF-alpha. *Am. J. Physiol.* **262**, C854–C861.

Martin, S., Maruta, K., Burkart, V., Gillis, S., and Kolb, H. (1988). IL-1 and IFN-gamma increase vascular permeability. *Immunology* **64**, 301–305.

May, L. T., Torcia, G., Cozzolino, F., Ray, A., Tatter, S. B., Santhanam, U., Sehgal, P. B., and Stern, D. (1989). Interleukin-6 gene expression in human endothelial cells: RNA start sites, multiple IL-6 proteins and inhibition of proliferation. *Biochem. Biophys. Res. Commun.* **159**, 991–998.

McDonagh, J., Fossel, E. T., Kradin, R. L., Dubinett, S. M., Laposata, M., and Hallaq, Y. A. (1992). Effects of tumor necrosis factor-alpha on peroxidation of plasma lipoprotein lipids in experimental animals and patients. *Blood* **80**, 3217–3226.

Mehta, J. L., Saldeen, T. G., and Rand, K. (1998). Interactive role of infection, inflammation and traditional risk factors in atherosclerosis and coronary artery disease. *J. Am. Coll. Cardiol.* **31**, 1217–1225.

Meier, R., Alessi, D. R., Cron, P., Andjelkovic, M., and Hemmings, B. A. (1997). Mitogenic activation, phosphorylation, and nuclear translocation of protein kinase Bbeta. *J. Biol. Chem.* **272**, 30491–30497.

Minshall, C., Arkins, S., Freund, G. G., and Kelley, K. W. (1996). Requirement for phosphatidylinositol 3′-kinase to protect hemopoietic progenitors against apoptosis depends upon the extracellular survival factor. *J. Immunol.* **156**, 939–947.

Minshall, C., Arkins, S., Straza, J., Conners, J., Dantzer, R., Freund, G. G., and Kelley, K. W. (1997). IL-4 and insulin-like growth factor-I inhibit the decline in Bcl-2 and promote the survival of IL-3-deprived myeloid progenitors. *J. Immunol.* **159**, 1225–1232.

Miura, A., Ishizuka, T., Kanoh, Y., Ishizawa, M., Itaya, S., Kimura, M., Kajita, K., and Yasuda, K. (1999). Effect of tumor necrosis factor-alpha on insulin signal transduction in rat adipocytes: Relation to PKCbeta and zeta translocation. *Biochim. Biophys. Acta* **1449**, 227–238.

Monaco, M. E., and Lippman, M. E. (1977). Insulin stimulation of fatty acid synthesis in human breast cancer in long term tissue culture. *Endocrinology* **101**, 1238–1246.

Monzillo, L. U., Hamdy, O., Horton, E. S., Ledbury, S., Mullooly, C., Jarema, C., Porter, S., Ovalle, K., Moussa, A., and Mantzoros, C. S. (2003). Effect of lifestyle modification on adipokine levels in obese subjects with insulin resistance. *Obes. Res.* **11**, 1048–1054.

Mooney, R. A., Senn, J., Cameron, S., Inamdar, N., Boivin, L. M., Shang, Y., and Furlanetto, R. W. (2001). Suppressors of cytokine signaling-1 and -6 associate with and inhibit the insulin receptor. A potential mechanism for cytokine-mediated insulin resistance. *J. Biol. Chem.* **276**, 25889–25893. Epub 22001 May 25887.

Mosser, D. M. (2003). The many faces of macrophage activation. *J. Leukoc. Biol.* **73**, 209–212.

Mrosovsky, N., Molony, L. A., Conn, C. A., and Kluger, M. J. (1989). Anorexic effects of interleukin 1 in the rat. *Am. J. Physiol.* **257**, R1315–R1321.

Mugridge, K. G., Perretti, M., Ghiara, P., and Parente, L. (1991). Alpha-melanocyte-stimulating hormone reduces interleukin-1 beta effects on rat stomach preparations possibly through interference with a type I receptor. *Eur. J. Pharmacol.* **197**, 151–155.

Myers, M. G., Jr., and White, M. F. (1996). Insulin signal transduction and the IRS proteins. *Annu. Rev. Pharmacol. Toxicol.* **36**, 615–658.

Nadkarni, G. B., and Chitnis, K. E. (1963). Effect of insulin on gluconeogenesis from glycine-2-C. *Arch. Biochem. Biophys.* **101**, 466–470.

Nakanishi, K., Yoshimoto, T., Tsutsui, H., and Okamura, H. (2001). Interleukin-18 regulates both Th1 and Th2 responses. *Annu. Rev. Immunol.* **19**, 423–474.

National Diabetes Fact Sheet. (2003). American Diabetes Association.

Nawroth, P. P., Bank, I., Handley, D., Cassimeris, J., Chess, L., and Stern, D. (1986). Tumor necrosis factor/cachectin interacts with endothelial cell receptors to induce release of interleukin 1. *J. Exp. Med.* **163**, 1363–1375.

Nelson, D. O., and Boulant, J. A. (1981). Altered CNS neuroanatomical organization of spontaneously hypertensive (SHR) rats. *Brain Res.* **226**, 119–130.

Nicoletti, F., Di Marco, R., Papaccio, G., Conget, I., Gomis, R., Bernardini, R., Sims, J. E., Shoenfeld, Y., and Bendtzen, K. (2003). Essential pathogenic role of endogenous IL-18 in murine diabetes induced by multiple low doses of streptozotocin. Prevention of hyperglycemia and insulitis by a recombinant IL-18-binding protein: Fc construct. *Eur. J. Immunol.* **33**, 2278–2286.

Nonogaki, K., Fuller, G. M., Fuentes, N. L., Moser, A. H., Staprans, I., Grunfeld, C., and Feingold, K. R. (1995). Interleukin-6 stimulates hepatic triglyceride secretion in rats. *Endocrinology* **136**, 2143–2149.

Nyui, N., Tamura, K., Yamaguchi, S., Nakamaru, M., Ishigami, T., Yabana, M., Kihara, M., Ochiai, H., Miyazaki, N., Umemura, S., and Ishii, M. (1997). Tissue angiotensinogen gene expression induced by lipopolysaccharide in hypertensive rats. *Hypertension* **30**, 859–867.

O'Connor, J. C., Satpathy, A., Hartman, M. E., Horvath, E. M., Kelley, K. W., Dantzer, R., Johnson, R. W., and Freund, G. G. (2005). IL-1beta-mediated innate immunity is amplified in the db/db mouse model of type 2 diabetes. *J. Immunol.* **174**, 4991–4997.

Okamoto, M., Hayashi, T., Kono, S., Inoue, G., Kubota, M., Okamoto, M., Kuzuya, H., and Imura, H. (1993). Specific activity of phosphatidylinositol 3-kinase is increased by insulin stimulation. *Biochem. J.* **290**, 327–333.

Okamura, H., Tsutsi, H., Komatsu, T., Yutsudo, M., Hakura, A., Tanimoto, T., Torigoe, K., Okura, T., Nukada, Y., Hattori, K., Akita, K., and Namba, M. (1995). Cloning of a new cytokine that induces IFN-gamma production by T cells. *Nature* **378**, 88–91.

Old, L. J. (1988). Tumor necrosis factor. *Sci. Am.* **258**, 59–60, 69–75.

O'Neill, T. J., Craparo, A., and Gustafson, T. A. (1994). Characterization of an interaction between insulin receptor substrate 1 and the insulin receptor by using the two-hybrid system. *Mol. Cell Biol.* **14**, 6433–6442.

Oral, E. A., Simha, V., Ruiz, E., Andewelt, A., Premkumar, A., Snell, P., Wagner, A. J., DePaoli, A. M., Reitman, M. L., Taylor, S. I., Gorden, P., and Garg, A. (2002). Leptin-replacement therapy for lipodystrophy. *N. Engl. J. Med.* **346**, 570–578.

Ozes, O. N., Akca, H., Mayo, L. D., Gustin, J. A., Maehama, T., Dixon, J. E., and Donner, D. B. (2001). A phosphatidylinositol 3-kinase/Akt/mTOR pathway mediates and PTEN antagonizes tumor necrosis factor inhibition of insulin signaling through insulin receptor substrate-1. *Proc. Natl. Acad. Sci. USA* **98**, 4640–4645. Epub 2001 Apr 4643.

Paquot, N., Castillo, M. J., Lefebvre, P. J., and Scheen, A. J. (2000). No increased insulin sensitivity after a single intravenous administration of a recombinant human tumor necrosis factor receptor: Fc fusion protein in obese insulin-resistant patients. *J. Clin. Endocrinol. Metab.* **85**, 1316–1319.

Park, C. R., and Johnson, L. H. (1955). Effect of insulin on transport of glucose and galactose into cells of rat muscle and brain. *Am. J. Physiol.* **182**, 17–23.

Pausova, Z., Deslauriers, B., Gaudet, D., Tremblay, J., Kotchen, T. A., Larochelle, P., Cowley, A. W., and Hamet, P. (2000). Role of tumor necrosis factor-alpha gene locus in obesity and obesity-associated hypertension in French Canadians. *Hypertension* **36**, 14–19.

Paz, K., Hemi, R., LeRoith, D., Karasik, A., Elhanany, E., Kanety, H., and Zick, Y. (1997). A molecular basis for insulin resistance. Elevated serine/threonine phosphorylation of IRS-1 and IRS-2 inhibits their binding to the juxtamembrane region of the insulin receptor and impairs their ability to undergo insulin-induced tyrosine phosphorylation. *J. Biol. Chem.* **272**, 29911–29918.

Pederson, T. M., Kramer, D. L., and Rondinone, C. M. (2001). Serine/threonine phosphorylation of IRS-1 triggers its degradation: Possible regulation by tyrosine phosphorylation. *Diabetes* **50**, 24–31.

Pickup, J. C. (2004). Inflammation and activated innate immunity in the pathogenesis of type 2 diabetes. *Diabetes Care* **27**, 813–823.

Pickup, J. C., Chusney, G. D., Thomas, S. M., and Burt, D. (2000). Plasma interleukin-6, tumour necrosis factor alpha and blood cytokine production in type 2 diabetes. *Life Sci.* **67**, 291–300.

Pinteaux, E., Parker, L. C., Rothwell, N. J., and Luheshi, G. N. (2002). Expression of interleukin-1 receptors and their role in interleukin-1 actions in murine microglial cells. *J. Neurochem.* **83**, 754–763.

Podor, T. J., Jirik, F. R., Loskutoff, D. J., Carson, D. A., and Lotz, M. (1989). Human endothelial cells produce IL-6. Lack of responses to exogenous IL-6. *Ann. NY Acad. Sci.* **557**, 374–385.

Prager, D., Gebremedhin, S., and Melmed, S. (1990). An insulin-induced DNA-binding protein for the human growth hormone gene. *J. Clin. Invest.* **85**, 1680–1685.

Rabinovitch, A., Sumoski, W., Rajotte, R. V., and Warnock, G. L. (1990). Cytotoxic effects of cytokines on human pancreatic islet cells in monolayer culture. *J. Clin. Endocrinol. Metab.* **71**, 152–156.

Rattazzi, M., Faggin, E., Bertipaglia, B., and Pauletto, P. (2005). Innate immunity and atherogenesis. *Lupus* **14**, 747–751.

Re, F., Muzio, M., De Rossi, M., Polentarutti, N., Giri, J. G., Mantovani, A., and Colotta, F. (1994). The type II "receptor" as a decoy target for interleukin 1 in polymorphonuclear leukocytes: Characterization of induction by dexamethasone and ligand binding properties of the released decoy receptor. *J. Exp. Med.* **179**, 739–743.

Renold, A. E., Marble, A., and Fawcett, D. W. (1950). Action of insulin on deposition of glycogen and storage of fat in adipose tissue. *Endocrinology* **46**, 55–66.

Resch, K., Martin, M., Lovett, D. H., Kyas, U., and Gemsa, D. (1986). The receptor for interleukin 1 in plasma membranes of the human leukemia cell K 562: Biological and biochemical characterization. *Immunobiology* **172**, 336–345.

Rice, K. M., Turnbow, M. A., and Garner, C. W. (1993). Insulin stimulates the degradation of IRS-1 in 3T3-L1 adipocytes. *Biochem. Biophys. Res. Commun.* **190**, 961–967.

Rickert, D. E., and Fischer, L. J. (1975). Cyproheptadine and beta cell function in the rat: Insulin secretion from pancreas segments *in vitro*. *Proc. Soc. Exp. Biol. Med.* **150**, 1–6.

Ricketts, W. A., Rose, D. W., Shoelson, S., and Olefsky, J. M. (1996). Functional roles of the Shc phosphotyrosine binding and Src homology 2 domains in insulin and epidermal growth factor signaling. *J. Biol. Chem.* **271**, 26165–26169.

Ricort, J. M., Tanti, J. F., Van Obberghen, E., and Le Marchand-Brustel, E. (1997). Cross talk between the platelet-derived growth factor and the insulin signaling pathways in 3T3-L1 adipocytes. *J. Biol. Chem.* **272**, 19814–19818.

Ridker, P. M., Hennekens, C. H., Buring, J. E., and Rifai, N. (2000a). C-reactive protein and other markers of inflammation in the prediction of cardiovascular disease in women. *N. Engl. J. Med.* **342**, 836–843.

Ridker, P. M., Rifai, N., Stampfer, M. J., and Hennekens, C. H. (2000b). Plasma concentration of interleukin-6 and the risk of future myocardial infarction among apparently healthy men. *Circulation* **101**, 1767–1772.

Ring, B. D., Scully, S., Davis, C. R., Baker, M. B., Cullen, M. J., Pelleymounter, M. A., and Danilenko, D. M. (2000). Systemically and topically administered leptin both accelerate wound healing in diabetic ob/ob mice. *Endocrinology* **141**, 446–449.

Ronnett, G. V., Knutson, V. P., and Lane, M. D. (1982). Insulin-induced down-regulation of insulin receptors in 3T3-L1 adipocytes. Altered rate of receptor inactivation. *J. Biol. Chem.* **257**, 4285–4291.

Rosic, N. K., Standaert, M. L., and Pollet, R. J. (1985). The mechanism of insulin stimulation of (Na^+,K^+)-ATPase transport activity in muscle. *J. Biol. Chem.* **260**, 6206–6212.

Rothe, H., Hausmann, A., Casteels, K., Okamura, H., Kurimoto, M., Burkart, V., Mathieu, C., and Kolb, H. (1999). IL-18 inhibits diabetes development in nonobese diabetic mice by counterregulation of Th1-dependent destructive insulitis. *J. Immunol.* **163**, 1230–1236.

Rotter Sopasakis, V., Larsson, B. M., Johansson, A., Holmang, A., and Smith, U. (2004). Short-term infusion of interleukin-6 does not induce insulin resistance *in vivo* or impair insulin signalling in rats. *Diabetologia* **47**, 1879–1887. Epub 2004 Nov 1817.

Rotter, V., Nagaev, I., and Smith, U. (2003). Interleukin-6 (IL-6) induces insulin resistance in 3T3-L1 adipocytes and is, like IL-8 and tumor necrosis factor-alpha, overexpressed in human fat cells from insulin-resistant subjects. *J. Biol. Chem.* **278**, 45777–45784. Epub 42003 Sep 45772.

Rui, L., Aguirre, V., Kim, J. K., Shulman, G. I., Lee, A., Corbould, A., Dunaif, A., and White, M. F. (2001). Insulin/IGF-1 and TNF-alpha stimulate phosphorylation of IRS-1 at inhibitory Ser307 via distinct pathways. *J. Clin. Invest.* **107**, 181–189.

Rui, L., Yuan, M., Frantz, D., Shoelson, S., and White, M. F. (2002). SOCS-1 and SOCS-3 block insulin signaling by ubiquitin-mediated degradation of IRS1 and IRS2. *J. Biol. Chem.* **277**, 42394–42398. Epub 42002 Sep 42312.

Sabers, C. J., Martin, M. M., Brunn, G. J., Williams, J. M., Dumont, F. J., Wiederrecht, G., and Abraham, R. T. (1995). Isolation of a protein target of the FKBP12-rapamycin complex in mammalian cells. *J. Biol. Chem.* **270**, 815–822.

Saltiel, A. R., and Kahn, C. R. (2001). Insulin signalling and the regulation of glucose and lipid metabolism. *Nature* **414**, 799–806.

Sanchez-Margalet, V., Goldfine, I. D., Vlahos, C. J., and Sung, C. K. (1994). Role of phosphatidylinositol-3-kinase in insulin receptor signaling: Studies with inhibitor, LY294002. *Biochem. Biophys. Res. Commun.* **204**, 446–452.

Sandler, S., Andersson, A., and Hellerstrom, C. (1987). Inhibitory effects of interleukin 1 on insulin secretion, insulin biosynthesis, and oxidative metabolism of isolated rat pancreatic islets. *Endocrinology* **121**, 1424–1431.

Sandler, S., Bendtzen, K., Eizirik, D. L., Sjoholm, A., and Welsh, N. (1989). Decreased cell replication and polyamine content in insulin-producing cells after exposure to human interleukin 1 beta. *Immunol Lett.* **22**, 267–272.

Sasaoka, T., Draznin, B., Leitner, J. W., Langlois, W. J., and Olefsky, J. M. (1994). Shc is the predominant signaling molecule coupling insulin receptors to activation of guanine nucleotide releasing factor and p21ras-GTP formation. *J. Biol. Chem.* **269**, 10734–10738.

Schmelzle, T., and Hall, M. N. (2000). TOR, a central controller of cell growth. *Cell* **103**, 253–262.

Schmidt, J. A. (1984). Purification and partial biochemical characterization of normal human interleukin 1. *J. Exp. Med.* **160**, 772–787.

Schwartz, C. J., Valente, A. J., Sprague, E. A., Kelley, J. L., Suenram, C. A., and Rozek, M. M. (1985). Atherosclerosis as an inflammatory process. The roles of the monocyte-macrophage. *Ann. NY Acad. Sci.* **454**, 115–120.

Shephard, R. J. (2002). Cytokine responses to physical activity, with particular reference to IL-6: Sources, actions, and clinical implications. *Crit. Rev. Immunol.* **22**, 165–182.

Siegall, C. B., Schwab, G., Nordan, R. P., FitzGerald, D. J., and Pastan, I. (1990). Expression of the interleukin 6 receptor and interleukin 6 in prostate carcinoma cells. *Cancer Res.* **50**, 7786–7788.

Sivitz, W. I., Walsh, S., Morgan, D., Donohoue, P., Haynes, W., and Leibel, R. L. (1998). Plasma leptin in diabetic and insulin-treated diabetic and normal rats. *Metabolism* **47**, 584–591.

Skoog, T., Dichtl, W., Boquist, S., Skoglund-Andersson, C., Karpe, F., Tang, R., Bond, M. G., de Faire, U., Nilsson, J., Eriksson, P., and Hamsten, A. (2002). Plasma tumour necrosis factor-alpha and early carotid atherosclerosis in healthy middle-aged men. *Eur. Heart. J.* **23**, 376–383.

Skundric, D. S., Dai, R., James, J., and Lisak, R. P. (2002). Activation of IL-1 signaling pathway in Schwann cells during diabetic neuropathy. *Ann. NY Acad. Sci.* **958**, 393–398.

Smithwick, R. H. (1951). The role of the sympathetic nervous system in essential hypertension in man. *Angiology* **2**, 227–242.

Soldevila, G., Buscema, M., Doshi, M., James, R. F., Bottazzo, G. F., and Pujol-Borrell, R. (1991). Cytotoxic effect of IFN-gamma plus TNF-alpha on human islet cells. *J. Autoimmun.* **4**, 291–306.

Southern, C., Schulster, D., and Green, I. C. (1990). Inhibition of insulin secretion by interleukin-1 beta and tumour necrosis factor-alpha via an L-arginine-dependent nitric oxide generating mechanism. *FEBS Lett.* **276**, 42–44.

Spriggs, M. K., Nevens, P. J., Grabstein, K., Dower, S. K., Cosman, D., Armitage, R. J., McMahan, C. J., and Sims, J. E. (1992). Molecular characterization of the interleukin-1 receptor (IL-1R) on monocytes and polymorphonuclear cells. *Cytokine* **4**, 90–95.

Stadtmauer, L., and Rosen, O. M. (1986). Increasing the cAMP content of IM-9 cells alters the phosphorylation state and protein kinase activity of the insulin receptor. *J. Biol. Chem.* **261**, 3402–3407.

Standaert, M. L., Bandyopadhyay, G., and Farese, R. V. (1995). Studies with wortmannin suggest a role for phosphatidylinositol 3-kinase in the activation of glycogen synthase and mitogen-activated protein kinase by insulin in rat adipocytes: Comparison of insulin and protein kinase C modulators. *Biochem. Biophys. Res. Commun.* **209**, 1082–1088.

Stenzel-Poore, M., Vale, W. W., and Rivier, C. (1993). Relationship between antigen-induced immune stimulation and activation of the hypothalamic-pituitary-adrenal axis in the rat. *Endocrinology* **132**, 1313–1318.

Stouthard, J. M., Romijn, J. A., Van der Poll, T., Endert, E., Klein, S., Bakker, P. J., Veenhof, C. H., and Sauerwein, H. P. (1995). Endocrinologic and metabolic effects of interleukin-6 in humans. *Am. J. Physiol.* **268**, E813–E819.

Sugiyama, F., Haraoka, S., Watanabe, T., Shiota, N., Taniguchi, K., Ueno, Y., Tanimoto, K., Murakami, K., Fukamizu, A., and Yagami, K. (1997). Acceleration of atherosclerotic lesions in transgenic mice with hypertension by the activated renin-angiotensin system. *Lab. Invest.* **76**, 835–842.

Sun, X. J., Rothenberg, P., Kahn, C. R., Backer, J. M., Araki, E., Wilden, P. A., Cahill, D. A., Goldstein, B. J., and White, M. F. (1991). Structure of the insulin receptor substrate IRS-1 defines a unique signal transduction protein. *Nature* **352,** 73–77.

Sun, X. J., Miralpeix, M., Myers, M. G., Jr., Glasheen, E. M., Backer, J. M., Kahn, C. R., and White, M. F. (1992). Expression and function of IRS-1 in insulin signal transmission. *J. Biol. Chem.* **267,** 22662–22672.

Sun, X. J., Wang, L. M., Zhang, Y., Yenush, L., Myers, M. G., Jr., Glasheen, E., Lane, W. S., Pierce, J. H., and White, M. F. (1995). Role of IRS-2 in insulin and cytokine signalling. *Nature* **377,** 173–177.

Sun, X. J., Goldberg, J. L., Qiao, L. Y., and Mitchell, J. J. (1999). Insulin-induced insulin receptor substrate-1 degradation is mediated by the proteasome degradation pathway. *Diabetes* **48,** 1359–1364.

Suzuki, S., Toyota, T., Suzuki, H., and Goto, Y. (1984). A putative second messenger of insulin action regulates hepatic microsomal glucose-6-phosphatase. *Biochem. Biophys. Res. Commun.* **118,** 40–46.

Takano, M., Itoh, N., Yayama, K., Yamano, M., Ohtani, R., and Okamoto, H. (1993). Interleukin-6 as a mediator responsible for inflammation-induced increase in plasma angiotensinogen. *Biochem. Pharmacol.* **45,** 201–206.

Takao, T., Tracey, D. E., Mitchell, W. M., and De Souza, E. B. (1990). Interleukin-1 receptors in mouse brain: Characterization and neuronal localization. *Endocrinology* **127,** 3070–3078.

Takayama, S., White, M. F., Lauris, V., and Kahn, C. R. (1984). Phorbol esters modulate insulin receptor phosphorylation and insulin action in cultured hepatoma cells. *Proc. Natl. Acad. Sci. USA* **81,** 7797–7801.

Takayama, S., White, M. F., and Kahn, C. R. (1988). Phorbol ester-induced serine phosphorylation of the insulin receptor decreases its tyrosine kinase activity. *J. Biol. Chem.* **263,** 3440–3447.

Tanti, J. F., Gremeaux, T., Van Obberghen, E., and Le Marchand-Brustel, E. (1991). Effects of okadaic acid, an inhibitor of protein phosphatases-1 and -2A, on glucose transport and metabolism in skeletal muscle. *J. Biol. Chem.* **266,** 2099–2103.

Tanti, J. F., Gremeaux, T., van Obberghen, E., and Le Marchand-Brustel, E. (1994). Serine/ threonine phosphorylation of insulin receptor substrate 1 modulates insulin receptor signaling. *J. Biol. Chem.* **269,** 6051–6057.

Tartaglia, L. A. (1997). The leptin receptor. *J. Biol. Chem.* **272,** 6093–6096.

Tartaglia, L. A., Dembski, M., Weng, X., Deng, N., Culpepper, J., Devos, R., Richards, G. J., Campfield, L. A., Clark, F. T., Deeds, J., Muir, C., Sanker, S., *et al.* (1995). Identification and expression cloning of a leptin receptor, OB-R. *Cell* **83,** 1263–1271.

Taub, R., Roy, A., Dieter, R., and Koontz, J. (1987). Insulin as a growth factor in rat hepatoma cells. Stimulation of proto-oncogene expression. *J. Biol. Chem.* **262,** 10893–10897.

Tengku-Muhammad, T. S., Hughes, T. R., Cryer, A., and Ramji, D. P. (1999). Involvement of both the tyrosine kinase and the phosphatidylinositol-3′ kinase signal transduction pathways in the regulation of lipoprotein lipase expression in J774.2 macrophages by cytokines and lipopolysaccharide. *Cytokine* **11,** 463–468.

Thenen, S. W., and Mayer, J. (1976). Hyperinsulinemia and fat cell glycerokinase activity in obese (ob/ob) and diabetic (db/db) mice. *Horm. Metab. Res.* **8,** 80–81.

Tornqvist, H. E., Pierce, M. W., Frackelton, A. R., Nemenoff, R. A., and Avruch, J. (1987). Identification of insulin receptor tyrosine residues autophosphorylated *in vitro. J. Biol. Chem.* **262,** 10212–10219.

Trayhurn, P., Thurlby, P. L., and James, W. P. (1977). Thermogenic defect in pre-obese ob/ob mice. *Nature* **266,** 60–62.

Tsakiridis, T., McDowell, H. E., Walker, T., Downes, C. P., Hundal, H. S., Vranic, M., and Klip, A. (1995). Multiple roles of phosphatidylinositol 3-kinase in regulation of glucose transport, amino acid transport, and glucose transporters in L6 skeletal muscle cells. *Endocrinology* **136**, 4315–4322.

Tuttle, H. A., Davis-Gorman, G., Goldman, S., Copeland, J. G., and McDonagh, P. F. (2004). Proinflammatory cytokines are increased in type 2 diabetic women with cardiovascular disease. *J. Diabetes Complications* **18**, 343–351.

Ueki, K., Kondo, T., and Kahn, C. R. (2004a). Suppressor of cytokine signaling 1 (SOCS-1) and SOCS-3 cause insulin resistance through inhibition of tyrosine phosphorylation of insulin receptor substrate proteins by discrete mechanisms. *Mol. Cell Biol.* **24**, 5434–5446.

Ueki, K., Kondo, T., Tseng, Y. H., and Kahn, C. R. (2004b). Central role of suppressors of cytokine signaling proteins in hepatic steatosis, insulin resistance, and the metabolic syndrome in the mouse. *Proc. Natl. Acad. Sci. USA* **101**, 10422–10427. Epub 12004 Jul 10426.

Uhari, M., Saukkonen, A. L., and Koskimies, O. (1979). Central nervous system involvement in severe arterial hypertension of childhood. *Eur. J. Pediatr.* **132**, 141–146.

Ullrich, A., and Schlessinger, J. (1990). Signal transduction by receptors with tyrosine kinase activity. *Cell* **61**, 203–212.

Van Damme, J., Van Beeumen, J., Decock, B., Van Snick, J., De Ley, M., and Billiau, A. (1988). Separation and comparison of two monokines with lymphocyte-activating factor activity: IL-1 beta and hybridoma growth factor (HGF). Identification of leukocyte-derived HGF as IL-6. *J. Immunol.* **140**, 1534–1541.

van den Brink, G. R., O'Toole, T., Hardwick, J. C., van den Boogaardt, D. E., Versteeg, H. H., van Deventer, S. J., and Peppelenbosch, M. P. (2000). Leptin signaling in human peripheral blood mononuclear cells, activation of p38 and p42/44 mitogen-activated protein (MAP) kinase and p70 S6 kinase. *Mol. Cell Biol. Res. Commun.* **4**, 144–150.

Vanhaesebroeck, B., and Alessi, D. R. (2000). The PI-3K-PDK1 connection: More than just a road to PKB. *Biochem. J.* **346**(Pt. 3), 561–576.

Vileisis, R. A., and Oh, W. (1983). Enhanced fatty acid synthesis in hyperinsulinemic rat fetuses. *J. Nutr.* **113**, 246–252.

Volpato, S., Guralnik, J. M., Ferrucci, L., Balfour, J., Chaves, P., Fried, L. P., and Harris, T. B. (2001). Cardiovascular disease, interleukin-6, and risk of mortality in older women: The women's health and aging study. *Circulation* **103**, 947–953.

Voros, G., Maquoi, E., Collen, D., and Lijnen, H. R. (2004). Influence of membrane-bound tumor necrosis factor (TNF)-alpha on obesity and glucose metabolism. *J. Thromb. Haemost.* **2**, 507–513.

Wagner, C. R., Vetto, R. M., and Burger, D. R. (1985). Expression of I-region-associated antigen (Ia) and interleukin 1 by subcultured human endothelial cells. *Cell Immunol.* **93**, 91–104.

Wang, B., Jenkins, J. R., and Trayhurn, P. (2005). Expression and secretion of inflammation-related adipokines by human adipocytes differentiated in culture: Integrated response to TNF-alpha. *Am. J. Physiol. Endocrinol. Metab.* **288**, E731–E740. Epub 2004 Nov 2023.

Wang, H. L., and Scott, R. E. (1991). Insulin-induced mitogenesis associated with transformation by the SV40 large T antigen. *J. Cell. Physiol.* **147**, 102–110.

Wang, L. M., Michieli, P., Lie, W. R., Liu, F., Lee, C. C., Minty, A., Sun, X. J., Levine, A., White, M. F., and Pierce, J. H. (1995). The insulin receptor substrate-1-related 4PS substrate but not the interleukin-2R gamma chain is involved in interleukin-13-mediated signal transduction. *Blood* **86**, 4218–4227.

Warren, R. S., Starnes, H. F., Jr., Gabrilove, J. L., Oettgen, H. F., and Brennan, M. F. (1987). The acute metabolic effects of tumor necrosis factor administration in humans. *Arch. Surg.* **122**, 1396–1400.

Welsh, N., Eizirik, D. L., Bendtzen, K., and Sandler, S. (1991). Interleukin-1 beta-induced nitric oxide production in isolated rat pancreatic islets requires gene transcription and may lead to inhibition of the Krebs cycle enzyme aconitase. *Endocrinology* **129**, 3167–3173.

Werner, E. D., Lee, J., Hansen, L., Yuan, M., and Shoelson, S. E. (2004). Insulin resistance due to phosphorylation of insulin receptor substrate-1 at serine 302. *J. Biol. Chem.* **279,** 35298–35305. Epub 32004 Jun 35214.

White, M. F. (1997). The insulin signalling system and the IRS proteins. *Diabetologia* **40**(Suppl. 2), S2–S17.

White, M. F. (1998). The IRS-signalling system: A network of docking proteins that mediate insulin action. *Mol. Cell Biochem.* **182,** 3–11.

White, M. F., Shoelson, S. E., Keutmann, H., and Kahn, C. R. (1988). A cascade of tyrosine autophosphorylation in the beta-subunit activates the phosphotransferase of the insulin receptor. *J. Biol. Chem.* **263,** 2969–2980.

Winkles, J. A., Alberts, G. F., Brogi, E., and Libby, P. (1993). Endothelin-1 and endothelin receptor mRNA expression in normal and atherosclerotic human arteries. *Biochem. Biophys. Res. Commun.* **191,** 1081–1088.

Wool, I. G., and Krahl, M. E. (1959). An effect of insulin on peptide synthesis independent of glucose or amino-acid transport. *Nature* **183,** 1399–1400.

Xanthoulea, S., Curfs, D. M., Hofker, M. H., and de Winther, M. P. (2005). Nuclear factor kappaB signaling in macrophage function and atherogenesis. *Curr. Opin. Lipidol.* **16,** 536–542.

Xing, Z., Jordana, M., Kirpalani, H., Driscoll, K. E., Schall, T. J., and Gauldie, J. (1994). Cytokine expression by neutrophils and macrophages *in vivo*: Endotoxin induces tumor necrosis factor-alpha, macrophage inflammatory protein-2, interleukin-1 beta, and interleukin-6 but not RANTES or transforming growth factor-beta 1 mRNA expression in acute lung inflammation. *Am. J. Respir. Cell Mol. Biol.* **10,** 148–153.

Yoshimura, A., Nishinakamura, H., Matsumura, Y., and Hanada, T. (2005). Negative regulation of cytokine signaling and immune responses by SOCS proteins. *Arthritis Res. Ther.* **7,** 100–110.

Zeiher, A. M., Ihling, C., Pistorius, K., Schachinger, V., and Schaefer, H. E. (1994). Increased tissue endothelin immunoreactivity in atherosclerotic lesions associated with acute coronary syndromes. *Lancet* **344,** 1405–1406.

Zhang, Y., Proenca, R., Maffei, M., Barone, M., Leopold, L., and Friedman, J. M. (1994). Positional cloning of the mouse obese gene and its human homologue. *Nature* **372,** 425–432.

Zhou, J. H., Broussard, S. R., Strle, K., Freund, G. G., Johnson, R. W., Dantzer, R., and Kelley, K. W. (2001). IL-10 inhibits apoptosis of promyeloid cells by activating insulin receptor substrate-2 and phosphatidylinositol 3′-kinase. *J. Immunol.* **167,** 4436–4442.

Zinman, B., Hanley, A. J., Harris, S. B., Kwan, J., and Fantus, I. G. (1999). Circulating tumor necrosis factor-alpha concentrations in a native Canadian population with high rates of type 2 diabetes mellitus. *J. Clin. Endocrinol. Metab.* **84,** 272–278.

Zisman, A., Peroni, O. D., Abel, E. D., Michael, M. D., Mauvais-Jarvis, F., Lowell, B. B., Wojtaszewski, J. F., Hirshman, M. F., Virkamaki, A., Goodyear, L. J., Kahn, C. R., and Kahn, B. B. (2000). Targeted disruption of the glucose transporter 4 selectively in muscle causes insulin resistance and glucose intolerance. *Nat. Med.* **6,** 924–928.

18

RELEASE OF INTERLEUKINS AND OTHER INFLAMMATORY CYTOKINES BY HUMAN ADIPOSE TISSUE IS ENHANCED IN OBESITY AND PRIMARILY DUE TO THE NONFAT CELLS

JOHN N. FAIN

Department of Molecular Sciences, College of Medicine
University of Tennessee Health Science Center
Memphis, Tennessee 38163

0083-6729/06 $35.00
DOI: 10.1016/S0083-6729(06)74018-3

The white adipose tissue, especially of humans, is now recognized as the central player in the mild inflammatory state that is characteristic of obesity. The question is how the increased accumulation of lipid seen in obesity causes an inflammatory state and how this is linked to the hypertension and type 2 diabetes that accompanies obesity. Once it was thought that adipose tissue was primarily a reservoir for excess calories that were stored in the adipocytes as triacylglycerols. In times of caloric deprivation these stored lipids were mobilized as free fatty acids and the insulin resistance of obesity was attributed to free fatty acids. It is now clear that in humans the expansion of adipose tissue seen in obesity results in more blood vessels, more connective tissue fibroblasts, and especially more macrophages. There is an enhanced secretion of some interleukins and inflammatory cytokines in adipose tissue of the obese as well as increased circulating levels of many cytokines. The central theme of this chapter is that human adipose tissue is a potent source of inflammatory interleukins plus other cytokines and that the majority of this release is due to the nonfat cells in the adipose tissue except for leptin and adiponectin that are primarily secreted by adipocytes. Human adipocytes secrete at least as much plasminogen activator inhibitor-1 (PAI-1), MCP-1,[1] interleukin-8 (IL-8), and IL-6 *in vitro* as they do leptin but the nonfat cells of adipose tissue secrete even more of these proteins. The secretion of leptin, on the other hand, by the nonfat cells is negligible. The amount of serum amyloid A proteins 1 & 2 (SAA 1 & 2), haptoglobin, nerve growth factor (NGF), macrophage migration inhibitory factor (MIF), and PAI-1 secreted by the adipocytes derived from a gram of adipose tissue is 144%, 75%, 72%, 37%, and 23%, respectively, of that by the nonfat cells derived from the same amount of human adipose tissue. However, the release of IL-8, MCP-1, vascular endothelial growth factor (VEGF), TGF-β1, IL-6, PGE$_2$, TNF-α, cathepsin S, hepatocyte growth factor (HGF), IL-1β, IL-10, resistin, C-reactive protein (CRP), and interleukin-1 receptor antagonist (IL-1Ra) by adipocytes is less than 12% of that by the nonfat cells present in human adipose tissue. Obesity markedly elevates the total release of TNF-α, IL-6, and IL-8 by adipose tissue but only that of TNF-α is enhanced in adipocytes. However, on a quantitative basis the vast majority of the TNF-α comes from the nonfat cells. Visceral adipose tissue also releases more VEGF, resistin, IL-6, PAI-1, TGF-β1, IL-8, and IL-10 per gram of tissue than does abdominal subcutaneous adipose tissue. In conclusion, there is an increasing recognition that adipose tissue is an endocrine organ that secretes leptin and adiponectin along with a host of other paracrine and endocrine factors in addition to free fatty acids.

[1]Abbreviations: BMI, body mass index; CRP, C reactive protein; HGF, hepatocyte growth factor; IL-1β, interleukin-1β; IL-6, interleukin-6; IL-8, interleukin-8; IL-10, interleukin-10; IL-1Ra, interleukin-1 receptor antagonist; MCP-1, monocyte chemoattractant protein 1; MIF, macrophage migration inhibitory factor; NGF, nerve growth factor; PGE$_2$, prostaglandin E$_2$; SAA 1 & 2, serum amyloid A proteins 1 & 2; SV, stromovascular; TGF-β1, transforming growth factor-β1; TNF-α, tumor necrosis factor-α; VEGF, vascular endothelial growth factor.

I. INTRODUCTION: MOST RELEASE OF ADIPOKINES/CYTOKINES BY ADIPOSE TISSUE IS DUE TO NONFAT CELLS

Adipose tissue is part of the connective tissue framework upon which epithelial tissues rest and within which muscle and nervous tissue are embedded. Adipocytes (fat cells) are specialized connective tissue cells that contain a single large internal fat droplet with only a thin rim of cytoplasm between the lipid droplet and the plasma membrane. Adipose tissue is essentially a specialized form of connective tissue that accumulates large numbers of adipocytes. Historically adipose tissue has been considered solely as a site for the synthesis and storage of lipid. However, the areolar or loose connective tissue that is known as adipose tissue also contains the cells involved in immunological defense. This is especially true in humans where there is a substantial amount of intercellular matrix consisting of collagen and elastic fibers. There are large numbers of fibroblasts, mast cells, macrophages, leukocytes, and other cells involved in inflammation embedded within the adipose tissue framework. The theme of this chapter is that the release of TNF-α, interleukin-8 (IL-8), IL-10, IL-6, and IL-1β by human adipose tissue is enhanced in obesity and primarily due to the nonfat cells in the adipose tissue rather than the adipocytes.

Obesity is a major health problem in this country that is largely responsible for the epidemic of type 2 diabetes and cardiovascular disease. Since the effects can be reversed by weight loss, which is essentially a reduction in adipose tissue mass, it is possible that the adverse effects of obesity are directly due to the massive accumulation of fat, especially visceral (omental) adipose tissue in the abdomen. Yudkin et al. (1999) suggested that obesity is associated with a low-level chronic inflammatory state that induces insulin resistance and endothelial dysfunction. Popular is the hypothesis that the mild inflammatory state of massively (morbidly) obese humans is linked to the altered release of cytokines by adipose tissue (Cottam et al., 2004; Fantuzzi, 2005; Hauner, 2005; Lau et al., 2005; Trayhurn, 2005; Wellen and Hotamisligil, 2005). In effect when you have too much fat what results is a proinflammatory, prothrombotic, and anti-insulin endocrine organ.

The source of the altered release of cytokines in obesity has generally been thought to be the adipocytes (Cottam et al., 2004; Rajala and Scherer, 2003; Trayhurn, 2005). While some refer to cytokines released by adipose tissue as adipokines that term should possibly be reserved for proteins, like leptin, that are released exclusively by mature adipocytes. Fain et al. (2004a) suggested that most of the factors released by adipose tissue from morbidly obese humans were derived from cells other than adipocytes. These nonfat cells are a large but understudied component of human adipose tissue. The increase in adipose tissue can account for over 50% of the total body weight in massively obese humans. Possibly the enhanced release of cytokines, such as IL-8 and TNF-α, by adipose tissue from massively obese humans [body mass index (BMI)$\geq$40] reflects a low-grade chronic inflammatory condition. This may be secondary to an expansion of the blood vessels and other supporting structures as the amount of adipose tissue enlarges in obesity. Equally important, or perhaps of greater significance, is the elevated content of inflammatory cells such as mast cells. Hellman *et al.* (1963) first demonstrated an enhanced accumulation of mast cells in the fat depots of obese mice. It was suggested that macrophages, whose content in human adipose tissue is elevated in obesity, might be of importance in the release of adipokines (Weisberg *et al.*, 2003; Xu *et al.*, 2003). There is also an increase in endothelial cells as well as adipocytes in obesity and both cells may have a common lineage (Hausman *et al.*, 1980).

II. COMPARISON OF RODENT VERSUS HUMAN ADIPOSE TISSUE

One of the problems that has retarded our understanding of the relative importance of adipocytes versus the nonfat cells of human adipose tissue is the enormous difference between rodent and human adipose tissue. Rodent adipose tissue depots are relatively small and contain far fewer blood vessels, connective tissue matrix, and nonfat cells than the large adipose tissue depots of humans. Furthermore, the difficulty in differentiating human preadipocytes into adipocytes and the lack of adipocyte cell lines of human origin has resulted in most investigators working with murine cell lines. It is easy to take a murine fibroblast cell line (3T3-L1) and differentiate them over several days into cells that accumulate large amounts of lipid. However, the fat droplets are multilocular while mature adipocytes are unilocular with a single large fat droplet. In many ways these cells are more like macrophages than adipocytes. Lin *et al.* (2000) demonstrated that 3T3-L1 adipocytes have a fully intact pathway of innate immunity and secrete immunomodulatory molecules. Furthermore, Charriere *et al.* (2003) found that the injection of 3T3-L1 cells into the peritoneal cavity of nude mice resulted in their conversion into macrophages. These data suggest that the 3T3-L1 cells have a protein profile as close to that of macrophages as to adipocytes.

Resistin is a protein whose expression is induced during differentiation of 3T3-L1 cells and has been postulated to be an adipokine secreted by adipocytes linking obesity to diabetes (Steppan *et al.*, 2001). However, resistin mRNA could not be found in human adipocytes but was readily detectable in circulating mononuclear cells (Savage *et al.*, 2001). Furthermore, resistin expression in human adipocytes or skeletal muscle did not correlate with type 2 diabetes (Nagaev and Smith, 2001). Fain *et al.* (2003) found that, while resistin was released by explants of human adipose tissue, it did not come from the adipocytes but rather from the nonfat cells present in the tissue.

From these data the author concludes that resistin is a cytokine, secreted by human immune cells rather than adipocytes.

Haptoglobin is the major protein secreted by 3T3-L1 adipocytes (Kratchmarova *et al.*, 2002) and inflammation in mice increases the expression of the haptoglobin gene by at least sixfold in adipose tissue (Friedrichs *et al.*, 1995). Haptoglobin is an acute-phase protein secreted by the liver whose circulating concentration is around 24×10^6 pmol/l (Putnam, 1975). However, Fain *et al.* (2004b) found that very little haptoglobin is released by human adipose tissue. These data indicate that haptoglobin, like resistin, is a protein secreted by 3T3-L1 cells but not by human adipocytes. Another example is the β3-catecholamine receptor that is present in rodent adipocytes but it does not appear to be involved in the regulation of lipolysis in human adipose tissue (Rosenbaum *et al.*, 1993). Thus while murine cell lines are very useful for mechanistic studies care must be taken in extrapolating data to human adipocytes since the multilocular 3T3-L1 adipocytes are as much like macrophages as they are unilocular adipocytes.

III. INTERLEUKIN RELEASE BY ADIPOSE TISSUE

A. IL-1β

IL-1β along with TNF-α is considered the prototypical proinflammatory cytokines. However, there have been no reports of effects of obesity on either circulating levels of IL-1β or the adipose tissue content of IL-1β. Fain *et al.* (2004a) reported that its total release by adipose tissue *in vitro* was 50% greater in tissue from obese individuals (Fig. 1). Massive obesity had far

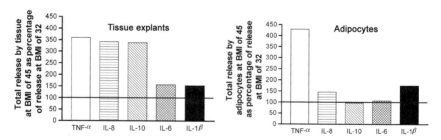

FIGURE 1. Comparison of total release by adipose tissue explants and adipocytes from 8 individuals with a BMI of 45 as compared to 8 with a BMI of 32. The total release of adipokines was obtained by averaging the data for release per gram of visceral (omental) and subcutaneous adipose tissue explants incubated in primary culture for 48 h. This was multiplied by the total body fat content, which was 56 kg in those with a BMI of 45 and 32 kg in those with a BMI of 32. Reproduced with permission from Fain *et al.* (2004a) Copyright 2004, The Endocrine Society.

greater effects on the release by human adipose tissue of IL-10 and IL-8 (Fig. 1) and the release of IL-1β was less than 0.001% of that for IL-6 or IL-8 (Fain *et al.*, 2004a). However, a neutralizing antibody against IL-1β in the presence of a soluble TNF-α receptor (etanercept) reduced the release of IL-6 by 39% and that of IL-8 by 46% over a 48 h incubation of human visceral adipose tissue explants (Fain *et al.*, 2005a). Neither antagonist alone had any significant effect on release of IL-6 or IL-8. These data suggest that endogenous release of both IL-1β and TNF-α by adipose tissue is involved in the upregulation of IL-6 and IL-8 release that is seen with human adipose tissue *in vitro* (Fain *et al.*, 2005a).

B. IL-6

IL-6 was postulated by Yudkin *et al.* (2000) to have a key role in the development of coronary heart disease. It has been known for some time that IL-6 has dramatic effects on the secretion of acute-phase proteins by the liver (Heinrich *et al.*, 1990). The acute-phase response can result in 10- to 100-fold increases in serum CRP and serum amyloid A proteins 1 & 2 (SAA 1 & 2) as well as somewhat smaller increases in haptoglobin. IL-6 turned out to be the major stimulatory factor for the production of these acute-phase proteins by the liver (Heinrich *et al.*, 1990). Obesity in humans results in elevations in circulating levels of IL-6 (Table I). Human obesity is also associated with elevated serum levels of SAA 1 & 2 (Poitou *et al.*, 2005; van Dielen *et al.*, 2001), haptoglobin (Hannerz *et al.*, 1995; Scriba *et al.*, 1979), and CRP (Engeli *et al.*, 2003; Festa *et al.*, 2001; Ouchi *et al.*, 2003; Pannacciulli *et al.*, 2001; van Dielen *et al.*, 2001). These correlations have led to the assumption that obesity results in enhanced release of IL-6 by visceral adipose tissue that in turn elevates IL-6 in the portal circulation. It is

TABLE I.   Effect of Bariatric Surgery on Circulating Levels of CRP, PAI-1, Leptin, TNF-α, and IL-6[a]

Hormone/factor	Controls BMI = 22	Bariatric surgery BMI = 45	Post-bariatric surgery BMI = 33	Percentage
CRP	109,500	462,000	228,000	49%
PAI-1	1710	3580	2180	61%
Leptin	375	2870	1120	39%
TNF-α	0.28	0.90	0.80	89%
IL-6	0.06	0.25	0.21	84%

[a]The data are in pmol/l and obtained by pooling those of Hanusch-Enserer *et al.*, 2003; Kopp *et al.*, 2003; Vazquez *et al.*, 2005; and Laimer *et al.*, 2002. The percentages are post-bariatric surgery values divided by pre-bariatric surgery values.

established that IL-6 enhances formation and release of CRP, haptoglobin, and amyloid protein by the liver. However, it is unclear how elevations of these acute-phase proteins are related to the induction of type 2 diabetes, hypertension, and atherosclerosis or even if IL-6 is the only cytokine involved in their regulation.

Enormous amounts of IL-6 are released by human adipose tissue both *in vivo* (Orban *et al.*, 1999) and *in vitro*, especially by visceral omental adipose tissue (Fain *et al.*, 2004a; Fried *et al.*, 1998). Furthermore, some of the IL-6 released by human subcutaneous adipose tissue appears in the bloodstream (Mohamed-Ali *et al.*, 1997). A positive correlation between circulating levels of IL-6 and *in vivo* insulin resistance was reported by Kern *et al.* (2001) while Bastard *et al.* (2002) found a positive correlation between adipose tissue IL-6 content and insulin resistance with respect to glucose uptake in humans. It is possible that these correlations have no causal relationship since there are many conditions, especially in muscle, where IL-6 enhances rather than inhibits glucose uptake (Carey and Febbraio, 2004; Pedersen *et al.*, 2003). However, in liver IL-6 impairs insulin signaling (Klover *et al.*, 2005), and Rotter Sopasakis *et al.* (2004) similarly found that the infusion over 2 h of large amounts of IL-6 into rats enhanced tyrosine phosphorylation of signal transducer and activator of transcription (STAT) 3 in liver, skeletal muscles, and adipose tissue without affecting insulin signaling in these tissues. One explanation for these conflicting results is that IL-6 itself does not interfere with insulin action but over time IL-6 stimulates the formation of anti-insulin factors.

C. IL-8

IL-8 is an inflammatory human chemokine involved in the recruitment of neutrophils from the blood to the site of its release (Reape and Groot, 1999). The murine IL-8 receptor binds macrophage inflammatory protein (MIP-2) as well as the N51 cytokine and these proteins are the murine homologs of IL-8 (Heinrich and Bravo, 1995). IL-8 may be more important in the low-grade inflammation of obesity than is IL-6 but has received relatively little attention to date. Elevated serum levels of IL-8 are associated with an increased risk of coronary artery disease (Boekholdt *et al.*, 2004). Furthermore, serum IL-8 levels are elevated in patients with type 1 or 2 diabetes (Zozulinska *et al.*, 1999). Obesity is also associated with elevated levels of IL-8 (Bruun *et al.*, 2003; Straczkowski *et al.*, 2002).

The total release of IL-8 by adipose tissue explants, but not that by adipocytes, from humans with a BMI of 45 was 2.5-fold greater than that by tissue from individuals with a BMI of 32 (Fig. 1). There was a positive correlation of 0.78 between release of IL-8 per gram of subcutaneous adipose tissue and the BMI (Bruun *et al.*, 2004). The ability of IL-8 to recruit neutrophils into adipose tissue, where they are converted to macrophages, may be responsible either wholly or in part for the enhanced accumulation of macrophages seen in adipose tissue of obese humans (Weisberg *et al.*, 2003; Xu *et al.*, 2003).

The elevation in IL-8 production in adipose tissue of obese humans could be secondary to enhanced release of IL-1β and/or TNF-α which stimulates IL-8 release by explants of human adipose tissue (Bruun *et al.*, 2001). Fain *et al.* (2005a) found that blocking the effects of endogenous IL-1β and TNF-α reduced the formation of IL-8 by 46% and of IL-6 by 39% over a 48 h incubation of explants of human visceral adipose tissue. However, neither the soluble TNF-α receptor (etanercept) nor the neutralizing antibody against IL-1β alone had any effect of IL-8 or IL-6 release (Fain *et al.*, 2005a). IL-8 thus appears to be an interleukin whose release by the nonfat cells of adipose tissue is enhanced in obesity and part of this release involves endogenous TNF-α and Il-1β.

D. IL-10

IL-10 is primarily an anti-inflammatory cytokine whose release appears to be coordinated with that of proinflammatory and chemoattractant cytokines (Mocellin *et al.*, 2003). The serum level of IL-10 is elevated in obese humans (Esposito *et al.*, 2003). However, Manigrasso *et al.* (2005) found that an 8-kg weight loss in obese women had no effect of the circulating levels of IL-10. The total release of IL-10 by adipose tissue from humans with a BMI of 45 was 2.5-fold greater than that by adipose tissue from individuals with a BMI of 32 and, on a percentage basis, comparable to the increase in release of IL-8 (Fig. 1). The author concludes that the *in vitro* release of IL-10 by adipose tissue is enhanced in obesity comes primarily from the nonfat cells of the tissue and that IL-10 may function as a feedback inhibitor of the effects of the inflammatory cytokines.

E. IL-18

Interleukin-18 shares structural homology with IL-1β and both are produced as 24-kDa inactive precursors that are cleaved by caspase-1 to generate the biologically active 18-kDa IL-18 protein (Gracie *et al.*, 2003; Reddy, 2004). There is a role for this interleukin in acquired and innate immunity but the exact position of IL-18 in the hierarchy of proinflammatory cytokines is still unclear. The specific role of IL-18 in the onset of type 1 diabetes is equally unclear. Serum levels of IL-18 are elevated during the early, subclinical stage of type 1 diabetes of humans (Nicoletti *et al.*, 2001). However, administration of IL-18 to diabetes-susceptible obese mice delayed the onset of autoimmune diabetes (Rothe *et al.*, 1999).

Elevated levels of serum IL-18 have been reported in humans with type 2 diabetes, 15 pmol/l versus 10 pmol/l in control subjects with similar BMIs, by Moriwaki *et al.* (2003). Esposito *et al.* (2002) reported that the mean IL-18 serum value was 14 pmol/l in obese women (BMI of 34) which was twice the value of 7 pmol/l seen in nonobese women (BMI of 24). The AtheroGene investigators have reported that serum IL-18 level is a predictor of death from cardiovascular causes in patients with coronary artery disease (Blankenberg *et al.*, 2002; Tiret *et al.*, 2005). These data suggest that IL-18 could be a link between obesity and increased risk of both diabetes and cardiovascular disease.

Skurk *et al.* (2005b) suggested that the elevated serum IL-18 seen in obese humans was due to elevated release by adipocytes. However, Fain *et al.* (2006) found a strong negative correlation ($r = -0.74$) between the fat mass of humans and the release of IL-18 by explants of human adipose tissue over 48 h of incubation. Approximately 80% of the IL-18 released by adipose tissue over 48 h was derived from the nonfat cells in human subcutaneous or visceral adipose tissue (Fain *et al.*, 2006). The release of IL-18 by explants of human adipose tissue was miniscule (0.2 fmol/kg/4 h) as compared to the release of IL-1β, IL-6, or IL-8, which were 18, 14,600, and 30,400 fmol/kg/4 h (Fain *et al.*, 2004a). In contrast, the serum IL-18 concentration (14 pmol/l) is much higher in obese individuals than that of IL-1β (0.07 pmol/l; Mirone *et al.*, 1996), IL-8 (0.4 pmol/l; Bruun *et al.*, 2003), or IL-6 (0.2 pmol/l in Table I). The author concludes that while IL-18 levels may be elevated in obesity the source of this increase is probably not adipose tissue. Furthermore, the small release of IL-18 by human adipose tissue is by nonfat cells rather than adipocytes.

F. IL-1Rᴀ

Interleukin-1 receptor antagonist (IL-1Ra) levels are elevated in human obesity (Juge-Aubry *et al.*, 2003; Meier *et al.*, 2002). This protein is a physiological antagonist of IL-1α and IL-1β effects since it competes with them for binding to their receptors. The IL-1Ra protein is induced by many of the same stimuli than enhance release of IL-1β in cells and by interferon-β, which is an anti-inflammatory protein. Insulin has been suggested as a possible regulator of IL-1Ra formation because of the positive association between serum insulin levels in obese individuals and IL-1Ra (Meier *et al.*, 2002). However, correlations do not prove causation. It was suggested that since the IL-1Ra protein is able to cross the blood–brain barrier and blocks hypothalamic signaling by leptin in rodents (Luheshi *et al.*, 1999), it might interfere with leptin effects in man (Meier *et al.*, 2002). In rodents it has been shown that leptin may mediate neuroimmune responses via actions in the brain dependent upon release of IL-1β and prostaglandins (Luheshi *et al.*, 1999). It is thought that IL-1β is involved in hypothalamic control of food intake and that leptin stimulates IL-1β gene expression while glucocorticoids have the opposite effect (Wisse *et al.*, 2004). The reason that

IL-1Ra levels are elevated in obesity is still unclear but could possibly involve termination of the IL-1β-induced inflammatory response in adipose tissue as well as in the hypothalamus. Since blocking the IL-1β signal in the hypothalamus may reduce the response to leptin, the elevated levels of this protein in obesity could also be involved in explaining the relative ineffectiveness of exogenous administration of leptin to reduce appetite in obese humans.

IV. EFFECT OF OBESITY ON CIRCULATING CYTOKINES AND RELEASE BY ADIPOSE TISSUE

The data in Table I summarize the findings from four studies where the circulating levels of CRP and TNF-α (all four studies), IL-6 (three studies), plasminogen activator inhibitor-1 (PAI-1), and leptin (one study for each) in the blood of normal controls with a mean BMI of 22 were compared to the levels in massively obese individuals before and after bariatric surgery. The circulating level of IL-6 was quite low and the same was true for TNF-α in nonobese individuals, but the levels of both were elevated in massively obese individuals and reduced by only a small extent after bariatric surgery (Table I). The circulating level of leptin, which is a hormone secreted by adipocytes, was at least a 1000-fold greater than that of the cytokines. PAI-1 was present at a 4.5-fold greater concentration in blood than was the case for leptin. The circulating level of CRP was almost 300-fold greater than that of leptin. The circulating levels of all five proteins were markedly elevated in morbidly obese individuals and reduced after bariatric surgery. However, the reduction of BMI from 45 to 33 reduced only PAI-1 to near normal levels.

Many studies on release of interleukins and other factors by human adipose tissue have utilized visceral or subcutaneous adipose tissue obtained during bariatric surgery from massively obese individuals with a BMI of 45 or from patients undergoing abdominoplasty approximately 1 year after bariatric surgery with an average BMI of 33. One way to examine the release of interleukins and other factors by human adipose tissue is to incubate explants or visceral or subcutaneous adipose tissue in primary culture for 48 h after removal from the donors. The total release of various factors by adipose tissue was compared using adipose tissue from humans at the time of bariatric surgery and approximately 1-year post-bariatric surgery when the total body fat content was 43% lower as shown in Fig. 1. These data were obtained by averaging the values for visceral and subcutaneous adipose tissue per kilogram of fat and multiplying by the total kilograms of fat (56 kg in individuals with a BMI of 45 and 32 in those with a BMI of 32). There was enhanced total release of TNF-α, IL-8, and IL-10 ($\sim$2.5-fold for each) as well as of IL-6 and IL-1β (~50% increase) in adipose tissue from individuals with 56 kg of fat as compared to release by tissue from individuals with 32 kg of body fat. It should be noted that total release of hepatocyte growth factor (HGF), PAI-1, and vascular endothelial growth factor (VEGF) was not enhanced in fat from humans with a BMI of 45 as compared to that by explants from donors with a BMI of 32 (Fain et al., 2004a). Only the release of TNF-α was enhanced in adipocytes from the morbidly obese individuals. These data indicate that the enhanced total release of cytokines seen in obesity is primarily by the nonfat cells of adipose tissue rather than the adipocytes except for TNF-α whose release was enhanced in adipocytes from morbidly obese humans. The enhanced total release of TNF-α by adipocytes may be a primary cause of the inflammatory cascade initiated by obesity (Fig. 1). A key role for TNF-α in obesity-linked insulin resistance was originally postulated by Hotamisligil et al. (1993) and reviewed by Warne (2003).

V. VISCERAL VERSUS SUBCUTANEOUS ADIPOSE TISSUE AS A SOURCE OF ADIPOKINES/CYTOKINES

Elevated visceral fat accumulation is a risk factor for cardiovascular disease, hypertension, and type 2 diabetes (Carr and Brunzell, 2004). The fat stored in the intra-abdominal cavity (visceral fat) is a more important predictor of myocardial infarction than is the total fat mass or BMI in women (Nicklas et al., 2004). The accumulation of visceral fat is also an especially important factor in the metabolic syndrome and insulin resistance (Goodpaster et al., 2005; Piche et al., 2005). It is unclear why elevated accumulation of visceral adipose tissue is a far greater health hazard than accumulation of fat in the subcutaneous regions of the hips and legs. The most likely reason could be the portal circulation, which results in a greater delivery of cytokines/adipokines, free fatty acids, and unknown substances to the liver from the visceral adipose tissue depots as compared to subcutaneous depots.

The release of VEGF, resistin, IL-6, PAI-1, TGF-β1, IL-8, and IL-10 as measured per gram of tissue over a 48 h incubation was anywhere from 2 to 4 times greater by visceral as compared to abdominal subcutaneous fat from individuals with an average BMI of 32 (Fig. 2). The visceral fat includes both omental and mesenteric adipose tissue but in our studies we used omental tissue because of its greater abundance. These increases in release were not found when adipocytes isolated from visceral adipose tissue were compared to those from subcutaneous adipose tissue (Fain et al., 2003, 2004a, 2005b). Furthermore, in the same experiments the release of leptin, adiponectin, TNF-α, and IL-1β per gram of visceral adipose tissue was not significantly different from that by subcutaneous adipose tissue explants (Fain et al., 2004a).

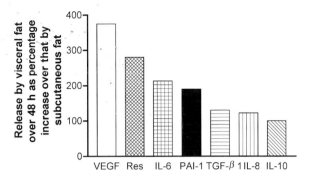

FIGURE 2. Comparison of release by visceral versus subcutaneous adipose tissue explants. The data are shown as the percentage increase in release per gram of visceral (omental) adipose tissue as compared to that by subcutaneous adipose tissue explants from the same individuals (BMI 32–35) incubated in primary culture for 48 h. The data for VEGF, IL-6, PAI-1, IL-8, and IL-10 are taken from Fain *et al.* (2004a) while those for resistin (Res) are from Fain *et al.* (2003) and those for TBF-β1 from Fain *et al.* (2005b).

PAI-1 formation was also greater by visceral explants than by explants of subcutaneous adipose tissue in the studies of Alessi *et al.* (1997).

The author concludes that there is enhanced release of some cytokines by the adipose tissue of massively obese humans, including IL-6, IL-8, and IL-10, which is due to the nonfat cells in the tissue. Whether the visceral fat has more mast cells, macrophages, and other inflammatory cells per gram of tissue or whether there is simply greater release is unclear. The nature of the primary signal also remains to be established with regard to the enhanced release of the interleukins and other factors from visceral adipose tissue of obese humans.

VI. FORMATION OF ADIPOKINES/CYTOKINES BY ADIPOSE TISSUE *IN VITRO* AS COMPARED TO CONNECTIVE TISSUE, THE NONFAT CELLS IN ADIPOSE TISSUE, AND ADIPOCYTES

The hypothesis that most of the interleukin release by adipose tissue is due to cells other than adipocytes is supported by the findings shown in Fig. 3. These data demonstrate that glucose conversion to lactate as well as release of IL-6, IL-8, TNF-α, and adiponectin was as great per gram weight of cut pieces of adipose tissue without enough lipid to float (connective tissue) as release by cut pieces of adipose tissue that floated. The one exception was leptin, an adipokine released exclusively by mature adipocytes, whose release by connective tissue was minimal (Fig. 3). In contrast, TNF-α, IL-8, and IL-6 were released in very small amounts by adipocytes.

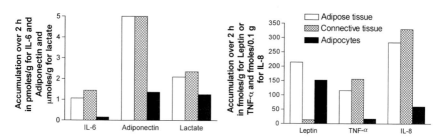

FIGURE 3. Comparison of short-term release by explants of human adipose tissue, connective tissue derived from adipose tissue and adipocytes. Freshly isolated explants of adipose tissue or connective tissue (the cut pieces of adipose tissue that did not float) were incubated for 2 h. Adipocytes were isolated from the individuals and subsequently incubated for 2 h. The values were based on averaging those for visceral (omental) and subcutaneous adipose tissue explants and are the net change in medium plus tissue for lactate, leptin, adiponectin, IL-6, IL-8 and TNF-α per gram based on wet weight of tissue or adipocytes from four humans (John N. Fain and Atul K. Madan, unpublished experiments).

Glucose conversion to lactate is shown to demonstrate that carbohydrate metabolism was similar in adipose tissue to that in connective tissue on a wet weight basis. The release of interleukins and other factors was measured over a short 2-h incubation to reduce the upregulation of cytokines that occurs in adipose tissue after its removal from the *in vivo* situation (Fain *et al.*, 2005a).

The hypothesis that most of the release of interleukins, as well as that of other cytokines, is by the nonfat cells present in human adipose tissue is supported by the data shown in Table II. The release of 13 proteins and PGE$_2$ by explants of adipose tissue over a 4-h incubation is ranked on a molar basis. There was an enormous release of IL-8 and IL-6 by tissue explants as compared to the release of leptin, which is the prototypical adipokine. Furthermore, the release of IL-8 and IL-6 by adipocytes was only 3–4% of that by tissue over 4 h. IL-10 was released by adipose tissue in amounts less than 0.6% of that for IL-8 and release by adipocytes was 4% of that value. Even less IL-1β was released by adipose tissue explants since over 4 h it was 0.06% of IL-8 release (Table II). The only substances released by adipocytes at levels more than 10% of that by tissue explants were PAI-1 at 12%, adiponectin at 24%, VEGF at 27%, IL-1β at 28%, and leptin at 39% of that by tissue.

If the low rate of interleukin release by adipocytes is due to either effects of collagenase digestion and/or the removal of adipocytes from the stimulatory influences of the nonfat cells in adipose tissue explants, one way to examine this possibility is to compare release by the three fractions obtained by collagenase digestion of human adipose tissue over 2 h versus 48 h incubations (Fig. 4). The tissue matrix is the tissue that is retained on a mesh filter after collagenase digestion and is the endothelial cells and smooth muscle cells of the blood vessels as well as other cells that are not released

TABLE II.   Comparison of Adipokine/Cytokine Release over 4 h by Human Adipose Tissue with that by Human Adipocytes[a]

	Release by tissue fmol/g/4 h	Release by adipocytes	
		fmol/g/4 h	Percentage of tissue
PGE$_2$	152,000 ± 40,000	4800 ± 1100	3%
IL-8	30,400 ± 16,000	1100 ± 500	4%
IL-6	14,600 ± 2600	505 ± 95	3%
MCP-1	7100 ± 1400	500 ± 100	7%
Adiponectin	6100 ± 1200	1445 ± 145	24%
PAI-1	1660 ± 220	200 ± 22	12%
HGF	746 ± 89	35 ± 9	5%
Leptin	595 ± 138	233 ± 5	39%
Resistin	310 ± 80	<1	0%
IL-1Ra	292 ± 30	16 ± 15	5%
TNF-α	200 ± 17	5 ± 5	2%
Haptoglobin	150 ± 25	12 ± 2	8%
VEGF	22 ± 2	6 ± 1	27%
IL-1β	18 ± 3	5 ± 1	28%

[a]Explants or adipocytes (100 mg/ml) from 8 to 12 individuals with an average BMI of 42 were incubated for 4 h. The values are shown as the mean ± SEM of pooled visceral (omental) and subcutaneous adipose tissue explants or adipocytes. Adipokine release to the medium is in fmol/g/4 h. The data are from Fain *et al.* (2004a) except for haptoglobin (Fain *et al.*, 2004b), resistin (Fain *et al.*, 2003), MCP-1 (Fain *et al.* 2005b), and IL-1Ra (Fain *et al.*, 2006).

by collagenase digestion. The SV cells are the cells that pass through a 200 μm filter and sediment after centrifugation while the adipocytes are those cells with sufficient lipid to float. The data are not corrected for losses due to lysis of cells, loss during washing of the three fractions, or upregulation due to effects of collagenase digestion. However, the total release of leptin, adiponectin, IL-8, and TNF-α by the fractions obtained after collagenase digestion ranged from 51% to 118% over a 48-h incubation of that by tissue explants from the same individuals and 73–154% after a 2-h incubation. Values over 100% represent upregulation while values of 73% probably represent the loss of components during digestion and washing.

Leptin was released primarily by adipocytes over either short- or long-term incubations while adiponectin was released by both tissue matrix and adipocytes. In contrast, IL-8 and TNF-α release was primarily by the SV and tissue matrix cells. The release of all factors by adipocytes as percentage of that by tissue was less over a 48-h incubation as compared to that over 2 h indicating either deleterious long-term effects of collagenase digestion and/or

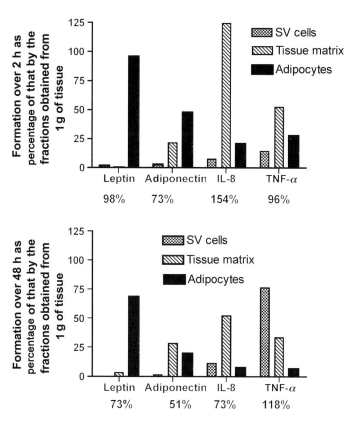

FIGURE 4. Comparison of relative release of leptin, adiponectin, IL-8, and TNF-α by the SV cells, tissue matrix, and adipocytes obtained by collagenase digestion of human adipose tissue. After a 2 h incubation of cut pieces of adipose tissue with bacterial collagenase the digest was filtered through 200-μm filter mesh that retained the undigested adipose tissue matrix and blood vessels. The filtered digest was centrifuged to separate the cells that float (adipocytes) from the rest of the cells liberated by collagenase (SV cells). The data are expressed as the release of the various substances per gram over 2 or 48 h of the minced adipose tissue in comparison to that by 1 g of cut pieces of adipose tissue from which the fractions were derived. The data for 48 h release are from Table 6 in the report by Fain *et al.* (2004a) while the 2 h values are from the experiments shown in Fig. 3. The percentage value under the legends for leptin, adiponectin, IL-8, and TNF-α represent the total recovery of release in all three fractions as compared to release by cut pieces of tissue from the same individuals.

the absence of stimulatory factors released by the nonfat cells in adipose tissue.

TNF-α release was unique in that the release by the SV fraction over 48 h was higher than that by the tissue matrix and may reflect a greater contribution of cells such as macrophages that are readily released from adipose tissue during collagenase digestion. In contrast, the release over 48 h of IL-8 was primarily by cells that were not released from adipose tissue during collagenase digestion.

The proteome profile for release of 22 proteins by the adipocytes as compared to release by the combined SV and tissue matrix fraction (nonfat cells) is shown in Tables III and IV. The 22 proteins were chosen since their circulating levels are elevated in human obesity except as follows.

TABLE III. Comparison of Adipokine/Cytokine Release by Adipocytes as Compared to the Other Cells in Adipose Tissue Ranked by Adipocyte Release[a]

Adipokine/cytokine	Formation by nonfat cells (pmol/g)	Formation by adipocytes (pmol/g)
PGE_2	1810	118
IL-8	1120	87
PAI-1	78	18
MCP-1	74	9.2
IL-6	66	5.1
Adiponectin	6	4.1
SAA 1 & 2	1.2	1.8
Leptin	0.1	1.8
MIF	2.8	1.0
Cathepsin S	4.4	0.26
IL-1Ra	4.1	0.14
HGF	2.8	0.11
Haptoglobin	0.08	0.06
Resistin	1.8	<0.04
IL-10	0.53	0.020
VEGF	0.30	0.020
VCAM-1	0.46	0.016
IL-1β	0.23	0.013
TNF-α	0.22	0.012
TGF-β1	0.17	0.009
NGF	0.006	0.005
CRP	0.010	0.001
IL-18	0.005	<0.001

[a]Pooled (subcutaneous and visceral) data (from 8 to 10 humans with a BMI of 32 and 8 to 12 humans with a BMI of 45) based on release over 48 h by nonfat cells (matrix plus SV cells) and fat cells. The data are from Fain et al. (2004a) except for haptoglobin (Fain et al., 2004b), resistin (Fain et al., 2003), MCP-1 (Fain and Madan, 2005b), TGFβ1 (Fain et al., 2005c), MIF, Cathepsin S, NGF, IL-1Ra, IL-18 (Fain et al., 2006), and CRP, VCAM-1, SAA 1 & 2 which are from unpublished experiments.

TABLE IV. Formation by Adipocytes as Percentage of that by Nonfat Cells (SV and Matrix Cells) of Human Adipose Tissue over 48 h[a]

Released to the medium exclusively by mature adipocytes			
Leptin	1800%		
Released by adipocytes at levels 64–144% of that by nonfat cells			
SAA 1 & 2 proteins	144%		
Haptoglobin	75%		
NGF	72%		
Adiponectin	64%		
Released by adipocytes at levels 12–37% of that by nonfat cells			
MIF	37%	PAI-1	23%
Lactate	30%	MCP-1	12%
Released by adipocytes at levels 9% or less of that by nonfat cells			
VEGF	8%	IL-1β	6%
IL-6	8%	TGF-β1	5%
IL-8	8%	IL-1Ra	5%
PGE$_2$	7%	HGF	4%
TNF-α	6%	IL-10	4%
Cathepsin S	6%	VCAM –1	3%

[a]The percentages are derived from the data shown in Table III. Release of IL-18, CRP, and resistin by adipocytes was too low for calculation.

Adiponectin is the one adipokine/cytokine released by human adipose tissue whose level goes down in obesity. There have been no reports on blood levels of IL-1β or nerve growth factor (NGF) in obesity. Resistin is included because of current interest in the role of this protein in obesity and insulin resistance (Sul, 2004). Data for PGE$_2$ whose release reflects the activity of cyclooxygenase (COX)-2 in human adipose tissue (Fain *et al.*, 2001, 2002) are included, but there is no evidence that circulating levels of PGE$_2$ are elevated in obesity (Curtis-Prior *et al.*, 1979).

The data shown in Table III are ranked by molar release over a 48-h incubation by adipocytes and demonstrate the enormous differences in release between IL-8 and IL-18, which was almost 100,000-fold. The release of the 22 proteins and PGE$_2$ by adipocytes as percentage of that by the nonfat cells fractions obtained by collagenase digestion is shown in Table IV. These data demonstrate that leptin is a true adipokine in that it is released exclusively by adipocytes.

Of the 22 proteins whose release to the medium was compared using human adipocytes versus nonfat cells, 15 were released over 48 h by adipocytes at levels

12% or less than by the nonfat cells (Table IV). Whether the release of these proteins by adipose tissue contributes to their circulating levels is unclear but if so, it is probably the nonfat cells that are responsible for the vast majority of their release by human adipose tissue.

A. HAPTOGLOBIN

Haptoglobin is released by adipocytes in amounts nearly equivalent to that by the nonfat cells (Tables III and IV). Circulating levels of haptoglobin are elevated in obese humans (Hannerz et al., 1995; Scriba et al., 1979) but the release of haptoglobin by adipose tissue is quite small in relationship to circulating levels and hepatic production (Fain et al., 2004b).

B. ADIPONECTIN

Adiponectin was released by adipocytes at only 64% of the release by nonfat cells (Table IV). The current paradigm is that adiponectin, like leptin, is exclusively made by adipocytes (Berg and Scherer, 2005; Scherer et al., 1995). However, adiponectin is also found in umbilical venous blood from human fetuses and expressed in fetal tissues of mesodermal and ectodermal origin (Corbetta et al., 2005). While the expression of adiponectin in non-adipose tissues shows a general decline during the progression of gestation, these data suggest that adiponectin is not an exclusive product of mature adipocytes or that adiponectin released by adipocytes is taken up and subsequently released by nonfat cells.

Adiponectin is unique among the proteins secreted by adipose tissue in that its expression in adipose tissue along with its serum level decreases in obesity (Berg and Scherer, 2005). Furthermore, it is now clear that in some, still unknown manner, low levels of adiponectin are associated with insulin resistance. It appears as if the larger the adipocyte the greater the formation of leptin and the lesser the formation of adiponectin. The mechanisms involved in these changes are incompletely understood much less whether decreases in adiponectin and increases in leptin have a role in the initiation of the inflammatory response seen in obesity. It may be that adiponectin is also produced by preadipocytes embedded in the adipose tissue matrix of human adipose tissue or other cells present in the adipose tissue matrix.

C. NGF

NGF has been described as an inflammatory response protein made by adipocytes (Peeraully et al., 2004). We have found that NGF is released by human visceral and subcutaneous adipose tissue explants in near equal amounts but its total release by adipose tissue explants in vitro is not enhanced in obesity (Fain et al., 2006).

D. PAI-1

Factors released by adipocytes in amounts 12–37% that by nonfat cells included PAI-1 (23%), macrophage migration inhibitory factor (MIF) (37%), CRP (14%), and MCP-1 (12%). The finding that lactate formation by adipocytes was only 30% of that by the nonfat cells derived from a gram of tissue indicates that glucose metabolism by tissue primarily involved the nonfat cells. Alessi *et al.* (1997) originally found that the production of PAI-1 by human adipocytes was between 14% and 34% of that by adipose tissue explants. The data indicate that MIF and PAI-1 are released by adipocytes as well as by nonfat cells in about the same relationship as lactate formation suggesting that they are equally expressed in all cells. Circulating PAI-1 levels as well as the content in adipose tissue are higher in obesity (Alessi *et al.*, 1997, 2000; Skurk and Hauner, 2004).

E. MCP-1

MCP-1, like IL-8, is a chemokine whose enhanced release by adipose tissue could enhance the recruitment of macrophage precursors, such as monocytes, into adipose tissue. MCP-1 is overexpressed in obese mice and white adipose tissue is a major source of MCP-1 in mice (Sartipy and Loskutoff, 2003; Takahashi *et al.*, 2003). Christiansen *et al.* (2005) reported that circulating MCP-1 and its content in adipose tissue are elevated in human obesity. Bruun *et al.* (2005) subsequently demonstrated that MCP-1 release was primarily by the nonfat cells present in adipose tissue and suggested that the greater release in obese subjects was due to macrophages. Fain and Madan (2005b) confirmed that the majority of MCP-1 release is due to the nonfat cells in human visceral adipose tissue. Furthermore, the release of MCP-1, which was upregulated over a 48-h incubation of adipose tissue explants, is partially dependent upon the release of endogenous TNF-α plus IL-1β and involves the p38MAPK and NF-κB pathways (Fain and Madan, 2005b).

F. MIF

MIF is a proinflammatory cytokine whose serum concentration is elevated in obesity (Dandona *et al.*, 2004). One unique feature of MIF is that its circulating concentration is at least 1000-fold higher than those of IL-6, IL-8, IL-10, or IL-1β. Church *et al.* (2005) found that in obese individuals with elevated circulating levels of MIF their participation in physical activity and a dietary-focused weight management resulted in reductions in both weight and MIF. The presence of MIF in the adipocytes of rodent adipose tissue was originally reported by Hirokawa *et al.* (1997). Skurk *et al.* (2005a) reported that both human preadipocytes and adipocytes release MIF.

The data shown in Table IV indicate that the nonfat cells and adipocytes present in a gram of human adipose tissue release lactate and MIF in roughly comparable amounts.

G. VEGF

VEGF is an angiogenic factor that induces migration and proliferation of endothelial cells as well as vascular permeability. The circulating level of VEGF is elevated in human obesity especially that associated with visceral fat accumulation (Miyazawa-Hoshimoto et al., 2003). The data shown in Fig. 2 indicate that of proteins examined to date, VEGF release is elevated in visceral adipose tissue to the greatest extent as compared to release by subcutaneous adipose tissue. The expression of VEGF mRNA is dramatically increased during the differentiation of murine 3T3 cells into adipocytes (Claffey et al., 1992). VEGF is secreted by rat adipocytes as well as human adipocytes and this secretion is enhanced by insulin (Fain and Madan, 2005a; Mick et al., 2002). VEGF is also secreted by the nonfat cells of human subcutaneous adipose tissue (Fain et al., 2004a; Rehman et al., 2004b). Over a 4-h incubation the release of VEGF by freshly isolated human adipocytes was 27% of that by explants of intact tissue (Table II). Over a 48-h incubation the release of VEGF was 8% of that by the nonfat cells of adipose tissue (Tables III and IV). Clearly most of the VEGF released by adipose tissue comes from the nonfat cells, but the ability of insulin to stimulate VEGF release by adipocytes may be of importance in accounting for some of the deleterious effects of the high levels of circulating insulin seen in obesity.

H. HGF

HGF levels in blood are elevated in obese subjects according to Rehman et al. (2004a) and Swierczynski et al. (2005) but not Silha et al. (2005). The data shown in Tables III and IV indicate that HGF is secreted by human adipose tissue in amounts comparable to those of leptin over a 48-h incubation of adipose tissue explants. However, 96% of the HGF secretion is by the nonfat cells of adipose tissue.

I. TGF-β1

A significant correlation has been reported between BMI of humans and circulating TGF-βl (Scaglione et al., 2003) or adipose tissue TGF-βl content (Alessi et al., 2000). In contrast, Corica et al. (1997) and Bastelica et al. (2002) found no correlation between BMI and circulating levels of TGF-βl. Fain et al. (2005b) found a positive correlation coefficient ($r = 0.7$) between calculated total release of TGF-β1 in vitro by adipose tissue explants and BMI.

The release of TGF-$\beta 1$ was primarily (at least 95%) by the nonfat cells present in human adipose tissue (Tables III and IV).

J. CATHEPSIN S

Cathepsin S is an elastolytic cysteine protease secreted by mononuclear cells (Reddy *et al.*, 1995) that is active at neutral pH (Liuzzo *et al.*, 1999; Vasiljeva *et al.*, 2005). Circulating levels of cathepsin S have a positive correlation with BMI and the level of cathepsin mRNA expression is elevated in subcutaneous adipose tissue from obese subjects (Taleb *et al.*, 2005). The elevated levels of cathepsin S in human obesity have been postulated to be a molecular link between obesity and atherosclerosis (Taleb *et al.*, 2005). The elevated expression of cathepsin S in the adipose tissue of obese individuals may reflect elevated levels of macrophages in the tissue (Weisberg *et al.*, 2003; Xu *et al.*, 2003). The data shown in Tables III and IV indicated that cathepsin S is released by human adipose tissue but that most of the release (94%) is by the nonfat cells as is expected of a macrophage marker.

K. RESISTIN

Circulating levels of resistin do not appear to be elevated in obese humans (Chen *et al.*, 2005; Hasegawa *et al.*, 2005; Iqbal *et al.*, 2005; Lee *et al.*, 2003). Resistin has been a molecule of interest in recent years since Steppan *et al.* (2001) postulated that it was secreted by adipose tissue and was the link between obesity and diabetes based on rodent studies. As noted earlier, resistin is made by murine adipocytes but in human adipose tissue more than 96% of its formation is due to the nonfat cells (Tables III and IV). Resistin may well have a role in inflammation, like TNF-α, as a paracrine factor that is released by macrophages and other nonfat cells in human adipose tissue.

L. CRP

CRP is an acute-phase protein present in large amounts in the circulation (Table I). Yudkin *et al.* (1999) reported that circulating levels of CRP, IL-6, as well as TNF-α are elevated in obesity. Similar findings for CRP and IL-6 were reported by Bastard *et al.* (1999) and by Hak *et al.* (1999) for CRP and PAI-1. Danesh *et al.* (1999) also found a positive correlation between the circulating levels of both CRP and SAA 1 & 2 with obesity. CRP is primarily secreted by the nonfat cells of human adipose tissue rather than the adipocytes (Tables III and IV) but total secretion by adipose tissue is miniscule in comparison to that by liver (see in a later section).

M. SAA 1 & 2

SAA 1 & 2 are acute-phase proteins made by the liver and in massively obese humans circulate at a concentration of around 500 nM (Holdstock *et al.*, 2005). Sjoholm *et al.* (2005) and Poitou *et al.* (2005) have suggested that since the adipocytes of human adipose tissue contain large amounts of the mRNA for serum SAA 1 & 2, the adipose tissue may contribute to serum SAA 1 & 2 values. The data in Tables III and IV indicate that SAA 1 & 2 are preferentially released by human adipocytes. If release *in vitro* by adipose tissue (Table III) is anywhere near that seen *in vivo*, over 24 h the amount of SAA 1 & 2 released by the total amount of fat (56 kg in morbidly obese individuals) would represent less than the amount present in 120 ml of plasma (Holdstock *et al.*, 2005). Similarly CRP is also made and released by human adipose tissue, primarily by nonfat cells, but the amount is so small that over 24 h the release of CRP by the adipose tissue of an individual with 56 kg of fat is equivalent to less than that found in 1 ml of plasma. These data suggest that the increases in circulating levels of the acute-phase proteins CRP and SAA 1 & 2 seen in obesity are primarily a reflection of elevated circulating levels of IL-6 and other inflammatory cytokines that stimulate hepatic production of these proteins. Of great interest, but still unanswered, are the questions of whether CRP and SAA 1 & 2 elevations in obesity contribute to insulin resistance. The SAA proteins are apolipoproteins that become components of the high-density lipoproteins and displace apolipoprotein A-1 as well as phospholipids from high-density lipoprotein particles (Miida *et al.*, 1999). SAA 1 & 2 have been reported to enhance the release of matrix metalloproteinases 2 and 3 by human synovial fibroblasts (Migita *et al.*, 1998). Whether these effects are relevant remains to be established.

N. TNF-α

The concentration of TNF-α, like that of IL-6, in blood is less than 1 pmol/l even in morbidly obese individuals (Table I) and only slightly affected by reduction of BMI from 45 to 33, but still markedly higher than in lean individuals. TNF-α is a pluripotent cytokine that is primarily released by macrophages and is thought to play a role in the insulin resistance of obesity. Hotamisligil *et al.* (1995) and Kern *et al.* (1995) reported that obese individuals have 2.5-fold more TNF-α in their adipose tissue as compared to lean controls. Kern *et al.* (1995) reported the presence of more TNF-α mRNA, based on RT-PCR, in adipocytes than in the isolated nonfat cells from human adipose tissue. Kern *et al.* (2001) subsequently reported that the expression of both TNF-α and IL-6 were elevated in the adipose tissue of humans with obesity-related insulin resistance.

The calculated total release of TNF-α by human adipose tissue explants was 2.5-fold greater in individuals with an average BMI or 45 as compared to that by tissue and adipocytes from individuals with a BMI of 32 (Fig. 1). The release of TNF-α by adipocytes may be important, since the 22 proteins listed in Table III, it was the only one whose total release was elevated in adipocytes from individuals with a total body fat content of 56 kg as compared to those with 32 kg. However, it should be noted that TNF-α release by adipocytes was less than 2% of that released by intact tissue over a 4-h (Table II) and 6% of that by nonfat cells of adipose tissue over a 48-h incubation (Table IV). Clearly most of the TNF-α release by adipose tissue is due to nonfat cells and the enhanced accumulation of macrophages suggest that TNF-α is a paracrine factor released by mast cells, macrophages, and other mononuclear cells that are involved in the insulin resistance of obesity. Di Gregorio et al. (2005) found a strong positive relationship between the accumulation of a macrophage marker mRNA (CD68) in the adipose tissue of humans and TNF-α secretion by the tissue.

O. LEPTIN

Leptin was reported in late 1994 to be the protein whose absence is the molecular basis of the infertility, obesity, and diabetes seen in the ob/ob mouse (Zhang et al., 1994). Leptin is secreted by the adipocytes of adipose tissue and it was hoped that obesity in humans might be due to a lack of this protein, whose blood level reflects the amount of adipose tissue. However, it was soon learned that nearly all obese humans, unlike the ob/ob mouse, have high levels of leptin and are relatively unresponsive to administration of leptin. The receptors for leptin are similar to those for cytokines and this protein circulates as a hormone released by adipocytes that interacts with receptors in hypothalamic nuclei (Fain and Bahouth, 2000). The mechanism by which release of leptin is enhanced as adipocytes enlarge is not yet understood but the leptin concentration in blood is apparently the primary signal by which the brain monitors the amount of adipose tissue in an organism. The data in Table IV indicate that leptin is the only protein measured to date whose release by cells in human adipose tissue is due exclusively to adipocytes. The amount of leptin released by adipocytes is far less than that of IL-8, PAI-1, MCP-1, adiponectin, or IL-6 (Table III). However, it is unclear whether these release rates reflect the in vivo situation since the release of leptin may be downregulated in primary culture while that of the proteins mentioned earlier is upregulated.

P. PGE$_2$

The circulating levels of prostaglandins in human females are very low and there is no effect of obesity (Curtis-Prior et al., 1979). Consequently, the role of PGE_2 or prostacyclin in the induction of the low-grade inflammatory response seen in adipose tissue from obese individuals has been relatively neglected. This is so despite the key role of prostaglandins in the inflammatory response and the knowledge that the most clinically useful anti-inflammatory agents are drugs that block the COX-2 enzyme or glucocorticoids that block COX-2 induction. The rate-limiting step in formation of prostaglandins is the COX-2 enzyme. Most of the prostaglandin formation by human adipose tissue measured as either PGE_2 or the prostacyclin metabolite 6-keto-PGF_1 is due to the nonfat cells and markedly reduced in the presence of a glucocorticoid such as dexamethasone (Fain et al., 2002). In human adipocytes there is a marked upregulation of COX-2 mRNA and protein over a 48-h incubation which is further enhanced in the presence of IL-1β (Fain et al., 2002). Furthermore, inhibition of endogenous release of either TNF-α or IL-1β inhibited the upregulation of PGE_2 release by explants of human visceral adipose tissue that is seen over a 48-h incubation (Fain and Madan, 2005b).

A role for COX-2-mediated overproduction of PGE_2 by stimulated monocytes in the inflammation and atherosclerosis associated with smoking and diabetes has been suggested by Beloqui et al. (2005). Helmersson et al. (2004) similarly suggested that type 2 diabetes in elderly men is related to COX-2-mediated inflammation. However, COX-2 expression in activated monocytes did not correlate with obesity (Beloqui et al., 2005). These data suggest, but by no means prove, that the enhanced COX-2 activity in activated macrophages is secondary to the greater release of inflammatory cytokines in smokers and type 2 diabetics.

VIII. PATHWAYS FOR UPREGULATION OF INTERLEUKIN RELEASE BY HUMAN ADIPOSE TISSUE

A. TNF-α AND IL-1β

One of the major problems is evaluating data obtained by in vitro incubations of human adipose tissue is the possibility of upregulation or downregulation of the release of adipokines/cytokines. In the case of TNF-α there is a marked downregulation over a 48-h incubation of either human adipose tissue or adipocytes (Fain et al., 2004c). In contrast, there is a marked upregulation of IL-8 and IL-6 mRNA as well as release within 3 h after the removal of visceral adipose tissue from humans (Fain et al., 2005a). This upregulation was the same whether one 200 mg piece of adipose tissue or minced adipose tissue was incubated for 5 h (Fain et al., 2005a).

Approximately half of the upregulation of IL-8 or IL-6 mRNA seen over a 5-h incubation of visceral adipose tissue explants was due to release of endogenous TNF-α plus IL-1β (Fain *et al.*, 2005a). This suggests that, in some unknown manner, the stress resulting from interruption of the blood supply to the adipose tissue releases TNF-α plus IL-1β or removes circulating inhibitors of these cytokines.

B. HYPOXIA

Adipose tissue blood flow is reduced in obese humans (Jansson *et al.*, 1992; Virtanen *et al.*, 2002) and obesity reduces perioperative tissue oxygenation (Kabon *et al.*, 2004). Trayhurn and Wood (2004) have postulated that the expansion of fat depots seen in obesity result in relative hypoxia in the parts of adipose tissue where expansion occurs in advance of angiogenesis. This is an attractive hypothesis and it is known that hypoxia upregulates IL-8 by a mechanism involving release of IL-1β in human astrocytes (Zhang *et al.*, 2000). The transient hypoxia and/or removal of the tissue from blood may initiate a series of stress responses culminating in activation of p38 MAPK and NF-κB pathways that regulate IL-8 and IL-6 mRNA.

C. ROLE OF P38 MAPK AND NF-κB IN REGULATION OF IL-8 MRNA

In macrophages the upregulation of IL-8 involves the ERK 1 and 2, Jun kinase (JNK), p38 mitogen-activated protein kinase (p38MAPK), and NF-κB pathways (Hoffmann *et al.*, 2002; Holtmann *et al.*, 1999). In explants of human adipose tissue it is primarily the p38MAPK and NF-κB pathways that are involved in IL-8 formation (Fain *et al.*, 2005a). Clearly in human adipose tissue there is a rapid upregulation of IL-8 and IL-6 formation after removal from the *in vivo* situation and the challenge will be to understand the mechanism by which this occurs. The primary signal is still unknown and the same can be said for what it is about obesity that induces a mild inflammatory state in adipose tissue.

In conclusion, it is becoming clear that obesity is a mild inflammatory state and that enhanced release of proinflammatory factors by adipose tissue may be as important, if not more so, than the release of fatty acids in the development of hypertension and type 2 diabetes in obese humans. However, while the lipids and leptin come from the adipocytes the nonfat cells of adipose tissue release most of the inflammatory factors. There is an enhanced accumulation of mast, cells, macrophages, and other cells involved in the immune response in adipose tissue of obese humans and these cells are probably involved in the enhanced cytokine release seen in adipose tissue of obese humans.

REFERENCES

Alessi, M. C., Peiretti, F., Morange, P., Henry, M., Nalbone, G., and Juhan-Vague, I. (1997). Production of plasminogen activator inhibitor 1 by human adipose tissue. *Diabetes* **46**, 860–867.

Alessi, M. C., Bastelica, D., Morange, P., Berthet, B., Leduc, I., Verdier, M., Geel, O., and Juhan-Vague, I. (2000). Plasminogen activator inhibitor 1, transforming growth factor-β1, and BMI are closely associated in human adipose tissue during morbid obesity. *Diabetes* **49**, 1374–1380.

Bastard, J.-P., Jardel, C., Delattre, J., Hainque, B., Brucker, E., and Oberlin, F. (1999). Evidence for a link between adipose tissue interleukin-6 content and serum C-reactive protein concentrations in obese subjects. *Circulation* **99**, 2221–2222.

Bastard, J.-P., Maachi, M., Van Nhieu, J. T., Jardel, C., Bruckert, E., Grimaldi, A., Robert, J.-J., Capeau, J., and Hainque, B. (2002). Adipose tissue IL-6 content correlates with resistance to insulin activation of glucose uptake both *in vivo* and *in vitro*. *J. Clin. Endocrinol. Metab.* **87**, 2084–2089.

Bastelica, D., Mavri, A., Verdierl, M., Berthet, B., Juhan-Vague, I., and Alessi, M. C. (2002). Relationships between fibrinolytic and inflammatory parameters in human adipose tissue: Strong contribution of TNFα receptors to PAI-1 levels. *Thromb. Haemost.* **88**, 481–487.

Beloqui, O., Paramo, J. A., Orbe, J., Benito, A., Colina, I., Monasterio, A., and Diez, J. (2005). Monocyte cyclooxygenase-2 overactivity: A new marker of subclinical atherosclerosis in asymptomatic subjects with cardiovascular risk factors? *Eur. Heart J.* **26**, 153–158.

Berg, A. H., and Scherer, P. E. (2005). Adipose tissue, inflammation, and cardiovascular disease. *Cir. Res.* **96**, 939–949.

Blankenberg, S., Tiret, L., Bickel, C., Peetz, D., Cambien, F., Meyer, J., and Rupprecht, H. J. (2002). Interleukin-18 is a strong predictor of cardiovascular death in stable and unstable angina. *Circulation* **106**, 24–30.

Boekholdt, S. M., Peters, R. J. G., Hack, C. E., Day, N. E., Luben, R., Bingham, S. A., Wareham, N. J., Reitsma, P. H., and Khaw, K.-T. (2004). IL-8 plasma concentrations and the risk of future coronary artery disease in apparently healthy men and women. *Arterioscler. Thromb. Vasc. Biol.* **24**, 1503–1508.

Bruun, J. M., Pedersen, S. B., and Richelsen, B. (2001). Regulation of Interleukin 8 production and gene expression in human adipose tissue *in vitro*. *J. Clin. Endocrinol. Metab.* **86**, 1267–1273.

Bruun, J. M., Verdich, C., Toubro, S., Astrup, A., and Richelsen, B. (2003). Association between measures of insulin sensitivity and circulating levels of interleukin-8, interleukin-6 and tumor necrosis factor-α. Effect of weight loss in obese men. *Eur. J. Endocrinol.* **148**, 535–542.

Bruun, J. M., Lihn, A. S., Madan, A. K., Pedersen, S. B., Schiott, K. M., Fain, J. N., and Richelsen, B. (2004). Higher production of IL-8 in visceral vs. subcutaneous adipose tissue. Implication of nonadipose cells in adipose tissue. *Am. J. Physiol. Endocrinol. Metab.* **286**, E8–E13.

Bruun, J. M., Lihn, A. S., Pedersen, S. B., and Richelsen, B. (2005). Monocyte chemoattractant protein-1 release is higher in visceral than subcutaneous human adipose tissue (AT): Implication of macrophages resident in the AT. *J. Clin. Endocrinol. Metab.* **90**, 2282–2289.

Carey, A. L., and Febbraio, M. A. (2004). Interleukin-6 and insulin sensitivity: Friend or foe? *Diabetologia* **47**, 1135–1142.

Carr, M. C., and Brunzell, J. D. (2004). Abdominal obesity and dyslipidemia in the metabolic syndrome: Importance of type 2 diabetes and familial combined hyperlipidemia in coronary artery disease risk. *J. Clin. Endocrinol. Metab.* **89**, 2601–2607.

Charriere, G., Cousin, B., Arnaud, E., Andre, M., Bacou, F., Penicaud, L., and Casteilla, L. (2003). Preadipocyte conversion to macrophage. Evidence of plasticity. *J. Biol. Chem.* **278**, 9850–9855.

Chen, C. C., Li, T. C., Li, C. I., Liu, C. S., Wang, J. J., and Lin, C. C. (2005). Serum resistin level among healthy subjects: Relationship to anthropometric and metabolic parameters. *Metabolism* **54**, 471–475.

Christiansen, T., Richelsen, B., and Bruun, J. M. (2005). Monocyte chemoattractant protein-1 is produced in isolated adipocytes, associated with adiposity and reduced after weight loss in morbid obese subjects. *Int. J. Obes. (Lond.)* **29**, 146–150.

Church, T. S., Willis, M. S., Priest, E. L., Lamonte, M. J., Earnest, C. P., Wilkinson, W. J., Wilson, D. A., and Giroir, B. P. (2005). Obesity, macrophage migration inhibitory factor, and weight loss. *Int. J. Obes. (Lond.)* **29**, 675–681.

Claffey, K. P., Wilkison, W. O., and Spiegelman, B. M. (1992). Vascular endothelial growth factor: Regulation by cell differentiation and activated second messenger pathways. *J. Biol. Chem.* **267**, 16317–16322.

Corbetta, S., Bulfamante, G., Cortelazzi, D., Barresi, V., Cetin, I., Mantovani, G., Bondioni, S., Beck-Peccoz, P., and Spada, A. (2005). Adiponectin expression in human fetal tissues during mid- and late gestation. *J. Clin. Endocrinol. Metab.* **90**, 2397–2402.

Corica, F., Allegra, A., Buemi, M., Corsonello, A., Bonanzinga, S., Rubino, F., Castagna, L., and Ceruso, D. (1997). Reduced plasma concentrations of transforming growth factor $\beta1$ (TGF-$\beta1$) in obese women. *Int. J. Obes. (Lond.)* **21**, 704–707.

Cottam, D. R., Mattar, S. G., Barinas-Mitchell, E., Eid, G., Kuller, L., Kelley, D. E., and Schauer, P. R. (2004). The chronic inflammatory hypothesis for the morbidity associated with morbid obesity: Implications and effects of weight loss. *Obes. Surg.* **14**, 589–600.

Curtis-Prior, P. B., Jenner, M., Smethurst, M., and Woodward, J. W. (1979). Plasma prostaglandin levels in fed and starved lean, normal and obese women. *Experientia* **35**, 911–912.

Dandona, P., Aljada, A., Ghanim, H., Mohanty, P., Tripathy, C., Hofmeyer, D., and Chaudhuri, A. (2004). Increased plasma concentration of macrophage migration factor (MIF) and MIF mRNA in monocuclear cells in the obese and the suppressive action of metformin. *J. Clin. Endocrinol. Metab.* **89**, 5043–5047.

Danesh, J., Muir, J., Wong, Y. K., Ward, M., Gallimore, J. R., and Pepys, M. B. (1999). Risk factors for coronary heart disease and acute-phase proteins. A population-based study. *Eur. Heart J.* **20**, 954–959.

Di Gregorio, G. B., Yao-Borengasser, A., Rasouli, N., Varma, V., Lu, T., Miles, L. M., Ranganathan, G., Peterson, C. A., McGehee, R. E., and Kern, P. A. (2005). Expression of CD68 and macrophase chemoattractant protein-1 genes in human adipose tissues: Association with cytokine expression, insulin resistance, and reduction by pioglitazone. *Diabetes* **54**, 2305–2313.

Engeli, S., Feldpausch, M., Gorzelniak, K., Hartwig, F., Heintze, U., Janke, J., Mohlig, M., Pfeiffer, A. F., Luft, F. C., and Sharma, A. M. (2003). Association between adiponectin and mediators of inflammation in obese women. *Diabetes* **52**, 942–947.

Esposito, K., Pontillo, A., Ciotola, M., di Paolo, C., Grella, E., Nicoletti, G., and Giugliano, D. (2002). Weight loss reduces interleukin-18 levels in obese women. *J. Clin. Endocrinol. Metab.* **87**, 3864–3866.

Esposito, K., Pontillo, A., Giugliano, F., Giugliano, G., Marfella, R., Nicoletti, G., and Giugliano, D. (2003). Association of low interleukin-10 levels with the metabolic syndrome in obese women. *J. Clin. Endocrinol. Metab.* **88**, 1055–1058.

Fain, J. N., and Bahouth, S. W. (2000). Regulation of leptin release by mammalian adipose tissue. *Biochem. Biophys. Res. Commun.* **274**, 571–575.

Fain, J. N., and Madan, A. K. (2005a). Insulin enhances VEGF, IL-8 and PAI-1 but not IL-6 release by human adipocytes. *Metabolism* **54**, 220–226.

Fain, J. N., and Madan, A. K. (2005b). Regulation of monocyte chomoattractant protein 1 (MCP-1) release by explants of human visceral adipose tissue. *Int. J. Obes. (Lond.)* **29**, 1299–1307.

Fain, J. N., Cowan, Jr., G. S. M., Buffington, C., Pouncey, L., and Bahouth, S. W. (2001). Stimulation of leptin release by arachidonic acid and PGE_2 in adipose tissue from obese humans. *Metabolism* **50**, 921–928.

Fain, J. N., Kanu, A., Bahouth, S. W., Cowan, Jr., G. S., Hiler, M. L., and Leffler, C. W. (2002). Comparison of PGE_2, prostacyclin and leptin release by human adipocytes versus explants of adipose tissue in primary culture. *Prostaglandins* **67**, 467–473.

Fain, J. N., Cheema, P. S., Bahouth, S. W., and Hiler, M. L. (2003). Resistin release by human adipose tissue explants in primary culture. *Biochem. Biophys. Res. Commun.* **300**, 674–678.

Fain, J. N., Madan, A. K., Hiler, M. L., Cheema, P., and Bahouth, S. W. (2004a). Comparison of the release of adipokines by adipose tissue, adipose tissue matrix and adipocytes from visceral and subcutaneous abdominal adipose tissues of obese humans. *Endocrinology* **145**, 2273–2282.

Fain, J. N., Bahouth, S. W., and Madan, A. K. (2004b). Haptoglobin release by human adipose tissue in primary culture. *J. Lipid Res.* **45**, 536–542.

Fain, J. N., Bahouth, S. W., and Madan, A. K. (2004c). TNFα release by the nonfat cells of human adipose tissue. *Intl. J. Obes. (Lond.)* **28**, 616–622.

Fain, J. N., Bahouth, S. W., and Madan, A. K. (2005a). Involvement of multiple signaling pathways in the post bariatric induction of IL-6 and IL-8 mRNA and release in human visceral adipose tissue. *Biochem. Pharmacol.* **69**, 1315–1324.

Fain, J. N., Tichansky, D. S., and Madan, A. K. (2005b). Transforming growth factor $\beta 1$ release by human adipose tissue is enhanced in obesity. *Metabolism* **54**, 1546–1551.

Fain, J. N., Tichansky, D. S., and Madan, A. K. (2006). The majority of the IL-1Ra, cathepsin S, MIF NGF, and IL-18 release by explants of human visceral adipose tissue is by the nonfat cells, not the adipocytes. *Metabolism* **55**, 1113–1121.

Fantuzzi, G. (2005). Adipose tissue, adipokines, and inflammation. *J. Allergy Clin. Immunol.* **115**, 911–919.

Festa, A., D'Agostino, Jr., R., Williams, K., Karter, A. J., Mayer-David, E. J., Tracy, R. P., and Haffner, S. M. (2001). The relation of body fat mass and distribution to markers of chronic inflammation. *Int. J. Obes. (Lond.)* **25**, 1407–1415.

Fried, S. K., Bunkin, D. A., and Greenberg, A. S. (1998). Omental and subcutaneous adipose tissues of obese subjects release interleukin-6: Depot difference and regulation by glucocorticoid. *J. Clin. Endocrinol. Metab.* **83**, 847–850.

Friedrichs, W. E., Navarijo-Ashbaugh, A. L., Bowman, B. H., and Yang, F. (1995). Expression and inflammatory regulation of haptoglobin gene in adipocytes. *Biochem. Biophys. Res. Commun.* **209**, 250–256.

Goodpaster, B. H., Krishnaswami, S., Harris, T. B., Katsiaras, A., Kritchevsky, S. B., Simonsick, E. M., Nevitt, M., Halvoet, P., and Newman, A. B. (2005). Obesity, regional body fat distribution, and the metabolic syndrome in older men and women. *Arch. Intern. Med.* **165**, 777–783.

Gracie, J. A., Robertson, S. E., and McInnes, I. B. (2003). Interleukin-18. *J. Leukoc. Biol.* **73**, 213–224.

Hak, A. E., Stehouwer, C. D., Bots, M. L., Polderman, K. H., Schalkwijk, C. G., Westendorp, I. C., Hofman, A., and Witteman, J. C. (1999). Associations of C-reactive protein with measures of obesity, insulin resistance, and subclinical atherosclerosis in healthy, middle-aged women. *Arterioscler. Thromb. Vasc. Biol.* **19**, 1986–1991.

Hannerz, J., Greitz, D., and Ericson, K. (1995). Is there a relationship between obesity and intracranial hypertension? *Int. J. Obes. (Lond.)* **19**, 762–763.

Hanusch-Enserer, U., Cauza, E., Spak, M., Dunky, A., Rosen, H. R., Wolf, H., Prager, R., and Eibl, M. M. (2003). Acute-phase response and immunological markers in morbid obese patients and patients following adjustable gastric banding. *Int. J. Obes. (Lond.)* **27**, 355–361.

Hasegawa, G., Ohta, M., Ichida, Y., Obayashi, H., Shigeta, M., Yamasaki, M., Fukui, M., Yoshikawa, T., and Nakamura, N. (2005). Increased serum resistin levels in patients with type 2 diabetes are not linked with markers of insulin resistance and adiposity. *Acta Diabetol.* **42**, 104–109.

Hauner, H. (2005). Secretory factors from human adipose tissue and their functional role. *Proc. Nutr. Soc.* **64**, 163–169.

Hausman, G. J., Campion, D. R., and Martin, R. J. (1980). Search for the adipocyte precursor cell and factors that promote its differentiation. *J. Lipid Res.* **21**, 657–670.

Heinrich, J. N., and Bravo, R. (1995). The orphan mouse receptor interleukin (IL)-8R beta binds N51. Structure-function analysis using N51/IL-8 chimeric molecules. *J. Biol. Chem.* **270**, 4987–4989.

Heinrich, P. C., Castell, J. V., and Andus, T. (1990). Interleukin-6 and the acute phase response. *Biochem. J.* **265**, 621–636.

Hellman, B., Larsson, S., and Westman, S. (1963). Mast cell content and fatty acid metabolism in the epididymal fat pad of obese mice. *Acta Physiol. Scand.* **58**, 255–262.

Helmersson, J., Vessby, B., Larsson, A., and Basu, S. (2004). Association of type 2 diabetes with cyclooxygenase-mediated inflammation and oxidative stress in an elderly population. *Circulation* **109**, 1729–1734.

Hirokawa, J., Sakaue, S., Tagami, S., Kawakami, Y., Sakai, M., Nishi, S., and Nishihira, J. (1997). Identification of macrophage migration inhibitory factor in adipose tissue and its induction by tumor necrosis factor-α. *Biochem. Biophys. Res. Commun.* **235**, 94–98.

Hoffmann, E., Dittrich-Breiholz, O., Holtmann, H., and Kracht, M. (2002). Multiple control of interleukin-8 gene expression. *J. Leukoc. Biol.* **72**, 847–855.

Holdstock, C., Lind, L., Engstrom, B. E., Ohrvall, M., Sundbom, M., Larsson, A., and Karlsson, F. A. (2005). CRP reduction following gastric bypass surgery is most pronounced in insulin-sensitive subjects. *Int. J. Obes.(Lond.)* **29**, 1275–1280.

Hotamisligil, G. S., Shargill, N. S., and Spiegelman, B. M. (1993). Adipose expression of tumor necrosis factor-α: Direct role in obesity-linked insulin resistance. *Science* **259**, 87–91.

Holtmann, H., Winzen, R., Holland, P., Eickemeier, S., Hoffman, E., Wallach, D., Malinin, N. L., Cooper, J. A., Resch, K., and Kracht, M. (1999). Induction of interleukin-8 synthesis integrates effects on transcription and mRNA degradation from at least three different cytokine- or stress-activated signal transduction pathways. *Mol. Cell Biol.* **19**, 6742–6753.

Hotamisligil, G. S., Arner, P., Caro, J. F., Atkinson, R. L., and Spiegelman, B. M. (1995). Increased adipose tissue expression of tumor necrosis factor-α in human obesity and insulin resistance. *J. Clin. Invest.* **95**, 2409–2415.

Iqbal, N., Seshadri, P., Stern, L., Loh, J., Kundu, S., Jafar, T., and Samaha, F. F. (2005). Serum resistin is not associated with obesity or insulin resistance in humans. *Eur. Rev. Med. Pharmacol. Sci.* **9**, 161–165.

Jansson, P.-A., Larsson, A., Smith, U., and Lonnroth, P. (1992). Glycerol production in subcutaneous adipose tissue in lean and obese humans. *J. Clin. Invest.* **89**, 1610–1617.

Juge-Aubry, C. E., Somm, E., Giusti, V., Pernin, A., Chicheportiche, R., Verdumo, C., Rohner-Jeanrenaud, F., Burger, D., Dayer, J. M., and Meier, C. A. (2003). Adipose tissue is a major source of interleukin-1 receptor antagonist: Upregulation in obesity and inflammation. *Diabetes* **52**, 1104–1110.

Kabon, B., Nagele, A., Reddy, D., Eagon, C., Fleshman, J. W., Sessler, D. I., and Kurz, A. (2004). Obesity decreases perioperative tissue oxygenation. *Anesthesiology* **100**, 274–280.

Kern, P. A., Saghizadeh, M., Ong, J. M., Bosch, R. J., Deem, R., and Simsolo, R. B. (1995). The expression of tumor necrosis factor in human adipose tissue. Regulation by obesity, weight loss, and relationship to lipoprotein lipase. *J. Clin. Invest.* **95**, 2111–2119.

Kern, P. A., Ranganathan, S., Li, C., Wood, L., and Ranganathan, G. (2001). Adipose tissue tumor necrosis factor and interleukin-6 expression in human obesity and insulin resistance. *Am. J. Physiol. Endocrinol. Metab.* **280**, E745–E751.

Klover, P. J., Clementi, A. H., and Mooney, R. A. (2005). Interleukin-6 depletion selectively improves hepatic insulin action in obesity. *Endocrinology* **146**, 3417–3427.

Kopp, H. P., Kopp, C. W., Festa, A., Krzyzanowska, K., Kriwanek, S., Minar, E., Roka, R., and Schernthaner, G. (2003). Impact of weight loss on inflammatory proteins and their association with the insulin resistance syndrome in morbidly obese patients. *Arterioscler. Thromb. Vasc. Biol.* **23**, 1042–1047.

Kratchmarova, I., Kalume, D. E., Blagoev, B., Scherer, P. E., Podtelejnikov, A. V., Molina, H., Bickel, P. E., Anderson, J. S., Fernandez, M. M., Bunkenborg, J., Roepstorff, P., Kristiansen, K., *et al.* (2002). A proteomic approach for identification of secreted proteins during the differentiation of 3T3-L1 preadipocytes to adipocytes. *Mol. Cell Proteomics* **1**, 213–222.

Laimer, M., Ebenbichler, C. F., Kaser, S., Sandhofer, A., Weiss, H., Nehoda, H., Aigner, F., and Patsch, J. R. (2002). Markers of chronic inflammation and obesity: A prospective study on the reversibility of this association in middle-aged women undergoing weight loss by surgical intervention. *Intl. J. Obes. (Lond.)* **26**, 659–662.

Lau, D. C., Dhillon, B., Yan, H., Szmitko, P. E., and Verma, S. (2005). Adipokines: Molecular links between obesity and atherosclerosis. *Am. J. Physiol. Heart Circ. Physiol.* **288**, H2031–H2041.

Lee, J. H., Chan, J. L., Yiannakouris, N., Kontogianni, M., Estrada, E., Seip, R., Orlova, C., and Mantzoros, C. S. (2003). Circulating resistin levels are not associated with obesity or insulin resistance in humans and are not regulated by fasting or leptin administration: Cross-sectional and interventional studies in normal, insulin-resistant, diabetic subjects. *J. Clin. Endocrinol. Metab.* **88**, 4848–4856.

Lin, Y., Lee, H., Berg, A. H., Lisanti, M. P., Shapiro, L., and Scherer, P. E. (2000). The lipopolysaccharide-activated toll-like receptor (TLR)-4 induces synthesis of the closely related receptor TLR-2 in adipocytes. *J. Biol. Chem.* **275**, 24255–24263.

Liuzzo, J. P., Petanceska, S. S., Moscatelli, D., and Devi, L. A. (1999). Inflammatory mediators regulate cathepsin S in macrophages and microglia: A role in attenuating heparan sulfate interactions. *Mol. Med.* **5**, 320–333.

Luheshi, G. N., Gardner, J. D., Rushforth, D. A., Loudon, A. S., and Rothwell, N. J. (1999). Leptin actions on food intake and body temperature are mediated by IL-1. *Proc. Natl. Acad. Sci. USA* **96**, 7047–7052.

Manigrasso, M. R., Ferroni, P., Santilli, F., Taraborelli, T., Guagnano, M. T., Michette, N., and Davi, G. (2005). Association between circulating adiponectin and interleukin-10 levels in android obesity. Effects of Weight. *J. Clin. Endocrinol. Metab.* **90**, 5876–5879.

Meier, C. A., Bobbioni, E., Gabay, C., Assimacopoulos-Jeannet, F., Golay, A., and Dayer, J. M. (2002). IL-1 receptor antagonist serum levels are increased in human obesity: A possible link to the resistance to leptin? *J. Clin. Endocrinol. Metab.* **87**, 1184–1188.

Mick, G. J., Wang, X., and McCormick, K. (2002). White adipocyte vascular endothelial growth factor: Regulation by insulin. *Endocrinology* **143**, 948–953.

Migita, K., Kawabe, Y., Tominaga, M., Origuchi, T., Aoyagi, T., and Eguchi, K. (1998). Serum amyloid A protein induces production of matrix metalloproteinases by human synovial fibroblasts. *Lab. Invest.* **78**, 535–539.

Miida, T., Yamada, T., Yamadera, T., Ozaki, K., Inano, K., and Okada, M. (1999). Serum amyloid A protein generates pre β1 high-density lipoprotein from α-migrating high-density lipoprotein. *Biochemistry* **38**, 16958–16962.

Mirone, L., Altomonte, L., D'Agostino, P., Zoli, A., Barini, A., and Magaro, M. (1996). A study of serum androgen and cortisol levels in female patients with rheumatoid arthritis. Correlation with disease activity. *Clin. Rheumatol.* **15**, 15–19.

Miyazawa-Hoshimoto, S., Takahashi, K., Bujo, H., Hashimoto, N., and Saito, Y. (2003). Elevated serum vascular endothelial growth factor is associated with visceral fat accumulation in human obese subjects. *Diabetologia* **46**, 1483–1488.

Mocellin, S., Panelli, M. C., Wang, E., Nagorsen, D., and Marincola, F. M. (2003). The dual role of IL-10. *Trends Immunol.* **24,** 36–43.

Mohamed-Ali, V., Goodrick, S., Rawesh, A., Katz, D. R., Miles, J. M., Yudkin, J. S., Klein, S., and Coppack, S. W. (1997). Subcutaneous adipose tissue releases interleukin-6, but not tumor necrosis factor-α, *in vivo. J. Clin. Endocrinol. Metab.* **82,** 4196–4200.

Moriwaki, Y., Yamamoto, T., Shibutani, Y., Aoki, E., Tsutsumi, Z., Takahashi, S., Okamura, H., Koga, M., Fukuchi, M., and Hada, T. (2003). Elevated levels of interleukin-18 and tumor necrosis factor-α in serum of patients with type 2 diabetes mellitus: Relationship with diabetic nephropathy. *Metabolism* **52,** 605–608.

Nagaev, I., and Smith, U. (2001). Insulin resistance and type 2 diabetes are not related to resistin expression in human fat cells or skeletal muscle. *Biochem. Biophys. Res. Commun.* **285,** 561–564.

Nicklas, B. J., Penninx, B. W., Cesari, M., Kritchevsky, S. B., Newman, A. B., Kanaya, A. M., Pahor, M., Jingzhong, D., and Harris, T. B. (2004). Association of visceral adipose tissue with incident myocardial infarction in older men and women. *Am. J. Epidemiol.* **160,** 741–749.

Nicoletti, F., Conget, I., Di Marco, R., Speciale, A. M., Morinigo, R., Bendtzen, K., and Gomis, R. (2001). Serum levels of the interferon-γ-inducing cytokine interleukin-18 are increased in individuals at high risk of developing type I diabetes. *Diabetologia* **44,** 309–311.

Orban, A., Remaley, A. T., Sampson, M., Trajanoski, Z., and Chrousos, G. P. (1999). The differential effect of food intake and β-adrenergic stimulation on adipose-derived hormones and cytokines in man. *J. Clin. Endocrinol. Metab.* **84,** 2126–2133.

Ouchi, N., Kihara, S., Funahashi, T., Nakamura, T., Nishida, M., Kumada, M., Okamoto, Y., Ohashi, K., Nagaretani, H., Kishida, K., Nishizawa, H., Maeda, N., *et al.* (2003). Reciprocal association of C-reactive protein with adiponectin in blood stream and adipose tissue. *Circulation* **107,** 671–674.

Pannacciulli, N., Cantatore, F. P., Minenna, A., Bellacicco, M., Giorgino, R., and De Pergola, G. (2001). C-reactive protein is independently associated with total body fat, central fat, and insulin resistance in adult women. *Int. J. Obes. (Lond.)* **25,** 1416–1420.

Pedersen, B. K., Steensberg, A., Fischer, C., Keller, C., Keller, P., Plomgaard, P., Febbraio, M., and Saltin, B. (2003). Searching for the exercise factor: Is IL-6 a candidate? *J. Muscle. Res. Cell. Motil.* **24,** 113–119.

Peeraully, M. R., Jenkins, J. R., and Trayhurn, P. (2004). NGF gene expression and secretion in white adipose tissue: Regulation in 3T3-L1 adipocytes by hormones and inflammatory cytokines. *Am. J. Physiol. Endocrinol. Metab.* **287,** E331–E339.

Piche, M. E., Weisnagel, S. J., Corneau, L., Nadeau, A., Bergeron, J., and Lemieux, S. (2005). Contribution of abdominal visceral obesity and insulin resistance to the cardiovascular risk profile of postmenopausal women. *Diabetes* **54,** 770–777.

Poitou, C., Viguerie, N., Cancello, R., De Matteis, R., Cinti, S., Stich, V., Coussieu, C., Gauthier, E., Courtine, M., Zucker, J. D., Barsh, G. S., Saris, W., *et al.* (2005). Serum amyloid A: Production by human white adipocytes and regulation by obesity and nutrition. *Diabetologia* **48,** 519–528.

Putnam, F. W. (1975). Haptoglobin. *In* "The Plasma Proteins Structure, Function, and Genetic Control" (F. W. Putnam, Ed.), 2nd ed., Vol II, pp. 2–50. Academic Press, New York.

Rajala, M. W., and Scherer, P. E. (2003). Minireview: The adipocyte-at the crossroads of energy homeostasis, inflammation, and atherosclerosis. *Endocrinology* **144,** 3765–3773.

Reape, T. J., and Groot, P. H. (1999). Chemokines and atherosclerosis. *Atherosclerosis* **147,** 213–225.

Reddy, P. (2004). Interleukin-18: Recent advances. *Curr. Opin. Hematol.* **11,** 405–410.

Reddy, V. Y., Zhang, Q. Y., and Weiss, S. J. (1995). Pericellular mobilization of the tissue-destructive cysteine proteinases, cathepsins, B, L, and S, by human monocyte-derived macrophages. *Proc. Natl. Acad. Sci. USA* **92,** 3849–3853.

Rehman, J., Considine, R. V., Bovenkerk, J. E., Li, J., Slavens, C. A., Jones, R. M., and March, K. L. (2004a). Obesity is associated with increased levels of circulating hepatocyte growth factor. *J. Am. Coll. Cardiol.* **41**, 1408–1413.

Rehman, J., Traktuev, D., Li, J., Merfeld-Clauss, S., Temm-Grove, C. J., Bovenkerk, J. E., Pell, C. L., Johnstone, B. H., Considine, R. V., and March, K. L. (2004b). Secretion of angiogenic and antiapoptotic factors by human adipose stromal cells. *Circulation* **109**, 1292–1298.

Rosenbaum, M., Malbon, C. C., Hirsch, J., and Leibel, R. L. (1993). Lack of β3-adrenergic effect on lipolysis in human subcutaneous adipose tissue. *J. Clin. Endocrinol. Metab.* **77**, 352–355.

Rothe, H., Hausmann, A, Casteels, K., Okamura, H., Kurimoto, M., Burkart, V., Mathieu, C., and Kolb, H. (1999). IL-18 inhibits diabetes development in nonobese diabetic mice by counterregulation of Th1-dependent destructive insulitis. *J. Immunol.* **163**, 1230–1236.

Rotter Sopasakis, V., Larsson, B. M., Johansson, A., Holmang, A, and Smith, U. (2004). Short-term infusion of interleukin-6 does not induce insulin resistance *in vivo* or impair insulin signaling in rats. *Diabetologia* **47**, 1879–1887.

Sartipy, P., and Loskutoff, D. J. (2003). Monocyte chemoattractant protein 1 in obesity and insulin resistance. *Proc. Natl. Acad. Sci. USA* **100**, 7265–7270.

Savage, D. B., Sewter, C. P., Klenk, E. S., Segal, D. G., Vidal-Puig, A., Considine, R. V., and O'Rahilly, S. (2001). Resistin/Fizz3 expression in relation to obesity and peroxisome proliferator-activated receptor-γ action in humans. *Diabetes* **50**, 2199–2202.

Scaglione, R., Argano, C., di Chiara, T., Colomba, D., Parrinello, G., Corrao, S., Avellone, G., and Licata, G. (2003). Central obesity and hypertensive renal disease: Association between higher levels of BMI, circulating transforming growth factor β1 and urinary albumin excretion. *Blood Press.* **12**, 269–276.

Scherer, P. E., Williams, S., Fogliano, M., Baldini, G., and Lodish, H. F. (1995). A novel serum protein similar to C1q, produced exclusively in adipocytes. *J. Biol. Chem.* **270**, 26746–26749.

Scriba, P. C., Bauer, M., Emmert, D., Fateh-Moghadam, A., Hoffman, G. G., Horn, K., and Pickardt, C. R. (1979). Effects of obesity, total fasting and re-alimentation on L-thyroxine (T4), 3,5,3'-L-triiodothyronine (T3), 3,3',5'-L-triiodothyronine (rT3), thyroxine binding globulin (TBG), cortisol, thyrotrophin, cortisol binding globulin (CBG), transferrin, α 2-haptoglobin and complement C'3 in serum. *Acta Endocrinol. (Copenh.)* **91**, 629–643.

Silha, J. V., Krsek, M., Sucharda, P., and Murphy, L. J. (2005). Angiogenic factors are elevated in overweight and obese individuals. *Int. J. Obes. (Lond.)* **29**, 1308–1314.

Sjoholm, K., Palming, J., Olofsson, L. E., Gummesson, A., Svensson, P. A., Lystig, T. C., Jennische, E., Brandberg, J., Torgerson, J. S., Carlsson, B., and Carlsson, L. M. (2005). A microarray search for genes predominantly expressed in human omental adipocytes: Adipose tissue as a major production site of serum amyloid A. *J. Clin. Endocrinol. Metab.* **90**, 2233–2239.

Skurk, T., and Hauner, H. (2004). Obesity and impaired fibrinolysis: Role of adipose production of plasminogen activator inhibitor-1. *Int. J. Obes. Relat. Metab. Disord.* **28**, 1357–1364.

Skurk, T., Herder, C., Kraft, I., Muller-Scholze, S., Hauner, H., and Kolb, H. (2005a). Production and release of macrophage migration inhibitory factor from human adipocytes. *Endocrinology* **146**, 1006–1011.

Skurk, T., Kolb, H., Muller-Scholze, S., Rohrig, K., Hauner, H., and Herder, C. (2005b). The proatherogenic cytokine interleukin-18 is secreted by human adipocytes. *Eur. J. Endocrinol.* **152**, 863–868.

Steppan, C. M., Bailey, S. T., Bhat, S., Brown, E. J., Banerjee, R. R., Wright, C. M., Patel, H. R., Ahima, R. S., and Lazar, M. A. (2001). The hormone resistin links obesity to diabetes. *Nature* **409**, 307–312.

Straczkowski, M., Dzienis-Straczkowska, S., Stepien, A., Kowalska, I., Szelachowska, M., and Kinalska, I. (2002). Plasma interleukin-8 concentrations are increased in obese subjects and related to fat mass and tumor necrosis factor-α system. *J. Clin. Endocrinol. Metab.* **87,** 4602–4606.

Sul, H. S. (2004). Resistin/ADSF/FIZZ3 in obesity and diabetes. *Trends Endocrinol. Metab.* **15,** 247–249.

Swierczynski, J., Korczynska, J., Goyke, E., Adrych, K., Raczynska, S., and Sledzinski, Z. (2005). Serum hepatocyte growth factor concentration in obese women decreases after vertical banded gastroplasty. *Obes. Surg.* **15,** 803–808.

Takahashi, K., Mizuarari, S., Araki, H., Mashiko, S., Ishihara, A., Kanatani, A., Itadani, H., and Kotani, H. (2003). Adiposity elevates plasma MCP-1 levels leading to the increased CD11b-positive monocytes in mice. *J. Biol. Chem.* **278,** 46654–46660.

Taleb, S., Lacasa, D., Bastard, J. P., Poitou, C., Cancello, R., Pelloux, V., Viguerie, N., Benis, A., Zucker, J. D., Bouillot, J. L., Coussieu, C., Basdevant, A., *et al.* (2005). Cathepsin S. A novel biomarker of adiposity: Relevance to atherogenesis. *FASEB J.* **19,** 1540–1542.

Tiret, L., Godefroy, T., Lubos, E., Nicaud, V., Tregouet, D. A., Barbaux, S., Schnabel, R., Bickel, C., Espinola-Klein, C., Poirier, O., Perret, C., Munzel, T., *et al.* (2005). Genetic analysis of the interleukin-18 system highlights the role of the interleukin-18 gene in cardiovascular disease. *Circulation* **112,** 643–650.

Trayhurn, P. (2005). Endocrine and signaling role of adipose tissue: New perspective on fat. *Acta Physiol. Scand.* **184,** 285–293.

Trayhurn, P., and Wood, I. S. (2004). Adipokines: Inflammation and the pleiotropic role of white adipose tissue. *Br. J. Nutrition* **92,** 347–355.

van Dielen, F. M., van't Veer, C., Schols, A. M., Soeters, P. B., Buurman, W. A., and Greve, J. W. (2001). Increased leptin concentrations correlate with increased concentrations of inflammatory markers in morbidly obese individuals. *Int. J. Obes. (Lond.)* **25,** 1759–1766.

Vasiljeva, O., Dolinar, M., Pungercar, J. R., Turk, V., and Turk, B. (2005). Recombinant human procathepsin S is capable of autocatalytic processing at neutral pH in the presence of glycosaminoglycans. *FEBS Lett.* **579,** 1285–1290.

Vazquez, L. A., Pazos, F., Berrazueta, J. R., Fernandez-Escalante, C., Garcia-Unzueta, M. T., Freijanes, J., and Amado, J. A. (2005). Effects of changes in body weight and insulin resistance on inflammation and endothelial function in morbid obesity after bariatric surgery. *J. Clin. Endocrinol. Metab.* **90,** 316–322.

Virtanen, K. A., Lonnroth, P., Parkkola, R., Peltoniemi, P., Asola, M., Viljanen, T., Tolvanen, T., Knuuti, J., Ronnemaa, T., Huupponen, R., and Nuutila, P. (2002). Glucose uptake and perfusion in subcutaneous and visceral adipose tissue during insulin stimulation in nonobese and obese humans. *J. Clin. Endocrinol. Metab.* **87,** 3902–3910.

Warne, J. P. (2003). Tumour necrosis factor α: A key regulator of adipose tissue mass. *J. Endocrinol.* **177,** 351–355.

Wellen, K. E., and Hotamisligil, G. S. (2005). Inflammation, stress, and diabetes. *J. Clin. Invest.* **115,** 1111–1119.

Weisberg, S. P., McCann, D., Desai, M., Rosenbaum, M., Leibel, R. L., and Ferrante, Jr., A. W. (2003). Obesity is associated with macrophage accumulation in adipose tissue. *J. Clin. Invest.* **112,** 1796–1808.

Wisse, B. E., Ogimoto, K., Morton, G. J., Wilkinson, C. W., Frayo, R. S., Cummings, D. E., and Schwartz, M. W. (2004). Physiological regulation of hypothalamic IL-1β gene expression by leptin and glucocorticoids: Implications for energy homeostasis. *Am. J. Physiol. Endocrinol. Metab.* **287,** E1107–E1113.

Xu, H., Barnes, G. T., Yang, Q., Tan, G., Yang, D., Chou, C. J., Sole, J., Nichols, A., Ross, J. S., Tartaglia, L. A., and Chen, H. (2003). Chronic inflammation in fat plays a crucial role in the development of obesity-related insulin resistance. *J. Clin. Invest.* **112,** 1821–1830.

Yudkin, J. S., Stehouwer, C. D., Emeis, J. J., and Coppack, S. W. (1999). C-reactive protein in healthy subjects: Associations with obesity, insulin resistance, and endothelial dysfunction: A potential role for cytokines originating from adipose tissue? *Arterioscler. Thromb. Vasc. Biol* **19,** 972–978.

Yudkin, J. S., Kumari, M., Humphries, S. E., and Mohamed-Ali, V. (2000). Inflammation, obesity, stress and coronary heart disease: Is interleukin-6 the link? *Atherosclerosis* **148,** 209–214.

Zhang, W., Smith, C., Howlett, C., and Stanimirovic, D. (2000). Inflammatory activation of human brain endothelial cells by hypoxic astrocytes *in vitro* is mediated by IL-1β. *J. Cereb. Blood Flow Metab.* **6,** 967–978.

Zhang, Y., Proenca, R., Maffei, M., Barone, M., Leopold, L., and Friedman, J. M. (1994). Positional cloning of the mouse obese gene and its human homologue. *Nature* **372,** 425–432.

Zozulinska, D., Majchrzak, A., Sobieska, M., Wiktorowicz, K., and Wierusz-Wysocka, B. (1999). Serum interleukin-8 level is increased in diabetic patients. *Diabetologia* **42,** 117–118.

19

ROLE OF INTERLEUKIN-13 IN CANCER, PULMONARY FIBROSIS, AND OTHER T$_H$2-TYPE DISEASES

BHARAT H. JOSHI,[*][†] CORY HOGABOAM,[*][‡]
PAMELA DOVER,[†] SYED R. HUSAIN,[†]
AND RAJ K. PURI[†]

[†]*Tumor Vaccines and Biotechnology Branch*
Division of Cellular and Gene Therapies
Center for Biologics Evaluation and Research
Food and Drug Administration, Bethesda, Maryland 20892
[‡]*Department of Pathology, University of Michigan Medical School*
Ann Arbor, Michigan 48109

*Bharat H. Joshi and Cory Hogaboam contributed equally to this chapter.

Vitamins and Hormones, Volume 74
Copyright 2006, Elsevier Inc. All rights reserved.

479

0083-6729/06 $35.00
DOI: 10.1016/S0083-6729(06)74019-5

Interleukin (IL)-13 plays a major role in various inflammatory diseases including cancer, asthma, and allergy. It mediates a variety of different effects on various cell types including B cells, monocytes, natural killer cells, endothelial cells, and fibroblasts. IL-13 binds to two primary receptor chains IL-13Rα1 and IL-13Rα2. The IL-13Rα2 but not IL-13Rα1 chain binds IL-13 with high affinity and is overexpressed in a variety of human cancer cells derived from glioma, squamous cell carcinoma of head and neck, and AIDS-associated Kaposi's sarcoma. We have also demonstrated that IL-13Rα2 expression is greatly increased in lung cells when mice were challenged intranasally with bleomycin or *Aspergillus fumigatus*. In addition, IL-13Rα2 increased in surgical lung biopsies from patients with usual interstitial pneumonia, nonspecific interstitial pneumonia, and respiratory bronchiolitic interstitial pneumonia of unknown origin. Based on various studies, it is concluded that IL-13Rα2-expressing cells are involved in various pulmonary pathological conditions. In contrast, normal tissues such as brain, lung, endothelial cells, and head and neck tissues express IL-13Rα1 chain, but show only marginal expression of IL-13Rα2 chain. Thus, IL-13Rα2 chain may serve as a novel biomarker for diseased cells such as cancer or fibrosis and a target for receptor-directed therapeutic agents. To target IL-13R, a recombinant fusion protein composed of IL-13 and a derivative of *Pseudomonas* exotoxin (PE) has been produced. This cytotoxin termed as IL-13PE38QQR or IL-13PE38, or IL-13PE is highly and specifically cytotoxic to a variety of human tumor cell lines. In preclinical models of human glioblastoma, head and neck and AIDS-associated Kaposi's cancer, IL-13PE has been found to have significant antitumor activity at a tolerated dose. Several phase I clinical trials have been completed in patients with recurrent malignant glioma. Recently a phase III clinical trial (PRECISE) in patients with recurrent malignant glioma has been completed recruiting a total of 294 patients. IL-13PE cytotoxin has also shown a significant therapeutic effect in preclinical bleomycin or *A. fumigatus* or *Schistosoma mansoni*–induced pulmonary pathology including granulomatous fibrosis in mouse models. A clinical study in these diseases has yet to be initiated. © 2006 Elsevier Inc.

I. INTRODUCTION

In this chapter, we will focus on the role of interleukin (IL)-13 and the expression of IL-13 receptors (IL-13R) in various cell types including human cancer cells and different pulmonary cells. We will describe the signaling events initiated by binding of IL-13 to its receptor. On the basis of receptor configuration present on different cell types including diseased cells, different types of receptors will be described. We will describe our observations that IL-13Rα2 chain is upregulated in cancer and pulmonary cells by various pathological states. We will also describe that human adrenomedullin, a calcitonin-growth-related peptide, upregulates IL-13Rα2 on cancer cells. The role and significance of IL-13R in IL-13PE cytotoxin-mediated cytotoxicity in cancer and pulmonary diseases *in vitro* and *in vivo* will be elucidated.

II. IL-13 AND ITS RECEPTORS

IL-13 is a 12-kDa lymphokine that was cloned from activated T cells (Brown *et al.*, 1989; Minty *et al.*, 1993). IL-13 protein has a 30% identity in the amino acid sequence to IL-4 protein (de Waal Malefyt *et al.*, 1995; Minty *et al.*, 1993). IL-13 inhibits the production of inflammatory cytokines (Aversa *et al.*, 1993; Minty *et al.*, 1993), upregulates major histocompatibility complex class II and CD23 expression on monocytes (de Waal Malefyt *et al.*, 1993), induces anti-CD40-dependent IgGE class switch, and induces IgG and IgM synthesis in B cells (Cocks *et al.*, 1993; Defrance *et al.*, 1994; McKenzie *et al.*, 1993; Minty *et al.*, 1993; Punnonen *et al.*, 1993). In contrast to IL-4, IL-13 does not affect resting or activated T cells (Punnonen *et al.*, 1993; Zurawski and de Vries, 1994a, Zurawski *et al.*, 1994b). Studies suggest that IL-13 is involved in induction of tissue fibrosis through transforming growth factor (TGF)-β1 and IL-13Rα2 pathway via tumor necrosis factor (TNF)-α production by macrophages (Fichtner-Feigl *et al.*, 2006). TGF-β1 regulates extracellular matrix formation and tissue remodeling *in vivo* (Kitani *et al.*, 2000, 2003; Lee *et al.*, 2001, 2004; Sanderson *et al.*, 1995). Tissue fibrosis is a main pathologic concern in many inflammatory diseases driven by T helper type 2 (T_H2) cells. These include *Schistosoma mansoni*, viral hepatitis, asthma, Crohn's disease, interstitial lung disease, and autoimmune diseases such as systemic sclerosis and ulcerative colitis (Fuss *et al.*, 2004; Hasegawa *et al.*, 1997; Ray and Cohn, 1999, 2000). Thus, IL-13 plays a central role in many pathological conditions.

In order to initiate a biological response, IL-13 must bind to its plasma membrane receptors. As IL-13 mediates biological effects in many cell types such as B cells, monocytes, and endothelial cells, it was predicted that these cells should express IL-13R. However, as receptor sites for IL-13 binding on these cells were extremely low, it was difficult to determine the structure of IL-13R.

In 1995, we discovered that human renal cell carcinoma (RCC) cell lines express IL-13R that allowed the study of receptor structure not only in RCC cells but also on malignant glioma cells and later cloning of these receptor chains (Debinski *et al.*, 1995a; Obiri *et al.*, 1997b). It is observed that IL-13R are overexpressed on AIDS-associated Kaposi's sarcoma (AIDS-KS) tumor cells, malignant glioma cells, renal cell carcinoma and squamous cell carcinoma of head and neck (SCCHN) (Debinski *et al.*, 1995b, 1996; Husain *et al.*, 1997; Joshi *et al.*, 2002; Kawakami *et al.*, 2000a, 2001b, 2005). Based on binding studies, we first demonstrated that ^{125}I-IL-13 cross-links to a dimer of 60–70-kDa proteins in RCC tumor cells (Obiri *et al.*, 1995, 1997a). Consistent with our hypothesis, two different chains of human IL-13R were cloned. One of the IL-13R chains was first cloned in murine and human cell systems and termed as IL-13Rα1 (also known as IL-13Rα') (Aman *et al.*, 1996; Hilton *et al.*, 1996). This chain forms a complex with primary IL-4-binding protein (IL-4Rα chain, also known as IL-4Rβ) for signal transduction (Obiri *et al.*, 1995). The second chain of IL-13R was cloned from RCC Caki cell line and later from human glioma cell lines. This chain migrated as a 70-kDa protein and showed a 50% sequence homology at the DNA level with IL-5Rα chain. This second chain was termed as IL-13Rα2 (also known as IL-13Rα) (Caput *et al.*, 1996; Kawakami *et al.*, 2000b). These two chains of IL-13R have no sequence homology with each other.

Based on binding, displacement, and cross-linking studies, IL-13R types were categorized as three different types as shown in Fig. 1. In type I IL-13R, IL-13Rα1 and IL-13Rα2 chains are expressed and IL-13Rα1 forms a complex with IL-4Rα chain. IL-13 binds to all three proteins while IL-4 binds to two proteins (IL-4Rα and IL-13Rα1). In this arrangement, IL-13 can displace ^{125}I-IL-13 binding while IL-4 cannot. However, ^{125}I-IL-4 binding would be displaced by both IL-4 and IL-13. This type of IL-13R has been found to be expressed on RCC, brain tumor cells, a majority of head and neck tumor cells, and AIDS-KS cells (Debinski *et al.*, 1995a, 1996; Husain *et al.*, 1997, Kawakami *et al.*, 2000a, 2001a,d, 2002; Obiri *et al.*, 1995). In type II IL-13R, IL-13Rα2 chain is not present, and IL-13 forms a complex with IL-13Rα1 and IL-4Rα chains. This type of IL-13 receptor is expressed in Colo 201, A 431, and Cos-7 cells. Because of the absence of IL-13Rα2 chain, ^{125}I-IL-13 and ^{125}I-IL-4 binding is displaced by both IL-4 and IL-13 (Murata *et al.*, 1995, 1998a; Obiri *et al.*, 1997a). In type III IL-13R, an additional component from IL-2R complex (termed as γC chain) is also present that may modulate IL-13 binding. These types of IL-13R are expressed on B cells, monocytes, and TF-1 cells (Obiri *et al.*, 1997; Vita *et al.*, 1995; Zurawski *et al.*, 1995). Even though γC chain does not appear to bind IL-13 it affects its binding and functionality in certain types of cells (Kuznetsov and Puri, 1999; Obiri *et al.*, 1997b). It is still not clear whether all three chains simultaneously form a productive IL-13R complex. The existence of various types of IL-13R has been confirmed by reconstitution studies (Kawakami *et al.*, 2001, 2002).

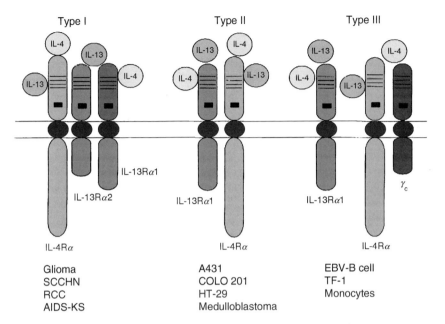

FIGURE 1.   IL-13 receptor types in human cancer cells.

III. IL-13R-MEDIATED SIGNAL TRANSDUCTION

IL-4R and IL-13R systems not only share two chains (IL-4α and IL-13α1) with each other, both IL-4 and IL-13 mediate signal transduction through Janus kinase (JAK)/signal transducer and activation of transcription (STAT) pathways. Both IL-13 and IL-4 phosphorylate and activate JAK1 and Tyk2 tyrosine kinases in hemapoietic cells, while they phosphorylate JAK1 and JAK2 tyrosine kinases in nonhemapoietic cells such as colon carcinoma and fibroblast cells (Murata *et al.*, 1996, 1998b). In contrast to IL-4, IL-13 cannot phosphorylate and activate JAK3 tyrosine kinase in any cell type (Murata *et al.*, 1997). JAK kinase phosphorylation by IL-13 leads to phosphorylation of IL-4Rα and 170-kDa insulin receptor substrate II (IRS-II) protein in hemapoietic cells and nonhemapoietic cells (Murata *et al.*, 1996; Smerz-Bertling and Duschl, 1995; Welham *et al.*, 1995). Although the signaling profile in hemapoietic and nonhemapoietic cells is different, IL-13 phosphorylates and activates STAT6 protein as does IL-4 (Kohler *et al.*, 1994, 1995; Lin *et al.*, 1995; Murata *et al.*, 1997). Various studies have reported that IL-13Rα2 chain does not seem to signal through STAT6 pathway but it inhibits signaling through STAT6 pathway by not only IL-13 but also by IL-4R (Murata *et al.*, 1997; Rahaman *et al.*, 2002, 2005; Wood, *et al.* 2003). It has also been reported that IL-13 can signal through IL-13Rα2 in a STAT6-independent, AP-1-dependent manner to induce activation of the TGFB1 promoter resulting in inflammation and fibrosis *in vivo* (Fichtner-Feigl *et al.*, 2006).

The specificity of IL-4 and IL-13 signaling seems restricted to the proximal JAK-signaling pathway. Therefore, the JAK-STAT-signaling pathway could serve as a useful target for pharmacologic intervention to interfere with the effects of both IL-4 and IL-13 (Kohler *et al.*, 1994; Lin *et al.*, 1995; Murata *et al.*, 1996). Alternatively, a molecule that can block the binding and signaling through both cytokines would be very useful. In that regard, we have generated a human IL-13 mutant (IL-13E13K), which is a powerful antagonist of IL-13, blocking the biological activities of IL-13 (Kioi *et al.*, 2004). It is also shown that IL-13E13K can competitively inhibit signaling and biological activities of IL-4 through IL-4R system (Kioi *et al.*, 2004a,b). Thus, IL-13E13K may be a useful agent for the treatment of diseases such as asthma, allergic rhinitis, and cancer, which are dependent on signaling through both IL-4 and IL-13 receptors.

IV. EFFECT OF IL-13 ON TUMOR CELLS

IL-13 inhibits cellular proliferation of three human RCC cell lines in a concentration-dependent manner (Obiri *et al.*, 1996). As IL-13 binds with IL-13Rα1 chain and recruits IL-4Rα for signaling, we determined whether blocking IL-4Rα by a specific antibody would inhibit IL-13 effect. Our data demonstrated that anti-IL-4Rα antibody did not block the effect of IL-13 indicating that these effects were IL-4Rα independent (Obiri *et al.*, 1995, 1996). We also demonstrated that although IL-13 did not impact the growth of human glioma tumor cell lines *in vitro*, IL-13 induced intercellular cell adhesion molecule (ICAM)-1 expression not only on glioma cells but also upregulated ICAM-1 in RCC cell lines indicating that IL-13R are functional (Kawakami *et al.*, 2000b, Obiri *et al.*, 1997a). In order to further examine the significance of IL-13R overexpression in tumor cells, sequencing and single nucleotide conformation polymorphism (SSCP) studies were undertaken (Kawakami *et al.*, 2000b). These studies were performed in human glioma cell lines, which demonstrated that IL-13R gene is neither mutated nor rearranged (Kawakami *et al.*, 2000b, 2005).

V. TARGETING IL-13R BY IL-13PE CYTOTOXIN

A. *IN VITRO* STUDIES

The discovery of overexpression of IL-13R on human RCC, glioma, and other tumor cell lines led us to develop an IL-13PE cytotoxin, which is a protein product of a chimeric gene IL-13 and mutated form of *Pseudomonas* exotoxin (PE) gene. The protein product is termed as IL-13PE, IL-13PE38, or IL-13PE38QQR. These fusion proteins were expressed in a prokaryotic (pET) expression system using ampicillin or kanamycin as a selection antibiotic (Debinski *et al.*, 1995a; Joshi and Puri, 2005; Joshi *et al.*, 2002). The recombinant protein was found to be highly cytotoxic (as determined by the inhibition of protein synthesis) to IL-13R-positive RCC cells at a very low concentration (Puri *et al.*, 1996). The properly refolded molecule was found to be highly cytotoxic to other IL-13R positive human solid tumor cell lines derived from malignant glioma, AIDS-KS, SCCHN, ovarian, prostate, and several human epithelial carcinomas such as colon and skin (Debinski *et al.*, 1995; Husain and Puri, 2000; Kawakami *et al.*, 2001c; Maini *et al.*, 1997; Puri *et al.*, 1996). The extent of cytotoxicity (IC$_{50}$, the concentration of the drug inhibiting protein synthesis by 50%) was dependent on the number of IL-13R on the cell surface. The level of cytotoxicity correlated with the number of receptor sites present on the tumor cell surface (Puri *et al.*, 1996). The cytotoxic activity of IL-13PE was mediated through IL-13R as cytotoxicity was blocked when an excess of human IL-13 was included in the assay. The mechanism of tumor cell killing by IL-13PE was investigated *in vitro* and *in vivo* in SCCHN and glioma tumors (Kawakami *et al.*, 2002b). IL-13PE induced apoptosis at least in part in these tumors and two pathways (classical and mitochondrial cytochrome C release) of apoptosis were operational *in vitro* and *in vivo* (Kawakami *et al.*, 2002b).

Interestingly, IL-13PE was highly selective in mediating cytotoxicity in certain tumor types. This was because these tumors preferentially express high levels of IL-13Rα2 (Kawakami *et al.*, 2001c; Obiri *et al.*, 1996). The role of IL-13Rα2 chain in IL-13PE-induced cytotoxicity in tumor cells was investigated by gene transfer studies and knock-down of IL-13Rα2 gene by RNAi (Kawakami *et al.*, 2005). Plasmid-mediated gene transfer of IL-13Rα2 highly sensitized previously insensitive pancreatic, breast, head and neck, prostate, and glioblastoma cell lines to IL-13PE *in vitro*. These *in vitro* data were confirmed by *in vivo* studies in a number of human tumor xenograft models (Kawakami *et al.*, 2000a, 2001b,c, 2002a). The *in vivo* studies also showed an evidence of activation of the innate immune response that mediated robust tumor response. This is a novel demonstration that an immunotoxin could induce cell killing in receptor positive tumors by recruiting the help of the innate immune response.

B. *IN VIVO* STUDIES

As IL-13PE was found to be highly cytotoxic to a variety of tumor types including malignant glioma cell lines *in vitro*, several studies were performed where the effect of IL-13PE against established human tumors was examined *in vivo*. Various human tumor models including glioblastoma, AIDS-KS, and SCCHN have been developed and tested (Husain and

Puri, 2000; Husain *et al.*, 1997, 2001; Kawakami *et al.*, 2000a, 2001b). IL-13PE cytotoxin mediated remarkable antitumor activity against these tumors when it was administered to subcutaneous tumor-bearing mice by different routes of administration. All mice in these tumor models tolerated the therapy well without any adverse effects. Intratumoral administration was the most effective route of administration followed by intraperitoneal administration. Their responses were remarkable and 100% of the animals showed complete regression of their tumors versus 36–54% complete response in mice treated by the intraperitoneal route (Husain and Puri, 2003). The complete responders remained disease free during the course of experiments. Although, the intravenous route was least effective among three routes of administration, 20% of animals achieved complete response.

Since glioblastoma is a localized intracranial disease, intratumoral administration of IL-13PE cytotoxin could be a practical approach to overcome intact blood–brain barrier. To study this, IL-13 cytotoxin was administered intratumorally in various subcutaneous tumors (Husain and Puri, 2000, 2003; Kawakami *et al.*, 2001b,c, 2002b). When drug levels were determined, it was found that a high level of IL-13PE remained in tumor without escaping into systemic circulation (Husain and Puri, 2000). This higher buildup of IL-13 cytotoxin by intratumoral route resulted in increased efficacy, which caused 100% complete regression of small tumors and 33% complete regression of three times larger tumors (Husain *et al.*, 2001). These observations indicate that IL-13PE cytotoxin can be useful in subjects with small and large glioblastoma tumors.

VI. SIGNIFICANCE OF IL-13Rα2 EXPRESSION

To study the significance of IL-13Rα2 in cancer biology, IL-13Rα2 gene was stably transfected into prostate, breast, and pancreatic tumor cell lines. These tumor cells were implanted subcutaneously in immunodeficient animals (Kawakami *et al.*, 2001a,b,c). Surprisingly, overexpression of the IL-13Rα2 chain in these tumor cells inhibited the growth of these tumors, while mock-transfected control tumor cells formed tumors which increased in size (Kawakami *et al.*, 2001a,b,c). IL-13Rα2 chain transfer also induced activation of the innate immune response and production of antiangiogenic factors at the tumor site. As IL-13 binds to IL-13Rα2 with high affinity, both IL-13 and IL-13R were hypothesized to be involved in tumorigenesis. A similar role of IL-13/IL-13R complex has also been reported by Terabe *et al.* (2000). Treatment of the host with an IL-13Rα2 extracellular domain, Fc-fusion protein repressed tumor regression in a tumor rejection–progression model indicating that IL-13 played a major role in tumor regrowth. Natural killer T (NKT) cells were found to produce IL-13, a key T_H2 cytokine, and therefore, believed to be involved in immunosurveillance.

VII. REGULATION OF IL-13Rα2 EXPRESSION

The molecular mechanism of IL-13Rα2 upregulation in humans or animals is unclear and it is known whether certain hormones, chemicals, or growth factors could act as positive or negative regulators of IL-13Rα2 chain. In this regard, we serendipitously discovered that adrenomedullin, a calcitonin growth-related peptide upregulates IL-13Rα2 gene in prostate cancer cell line PC-3 (Gonzalez-Moreno et al., 2005). The stable transfection of adrenomedullin in this cell line resulted into over expression of IL-13Rα2 chain, which increased its sensitivity to IL-13PE (Gonzalez-Moreno et al., 2005). These observations have provided new mechanistic insights into the regulation of IL-13Rα2 expression and potentially important therapeutic applications in sensitizing nonresponsive tumors to IL-13PE-based therapy. Certain other cytokines such as interferon (IFN)-γ, TNF-α, and IL-4 are reported to either mobilize or upregulate the intracellular pool of IL-13R in immortalized monocytic macrophagic U937, A549 respiratory epithelial cell line, elutriated human monocytes, and human fibroblasts (Daines and Hershey, 2002; David et al., 2002; Yoshikawa et al., 2003).

VIII. CLINICAL STUDIES WITH IL-13PE CYTOTOXIN

On the basis of preclinical results, several phase I/II clinical trials were initiated at various medical centers to determine safety and tolerability of IL-13PE in patients with malignant brain tumors (Croteau et al., 2006; Krieg et al., 1998; Kunwar et al., 1993, 2003, 2005a,b; Lang et al., 2002; Parney et al., 2005; Prados et al., 2001, 2002a,b, 2005; Sampson et al., 2004; Weingart et al., 2001a,b, 2003). In these studies, IL-13PE cytotoxin has been administered by convection-enhanced delivery via intratumoral or peritumoral catheters. In the first trial, the IL-13PE cytotoxin was administered directly into the tumors, and the concentration of IL-13PE was increased in cohorts of 3 patients to determine the maximum tolerated dose (MTD) and dose limiting toxicity (DLT). The second trial (Lang et al., 2002; Prados et al., 2001, 2002a,b) was initiated to determine the histologically effective concentration of IL-13PE cytotoxin that might show an evidence of cytotoxicity to tumor. In stage 1 of the study, IL-13PE cytotoxin was infused for 2 days by intratumoral convection-enhanced delivery (CED) into recurrent malignant glioma prior to surgical resection. Another aim was to determine the toxicity of the drug infused via catheter into brain adjacent to tumor resection site after surgical resection. The secondary objective of the trial was to monitor the disease progression and survival of the patients. In the third phase I clinical study, the primary objective was to determine the MTD in terms of duration of infusion and drug concentration of IL-13PE cytotoxin delivered by CED via one or two intratumoral catheters into recurrent or progressive malignant glioma prior to surgical resection. All three studies demonstrate that intratumoral and peritumoral infusion of IL-13PE is well tolerated. Based on these results, a phase III study was initiated in which two to three catheters were placed peritumorally, and IL-13PE at a concentration of 0.5 μg/ml was infused (Prados *et al.*, 2005). This multicenter trial has been completed. The efficacy of IL-13PE will be evaluated by assessing the overall survival of treated patients when compared with standard Gliadel treatment.

We also performed a phase I study in patients with advanced RCC in which IL-13PE was administered intravenously. A total of 12 patients with metastatic disease, which had been previously treated with standard therapeutic regimens and who had adequate vital organ function, were recruited in this study. The first cohort of three patients was dosed with IL-13PE cytotoxin at 8 μg/kg i.v. bolus daily for five consecutive days. Two patients at this dose showed reversible platelet consumption (decline>100 K) with rebound above baseline at day 8. One of three patients developed acute renal failure (ARF) requiring dialysis after five doses of IL-13PE cytotoxin and the second patient developed ARF after three doses. This patient did not require dialysis. The renal biopsies from these two patients showed endothelial swelling, thrombotic glomerulopathy, and tubular necrosis. One of these two patients also developed transient Grade 3 liver enzymes (AST/ALT) elevation and erythematous rash. Nonetheless, the third patient did not show any renal toxicity. It was found that the third patient had preexisting antibody to *Pseudomonas* exotoxin, which neutralized the IL-13PE cytotoxin effect (Kuzel *et al.*, 2002). Because of this unanticipated renal toxicity, which was not observed in any preclinical studies, IL-13PE cytotoxin doses were reduced to 4 μg/kg every alternate day for three doses. Adverse events in these patients noticed were grade 1/2 fever, chills, nausea, fatigue, edema, and headache, but no platelet consumption was observed. Of two patients treated at the 4 μg/kg dose, one had no nephrotoxicity; however the other patient, despite weakly positive preexisting antibody, had Grade 4 ARF with marked platelet decrease and schistocytes on peripheral blood smear, unresponsive to plasmapheresis. Therefore, the next cohorts of seven patients received 1 or 2 μg/kg of IL-13PE cytotoxin daily for three alternate days. These patients did not show any renal or other toxicity indicating the 2 μg/kg dose to be the maximum tolerated dose.

Pharmacokinetics studies in anti-PE antibody-negative patients after 1, 2, 4, and 8 μg/kg doses on day 1 showed mean peak serum IL-13PE levels of 4, 8, 13, and 79 ng/ml, respectively, with $t_{1/2\beta}$ of 30 min. The half-life is shorter compared to murine and monkey pharmacokinetic studies although the dose regimens were different. At 8 μg/kg dose, however, the mean peak level was 79 ng/ml with delayed clearance. All patients developed antibody to IL-13PE cytotoxin, and subsequent serum levels of the drug (if any) were markedly reduced.

The mechanism of IL-13PE cytotoxin-induced ARF is not known. ARF occurrence in 3 of 12 patients may be because of IL-13 receptor expression in normal kidney cells or renal endothelium of these patients. As normal monkeys and mice did not show this toxicity and they did not have RCC, it is possible that the presence of RCC in kidney may activate IL13R in normal kidney cells. Finally, since IL-13PE cytotoxin can eliminate 100% RCC cells *in vitro* at <1 ng/ml and the peak serum level of IL-13PE cytotoxin at 2 μg/kg is well tolerated, it is possible that this dose level will mediate an antitumor effect. In addition, other schedules or routes of administration, for example, intratumoral, may be tested that will avoid this side effect and may be beneficial to patients with RCC (Kuzel *et al.*, 2002).

IX. IL-13 AND CHRONIC LUNG DISEASE

Since its recognition as a T cell–derived factor that modulates the synthesis of inflammatory cytokines by immune cells (D'Andrea *et al.*, 1995, Doyle *et al.*, 1994), the role of IL-13 has expanded tremendously. Although this cytokine is often grouped with other T$_H$2-type cytokines including IL-4 and IL-5, IL-13 possesses unique qualities that distinguish it particularly from its sister cytokine IL-4 (Zund *et al.*, 1996). Although IL-4 and IL-13 share many molecular and cellular properties, IL-13, to a greater extent than IL-4, has been shown to play a major role in the several biological processes including airway hyperresponsiveness, allergic inflammation, tissue eosinophilia, parasite elimination, mast cell hyperplasia, IgE antibody synthesis, goblet cell metaplasia, tissue remodeling, and fibrosis (Brombacher, 2000; Wynn, 2003). A major target organ of the pathological effects of IL-13 is the lung and the list of pulmonary diseases now includes acute lung injury, allergy, asthma, COPD, and pulmonary fibrosis. The recognition that IL-13 is a major target in all of these diseases has certainly motivated attempts to identify therapeutics with the ability to block its effects in the lung and elsewhere.

While IL-13 does not drive T$_H$2 cell development like IL-4 because T cells only express the IL-4-specific or type I IL-4 receptor (composed of the common γ-chain and IL-4Rα), it has a major role in the activation of both immune and nonimmune cells in the lung during disease (Brubaker and Montaner, 2001). Cellular examples include eosinophils, mast cells, mucus cells, airway epithelium, smooth muscle cells, and fibroblasts. All of these cells appear to express the major IL-13 receptor subunits, namely IL-13Rα1 and IL-13Rα2, under inflammatory conditions when IL-13 levels are increased. The latter receptor subunit was thought to be an endogenous regulator of IL-13 function given its high affinity and its postulated lack of signaling due to its structure. However, studies clearly demonstrate that IL-13 promotes TGF-β and tissue fibrosis via IL-13Rα2 signaling (Fichtner-Feigl *et al.*, 2006).

This latter finding is very interesting because the expression of IL-13Rα2 is dramatically increased in the context of IL-13-driven diseases (Mentink-Kane and Wynn, 2004).

Experimental studies have relied on four strategies for attenuating IL-13 effects: (1) targeted gene deletion (McKenzie *et al.*, 1998, 1999) or transgene insertion (Zhu *et al.*, 1999) (2) neutralization of IL-13 with polyclonal (Blease *et al.*, 2001b; Kolodsick *et al.*, 2004) or monoclonal antibodies (Yang *et al.*, 2005) (3) the neutralization of IL-13 with a soluble version of the IL-13Rα2-Fc subunit (Grunig *et al.*, 1998; Wills-Karp *et al.*, 1998), and (4) a strategy intensively studied by the contributors to this chapter, chimeric protein composed of human IL-13 and a truncated form of *Pseudomonas* exotoxin. IL-13PE uniquely targets cells that are responsive to IL-4 and IL-13, thereby eliminating these cells from diseased tissues.

While targeted gene deletion is simply not an option for treating clinical diseases, considerable attention has been directed toward neutralizing the effects of IL-13 with antibodies or soluble receptors in diseases such as asthma (Blease *et al.*, 2003), allergy, and certain infectious disorders (Brombacher, 2000).

X. ACTIVITY OF IL-13PE IN PULMONARY DISEASES

The utility of IL-13PE cytotoxin in targeting lung disease has been the subject of investigation in our laboratories. Unlike most other organs, drug delivery to the lung is less problematic in that it is possible to deliver drugs in an inhaled or aerosolized form. This fact has aided in examining the therapeutic effects of intranasally delivered IL-13PE cytotoxin in experimental lung disease. The intranasal delivery of IL-13PE cytotoxin has proved to be effective in the treatment of several experimental lung diseases including fungal asthma, *S. mansoni* egg-induced granuloma, and bleomycin-induced pulmonary fibrosis. This therapeutic has also been used to target human cells, particularly fibroblasts, and it is thus being considered as a putative therapeutic in the treatment of human fibrotic lung diseases driven by IL-4 and IL-13.

XA. ASTHMA AND ALLERGY

Concerted clinical and basic research over the past 20 years has led to the recognition that asthma is characterized by airway hyperresponsiveness, eosinophilic inflammation, mucus hypersecretion, peribronchial fibrosis, and increased IgE levels. Postmortem studies reveal that airway wall thickening (due to peribronchial fibrosis, increased muscle mass, and increased mucus producing cells) is present in asthmatic patients, and this histological obser- vation appears to correlate to the severity of airway hyperresponsiveness and airflow obstruction. A growing subset of asthmatics experience persistent symptoms including permanent airway obstruction despite maximal anti- inflammatory therapy (Backman *et al.* 1997; Ollerenshaw and Woolcock, 1992). Consequently, novel therapeutic approaches are required for the treatment of asthma.

Clinical and experimental studies have revealed the prominent expression of the type 2 cytokines such as IL-4 and IL-13 in asthma and allergic airway disease (Huang *et al.*, 1997; Kotsimbos *et al.*, 1996). The major cellular source of both cytokines is the activated CD4(+) T$_H$2 cell (Devouassoux *et al.*, 1999), a primary effector cell in chronic allergic and asthmatic diseases (Umetsu and DeKruyff, 1997). Our previous studies have revealed distinct but synergistic roles for IL-4 and IL-13 during chronic fungal asthma (Blease *et al.*, 2001a), suggesting the importance of negating the actions of both cytokines during allergic or asthmatic responses. Targeting of IL-4 and IL-13 is possible because IL-4 shares a receptor component and signaling pathways with IL-13, including the alpha chain of the IL-4 receptor (Hilton *et al.*, 1996). Using a well-established model of chronic fungal asthma (Hogaboam *et al.*, 2000), we have investigated the therapeutic potential of IL-13PE (Blease *et al.*, 2001a). *Aspergillus fumigatus*–sensitized mice challenged with *A. fumigatus* spores, or conidia received 50, 100, or 200 ng of IL-13PE or diluent alone (i.e., control group) on alternate days from day 14 to day 28 after the conidia challenge. The control group of mice (i.e., *A. fumigatus*–sensitized and conidia-challenged mice) exhibited significant airway hyperreactivity, goblet cell hyperplasia, and peribronchial fibrosis at day 28 after conidia. Although the two lower doses of IL-13PE had limited therapeutic effects in mice with fungal-induced allergic airway disease, the highest dose of IL-13PE cytotoxin (i.e., 200 ng/dose) tested significantly reduced all features of airway disease compared with the control group. Whole lung mRNA expression of IL-4Rα and IL-13Rα1 was markedly reduced, whereas bronchoalveolar lavage and whole lung levels of IFN-γ were significantly elevated in mice treated with 200 ng of IL-13PE cytotoxin compared with the control group. We have also observed that IL-13PE cytotoxin at this dose also attenuates chronic fungal asthma in the context of STAT6 deficiency demonstrating that the targeting of IL-4- and IL-13-responsive cells in the lung ameliorates established fungal-induced allergic airway disease in mice regardless of the intracellular signaling molecule(s) mediating the effects of these T$_H$2 cytokines (Blease *et al.*, 2002). Importantly, from other studies it was shown that nonallergic mice did not exhibit any adverse effects from prolonged systemic *in vivo* administration of IL-13PE during tumor treatment (Husain and Puri, 2000).

Xʙ. *S. MANSONI* GRANULOMA FORMATION

Like all extracellular parasites, *S. mansoni* induces a strong T$_H$2 response that culminates in profound tissue remodeling and fibrosis, particularly around the eggs released by *S. mansoni*. Classic granuloma responses form around tissue resident *S. mansoni* eggs and this pathologic process requires the actions of IL-4 and IL-13 (Wynn, 2003). Because receptors for IL-4 and IL-13 share chains, we examined the effect of IL-13PE on the development of pulmonary granulomas in mice (Jakubzick *et al.*, 2002). At day 8 after an intravenous injection of live *S. mansoni* eggs, whole lung samples from IL-13PE-treated mice exhibited significantly lower IL-4 and IL-13 gene expression, smaller granulomas (Fig. 2), decreased collagen levels, and increased IL-13Rα2 gene expression compared to controls. The therapeutic effects of IL-13PE were also observed at day 16 despite the termination of IL-13PE treatment at day 8. The persistent therapeutic effects of IL-13PE were related to the ability of this therapeutic to eliminate IL-13-responsive cells in the respiratory system. These IL-13-responsive cells included macrophages, NK cells, B cells, and, most importantly, fibroblasts (Jakubzick *et al.*, 2002, 2003a). The absence of these cells was critical since the withdrawal of IL-13PE from mice with *S. mansoni* egg granulomas was associated with a persistent attenuation in granuloma cellularity and collagen content. We have shown that chemokine receptor 4 (CCR4)-responsive cells such as NK cells and macrophages have a major role in the development and maintenance of granulomatous responses in the mouse (Jakubzick *et al.*, 2004e). IL-13PE significantly decreased the presence of CCR4-positive cells (Fig. 3) in granulomas showing that this therapeutic may modulate the presence of other

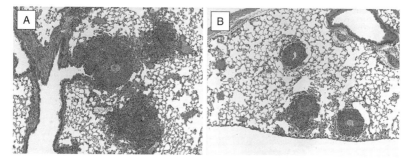

FIGURE 2. Histological appearance of *S. mansoni* egg granulomas at day 32 after intranasal vehicle (Panel A) or IL13-PE (1000 ng/dose; Panel B). Vehicle or IL-13PE was administered every other day from day 8 to day 16 after the intravenous injection of 3000 live *S. mansoni* eggs into mice that had been previously sensitized to *S. mansoni* antigens. The IL-13PE treatment significantly decreased the size (i.e., cellularity) and remodeling (i.e., degreed of fibrosis) of the egg granulomas. The cessation of the IL-13PE treatment was not associated with a resumption of the granulomatous response in IL-13PE-treated mice. Original magnification was 100×. (See Color Insert.)

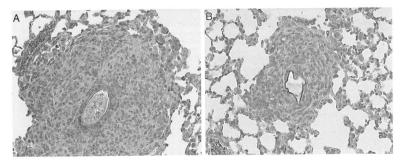

FIGURE 3. Immunohistochemical staining for CCR4 (red staining) in *S. mansoni* egg granulomas at day 8 after intranasal vehicle (Panel A) or IL-13PE (1000 ng/dose; Panel B). Vehicle or IL-13PE was administered by intranasal instillation every other day from day 0 to day 8 after the intravenous injection of 3000 live *S. mansoni* eggs into naïve mice. The IL-13PE treatment significantly decreased the size (i.e., cellularity), remodeling (i.e., degreed of fibrosis), and the presence of CCR4-positive cells in egg granulomas. Original magnification was 400×. (See Color Insert.)

factors that contribute to pathological processes in the granulomatous lung. This persistent attenuation was not observed in the context of the withdrawal of neutralizing antibodies directed against IL-13 (unpublished data). Together, these studies demonstrate that targeting IL-4- and IL-13-responsive cells with IL-13PE effectively arrests *S. mansoni* egg granuloma formation and the pathologic fibrotic response associated with this lesion.

Xc. PULMONARY FIBROSIS

Chronic pulmonary interstitial (or alveolar) fibrosis of known and idiopathic origin presents extraordinary clinical challenges for which treatment options show limited effectiveness (Douglas *et al.*, 2000) or toxicity (Hampton *et al.*, 1994), and the median survival rate following diagnosis have changed a little (Lasky and Brody, 2000; Ryu *et al.*, 1998). At least 140 known profibrotic stimuli have been identified such as radiation, inhaled mineral and organic particles, gaseous oxidants, pharmaceutics, and infectious organisms (Kuwano *et al.*, 2001). Nevertheless, a significant proportion of patients exhibit fibrosis due to unknown or idiopathic causes, and these diseases are collectively referred to as idiopathic interstitial pneumonias (IIPs).

Severe forms of IIP, such as usual interstitial pneumonia (UIP), can be impervious to modern steroid and immunosuppressive treatment regimens, thereby emphasizing the need for novel effective therapies. Consequently, we focused on cytokine networks that may affect fibroblast activation and, hence, the progression of certain IIPs. We investigated whether the specific targeting of resident lung cells responsive to IL-4 and IL-13 exerted a therapeutic effect in an experimental model of IIP, namely the bleomycin-induced model of pulmonary fibrosis. Accordingly, IL-4, IL-13, and their corresponding receptor subunits, IL-4Rα, IL-13Rα1, and IL-13Rα2, were maximally expressed at the mRNA and protein levels in whole lung samples on day 21 or 28 after an intratracheal bleomycin challenge. The intranasal administration of IL-13PE from days 21–28, but not for 1-week period at earlier times, after bleomycin challenge had a significant therapeutic effect on histological and biochemical parameters of bleomycin-induced pulmonary fibrosis compared with the control group. The intranasal IL-13PE therapy significantly reduced the numbers of IL-4 and IL-13 receptor-positive mononuclear cells and macrophages and the levels of profibrotic cytokine and chemokine in the lungs of bleomycin-challenged mice on day 28. Thus, this study demonstrated that IL-4- and/or IL-13-binding cells are required for the maintenance of pulmonary fibrosis induced by bleomycin (Jakubzick et al., 2003b).

Furthermore, we examined the expression of IL-4, IL-13, and their corresponding receptor subunits in the various forms of IIP and normal patient groups. Molecular and immunohistochemical analysis of IL-4, IFN-γ, IL-13, IL-4R, and IL-13R subunits in surgical lung biopsies (SLBs) from 39 patients (21 UIP), 6 nonspecific interstitial pneumonia (NSIP), 8 respiratory bronchiolitic interstitial lung disease (RBILD), and 5 normal controls were performed. These analyses demonstrated that IL-13Rα2, IL-13Rα1, and IL-4Rα were present in a greater proportion of upper and lower lobe biopsies from patients with UIP than patients with NSIP and RBILD. Immunohistochemical analysis of patients with UIP, NSIP, and RBILD revealed interstitial staining for all three receptor subunits, whereas such staining was only seen in mononuclear cells present in normal SLBs. Fibroblastic foci in patients with UIP strongly stained for IL-4Rα and IL-13Rα2. Localized expression of IL-4Rα was also seen in SLBs from patients with NSIP but not in other groups. Thus, some histological subtypes of IIP are associated with increased pulmonary expression of receptor subunits responsive to IL-4 and IL-13 (Jakubzick et al., 2004a,b). Abnormal proliferation of pulmonary fibroblasts is a prominent feature of chronic pulmonary fibrotic diseases such as IIP, but it was not presently clear how this proliferative response by lung fibroblasts can be therapeutically modulated. We therefore examined whether it was possible to selectively target primary human pulmonary fibroblasts grown out of SLBs from IIP patients based on their expression of IL-4R and IL-13R subunits. Pulmonary fibroblast lines cultured from patients with the severest form of IIP, namely usual interstitial pneumonia, exhibited the greatest gene and protein expression of IL-4Rα, IL-13Rα1, and IL-13Rα2 compared with primary pulmonary fibroblast lines grown from other IIP SLBs and normal SLBs. When exposed to increasing concentrations of IL-13PE, the proliferation of primary UIP fibroblasts was inhibited to a much greater extent compared with fibroblast lines from NSIP and RBILD patient groups. Fibroblasts from normal patients exhibited minimal susceptibility to the cytotoxic effect of IL-13PE. Thus, these data suggest that the abnormal proliferative properties of human lung fibroblasts from certain IIP patient groups can be modulated in a manner that is dependent on the IL-4 and IL-13 receptor subunit expression by these cells (Jakubzick *et al.*, 2004a,b).

Future directions in the therapeutic use of IL-13PE will focus on the safety and optimization of pulmonary delivery of this therapeutic. Toxicology studies are forthcoming in nonhuman primates, where nebulization techniques will also be tested for the efficiency of therapeutic delivery of IL-13PE.

XI. CONCLUDING REMARKS

IL-13 has evolved as an important cytokine in inflammatory and neoplastic diseases. IL-13 plays a major role in cancer, pulmonary asthma, pulmonary fibrosis, *S. mansoni* infection, ulcerative colitis, and Crohn's disease. Consistent with biological activity of IL-13, the receptors for IL-13 have been found to be overexpressed on a variety of diseased cell types. A majority of human tumors express type II IL-13R, while a minority of tumors express type I IL-13R. IL-13Rα2 chain is uniquely expressed on cancer and diseased cells and serves as an efficient target for IL-13 cytotoxin *in vivo*. It sensitizes cells to the cytotoxic effect of IL-13PE cytotoxin. Normal cells that express low levels of IL-13Rα2 or not expressed at all are considerably less sensitive or not sensitive to IL-13PE cytotoxin.

These data suggest that IL-13Rα2 chain can improve sensitivity of tumors to IL-13PE. Consistent with *in vitro* cytotoxic activity of IL-13PE cytotoxin in IL-13Rα2-positive tumors, IL-13PE cytotoxin mediates remarkable anti-tumor activity in various animal models of human cancer (e.g., gliomas, squamous cell carcinoma, RCC, and AIDS-KS) without any evidence of visible toxicity. Among three different routes of administration, intratumoral administration of IL-13PE cytotoxin mediated complete eradication of established tumors. Based on these preclinical studies, several phase I/II clinical trials have been completed, which investigated safety, tolerability, and activity of IL-13PE cytotoxin in patients with recurrent glioblastoma multiforme and RCC. These promising activities of IL-13PE have resulted into phase III clinical study (PRECISE) in patients with recurrent glioblastoma. This phase III clinical trial has recently completed. In addition to cancer, IL-13PE cytotoxin has been found to have therapeutic effects in various animal models of airway diseases including pulmonary asthma and fibrosis induced by chemical drug or *S. mansoni*. Further evaluation of IL-13PE cytotoxin should be performed in these inflammatory diseases.

ACKNOWLEDGMENTS

These studies were conducted as part of collaboration between the Food and Drug Administration and NeoPharm Inc. under the Cooperative Research and Development Agreement (CRADA). The views presented in this chapter do not necessarily reflect those of the Food and Drug Administration. We thank Dr. Brenton McCright of Division of Cellular and Gene Therapies, Center for Biologics Evaluation and Research, Food and Drug Administration for critical reading of the chapter and members of Tumor Vaccines and Biotechnology Branch for their support and help.

REFERENCES

Aman, M. J., Tayebi, N., Obiri, N. I., Puri, R. K., Modi, W. S., and Leonard, W. J. (1996). cDNA cloning and characterization of the human interleukin 13 receptor alpha chain. *J. Biol. Chem.* **271**, 29265–29270.

Aversa, G., Punnonen, J., Cocks, B. G., de Waal Malefyt, R., Vega, F., Jr., Zurawski, S. M., Zurawski, G., and de Vries, J. E. (1993). An interleukin 4 (IL-4) mutant protein inhibits both IL-4 or IL-13-induced human immunoglobulin G4 (IgG4) and IgE synthesis and B cell proliferation: Support for a common component shared by IL-4 and IL-13 receptors. *J. Exp. Med.* **178**, 2213–2218.

Backman, K. S., Greenberger, P. A., and Patterson, R. (1997). Airways obstruction in patients with long-term asthma consistent with 'irreversible asthma.' *Chest* **112**, 1234–1240.

Blease, K., Jakubzick, C., Schuh, J. M., Joshi, B. H., Puri, R. K., and Hogaboam, C. M. (2001a). IL-13 fusion cytotoxin ameliorates chronic fungal-induced allergic airway disease in mice. *J. Immunol.* **167**, 6583–6592.

Blease, K., Jakubzick, C., Westwick, J., Lukacs, N., Kunkel, S. L., and Hogaboam, C. M. (2001b). Therapeutic effect of IL-13 immunoneutralization during chronic experimental fungal asthma. *J. Immunol.* **166**, 5219–5224.

Blease, K., Schuh, J. M., Jakubzick, C., Lukacs, N. W., Kunkel, S. L., Joshi, B. H., Puri, R. K., Kaplan, M. H., and Hogaboam, C. M. (2002). Stat6-deficient mice develop airway hyperresponsiveness and peribronchial fibrosis during chronic fungal asthma. *Am. J. Pathol.* **160**, 481–490.

Blease, K., Lewis, A., and Raymon, H. K. (2003). Emerging treatments for asthma. *Expert Opin. Emerg. Drugs* **8**, 71–81.

Brombacher, F. (2000). The role of interleukin-13 in infectious diseases and allergy. *Bioessays* **22**, 646–656.

Brown, K. D., Zurawski, S. M., Mosmann, T. R., and Zurawski, G. (1989). A family of small inducible proteins secreted by leukocytes are members of a new superfamily that includes leukocyte and fibroblast-derived inflammatory agents, growth factors, and indicators of various activation processes. *J. Immunol.* **142**, 679–687.

Brubaker, J. O., and Montaner, L. J. (2001). Role of interleukin-13 in innate and adaptive immunity. *Cell Mol. Biol. (Noisy-le-grand)* **47**, 637–651.

Caput, D., Laurent, P., Kaghad, M., Lelias, J. M., Lefort, S., Vita, N., and Ferrara, P. (1996). Cloning and characterization of a specific interleukin (IL)-13 binding protein structurally related to the IL-5 receptor alpha chain. *J. Biol. Chem.* **271**, 16921–16926.

Cocks, B. G., de Waal Malefyt, R., Galizzi, J. P., de Vries, J. E., and Aversa, G. (1993). IL-13 induces proliferation and differentiation of human B cells activated by the CD40 ligand. *Int. Immunol.* **5**, 657–663.

Croteau, D., Kunwar, S., Ram, Z., Sampson, J. H., Prados, M., Chang, S. M., Lang, F., Piepmeier, J., Gutin, P., Sherman, J., Dul, J., Grahn, A., *et al.* (2006). A cytokine Tumor

Targeting Agent, IL-13PE38QQR (Cintredekin Besudotox), Administered by Intraparenchymal Convection-Enhanced delivery (CED) for the Treatment of Recurrent Malignant Glioma (MG) Brain Tumors Presented at Cytokines and Inflammation, San Diego, CA.

Daines, M. O., and Hershey, G. K. (2002). A novel mechanism by which interferon-gamma can regulate interleukin (IL)-13 responses. Evidence for intracellular stores of IL-13 receptor alpha-2 and their rapid mobilization by interferon-gamma. *J. Biol. Chem.* **277,** 10387–10393.

D'Andrea, A., Ma, X., Aste-Amezaga, M., Paganin, C., and Trinchieri, G. (1995). Stimulatory and inhibitory effects of interleukin (IL)-4 and IL-13 on the production of cytokines by human peripheral blood mononuclear cells: Priming for IL-12 and tumor necrosis factor alpha production. *J. Exp. Med.* **181,** 537–546.

David, M., Bertoglio, J., and Pierre, J. (2002). TNF-alpha potentiates IL-4/IL-13-induced IL-13Ralpha2 expression. *Ann. NY Acad. Sci.* **973,** 207 209.

de Waal Malefyt, R., Figdor, C. G., Huijbens, R., Mohan-Peterson, S., Bennett, B., Culpepper, J., Dang, W., Zurawski, G., and de Vries, J. E. (1993). Effects of IL-13 on phenotype, cytokine production, and cytotoxic function of human monocytes. Comparison with IL-4 and modulation by IFN-gamma or IL-10. *J. Immunol.* **151,** 6370–6381.

de Waal Malefyt, R., Abrams, J. S., Zurawski, S. M., Lecron, J. C., Mohan-Peterson, S., Sanjanwala, B., Bennett, B., Silver, J., de Vries, J. E., and Yssel, H. (1995). Differential regulation of IL-13 and IL-4 production by human CD8+ and CD4+ Th0, Th1 and Th2 T cell clones and EBV-transformed B cells. *Int. Immunol.* **7,** 1405–1416.

Debinski, W., Obiri, N. I., Pastan, I., and Puri, R. K. (1995a). A novel chimeric protein composed of interleukin 13 and Pseudomonas exotoxin is highly cytotoxic to human carcinoma cells expressing receptors for interleukin 13 and interleukin 4. *J. Biol. Chem.* **270,** 16775–16780.

Debinski, W., Obiri, N. I., Powers, S. K., Pastan, I., and Puri, R. K. (1995b). Human glioma cells overexpress receptors for interleukin 13 and are extremely sensitive to a novel chimeric protein composed of interleukin 13 and pseudomonas exotoxin. *Clin. Cancer. Res.* **1,** 1253–1258.

Debinski, W., Miner, R., Leland, P., Obiri, N. I., and Puri, R. K. (1996). Receptor for interleukin (IL) 13 does not interact with IL4 but receptor for IL4 interacts with IL13 on human glioma cells. *J. Biol. Chem.* **271,** 22428–22433.

Defrance, T., Carayon, P., Billian, G., Guillemot, J. C., Minty, A., Caput, D., and Ferrara, P. (1994). Interleukin 13 is a B cell stimulating factor. *J. Exp. Med.* **179,** 135–143.

Devouassoux, G., Foster, B., Scott, L. M., Metcalfe, D. D., and Prussin, C. (1999). Frequency and characterization of antigen-specific IL-4- and IL-13-producing basophils and T cells in peripheral blood of healthy and asthmatic subjects. *J. Allergy Clin. Immunol.* **104,** 811–819.

Douglas, W. W., Ryu, J. H., and Schroeder, D. R. (2000). Idiopathic pulmonary fibrosis: Impact of oxygen and colchicine, prednisone, or no therapy on survival. *Am. J. Respir. Crit. Care Med.* **161,** 1172–1178.

Doyle, A. G., Herbein, G., Montaner, L. J., Minty, A. J., Caput, D., Ferrara, P., and Gordon, S. (1994). Interleukin-13 alters the activation state of murine macrophages *in vitro*: Comparison with interleukin-4 and interferon-gamma. *Eur. J. Immunol.* **24,** 1441–1445.

Fichtner-Feigl, S., Strober, W., Kawakami, K., Puri, R. K., and Kitani, A. (2006). IL-13 signaling through the IL-13alpha(2) receptor is involved in induction of TGF-beta(1) production and fibrosis. *Nat. Med.* **12,** 99–106.

Fuss, I. J., Heller, F., Boirivant, M., Leon, F., Yoshida, M., Fichtner-Feigl, S., Yang, Z., Exley, M., Kitani, A., Blumberg, R. S., Mannon, P., and Strober, W. (2004). Nonclassical CD1d-restricted NK T cells that produce IL-13 characterize an atypical Th2 response in ulcerative colitis. *J. Clin. Invest.* **113,** 1490–1497.

Gonzalez-Moreno, O., Calvo, A., Joshi, B. H., Abasolo, I., Leland, P., Wang, Z., Montuenga, L., Puri, R..K., and Green, J. E. (2005). Gene expression profiling identifies IL-13 receptor alpha

2 chain as a therapeutic target in prostate tumor cells overexpressing adrenomedullin. *Int. J. Cancer* **114,** 870–878.

Grunig, G., Warnock, M., Wakil, A. E., Venkayya, R., Brombacher, F., Rennick, D. M., Sheppard, D., Mohrs, M., Donaldson, D. D., Locksley, R. M., and Corry, D. B. (1998). Requirement for IL-13 independently of IL-4 in experimental asthma. *Science* **282,** 2261–2263.

Hampton, J., Martinez, F. J., Oren, J., Toews, G. B., and Lynch, J., III (1994). Corticosteroids in idiopathic pulmonary fibrosis (IPF): Toxicity may outweigh benefits. *Am. J. Respir. Crit. Care Med.* **149,** A878.

Hasegawa, M., Fujimoto, M., Kikuchi, K., and Takehara, K. (1997). Elevated serum levels of interleukin 4 (IL-4), IL-10, and IL-13 in patients with systemic sclerosis. *J. Rheumatol.* **24,** 328–332.

Hilton, D. J., Zhang, J. G., Metcalf, D., Alexander, W. S., Nicola, N. A., and Willson, T. A. (1996). Cloning and characterization of a binding subunit of the interleukin 13 receptor that is also a component of the interleukin 4 receptor. *Proc. Natl. Acad. Sci. USA* **93,** 497–501.

Hogaboam, C. M., Blease, K., Mehrad, B., Steinhauser, M. L., Standiford, T. J., Kunkel, S. L., and Lukacs, N. W. (2000). Chronic airway hyperreactivity, goblet cell hyperplasia, and peribronchial fibrosis during allergic airway disease induced by *Aspergillus fumigatus. Am. J. Pathol.* **156,** 723–732.

Huang, H., Hu-Li, J., Chen, H., Ben-Sasson, S. Z., and Paul, W. E. (1997). IL-4 and IL-13 production in differentiated T helper type 2 cells is not IL-4 dependent. *J. Immunol.* **159,** 3731–3738.

Husain, S. R., and Puri, R. K. (2000). Interleukin-13 fusion cytotoxin as a potent targeted agent for AIDS-Kaposi's sarcoma xenograft. *Blood* **95,** 3506–3513.

Husain, S. R., and Puri, R. K. (2003). Interleukin-13 receptor-directed cytotoxin for malignant glioma therapy: From bench to bedside. *J. Neuro-Oncology* **65,** 37–48.

Husain, S. R., Obiri, N. I., Gill, P., Zheng, T., Pastan, I., Debinski, W., and Puri, R. K. (1997). Receptor for interleukin 13 on AIDS-associated Kaposi's sarcoma cells serves as a new target for a potent Pseudomonas exotoxin-based chimeric toxin protein. *Clin. Cancer Res.* **3,** 151–156.

Husain, S. R., Joshi, B. H., and Puri, R. K. (2001). Interleukin-13 receptor as a unique target for anti-glioblastoma therapy. *Int. J. Cancer* **92,** 168–175.

Jakubzick, C., Kunkel, S. L., Joshi, B. H., Puri, R. K., and Hogaboam, C. M. (2002). Interleukin-13 fusion cytotoxin arrests *Schistosoma mansoni* egg-induced pulmonary granuloma formation in mice. *Am. J. Pathol.* **161,** 1283–1297.

Jakubzick, C., Choi, E. S., Joshi, B. H., Keane, M. P., Kunkel, S. L., Puri, R. K., and Hogaboam, C. M. (2003a). Therapeutic attenuation of pulmonary fibrosis via targeting of IL-4- and IL-13-responsive cells. *J. Immunol.* **171,** 2684–2693.

Jakubzick, C., Choi, E. S., Kunkel, S. L., Joshi, B. H., Puri, R. K., and Hogaboam, C. M. (2003b). Impact of interleukin-13 responsiveness on the synthetic and proliferative properties of Th1- and Th2-type pulmonary granuloma fibroblasts. *Am. J. Pathol.* **162,** 1475–1486.

Jakubzick, C., Choi, E. S., Carpenter, K. J., Kunkel, S. L., Evanoff, H., Martinez, F. J., Flaherty, K. R., Toews, G. B., Colby, T. V., Travis, W. D., Joshi, B. H., Puri, R. K., *et al.* (2004a). Human pulmonary fibroblasts exhibit altered interleukin-4 and interleukin-13 receptor subunit expression in idiopathic interstitial pneumonia. *Am. J. Pathol.* **164,** 1989–2001.

Jakubzick, C., Choi, E. S., Kunkel, S. L., Evanoff, H., Martinez, F. J., Puri, R. K., Flaherty, K. R., Toews, G. B., Colby, T. V., Kazerooni, E. A., Gross, B. H., Travis, W. D., *et al.* (2004b). Augmented pulmonary IL-4 and IL-13 receptor subunit expression in idiopathic interstitial pneumonia. *J. Clin. Pathol.* **57,** 477–486.

Jakubzick, C., Wen, H., Matsukawa, A., Keller, M., Kunkel, S. L., and Hogaboam, C. M. (2004c). Role of CCR4 ligands, CCL17 and CCL22, during *Schistosoma mansoni* egg-induced pulmonary granuloma formation in mice. *Am. J. Pathol.* **165**, 1211–1221.

Joshi, B. H., and Puri, R. K. (2005). Optimization of expression and purification of two biologically active chimeric fusion proteins that consist of human interleukin-13 and Pseudomonas exotoxin in *Escherichia coli. Protein Expr. Purif.* **39**, 189–198.

Joshi, B. H., Kawakami, K., Leland, P., and Puri, R. K. (2002). Heterogeneity in interleukin-13 receptor expression and subunit structure in squamous cell carcinoma of head and neck: Differential sensitivity to chimeric fusion proteins comprised of interleukin-13 and a mutated form of Pseudomonas exotoxin. *Clin. Cancer Res.* **8**, 1948–1956.

Kawakami, K., Joshi, B. H., and Puri, R. K. (2000). Sensitization of cancer cells to interleukin 13-pseudomonas exotoxin- induced cell death by gene transfer of interleukin 13 receptor alpha chain [In Process Citation]. *Hum. Gene Ther.* **11**, 1829–1835.

Kawakami, K., Husain, S. R., Bright, R. K., and Puri, R. K. (2001a). Gene transfer of interleukin 13 receptor alpha2 chain dramatically enhances the antitumor effect of IL-13 receptor-targeted cytotoxin in human prostate cancer xenografts. *Cancer Gene Ther.* **8**, 861–868.

Kawakami, K., Kawakami, M., Joshi, B. H., and Puri, R. K. (2001b). Interleukin-13 receptor-targeted cancer therapy in an immunodeficient animal model of human head and neck cancer. *Cancer Res.* **61**, 6194–6200.

Kawakami, K., Kawakami, M., Snoy, P. J., Husain, S. R., and Puri, R. K. (2001c). *In vivo* overexpression of IL-13 receptor alpha2 chain inhibits tumorigenicity of human breast and pancreatic tumors in immunodeficient mice. *J. Exp. Med.* **194**, 1743–1754.

Kawakami, K., Taguchi, J., Murata, T., and Puri, R. K. (2001d). The interleukin-13 receptor alpha2 chain: An essential component for binding and internalization but not for interleukin-13-induced signal transduction through the STAT6 pathway. *Blood* **97**, 2673–2679.

Kawakami, K., Husain, S. R., Kawakami, M., and Puri, R. K. (2002). Improved anti-tumor activity and safety of interleukin-13 receptor targeted cytotoxin by systemic continuous administration in head and neck cancer xenograft model. *Mol. Med.* **8**, 487–494.

Kawakami, M., Leland, P., Kawakami, K., and Puri, R. K. (2000). Mutation and functional analysis of IL-13 receptors in human malignant glioma cells. *Oncol. Res.* **12**, 459–467.

Kawakami, K., Kioi, M., Liu, Q., Kawakami, M., and Puri, R. K. (2005). Evidence that IL-13R alpha2 chain in human glioma cells is responsible for the antitumor activity mediated by receptor-directed cytotoxin therapy. *J. Immunother.* **28**, 193–202.

Kawakami, M., Kawakami, K., and Puri, R. K. (2002a). Apoptotic pathways of cell death induced by an interleukin-13 receptor-targeted recombinant cytotoxin in head and neck cancer cells. *Cancer Immunol. Immunother.* **50**, 691–700.

Kawakami, M., Kawakami, K., and Puri, R. K. (2002b). Intratumor administration of interleukin 13 receptor-targeted cytotoxin induces apoptotic cell death in human malignant glioma tumor xenografts. *Mol. Cancer Ther.* **1**, 999–1007.

Kioi, M., Kawakami, K., and Puri, R. K. (2004a). Analysis of antitumor activity of an interleukin-13 (IL-13) receptor-targeted cytotoxin composed of IL-13 antagonist and Pseudomonas exotoxin. *Clin. Cancer Res.* **10**, 6231–6238.

Kioi, M., Kawakami, K., and Puri, R. K. (2004b). Mechanism of action of interleukin-13 antagonist (IL-13E13K) in cells expressing various types of IL-4R. *Cell Immunol.* **229**, 41–51.

Kitani, A., Fuss, I. J., Nakamura, K., Schwartz, O. M., Usui, T., and Strober, W. (2000). Treatment of experimental (Trinitrobenzene sulfonic acid) colitis by intranasal administration of transforming growth factor (TGF)-beta1 plasmid: TGF-beta1-mediated suppression of T helper cell type 1 response occurs by interleukin (IL)-10 induction and IL-12 receptor beta2 chain downregulation. *J. Exp. Med.* **192**, 41–52.

Kitani, A., Fuss, I., Nakamura, K., Kumaki, F., Usui, T., and Strober, W. (2003). Transforming growth factor (TGF)-beta1-producing regulatory T cells induce Smad-mediated interleukin 10 secretion that facilitates coordinated immunoregulatory activity and amelioration of TGF-beta1-mediated fibrosis. *J. Exp. Med.* **198**, 1179–1188.

Kohler, I., Alliger, P., Minty, A., Caput, D., Ferrara, P., Holl-Neugebauer, B., Rank, G., and Rieber, E. P. (1994). Human interleukin-13 activates the interleukin-4-dependent transcription factor NF-IL4 sharing a DNA binding motif with an interferon-gamma-induced nuclear binding factor. *FEBS Lett.* **345**, 187–192.

Kohler, I., Alliger, P., and Rieber, E. P. (1995). Activation of gene transcription by IL-4, IL-13 and IFN-gamma through a shared DNA binding motif. *Behring Inst. Mitt.* **96**, 78–86.

Kolodsick, J. E., Toews, G. B., Jakubzick, C., Hogaboam, C., Moore, T. A., McKenzie, A., Wilke, C. A., Chrisman, C. J., and Moore, B. B. (2004). Protection from fluorescein isothiocyanate-induced fibrosis in IL-13-deficient, but not IL-4-deficient, mice results from impaired collagen synthesis by fibroblasts. *J. Immunol.* **172**, 4068–4076.

Kotsimbos, T. C., Ernst, P., and Hamid, Q. A. (1996). Interleukin-13 and interleukin-4 are coexpressed in atopic asthma. *Proc. Assoc. Am. Physicians* **108**, 368–373.

Krieg, M., Marti, H. H., and Plate, K. H. (1998). Coexpression of erythropoietin and vascular endothelial growth factor in nervous system tumors associated with von Hippel-Lindau tumor suppressor gene loss of function. *Blood* **92**, 3388–3393.

Kunwar, S., Pai, L. H., and Pastan, I. (1993). Cytotoxicity and antitumor effects of growth factor-toxin fusion proteins on human glioblastoma multiforme cells. *J. Neurosurg.* **79**, 569–576.

Kunwar, S., Prados, M., Lang, F., Fleming, C., Croteau, D., Aldape, K., Gutin, P., Piepmeier, J., Berger, M. S., McDermott, M., and Puri, R. (2003). Intracerebral convection-enhanced delivery (CED) of IL-13PE38QQR, a recombinant tumor-targeted cytotoxin, in recurrent malignant glioma in recurrent malignant glioma: A Phase I. *Neuro-oncology* **5**, 387.

Kunwar, S., Prados, M., Chang, S. M., Lang, F., Aldape, K., Piepmeier, J., Gutin, P., Croteau, D., and Puri, R. (2005a). Convection-Enhanced Delivery of IL-13PE38QQR: Results of a Multicenter Phase I study in Recurrent Malignant Glioma. Presented at AANS, New Orleans, La.

Kunwar, S., Ram, Z., Sampson, J. H., Prados, M., Chang, S. M., Lang, F., Piepmeier, J., Gutin, P., Croteau, D., and Puri, R. (2005b). Peritumoral convection-enhanced delivery (CED) of IL-13PE38QQR (IL13PE): Results of multicenter phase 1 studies in recurrent high grade glioma (HGG). *Neuro-oncology* **7**, 114.

Kuwano, K., Hagimoto, N., and Hara, N. (2001). Molecular mechanisms of pulmonary fibrosis and current treatment. *Curr. Mol. Med.* **1**, 551–573.

Kuzel, T., Smith, J, II., Urba, W., Fox, B., Moudgil, T., Strauss, L., Joshi, B., and Puri, R. (2002). *IL13-PE38QQR cytototxind in advanced renal cell carcinoma (RCC): Phase 1 and pharmacokinetic study.* Presented at American Society of Clinical Oncology (ASCO), San Franscisco, CA.

Kuznetsov, V. A., and Puri, R. K. (1999). Kinetic analysis of high affinity forms of interleukin (IL)-13 receptors: Suppression of IL-13 binding by IL-2 receptor gamma chain. *Biophys. J.* **77**, 154–172.

Lang, F., Kunwar, S., Strauss, L., Piepmeier, J., McDermott, M., Fleming, C., Sherman, J., Raizer, J., Alalpe, K., Yung, W. K., Husain, S. R., Chang, S. M., *et al.* (2002). "A clinical study of convection-enhanced delivery of IL-13PE38QQR cytotoxin pre- and post-resection of recurrent GBM." American Society of Neuro-Oncologists, Chicago.

Lasky, J. A., and Brody, A. R. (2000). Interstitial fibrosis and growth factors. *Environ. Health Perspect.* **108**(Suppl. 4), 751–762.

Lee, C. G., Homer, R. J., Zhu, Z., Lanone, S., Wang, X., Koteliansky, V., Shipley, J. M., Gotwals, P., Noble, P., Chen, Q., Senior, R. M., and Elias, J. A. (2001). Interleukin-13 induces tissue fibrosis by selectively stimulating and activating transforming growth factor beta(1). *J. Exp. Med.* **194**, 809–821.

Lee, C. G., Cho, S. J., Kang, M. J., Chapoval, S. P., Lee, P. J., Noble, P. W., Yehualaeshet, T., Lu, B., Flavell, R. A., Milbrandt, J., Homer, R. J., and Elias, J. A. (2004). Early growth response gene 1-mediated apoptosis is essential for transforming growth factor beta1-induced pulmonary fibrosis. *J. Exp. Med.* **200**, 377–389.

Lin, J. X., Migone, T. S., Tsang, M., Friedmann, M., Weatherbee, J. A., Zhou, L., Yamauchi, A., Bloom, E. T., Mietz, J., John, S., and Leonard, W. J. (1995). The role of shared receptor motifs and common Stat proteins in the generation of cytokine pleiotropy and redundancy by IL-2, IL-4, IL-7, IL-13, and IL-15. *Immunity* **2**, 331–339.

Maini, A., Hillman, G., Haas, G. P., Wang, C. Y., Montecillo, E., Hamzavi, F., Pontes, J. E., Leland, P., Pastan, I., Debinski, W., and Puri, R. K. (1997). Interleukin-13 receptors on human prostate carcinoma cell lines represent a novel target for a chimeric protein composed of IL-13 and a mutated form of Pseudomonas exotoxin. *J. Urol.* **158**, 948–953.

McKenzie, A. N., Culpepper, J. A., de Waal Malefyt, R., Briere, F., Punnonen, J., Aversa, G., Sato, A., Dang, W., Cocks, B. G., Menon, S., de Vries, J. E., Banchereau, J., *et al.* (1993). Interleukin 13, a T-cell-derived cytokine that regulates human monocyte and B-cell function. *Proc. Natl. Acad. Sci. USA* **90**, 3735–3739.

McKenzie, G. J., Emson, C. L., Bell, S. E., Anderson, S., Fallon, P., Zurawski, G., Murray, R., Grencis, R., and McKenzie, A. N. (1998). Impaired development of Th2 cells in IL-13-deficient mice. *Immunity* **9**, 423–432.

McKenzie, G. J., Fallon, P. G., Emson, C. L., Grencis, R. K., and McKenzie, A. N. (1999). Simultaneous disruption of interleukin (IL)-4 and IL-13 defines individual roles in T helper cell type 2-mediated responses. *J. Exp. Med.* **189**, 1565–1572.

Mentink-Kane, M. M., and Wynn, T. A. (2004). Opposing roles for IL-13 and IL-13 receptor alpha 2 in health and disease. *Immunol Rev.* **202**, 191–202.

Minty, A., Chalon, P., Derocq, J. M., Dumont, X., Guillemot, J. C., Kaghad, M., Labit, C., Leplatois, P., Liauzun, P., Miloux, B., Minty, C., Casellas, P., *et al.* (1993). Interleukin-13 is a new human lymphokine regulating inflammatory and immune responses. *Nature* **362**, 248–250.

Murata, T., and Puri, R. K. (1997). Comparison of IL-13- and IL-4-induced signaling in EBV-immortalized human B cells. *Cellullar Immunology* **175**, 33–40.

Murata, T., Noguchi, P. D., and Puri, R. K. (1995). Receptors for interleukin (IL)-4 do not associate with the common gamma chain, and IL-4 induces the phosphorylation of JAK2 tyrosine kinase in human colon carcinoma cells. *J. Biol. Chem.* **270**, 30829–30836.

Murata, T., Noguchi, P. D., and Puri, R. K. (1996). IL-13 induces phosphorylation and activation of JAK2 Janus kinase in human colon carcinoma cell lines: Similarities between IL-4 and IL-13 signaling. *J. Immunol.* **156**, 2972–2978.

Murata, T., Obiri, N. I., and Puri, R. K. (1997). Human ovarian-carcinoma cell lines express IL-4 and IL-13 receptors: Comparison between IL-4- and IL-13-induced signal transduction. *Int. J. Cancer* **70**, 230–240.

Murata, T., Husain, S. R., Mohri, H., and Puri, R. K. (1998a). Two different IL-13 receptor chains are expressed in normal human skin fibroblasts, and IL-4 and IL-13 mediate signal transduction through a common pathway. *Int. Immunol.* **10**, 1103–1110.

Murata, T., Obiri, N. I., and Puri, R. K. (1998b). Structure of and signal transduction through interleukin-4 and interleukin-13 receptors (review). *Int J Mol Med* **1**, 551–557.

Obiri, N. I., Debinski, W., Leonard, W. J., and Puri, R. K. (1995). Receptor for interleukin 13. Interaction with interleukin 4 by a mechanism that does not involve the common gamma chain shared by receptors for interleukins 2, 4, 7, 9, and 15. *J. Biol. Chem.* **270**, 8797–8804.

Obiri, N. I., Husain, S. R., Debinski, W., and Puri, R. K. (1996). Interleukin 13 inhibits growth of human renal cell carcinoma cells independently of the p140 interleukin 4 receptor chain. *Clin. Cancer Res.* **2**, 1743–1749.

Obiri, N. I., Leland, P., Murata, T., Debinski, W., and Puri, R. K. (1997a). The IL-13 receptor structure differs on various cell types and may share more than one component with IL-4 receptor. *J. Immunol.* **158**, 756–764.

Obiri, N. I., Murata, T., Debinski, W., and Puri, R. K. (1997b). Modulation of interleukin (IL)-13 binding and signaling by the gamma c chain of the IL-2 receptor. *J. Biol. Chem.* **272**, 20251–20258.

Ollerenshaw, S. L., and Woolcock, A. J. (1992). Characteristics of the inflammation in biopsies from large airways of subjects with asthma and subjects with chronic airflow limitation. *Am. Rev. Respir. Dis.* **145**, 922–927.

Parney, I. F., Kunwar, S., McDermott, M., Berger, M., Prados, M., Cha, S., Croteau, D., Puri, R. K., and Chang, S. M. (2005). Neuroradiographic changes following convection-enhanced delivery of the recombinant cytotoxin interleukin 13-PE38QQR for recurrent malignant glioma. *J. Neurosurg.* **102**, 267–275.

Prados, M., Lang, F., Strauss, L., Fleming, C., Aldape, K., Kunwar, S., Yung, W. K. A., Husain, S. R., Chang, S. M., Gutin, P., Raizer, J., Piepmeier, J., et al. (2001). Pre and post-resection interstitial infusions of IL13-PE38QQR cytotoxin: Phase I study in recurrent respectable malignant glioma. Presented at First Quadrennial Meeting—World Federation of Neuro-Oncology, Washington, DC.

Prados, M., Lang, F., Sherman, J., Strauss, L., Fleming, C., Alalpe, K., Kunwar, S., Yung, W. K., Chang, S. M., Husain, S. R., Gutin, P., Raizer, J., et al. (2002a). Convection-enhanced delivery (CED) by positive pressure infusion for intra-tumoral and peri-tumoral administration of IL-13PE38QQR a recombinant tumor-targeted cytotoxin in recurrent malignant glioma. *J. Neuro-Oncology* **4**, S78.

Prados, M., Lang, F., Strauss, L., Fleming, C., Alalpe, K., Kunwar, S., Yung, W. K., Chang, S. M., Husain, S. R., Gutin, P., Raizer, J., Piepmeier, J., et al. (2002b). Intratumoral and intracerebral microinfusion of Il13-PE38QQR cytotoxin: Phase I/II study of pre- and post-resection infusions in recurrent resectable malignant glioma. *Am. Soc. Clin. Oncol.*

Prados, M., Kunwar, S., Lang, F., Ram, Z., Westphal, M., Barnett, G. H., Sampson, J. H., Croteau, D., and Puri, R. K. (2005). Final results of PhaseI/II studies of IL-13PE38QQR administered intratumorally (IT) and/or peritumorally (PT) via convection-enhanced delivery (CED) in patients undergoing tumor resection for recurrent malignant glioma. *J. Clin. Oncol.* **23**, 115S.

Punnonen, J., Aversa, G., Cocks, B. G., McKenzie, A. N., Menon, S., Zurawski, G., de Waal Malefyt, R., and de Vries, J. E. (1993). Interleukin 13 induces interleukin 4-independent IgG4 and IgE synthesis and CD23 expression by human B cells. *Proc. Natl. Acad. Sci. USA* **90**, 3730–3734.

Puri, R. K., Leland, P., Obiri, N. I., Husain, S. R., Kreitman, R. J., Haas, G. P., Pastan, I., and Debinski, W. (1996). Targeting of interleukin-13 receptor on human renal cell carcinoma cells by a recombinant chimeric protein composed of interleukin-13 and a truncated form of Pseudomonas exotoxin A (PE38QQR). *Blood* **87**, 4333–4339.

Rahaman, S. O., Sharma, P., Harbor, P. C., Aman, M. J., Vogelbaum, M. A., and Haque, S. J. (2002). IL-13R(alpha)2, a decoy receptor for IL-13 acts as an inhibitor of IL-4-dependent signal transduction in glioblastoma cells. *Cancer Res.* **62**, 1103–1109.

Rahaman, S. O., Vogelbaum, M. A., and Haque, S. J. (2005). Aberrant Stat3 signaling by interleukin-4 in malignant glioma cells: Involvement of IL-13Ralpha2. *Cancer Res.* **65**, 2956–2963.

Ray, A., and Cohn, L. (1999). Th2 cells and GATA-3 in asthma: New insights into the regulation of airway inflammation. *J. Clin. Invest.* **104**, 985–993.

Ray, A., and Cohn, L. (2000). Altering the Th1/Th2 balance as a therapeutic strategy in asthmatic diseases. *Curr. Opin. Investig. Drugs* **1**, 442–448.

Ryu, J. H., Colby, T. V., and Hartman, T. E. (1998). Idiopathic pulmonary fibrosis: Current concepts. *Mayo Clin. Proc.* **73**, 1085–1101.

Sampson, J. H., Friedman, A. H., Reardon, D. A., Friedman, H. S., Provenzale, J. M., Bigner, D. D., Brady, M., Raghavan, R., Pedain, C., Archer, G. E., Lally-Batts, D., Grahan, A., et al. (2004). Convection-Enhanced Delivery of IL-13PE38QQR in Malignant Glioma: Effect of Catheter Placement on Drug Distribution.

Sanderson, N., Factor, V., Nagy, P., Kopp, J., Kondaiah, P., Wakefield, L., Roberts, A. B., Sporn, M. B., and Thorgeirsson, S. S. (1995). Hepatic expression of mature transforming growth factor beta 1 in transgenic mice results in multiple tissue lesions. *Proc. Natl. Acad. Sci. USA* **92**, 2572–2576.

Smerz-Bertling, C., and Duschl, A. (1995). Both interleukin 4 and interleukin 13 induce tyrosine phosphorylation of the 140-kDa subunit of the interleukin 4 receptor. *J. Biol. Chem.* **270**, 966–970.

Terabe, M., Matsui, S., Noben-Truath, N., Chen, H., Watson, C., Donaldson, D. D., Carbone, D. P., Paul, W. E., and Berzofsky, J. A. (2000). NKT cell-mediated repression of tumor immunosurveillance by IL-13 and the IL-4R-STAT6 pathway. *Nat. Immunol.* **1**, 515–520.

Umetsu, D. T., and De Kruyff, R. H. (1997). Th1 and Th2 CD4+cells in the pathogenesis of allergic diseases. *Proc. Soc. Exp. Biol. Med.* **215**, 11–20.

Vita, N., Lefort, S., Laurent, P., Caput, D., and Ferrara, P. (1995). Characterization and comparison of the interleukin 13 receptor with the interleukin 4 receptor on several cell types. *J. Biol. Chem.* **270**, 3512–3517.

Weingart, J., Grossman, S. A., Bohan, E., Fisher, J. D., Strauss, L., and Puri, R. K. (2001a). Phase I/II study of interstitial infusion of IL13-PE38QQR cytotoxin in recurrent malignant glioma. Presented at First Qudrennial Meeting—World Federation of Neuro-Oncology, Washington, DC.

Weingart, J., Strauss, L., Grossman, S. A., Markett, J., Tatter, S., Fisher, J. D., Fleming, C., and Puri, R. K. (2001b). Phase I/II study: Intra-tumoral infusion of IL13-PE38QQR cytotoxin for recurrent supratentorial malignat.

Weingart, J., Tatter, S. S. R., Mikkelsen, T., Barnett, G., Fisher, J., Grossman, S. A., Croteau, D., Grahan, A., Sherman, J., and Puri, R. (2003). Intratumoral convection-enhanced delivery of IL-13PE38QQR cytototxin for recurrent malignant glioma without planned resection: A Phase I/II study. Presented at 8th Annual Meeting of the Society for Neuro-Oncology, Keystone, CO.

Welham, M. J., Learmonth, L., Bone, H., and Schrader, J. W. (1995). Interleukin-13 signal transduction in lymphohemopoietic cells. Similarities and differences in signal transduction with interleukin-4 and insulin. *J. Biol. Chem.* **270**, 12286–12296.

Wills-Karp, M., Luyimbazi, J., Xu, X., Schofield, B., Neben, T. Y., Karp, C. L., and Donaldson, D. D. (1998). Interleukin-13: Central mediator of allergic asthma. *Science* **282**, 2258–2261.

Wood, N., Whitters, M. J., Jacobson, B. A., Witek, J., Sypek, J. P., Kasaian, M., Eppihimer, M. J., Unger, M., Tanaka, T., Goldman, S. J., Collins, M., Donaldson, D., et al. (2003). Enhanced interleukin (IL)-13 responses in mice lacking IL-13 receptor alpha 2. *J. Exp. Med.* **197**, 703–709.

Wynn, T. A. (2003). IL-13 effector functions. *Annu. Rev. Immunol.* **21**, 425–456.

Yang, G., Li, L., Volk, A., Emmell, E., Petley, T., Giles-Komar, J., Rafferty, P., Lakshminarayanan, M., Griswold, D. E., Bugelski, P. J., and Das, A. M. (2005). Therapeutic dosing with anti-interleukin-13 monoclonal antibody inhibits asthma progression in mice. *J. Pharmacol. Exp. Ther.* **313**, 8–15.

Yoshikawa, M., Nakajima, T., Tsukidate, T., Matsumoto, K., Iida, M., Otori, N., Haruna, S., Moriyama, H., and Saito, H. (2003). TNF-alpha and IL-4 regulate expression of IL-13 receptor alpha2 on human fibroblasts. *Biochem. Biophys. Res. Commun.* **312,** 1248–1255.

Zhu, Z., Homer, R. J., Wang, Z., Chen, Q., Geba, G. P., Wang, J., Zhang, Y., and Elias, J. A. (1999). Pulmonary expression of interleukin-13 causes inflammation, mucus hypersecretion, subepithelial fibrosis, physiologic abnormalities, and eotaxin production. *J. Clin. Invest.* **103,** 779–788.

Zund, G., Madara, J. L., Dzus, A. L., Awtrey, C. S., and Colgan, S. P. (1996). Interleukin-4 and interleukin-13 differentially regulate epithelial chloride secretion. *J. Biol. Chem.* **271,** 7460–7464.

Zurawski, G., and de Vries, J. E. (1994a). Interleukin 13 elicits a subset of the activities of its close relative interleukin 4. *Stem Cells* **12,** 169–174.

Zurawski, G., and de Vries, J. E. (1994b). Interleukin 13, an interleukin 4-like cytokine that acts on monocytes and B cells, but not on T cells. *Immunol Today* **15,** 19–26.

Zurawski, S. M., Chomarat, P., Djossou, O., Bidaud, C., McKenzie, A. N., Miossec, P., Banchereau, J., and Zurawski, G. (1995). The primary binding subunit of the human interleukin-4 receptor is also a component of the interleukin-13 receptor. *J. Biol. Chem.* **270,** 13869–13878.

20

INTERLEUKINS, INFLAMMATION, AND MECHANISMS OF ALZHEIMER'S DISEASE

DAVID WEISMAN,*,† EDWIN HAKIMIAN,*
AND GILBERT J. HO*,†

*Department of Neurosciences and the Alzheimer's Disease Research Center
University of California, San Diego, California 92093
†Neurology Service, Department of Veterans Affairs Medical Center
San Diego, California 92161

Alzheimer's disease (AD) is the most common progressive neurodegenerative form of dementia in the elderly and is characterized neuropathologically by neurofibrillary tangles (NFT), amyloid neuritic plaques (NP), and prominent synaptic and eventually neuronal loss. Although the molecular basis of AD is not clearly understood, a neuroinflammatory process, triggered by $A\beta42$, plays a central role in the neurodegenerative process. This inflammatory process is driven by activated microglia, astrocytes and the induction of proinflammatory molecules and related signaling pathways, leading to both synaptic and neuronal damage as well as further inflammatory cell activation. Epidemiologic data as well as clinical trial evidence suggest that nonsteroidal anti-inflammatory drug (NSAID) use may decrease the incidence of AD, further supporting a role for inflammation in AD pathogenesis. Although the precise molecular and cellular relationship between AD and inflammation remains unclear, interleukins and cytokines might induce activation of signaling pathways leading to futher inflammation and neuronal injury. This chapter will discuss the association between interleukins and neurodegeneration in AD and highlight the significance of genetic and clinical aspects of interleukins in disease expression and progression. As part of an emerging inflammatory signaling network underlying AD pathogenesis, β-amyloid ($A\beta$) stimulates the glial and microglial production of interleukins and other cytokines, leading to an ongoing inflammatory cascade and contributing to synaptic dysfunction and loss, and later, neuronal death. Inflammatory pathways involving interleukin and cytokine signaling might suggest potential targets for intervention and influence the development of novel therapies to circumvent synaptic and neuronal dysfunction ultimately leading to AD neurodegeneration. © 2006 Elsevier Inc.

I. INTRODUCTION

Alzheimer's disease (AD) is the most common cause of progressive neurodegenerative dementia in the elderly and is characterized clinically by the insidious onset of memory loss accompanied by dysfunction affecting other additional cognitive domains. Because of progressive widespread cortical involvement, AD eventually leads to loss of functional abilities and the emergence of behavioral abnormalities such as hallucinations and delusions. Neuropathological findings of AD include amyloid-containing neuritic plaques (NP), tau-bearing neurofibrillary tangles (NFT), synaptic loss, and eventually neuronal damage. Significant neuronal loss occurs in the cholinergic nuclei of the basal forebrain, which project widely to cortical areas and account for observed cholinergic neurotransmission deficits that contribute, in part, to memory decline.

Plaques are recognized as one of the hallmark lesions of AD brain and undergo morphologic evolution over several stages. As with other proteins centrally related to neurodegeneration, β-amyloid (Aβ) tends to self-aggregate, forming large insoluble β-pleated sheet structures. Increased production of extracellular Aβ coupled with decreased clearance, leads to its aggregation and deposition, forming diffuse plaques. Plaques then coalesce and mature with the further accumulation of insoluble fibrillar Aβ and subsequently form senile plaques or NPs in later stages with the appearance of abnormal Aβ-induced neuritic dystrophy and reactive sprouting. NPs also become associated with numerous activated inflammatory cells, cytokines, acute-phase reactants such as the protease inhibitor, α-1-antichymotrypsin (α-1-ACT), and other inflammatory markers. Eventually, as the disease progresses in severity and plaques become "burnt out," severe neocortical neuronal loss is observed in surrounding brain tissue (Ho et al., 2005a).

Aβ in AD brain is derived intracellularly from proteolytic cleavage of a larger amyloid precursor protein (APP) through the concerted action of both β-secretase and γ-secretase complex [presenilin 1 (PS1)]. APP cleavage to Aβ occurs intramembranously by a unique and previously unknown intramembranous catalytic mechanism (Brunkan and Goate, 2005; De Strooper, 2003). Following proteolysis, subsequent intracellular trafficking of Aβ via trans-Golgi network occurs and results in packaging of the peptide into secretory vesicles for eventual release into the extracellular environment (Selkoe et al., 1996). Aβ overproduction, and the above mechanisms, appear central to the clinical expression of AD, both in sporadic and familial, early-onset cases. Of several species of Aβ found in AD, Aβ42, rather than Aβ40, represents the predominant form of the peptide deposited in NPs, whereas Aβ40 is likely more involved in vascular amyloid deposition.

NFT, the other major well-recognized pathological hallmark of AD, accumulate early in AD brain as well as in other neurodegenerative diseases, including so-called tauopathies such as frontotemporal dementia (Neary et al., 2005). Caused by abnormal hyperphosphorylation of tau by the putative tau kinases, glycogen synthase kinase-3β (GSK-3β) and cyclin-dependent kinase 5 (cdk5), NFTs accumulate intracellularly in the neuronal cytoplasm. Tau normally binds to microtubules to facilitate microtubular and cytoskeletal stability, but hyperphosphorylated tau displays a strong tendency to aggregate abnormally, leading initially to formation of paired helical filaments and then larger NFTs. Subsequently, microtubular and cytoskeletal instability leads to impaired axonal transport to presynaptic and postsynaptic terminals, causing energy and nutritional depletion at these sites. Studies visualizing axonal transport using in vitro models harboring tau mutations show that transport is impaired (Mandelkow et al., 2003).

Despite their prominence as neuropathological hallmarks of AD brain, the importance of NP and NFT to the pathogenesis of AD is not entirely clear.

Although NFTs have been shown to correlate with cognitive dysfunction in AD (Terwel *et al.*, 2002), the role of NP remains controversial because of their consistently poor association with cognitive measures. It is now believed that amyloid accumulation within plaques may represent an extraneuronal protective response to neuronal injury and amyloid overproduction or simply an epiphenomenon of the disease process (Carter and Lippa, 2001). Even though not directly involved in neuronal damage, NPs do provide evidence of amyloid-related induction of the inflammation in AD brain due to the sequestration of inflammatory and acute-phase proteins. Recent evidence suggests that synaptotoxicity and neurotoxicity might actually be due to formation of soluble oligomeric Aβ rather than the larger and insoluble fibrillar Aβ found within NPs (Walsh *et al.*, 2002), and inflammatory processes could mediate Aβ oligomer toxicity (White *et al.*, 2005). Of the key neuropathological changes in AD, the loss of neocortical presynaptic terminals, the structural alteration that best correlates with cognitive decline, appears to be most important (DeKosky and Scheff, 1990; Terry *et al.*, 1991). Thus, the clinical expression of AD is also related to early neocortical synaptic injury and loss, followed later by more overt neuronal dropout.

II. THE INFLAMMATORY RESPONSE IN AD

Activated central nervous system (CNS) microglia as well as astrocytes play critical roles in promoting and perhaps sustaining cellular injury. As cells of monocyte lineage residing within the CNS, microglia are important for normal brain immunological function by supporting neurons through immune surveillance, antigen presentation, phagocytosis of debris, and the secretion of immune effectors such as cytokines, complement components, excitatory amino acids, oxygen radicals, and neurotrophins which can regulate glial proliferation and phagocytic activity (Elkabes *et al.*, 1996; Morgan *et al.*, 2005). Stimulated by foreign epitopes and other immunologically active molecules, microglia transform rapidly from a ramified, resting state into an active macrophagelike morphology, and once activated, microglia migrate to sites of neuronal injury to remove injured cells and accumulating debris by phagocytosis (Bruce-Keller, 1999).

Perhaps not as well emphasized as microglia, astrocytes are equally important in brain immunologic defense and in the response to injury. Well known is the association of CNS astrocytes with the vascular endothelium to form the blood–brain barrier, an essential structure limiting the entry of injurious substances into the brain (Dong and Benveniste, 2001). Yet, astrocytes also act as antigen-presenting cells (Girvin *et al.*, 2002), displaying class I and II major histocompatibility antigen (MHC; Dong and Benveniste, 2001), as well as providing structural and nutritive support to the surrounding neurons. With relevance to AD, they are also active in synaptic maintenance and can augment the number of functional synapses (Ullian *et al.*, 2001). In the presence of injury, glial activation and proliferation occurs with characteristic biochemical and cellular alterations. By producing soluble factors, such as cytokines and inflammatory mediators, activated astrocytes, neurons and microglia engage in a complex interaction, ultimately leading to microglial release of proinflammatory substances, excitotoxins, and other substances that may in turn further activate astrocytes and induce neuronal damage (Giulian and Baker, 1985).

When compared to normal controls, brains with AD pathology show more activated microglia diffusely and in physical proximity to plaques, where they are found clustering both in and around these lesions. The colocalization of microglia and astrocytes with NPs suggests that they are activated by direct contact with fibrillar $A\beta$, but soluble $A\beta$ has also been shown to stimulate microglial secretion of proinflammatory cytokines such as chemokines, complement components, and free radicals (McGeer and McGeer, 2001). $A\beta$ is believed to activate microglia via direct stimulation and autocrine processes involving heat-shock proteins (Kakimura *et al.*, 2002). Normally, microglia effectively contributes to the balance between $A\beta$ production and clearance through their scavenging of extracellular $A\beta$ and the $A\beta$ in early diffuse plaques. Yet, with the formation of insoluble $A\beta$ aggregates in NPs, markedly increased activation and migration of microglia into and around NPs is triggered, followed by the induction of microglial proinflammatory surface markers CD45, CD36, and CD40. With CD40 expression and subsequent cytokine production, plaque-associated microglia, despite their increased activity, become highly ineffective in phagocytizing insoluble $A\beta$, allowing for further abnormal $A\beta$ accumulation in plaques. The expression of MHC class II, further release of oxygen radicals which provoke oxidative damage, as well as the release of a host of compounds including complement and interleukins, all accelerate the inflammation and neuronal damage (Town *et al.*, 2005; Townsend *et al.*, 2005). Beyond this, another hypothesis suggests that microglia, because of their ability to sequester $A\beta$, might actually directly accelerate the conversion of oligomeric $A\beta$ to fibrillar $A\beta$ and its depostion in NPs (Nagele *et al.*, 2003).

Astrocytes are also involved in the clearance of debris and other extraneous material from the interstitial space, and gliosis surrounding NPs in AD brain reflects an attempt by astrocytes to remove accumulating $A\beta$, which then is contained within the astrocytic cytoplasmic space. Yet, evidence suggests that in AD brain, this process may actually contribute to plaque formation rather than reduction. Astrocytes, because of limited capacity to retain $A\beta$, may actually undergo lysis and release large amounts of $A\beta$ back into the extracellular space, promoting plaque development (Nagele *et al.*, 2003).

III. INTERLEUKINS AS CNS MODULATORS
OF INFLAMMATION

Cytokines act in both an autocrine and a paracrine fashion to affect, among other processes, inflammation. The biological activity of cytokines is extremely complex and depends on target cell type and state of activation, the local cytokine concentration, receptor type, and interaction with other cytokine mediators, and because of this, the precise effect of cytokines on specific tissue types may be difficult to predict. In general, during peripheral inflammation, cytokines released by activated macrophages play a role in immunomodulation, either by activating other inflammatory cells or by inhibiting their function, thereby establishing a balance of these influences (Fujiwara and Kobayashi, 2005). Failure of coordinated activity of cytokines, inflammatory cells, and other inflammatory triggers leads to inflammatory disorders. Interleukins are an important class of inflammatory cytokines in many organs and tissues. Initially studied in macrophages, blood leukocytes, and other bone marrow origin cells (Balkwill, 1988), interleukins act as cell messengers, facilitating communication between cells within the peripheral immune system, and are now recognized to act as mediators between the immune system and the CNS (Fujiwara and Kobayashi, 2005). They direct the inflammatory response within the CNS by activating several intracellular signaling pathways within multiple CNS cell types, as well as coordinating signaling between neurons and astrocytes.

IV. INTERLEUKINS AND THE
CLINICOPATHOLOGIC
CHARACTERISTICS OF AD

A. INTERLEUKIN-1 AND AD PATHOGENESIS

Several cytokines thought to be important in AD pathogenesis have been identified in vulnerable areas in the AD brain and cytokine expression is upregulated in AD brain, especially within areas closely apposed to AD lesions. As summarized in Table I, these include interleukin-1α (IL-1α), IL-1β, IL-6, IL-4, IL-8, IL-10, IL-13, and tumor necrosis factor-α (TNF-α), many of which are likely derived from activated microglia (Akiyama et al., 2000; McGeer and McGeer, 2001).

IL-1, a potent proinflammatory cytokine, is increased in microglia associated with NPs compared to those found in diffuse amyloid plaques (Griffin et al., 1995) and is overexpressed by sixfold in AD brain tissue compared with normal brain (Griffin et al., 1989). IL-1β levels are highest in frontal cortex in AD brain but are also significantly elevated in parietal cortex,

TABLE 1. Key Interleukins Associated with AD Pathogenesis[a]

Interleukin	Biological action in AD	Receptor involved	Antagonist(s)	Detected in human sample	Genes associated with AD risk	Relevance to AD pathogenesis
IL-1	↑ Inflammation	sIL-1R	sIL-1RII (decoy), sIL-1Ra	Brain (NP), CSF, plasma	IL-1α (−899), IL-1β (−511), IL-1β (+3953), IL-1Ra (+2018)	Primary inflammatory IL in AD; possible increased AD risk; association with ↑ amyloid, abnormal tau, synapse loss
IL-4	↓ Inflammation	sIL-4R (Th2-type cytokine receptor)	Unknown	Brain (IL-4 mRNA), blood monocytes	IL-4 (+33)—lacks association with AD risk	Anti-inflammatory; ? decreased in AD; peripherally, may be induced by AChE inhibitors and decrease peripheral IL-1
IL-6	↑ Inflammation	sIL-6R, gp130	Unknown	Brain (DP), CSF, plasma	IL-6 (−174), IL-6 VNTR	Proinflammatory; may act in early plaque development; association with abnormal tau and ↓ synapse function
IL-8	↑ Inflammation	IL-8RB/CXCR2	Unknown	IL-8RB in brain (NP)	Unknown	Potent chemokine, possibly recruits microglia/glia into NP
IL-10	↓ Inflammation	sIL-10Rα chain	Unknown	Brain (IL-10 mRNA), blood monocytes	IL-10 (−1082), IL-10 (−819), IL-10 (−592)	Potent anti-inflammatory effect; ? decreased in AD; may block Aβ-induced IL-1 expression
IL-13	↓ Inflammation	IL-13Rα1, IL-4Rα	IL-13Rα2 (decoy)	Brain (IL-13 mRNA)	Unknown	Anti-inflammatory; ? decreased in AD; may also prevent IL-1 expression

[a]IL, interleukin; NP, neuritic plaques; DP, diffuse plaques; CSF, cerebrospinal fluid; AChE, acetylcholinesterase; VNTR, variable number tandem repeat.

temporal cortex, thalamus, hypothalamus, and other areas compared to vascular dementia and normal brain (Cacabelos et al., 1994). IL-1 receptor antagonist (IL-1Ra) protein immunoreactivity is also greatly increased in neurons,
especially around plaques in AD brain compared to control brain (Yasuhara
et al., 1997). During plaque development, IL-1-positive microglia appear
early, but their presence varies according to the degree of neuritic pathology,
disappearing ultimately with plaque "burn-out," suggesting that IL-1 may be
important in driving plaque-associated neuritic pathology and neuronal dystrophy in AD (Griffin et al., 1995). IL-1 is also associated with α-1-ACT, an
acute-phase reactant in NPs, and induces another neurotrophic cytokine,
S100B, which is elevated in AD brain (Marshak et al., 1992), both contributing to further neuronal dystrophy. Evidence also suggests that p38 mitogen-
activated protein kinase (p38 MAPK) signaling may play a role in neuronal
injury associated with IL-1. In AD brain, IL-1-overexpressing microglia
are frequently associated with neurons bearing both p38 MAPK and hyperphosphorylated tau immunoreactivity, and p38 MAPK immunoreactivity
correlates significantly with hyperphosphorylated tau (Sheng et al., 2001a).

Studies examining cerebrospinal fluid (CSF) and plasma levels of IL-1
signaling components provide conflicting results. IL-1 levels are increased in
CSF in some studies (Blum-Degen et al., 1995; Cacabelos et al., 1991a;
Garlind et al., 1999) but are unchanged in others (Pirttila et al., 1994).
Differing results are similarly found with the measurement of IL-1 plasma
levels in AD, with both increased levels found (Licastro et al., 2000a), as well
as unchanged levels among normal control, AD, and vascular dementia
subjects (Cacabelos et al., 1991b). Moreover, levels of molecules related to
the IL-1 family and IL-1 function, including naturally occurring IL-1 soluble
receptor antagonist type II (sIL-1RII) and IL-1Ra were examined. Mecha-
nistically, sIL-1RII acts as a signaling "decoy" preventing stimulation of the
active type I receptor that mediates intracellular signaling, while IL-1Ra directly inhibits IL-1 receptor function. Such antagonism of IL-1 activity likely serves
as a regulatory mechanism against overactivity of IL-1-induced signaling,
thereby neutralizing and balancing proinflammatory effects. Altered levels of
these factors might suggest a tendency for increased neuroinflammation. In
AD, some studies demonstrated elevated CSF levels of sIL-1RII in mild/
moderate stage disease (Garlind et al., 1999), decreased CSF levels of IL-
1Ra (Tarkowski et al., 2001), or no difference in serum and CSF IL-1Ra
(Lanzrein et al., 1998). sIL-1RII levels were unchanged in mild cognitive
impairment and in late AD stage subjects, suggesting that IL-1-related inflammation is not related to early AD pathogenesis or late AD where extensive neurodegeneration already exists (Lindberg et al., 2005a). Many of these
studies, however, are limited by small sample size and methodological diffi-
culties in detecting lower levels of these factors. Certainly, the utility of CSF
or peripheral levels of IL-1, sIL-1RII, and IL-1Ra as diagnostic biomarkers
for AD remains unclear.

There is, however, mounting evidence for a genetic association between IL-1 and AD risk. Essentially, several polymorphisms of the IL-1 genes, including IL-1α (−899), IL-β (−511), and IL-β (+3953) may be important in determining the risk of developing AD. For instance, polymorphisms in −889 region of the IL-1α gene, allele 2, are linked to increased AD risk, especially in later onset patients, with an odds ratio of 1.68 in heterozygous gene carriers and 7.2 in those homozygous for the gene (Du et al., 2000). This is consistent with findings from a series of neuropathologically confirmed AD cases (Nicoll et al., 2000). Similarly, polymorphisms at IL-1β (−551) and IL-1Ra (+2018) also show increased AD risk (Yucesoy et al., 2005). Patients homozygous for the IL-1α (−899) allele 1 polymorphism declined more rapidly by mini-mental state examination (MMSE) than those homozygous for IL-1α −899 allele 2 or heterozygous subjects (Murphy et al., 2001). Furthermore, age at onset of AD is influenced by the presence of several polymorphisms. Earlier disease onset was found in patients with IL-1α (−889) T/T genotype (odds ratio 4.89; Grimaldi et al., 2000) and with IL-1β (+3953) CT or TT (Sciacca et al., 2003), and disease onset in the (+3953) group was further hastened by the co-occurrence of IL-1α T/T genotype. IL-1β T/T genotype, which was also linked to earlier onset, was associated with higher IL-1β plasma levels (Licastro et al., 2000b), but curiously, in the absence of ApoE4, conferred lower NP and NFT burden and delayed ages at onset and death (Licastro et al., 2004). Thus, evidence supports the concept that IL-1 polymorphisms may increase AD risk, alter disease onset or progression, or influence the neuropathological features of AD.

B. ROLE OF IL-6 IN AD

Unlike IL-1 where proinflammatory effects dominate, the actions of IL-6 generally depend on cellular and enviromental conditions, where the cytokine may exert either a damaging, proinflammatory effect in the CNS or an anti-inflammatory, neuroprotective, and immunosuppressive effect necessary for normal neuronal growth and function (Akiyama et al., 2000). The precise role of IL-6 in AD pathogenesis remains elusive, but proinflammatory influences appear to dominate as well. IL-6 is also produced by microglia in response to Aβ-induced injury and promotes further plaque progression (Meda et al., 1999). IL-6 and its soluble receptors, IL-6R and glycoprotein 130 (gp130), have been detected in AD brain (Strauss et al., 1992), and these complexes are localized to astrocytes in AD frontal, temporal, parietal, and occipital cortices from rapid autopsies (Hampel et al., 2005). In NPs, IL-6 is strongly colocalized with α-2-macroglobulin, an acute-phase reactant (Bauer et al., 1991), and IL-6 is found in a significantly larger proportion of diffuse plaques than other plaque types in AD brain, suggesting that it may be important in driving the earlier development of NP

(Huell *et al.*, 1995; Hull *et al.*, 1996). Also, in rapid autopsies of Braak IV and V (later stage), AD patients showed increased IL-6 expression in parietal cortex and decreased expression in occipital cortex compared with control brains, whereas sIL-6R immunolabeling was significantly increased in frontal and occipital cortex (Hampel *et al.*, 2005). In nondemented elderly, IL-6 mRNA is normally expressed in the entorhinal cortex and superior temporal gyrus, areas important in AD pathogenesis, and in severe AD subjects, IL-6 mRNA is elevated in these brain regions (Luterman *et al.*, 2000). When stratified by criteria from the Consortium to Establish a Registry for AD (CERAD; Mirra *et al.*, 1991), IL-6 mRNA in AD brain is also significantly correlated with NFTs but not with NPs (Luterman *et al.*, 2000). Overall, the data might suggest that IL-6 participates in plaque development and accelerate NFT pathology in vulnerable brain regions of the AD brain.

Similar to IL-1, measurement of IL-6 in CSF and serum samples in AD patients yields inconsistent results among the various studies. In AD, CSF levels of IL-6 are increased and may correlate to levels of soluble Fas, an apoptotic and cell injury factor (Martinez *et al.*, 2000). Serum IL-6 levels were also correlated with IL-6 in matched CSF samples from probable AD subjects (Sun *et al.*, 2003), and soluble CSF IL-6R levels, which reflect changes in IL-6 signaling, are decreased in AD, suggesting perhaps a compensatory down-regulation of aberrant IL-6 activation (Hampel *et al.*, 1998). Increased CSF IL-6 levels are also found in vascular dementia, which may have some overlap with AD (Wada-Isoe *et al.*, 2004). Peripherally, significantly increased serum IL-6 levels have been reported to correlate with disease severity (Kalman *et al.*, 1997; Licastro *et al.*, 2000a). In the "metabolic syndrome," high serum IL-6 and C-reactive protein levels are significantly associated with cognitive decline in elderly individuals (Yaffe *et al.*, 2004). Still, other studies demonstrate no increase in CSF IL-6 or CSF soluble IL-6R (Marz *et al.*, 1997) levels in AD compared with normal control CSF.

Differences in IL-6 gene polymorphisms have been identified which might influence IL-6 expression both in the CNS and peripherally. Licastro *et al* (2003) found a significant overrepresentation of the IL-6 (−174) C allele in the IL-6 gene promoter region and of the D allele in the IL-6 gene variable number tandem repeat (VNTR), both of which are associated with increases AD risk and serum and brain levels of IL-6. On the contrary, the frequency of the IL-6 gene VNTR C allele is significantly decreased in AD patients compared to normal controls and confers an inverse risk of developing AD. Others show that IL-6 (−174) C allele frequency was significantly higher and the frequency of IL-6 (−174) G allele significantly lower in perirpheral blood mononuclear cells from patients with AD (Arosio *et al.*, 2004). Another study, however, found that overrepresentation of the C allele may delay in age at onset of the disease, thus reducing AD risk (Papassotiropoulos *et al.*, 1999). In a large community sample from the United Kingdom, the IL-6 C (−174) G polymorphism was not related to AD risk or associated with age at onset of the disease, brain amyloid or tau levels, or the number of microglia or reactive astrocytes (Zhang *et al.*, 2004). It is proposed that differences in findings regarding the impact of IL-6 gene (−174) polymorphisms on AD are due to regional geographic differences in genotype and allele frequency (Capurso *et al.*, 2004).

C. OTHER INTERLEUKINS AND CYTOKINES LINKED TO AD

1. IL-4

Several other interleukins have been implicated in AD pathogenesis, but due to relatively limited evidence, their role remains unclear at present. IL-4, IL-8, IL-10, and IL-13, which appear largely anti-inflammatory in the context of AD, have all been associated with the disease, either by genetic association, identification in AD brain, CSF, plasma, or from *in vitro* culture studies. IL-4 is a potent anti-inflammatory cytokine and is thought to modulate the neuroinflammatory process in AD by antagonizing the proinflammatory activity of IL-1β. Conceivably, decreased expression or decreased function of the anti-inflammatory interleukins, IL-4, IL-10, and IL-13, during AD pathogenesis, might contribute to further neuronal and synaptic injury by allowing neuroinflammation to dominate unchallenged. Levels of IL-4, which is expressed in normal brain (Szczepanik *et al.*, 2001), but not yet shown to be altered in AD brain, appear to be influenced by the action of cholinergic agents used to treat AD. Two studies found that AD patients treated with donepezil, a cholinesterase inhibitor commonly used to delay symptom progression, generate significantly increased IL-4 levels in peripheral monocytes compared with untreated AD patients and nondemented subjects (Gambi *et al.*, 2004; Lugaresi *et al.*, 2004). Furthermore, monocyte IL-1β levels were significantly decreased in the donepezil-treated AD subjects (Gambi *et al.*, 2004), and these changes were independent of age, gender, and other comorbidities (Lugaresi *et al.*, 2004). This implies that cholinesterase inhibitors may have a secondary effect in altering AD progression by modifying IL-1-induced inflammation through IL-4. No clear genetic associations have been established, and Shibata *et al.* (2002) failed to show association of the IL-4 gene promoter polymorphism, IL-4 C(+33)T, with AD risk or IL-4 plasma concentration.

2. IL-10

Similarly, IL-10 is a potent anti-inflammatory cytokine in the CNS that may function to decrease inflammation during AD. As with IL-4, IL-10 mRNA is expressed in normal brain, but little to no neuropathological data exist on IL-10 expression, distribution, and alteration in AD brain (Szczepanik *et al.*, 2001). Rather, microglial culture data indicate that IL-10, IL-4, and IL-13 can effectively suppress activity of Aβ and lipopolysaccharide (LPS)-induced proinflammatory interleukins, including IL-1α, IL-1β, IL-6 as well as other cytokines and chemokines (Szczepanik *et al.*, 2001). Peripherally, however, IL-10 levels were unaltered in blood cells from AD patients following LPS stimulation but were decreased in individuals with vascular dementia (De Luigi *et al.*, 2002). Moreover, several polymorphisms in the IL-10 gene promoter region, which presumably reduce IL-10 expression and activity, may be linked to AD risk, including IL-10 G (−1082) A, T (−819) C, and C (−592) A (Arosio *et al.*, 2004; Lio *et al.*, 2003; Ma *et al.*, 2005; Scassellati *et al.*, 2004). There is agreement among investigators that the G (−1082) A polymorphism is associated with increase AD risk. Scassellati *et al.* (2004) reported that the GCC/ACC haplotype combination was overrepresented in Italian AD patients (OR 1.91), while others find the IL-10 (−819) C/T polymorphism to be increased in AD (Lio *et al.*, 2003). In a Chinese population sample, IL-10 (−592) C and IL-10 (−819) C, which are in complete linkage disequilibrium, are strongly associated with AD and are directly related to plasma IL-10 levels (Ma *et al.*, 2005). Overall, however, it remains unclear whether impaired anti-inflammatory interleukin function, from abnormally decreased levels or activity of IL-4 and IL-10, might contribute significantly to AD neurodegeneration.

3. IL-8

As a response to neuronal injury in the AD brain, activation and recruitment of neuroinflammatory cells, such as microglia, is important in fueling inflammation. Among many secreted factors that act as microglial chemoattractants in the CNS, chemokines or chemotatic cytokines are most prominent and are thought to play an increasing role not only in AD but also in other neurologic disorders such as HIV dementia and multiple sclerosis (Cross and Woodroofe, 1999). IL-8, a microglia-derived chemokine produced in response to proinflammatory signals, such as amyloid (Ehrlich *et al.*, 1998), could be important in recruiting further activated microglia into areas of damage in AD brain, and *in vitro*, IL-8 mRNA expression is induced by both Aβ25-35 and Aβ42 (Nagai *et al.*, 2001). Also, IL-8 potentiates Aβ-associated release of IL-1β, IL-6, TNF-α, and cyclooxygenase-2 (COX-2) in microglial culture (Franciosi *et al.*, 2005). Although IL-8 itself has not been demonstrated in AD brain, immunoreactivity against IL-8 receptor B (IL-8RB), also known as CXCR2, is localized to dystrophic neurites within mature NPs, suggesting that IL-8 may mediate glial and microglial interactions with neurons, contributing to neuronal damage and reactive neuronal sprouting (Xia *et al.*, 1997).

4. TNF-α

TNF-α, a noninterleukin cytokine, is also produced in response to amyloid and IL-1 during AD, and interacts with interleukins to induce neuronal injury. TNF-α, a significant mediator of Aβ-induced microglial neurotox-city, binds to receptors expressed on neurons, microglia, and astrocytes, allowing for activation of inflammation signaling in multiple cell types (Bamberger and Landreth, 2001), and NP-induced TNF-α causes in neuronal death in tissue culture models (Giulian *et al.*, 1996). Furthermore, TNF-α-induced neurotoxicity requires the participation of other cytokines, the generation of neurotoxic reactive oxygen species (ROS), and neuronal and microglial production of nitric oxide via activation of inducible nitric oxide synthase (iNOS) (Ishii *et al.*, 2000; Klegeris and McGeer, 1997).

V. β-AMYLOID, INTERLEUKINS, AND INFLAMMATORY SIGNALING IN AD

As illustrated in Fig. 1, interleukins mediate a self-perpetuating cycle of neuroinflammation in AD, in which Aβ appears to be the central trigger, causing glial activation and neurodegeneration. As previously mentioned, IL-1 (IL-1α and IL-1β) and to a lesser extent, IL-6, are the predominant proinflammatory factors which, when aberrantly overactivated, contribute to the damage and injury observed. Despite work indicating that the physiologic expression of IL-1R1 mRNA is highly limited to ventricular-associated areas, amygdala, arcuate nucleus, trigeminal, and hypoglossal motor nuclei, marked upregulation of IL-1 signaling is observed widely throughout the brain in response to injury of any type (Ericsson *et al.*, 1995). Reflecting this sensitivity to brain injury states, a wide variety of molecules and signals associated with early injury can induce the transcription and expression of IL-1 mRNA, including the immediate early genes, *c-Jun* and *c-Fos*, as well as NF-κB, CCAAT/enhancer binding protein-β (CEBP-β) and perhaps others (Basu *et al.*, 2004; Gao *et al.*, 2002). Produced by activated microglia and astrocytes, IL-1 initiates cell signaling by binding to IL-1R1, which then complexes with the accessory protein IL-1RAcP (Greenfeder *et al.*, 1995), and in turn activates the specific receptor. Alternatively, IL-1 is antagonized by the nonfunctional inhibitory receptor, IL-1RII, and by IL-1Ra, to prevent over-activation (Arend, 2002; Colotta *et al.*, 1996). Evidence from peripheral cell types indicates that IL-1R and Toll-like receptors (TLR) are members of a superfamily of related molecules, which, following activation, induce intracellular assembly of myeloid differentiation primary response gene (MyD88), IL-1-associated receptor kinase (IRAK), TNF-associated factor (TRAF6), and Toll/IL-1 receptor domain-containing adapter protein (TIRAP) into an IL-1 signaling complex, leading eventually to Jun kinase (JNK) and MAPK pathway activation, IL-6 production, and propagation of inflammation (Huang *et al.*, 2004). IL-6 signaling, which has been partially elucidated, can promote cellular growth and differentiation, as well as inflammation, through interaction with the sIL-6R, leading to homodimerization of

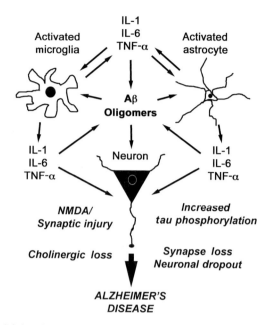

FIGURE 1. Aβ, interleukins, and neurodegeneration in AD. Key aspects of interleukin-mediated damage in AD are emphasized in this diagram. Increased production and subsequent misfolding of Aβ42 leads to increased Aβ oligomers as well as Aβ sequestered in NPs. Collectively, they induce inflammation and activation of microglia and astrocytes. IL-1, IL-6, and TNF-α release further perpetuates this cycle, but more importantly, directly contributes to increased tau abnormalities and tangle formation, synaptic transmission defects leading to synapse loss, cholinergic deficits, and eventually neuron dropout characteristic of AD.

the gp130 subunit and activation of receptor-associated Janus kinases (JAK). The consequence of JAK activation is tyrosine phosphorylation of the signal transducer and activator of transcription (STAT) family of proteins, subsequent nuclear translocation of STAT, and transcriptional activation of target genes directed toward inflammation and presumably tissue injury (Ishihara and Hirano, 2002).

Abundant evidence from transgenic models and *in vitro* cell culture has provided insight into the role of interleukins and relevant mechanisms underlying amyloid-induced inflammation in AD. Increased IL-1 expression is observed in rat brain microglia and astrocytes, after cortical injection with aggregated Aβ42 (Heneka *et al.*, 2002). Also, Aβ42 treatment results in microglial transformation and elevated IL-1 secretion in glial cell cultures (Araujo and Cotman, 1992). Of significance, soluble Aβ oligomers, which exert greater toxicity than other forms of Aβ (Walsh *et al.*, 2002), have been shown to cause markedly increased IL-1β secretion in cultured rat astrocytes and in cultured microglia, as compared with fibrillar Aβ (Lindberg *et al.*, 2005b; White *et al.*, 2005). Soluble oligomers of aggregating molecules, such as Aβ, appear to be critically important in causing synaptic and neuronal damage by activating aberrant signaling pathways. In the case of Aβ oligomers, signaling complexes likely involve p59 Fyn kinase, are likely activated within neuronal membrane lipid raft domains, causing synaptic loss and perhaps promoting NFT formation (Ho *et al.*, 2005b).

Conversely, IL-1 signaling also stimulates further cellular APP production, leading to even greater pathologic accumulation of Aβ. In cultured neurons and endothelial cells (Forloni *et al.*, 1992), as well as in primary human astrocytes and neuroblastoma cells (Rogers *et al.*, 1999), IL-1 significantly increases levels of APP mRNA transcription and expression, and in a transient *in vitro* assay system, IL-1 induces expression of the APP promoter (Donnelly *et al.*, 1990; Yang *et al.*, 1998). Liao *et al.* (2004) demonstrated elegantly that IL-1 can augment APP proteolysis to form Aβ. Using HEK293 cells cotransfected with a luciferase reporter gene and Gal4/VP16-tagged C-terminal fragment of APP, it was shown that IL-1 treatment significantly increased γ-secretase cleavage of C99 fragment, resulting in increase in luciferase expression, and concomitant increases in the production of Aβ and AICD, the intracellular domain of APP. Also, these phenomena appear to be dependent on JNK activation and signal transduction, suggesting that well-established IL-1 signaling pathways found in the peripheral cells are also responsible for the increased APP production and proteolytic cleavage to Aβ. Finally, IL-6 mRNA levels were increased in the cortex and hippocampus of Tg2576 APP transgenic mice (Tehranian *et al.*, 2001). Together, these findings indicate that Aβ and interleukins are linked in a self-perpetuating cycle, in which each augments the production of the other, ultimately leading to increased neuronal damage and synaptotoxicity.

Aside from Aβ-mediated neurotoxicity, interleukins in AD brain may cause injury via other, alternate modes of neuronal dysfunction. For instance, when conditioned medium from glutamate-treated neurons and PC12 cells containing elevated secreted sAPPα are added to cocultures of microglia and naïve PC12 cells, IL-1 production is increased, accompanied by increases in AChE mRNA levels and activity, and IL-1 pellet implantation into rat cortex induced similar AChE mRNA increases (Li *et al.*, 2000). This suggests that one important aspect of AD, cholinergic dysfunction, may be due in part to the action of interleukins. In APPV717F transgenic mice, which form brain Aβ plaques similar to AD, increased expression of IL-1β converting enzyme, a cysteine protease that cleaves inactive pro-IL-1β to active IL-1β, and increased neuronal DNA damage by terminal deoxynucleotidyl transferase (TdT)-mediated dUTP nick end labeling (TUNEL) are both observed (Sheng *et al.*, 2001b). IL-1 may also promote tau hyperphosphorylation and accelerate the formation of NFTs, leading to neuronal transport dysfunction and synaptic damage. In AD brain as well as in IL-1 pellet-implanted rats, significantly elevated levels of p38 MAPK are observed, which, when coupled with the finding in AD brain that IL-1 immunoreactive microglia correlate strongly with immunoreactivity for both hyperphosphorylated tau and p38 MAPK-immunoreactive neurons, suggest that an IL-1 and p38 MAPK signal transduction pathway contributes to NFT formation (Sheng *et al.*, 2001a). This notion is further supported by the *in vitro* finding that either coculturing sAPPα-stimulated microglia, which overexpress inflammatory cytokines, with neurons or adding IL-1β directly to neuronal culture, both markedly increase neuronal tau hyperphosphorylation and decrease levels of synaptophysin. Moreover, these phenomena are attenuated by IL-1Ra and anti-IL-1 antibody, suggesting IL-1 is important in NFT formation (Li *et al.*, 2003). Finally, IL-6 also promotes tau hyperphosphorylation by increasing p35 levels and activating cdk5, a key serine/threonine kinase implicated in abnormal tau phosphorylation (Quintanilla *et al.*, 2004).

Early synaptic damage and loss is perhaps one of the most important structural alterations in AD brain, and the precise nature and mechanisms of this dysfunction are actively being investigated. An exciting concept has emerged in AD research, involving the direct impact of interleukins on synaptic function and transmission (Lynch, 2002). Overactivity of *N*-methyl-D-aspartate (NMDA) ligand-gated channels is important in excitotoxicity and neuronal damage, and it was found that the combined action of chronic IL-6 and Aβ treatment in cultured neurons, with acute NMDA treatment, resulted in loss of neuronal viability (Qiu and Gruol, 2003). Moreover, in NMDA-lesioned hippocampal slice culture, IL-1 enhanced neuronal damage by microglial activation and proliferation, which was inhibited by IL-1Ra (Hailer *et al.*, 2005). From the electrophysiological aspect, IL-1β at ng/ml concentrations, directly decreased the frequency of excitatory postsynaptic potentials and significantly increased the L-type voltage-gated Ca^{+2} current (Yang *et al.*, 2005). Aβ and IL-1β-induced inhibition of long-term potentiation, which is important for memory and learning, is dependent on JNK activation (Minogue *et al.*, 2003). Also, NMDA treatment inhibits IL-8/CXCR2-mediated protection of neurons from Aβ toxicity, and the mechanism involves altered NMDA receptor activity and phosphorylation of CXCR2 (Luo *et al.*, 2005). Thus, it appears that alteration of NMDA-mediated synaptic transmission might be another mechanism by which interleukins contribute to neurodegeneration and cognitive decline in AD.

VI. INTERLEUKINS: THERAPEUTIC IMPLICATIONS FOR AD

Much of the impetus for investigating aspects of interleukin and cytokine biology with relevance to AD pathogenesis originated from epidemiologic evidence which links the use of anti-inflammatory agents to significantly decrease risk of incident AD. Many agents have been examined, including corticosteroids, NSAIDS, aspirin, COX-2 inhibitors, which block interleukin production locally. Epidemiological evidence indicates decreased AD risk in higher dose NSAID with rheumatoid arthritis [see meta-analysis by McGeer *et al.* (1996) and review by Ho *et al.* (2005a)]. In addition, clinical trial experience finds that high-dose NSAIDs, such as indomethacin, for example, might slow disease progression (Rogers *et al.*, 1993). Depending on the anti-inflammatory agent, there may be multiple mechanisms of action leading to reduced inflammation, and one mechanism may be the modulation of proinflammatory factors such as interleukins. In Tg2576 APP transgenic mice, after 6 months of chronic ibuprofen treatment, showed reduced amyloid deposition, glial activation, IL-1β levels, and α-1-ACT levels, indicating that reduction in amyloid pathology is due to a modulation of brain inflammation (Lim *et al.*, 2000; Morihara *et al.*, 2005). In mice challenged acutely with intracerebral Aβ42 injection, concomitant prenisolone, dexamethasone, or IL-10 treatment prevented time- and dose-dependent increases in IL-1, IL-6, and MCP-1 (Szczepanik and Ringheim, 2003). Furthermore, rats chronically treated with sulindac, a nonselective COX inhibitor, not only showed inhibition of age-related increases in hippocampal IL-1β levels and age-related decreases in NR1 and NR2 NMDA subunits, but also lacked any decline in learning and memory (Mesches *et al.*, 2004). Thus, one rationale for using anti-inflammatory agents in AD is to interrupt the cycles of glial and microglial activation by reducing interleukin overexpression and amyloid pathology, ultimately decreasing neuronal and synaptic damage.

Additionally, an exciting novel mechanism has been elucidated in a certain subset of NSAIDs that effectively inhibit Aβ production and prevent some aspects of AD-related neuroinflammation. It is well known that the majority of NSAIDs inhibit COX, which has the disadvantage of increased gastrointestinal toxicity, especially at higher doses potentially needed for effective decreases in Aβ. Yet, it was found that NSAIDs, such as ibuprofen, indomethacin, and sulindac, may also directly reduce Aβ production in tissue culture in a COX-independent manner (Weggen *et al.*, 2001), and *in vitro*, NSAIDs may reduce Aβ production by directly altering presenilin 1 (PS1) and γ-secretase activity (Weggen *et al.*, 2003). Inhibition of NF-κB is implicated as a mechanism by which NSAIDs lower Aβ levels, but other NF-κB inhibitors do not appear to affect the generation of Aβ (Morihara *et al.*, 2002). Widely used COX inhibitors are a racemic mixture of *R*- and *S*-enantiomers, but the *S*-enantiomers appear to confer the major toxicities associated with NSAIDs. Thus, studies have focused on the development of *R*-enantiomers, such as *R*-flurbiprofen, which are as effective as other forms in preventing Aβ generation, but lack undesirable NSAID-related toxicities. A nitric oxide–releasing derivative of flurbiprofen, NCX-2216, was recently shown to reduce brain amyloid deposition and numbers of MHC-II-positive activated microglia in APP and PS1 doubly-transgenic mice (Jantzen *et al.*, 2002). *R*-flurbiprofen, which is currently being investigated in human clinical trials, and similar NSAID compounds are therefore being developed as potential therapies for AD.

Immunotherapies to prevent amyloid deposition may attenuate the subsequent neuroinflammatory response observed in AD. Active vaccinations using peripheral injection of Aβ peptide, in combination with an adjuvant, were developed for this purpose and generated a robust antibody response. Promising initial studies demonstrated the impressive effectiveness of this method in reducing amyloid deposition, likely through increased Fc-mediated microglial phagocytosis of Aβ, as well as decreasing gliosis and dystrophic neurites in PDAPP transgenic mice overexpressing mutant human APP (Schenk *et al.*, 1999). Intranasal delivery of active synthetic human Aβ peptide vaccine, which has a potent systemic impact in PDAPP mice, reduced not only Aβ plaque burden but also showed a modest increase in brain mononuclear cells immunoreactive for the anti-inflammatory cytokines, IL-4 and IL-10 (Weiner *et al.*, 2000). This might suggest that strategies that prevent Aβ deposition, and potentially those that also decrease Aβ production, can attenuate neuroinflammation in AD. Yet, one important consideration is that such therapies should be administered sufficiently early in the course of AD pathogenesis before the establishment of AD pathology and also before significant, irreversible synaptic loss has occurred. Unfortunately, human clinical trials of active Aβ vaccination in AD subjects, albeit effective, resulted in unexpected fatal T cell–mediated meningoencephalitis in several patients (Nicoll *et al.*, 2003). Certainly, further investigation is needed to better understand the impact of Aβ immunotherapy on the neuroimmune system in both AD and normal physiologic conditions.

VII. CONCLUSIONS: FUTURE DIRECTIONS

Because of the increasing importance of unregulated inflammatory response in AD brain, interleukins will undoubtedly play an ever-expanding role in the pathogenesis of the disease and in the process of neurodegeneration. Because their prinicipal function is in modulatory control of immune activities and responses in the CNS, interleukins are involved in complex intercellular interactions among neurons, microglia, and astrocytes, as well as intracellular signal transduction events, which are necessary to promote the inflammatory cascade characteristic of AD neuropathology. Normally, during immune surveillance, a balance is maintained between proinflammatory and anti-inflammatory influences. Yet, during AD, the abnormal accumulation of soluble amyloid oligomers triggers excessive release of proinflammatory factors, such as IL-1, IL-6, cytokines, and other acute-phase reactants, out of proportion to the regulatory components, such as IL-4, IL-10, receptor antagonists, interleukin inhibitors and others, ultimately leading to neuronal and synaptic inury and loss and cognitive decline. Future efforts toward reducing AD inflammation will likely to continue to focus on amyloid reduction strategies as well as efforts to augment the production of innate anti-inflammatory cytokines and interleukin inhibitors. Futhermore, novel effective methods will be engineered to inhibit proinflammatory interleukins, possibly downregulation by small interfering RNAs, and to therapeutically target individual components of the interleukin signaling system in AD.

REFERENCES

Akiyama, H., Barger, S., Barnum, S., Bradt, B., Bauer, J., Cole, G. M., Cooper, N. R., Eikelenboom, P., Emmerling, M., Fiebich, B. L., Finch, C. E., Frautschy, S., *et al.* (2000). Inflammation and Alzheimer's disease. *Neurobiol. Aging* **21**, 383–421.

Araujo, D. M., and Cotman, C. W. (1992). Beta-amyloid stimulates glial cells *in vitro* to produce growth factors that accumulate in senile plaques in Alzheimer's disease. *Brain Res.* **569**, 141–145.

Arend, W. P. (2002). The balance between IL-1 and IL-1Ra in disease. *Cytokine Growth Factor Rev.* **13**, 323–340.

Arosio, B., Trabattoni, D., Galimberti, L., Bucciarelli, P., Fasano, F., Calabresi, C., Cazzullo, C. L., Vergani, C., Annoni, G., and Clerici, M. (2004). Interleukin-10 and interleukin-6 gene polymorphisms as risk factors for Alzheimer's disease. *Neurobiol. Aging* **25**, 1009–1015.

Balkwill, F. (1988). Cytokines–soluble factors in immune responses. *Curr. Opin. Immunol.* **1**, 241–249.

Bamberger, M. E., and Landreth, G. E. (2001). Microglial interaction with beta-amyloid: Implications for the pathogenesis of Alzheimer's disease. *Microsc. Res. Tech.* **54**, 59–70.

Basu, A., Krady, J. K., and Levison, S. W. (2004). Interleukin-1: A master regulator of neuroinflammation. *J Neurosci. Res.* **78**, 151–156.

Bauer, J., Strauss, S., Schreiter-Gasser, U., Ganter, U., Schlegel, P., Witt, I., Yolk, B., and Berger, M. (1991). Interleukin-6 and alpha-2-macroglobulin indicate an acute-phase state in Alzheimer's disease cortices. *FEBS Lett.* **285**, 111–114.

Blum-Degen, D., Muller, T., Kuhn, W., Gerlach, M., Przuntek, H., and Riederer, P. (1995). Interleukin-1 beta and interleukin-6 are elevated in the cerebrospinal fluid of Alzheimer's and *de novo* Parkinson's disease patients. *Neurosci. Lett.* **202**, 17–20.

Bruce-Keller, A. J. (1999). Microglial-neuronal interactions in synaptic damage and recovery. *J. Neurosci. Res.* **58**, 191–201.

Brunkan, A. L., and Goate, A. M. (2005). Presenilin function and gamma-secretase activity. *J. Neurochem.* **93**, 769–792.

Cacabelos, R., Barquero, M., Garcia, P., Alvarez, X. A., and Varela de Seijas, E. (1991a). Cerebrospinal fluid interleukin-1 beta (IL-1 beta) in Alzheimer's disease and neurological disorders. *Methods Find. Exp. Clin. Pharmacol.* **13**, 455–458.

Cacabelos, R., Franco-Maside, A., and Alvarez, X. A. (1991b). Interleukin-1 in Alzheimer's disease and multi-infarct dementia: Neuropsychological correlations. *Methods Find. Exp. Clin. Pharmacol.* **13**, 703–708.

Cacabelos, R., Alvarez, X. A., Fernandez-Novoa, L., Franco, A., Mangues, R., Pellicer, A., and Nishimura, T. (1994). Brain interleukin-1 beta in Alzheimer's disease and vascular dementia. *Methods Find. Exp. Clin. Pharmacol.* **16**, 141–151.

Capurso, C., Solfrizzi, V., D' Introno, A., Colacicco, A. M., Capurso, S. A., Capurso, A., and Panza, F. (2004). Interleukin 6-174 G/C promoter gene polymorphism and sporadic Alzheimer's disease: Geographic allele and genotype variations in Europe. *Exp. Gerontol.* **39,** 1567–1573.

Carter, J., and Lippa, C. F. (2001). Beta-amyloid, neuronal death and Alzheimer's disease. *Curr. Mol. Med.* **1,** 733–737.

Colotta, F., Saccani, S., Giri, J. G., Dower, S. K., Sims, J. E., Introna, M., and Mantovani, A. (1996). Regulated expression and release of the IL-1 decoy receptor in human mononuclear phagocytes. *J. Immunol.* **156,** 2534–2541.

Cross, A. K., and Woodroofe, M. N. (1999). Chemokines induce migration and changes in actin polymerization in adult rat brain microglia and a human fetal microglial cell line *in vitro*. *J. Neurosci. Res.* **55,** 17–23.

De Luigi, A., Pizzimenti, S., Quadri, P., Lucca, U., Tettamanti, M., Fragiacomo, C., and De Simoni, M. G. (2002). Peripheral inflammatory response in Alzheimer's disease and multiinfarct dementia. *Neurobiol. Dis.* **11,** 308–314.

De Strooper, B. (2003). Aph-1, Pen-2, and Nicastrin with Presenilin generate an active gamma-Secretase complex. *Neuron* **38,** 9–12.

DeKosky, S. T., and Scheff, S. W. (1990). Synapse loss in frontal cortex biopsies in Alzheimer's disease: Correlation with cognitive severity. *Ann. Neurol.* **27,** 457–464.

Dong, Y., and Benveniste, E. N. (2001). Immune function of astrocytes. *Glia* **36,** 180–190.

Donnelly, R. J., Friedhoff, A. J., Beer, B., Blume, A. J., and Vitek, M. P. (1990). Interleukin-1 stimulates the beta-amyloid precursor protein promoter. *Cell Mol. Neurobiol.* **10,** 485–495.

Du, Y., Dodel, R. C., Eastwood, B. J., Bales, K. R., Gao, F., Lohmuller, F., Muller, U., Kurz, A., Zimmer, R., Evans, R. M., Hake, A., Gasser, T., *et al.* (2000). Association of an interleukin 1 alpha polymorphism with Alzheimer's disease. *Neurology* **55,** 480–483.

Ehrlich, L. C., Hu, S., Sheng, W. S., Sutton, R. L., Rockswold, G. L., Peterson, P. K., and Chao, C. C. (1998). Cytokine regulation of human microglial cell IL-8 production. *J. Immunol.* **160,** 1944–1948.

Elkabes, S., DiCicco-Bloom, E. M., and Black, I. B. (1996). Brain microglia/macrophages express neurotrophins that selectively regulate microglial proliferation and function. *J. Neurosci.* **16,** 2508–2521.

Ericsson, A., Liu, C., Hart, R. P., and Sawchenko, P. E. (1995). Type 1 interleukin-1 receptor in the rat brain: Distribution, regulation, and relationship to sites of IL-1-induced cellular activation. *J. Comp. Neurol.* **361,** 681–698.

Forloni, G., Demicheli, F., Giorgi, S., Bendotti, C., and Angeretti, N. (1992). Expression of amyloid precursor protein mRNAs in endothelial, neuronal and glial cells: Modulation by interleukin-1. *Brain Res. Mol. Brain Res.* **16,** 128–134.

Franciosi, S., Choi, H. B., Kim, S. U., and McLarnon, J. G. (2005). IL-8 enhancement of amyloid-beta (Abeta 1-42)-induced expression and production of pro-inflammatory cytokines and COX-2 in cultured human microglia. *J. Neuroimmunol.* **159,** 66–74.

Fujiwara, N., and Kobayashi, K. (2005). Macrophages in inflammation. *Curr. Drug Targets Inflamm. Allergy.* **4,** 281–286.

Gambi, F., Reale, M., Iarlori, C., Salone, A., Toma, L., Paladini, C., De Luca, G., Feliciani, C., Salvatore, M., Salerno, R. M., Theoharides, T. C., Conti, P., *et al.* (2004). Alzheimer patients treated with an AchE inhibitor show higher IL-4 and lower IL-1 beta levels and expression in peripheral blood mononuclear cells. *J. Clin. Psychopharmacol.* **24,** 314–321.

Gao, F., Bales, K. R., Dodel, R. C., Liu, J., Chen, X., Hample, H., Farlow, M. R., Paul, S. M., and Du, Y. (2002). NF-kappaB mediates IL-1beta-induced synthesis/release of alpha2-macroglobulin in a human glial cell line. *Brain Res. Mol. Brain Res.* **105,** 108–114.

Garlind, A., Brauner, A., Hojeberg, B., Basun, H., and Schultzberg, M. (1999). Soluble interleukin-1 receptor type II levels are elevated in cerebrospinal fluid in Alzheimer's disease patients. *Brain Res.* **826,** 112–116.

Girvin, A. M., Gordon, K. B., Welsh, C. J., Clipstone, N. A., and Miller, S. D. (2002). Differential abilities of central nervous system resident endothelial cells and astrocytes to serve as inducible antigen-presenting cells. *Blood* **99,** 3692–3701.

Giulian, D., and Baker, T. J. (1985). Peptides released by ameboid microglia regulate astroglial proliferation. *J. Cell Biol.* **101,** 2411–2415.

Giulian, D., Haverkamp, L. J., Yu, J. H., Karshin, W., Tom, D., Li, J., Kirkpatrick, J., Kuo, L. M., and Roher, A. E. (1996). Specific domains of beta-amyloid from Alzheimer plaque elicit neuron killing in human microglia. *J. Neurosci.* **16,** 6021–6037.

Greenfeder, S. A., Nunes, P., Kwee, L., Labow, M., Chizzonite, R. A., and Ju, G. (1995). Molecular cloning and characterization of a second subunit of the interleukin 1 receptor complex. *J. Biol. Chem.* **270,** 13757–13765.

Griffin, W. S., Stanley, L. C., Ling, C., White, L., MacLeod, V., Perrot, L. J., White, C. L., III, and Araoz, C. (1989). Brain interleukin 1 and S-100 immunoreactivity are elevated in Down syndrome and Alzheimer disease. *Proc. Natl. Acad. Sci. USA* **86,** 7611–7615.

Griffin, W. S., Sheng, J. G., Roberts, G. W., and Mrak, R. E. (1995). Interleukin-1 expression in different plaque types in Alzheimer's disease: Significance in plaque evolution. *J. Neuropathol. Exp. Neurol.* **54,** 276–281.

Grimaldi, L. M., Casadei, V. M., Ferri, C., Veglia, F., Licastro, F., Annoni, G., Biunno, I., De Bellis, G., Sorbi, S., Mariani, C., Canal, N., Griffin, W. S., *et al.* (2000). Association of early-onset Alzheimer's disease with an interleukin-1alpha gene polymorphism. *Ann. Neurol.* **47,** 361–365.

Hailer, N. P., Vogt, C., Korf, H. W., and Dehghani, F. (2005). Interleukin-1beta exacerbates and interleukin-1 receptor antagonist attenuates neuronal injury and microglial activation after excitotoxic damage in organotypic hippocampal slice cultures. *Eur. J. Neurosci.* **21,** 2347–2360.

Hampel, H., Sunderland, T., Kotter, H. U., Schneider, C., Teipel, S. J., Padberg, F., Dukoff, R., Levy, J., and Moller, H. J. (1998). Decreased soluble interleukin-6 receptor in cerebrospinal fluid of patients with Alzheimer's disease. *Brain Res.* **780,** 356–359.

Hampel, H., Haslinger, A., Scheloske, M., Padberg, F., Fischer, P., Unger, J., Teipel, S. J., Neumann, M., Rosenberg, C., Oshida, R., Hulette, C., Pongratz, D., *et al.* (2005). Pattern of interleukin-6 receptor complex immunoreactivity between cortical regions of rapid autopsy normal and Alzheimer's disease brain. *Eur. Arch. Psychiatry Clin. Neurosci.* **255,** 269–278.

Heneka, M. T., Galea, E., Gavriluyk, V., Dumitrescu-Ozimek, L., Daeschner, J., O' Banion, M. K., Weinberg, G., Klockgether, T., and Feinstein, D. L. (2002). Noradrenergic depletion potentiates beta-amyloid-induced cortical inflammation: Implications for Alzheimer's disease. *J. Neurosci.* **22,** 2434–2442.

Ho, G. J., Drego, R., Hakimian, E., and Masliah, E. (2005a). Mechanisms of cell signaling and inflammation in Alzheimer's disease. *Curr. Drug Targets Inflamm. Allergy* **4,** 247–256.

Ho, G. J., Hashimoto, M., Adame, A., Izu, M., Alford, M. F., Thal, L. J., Hansen, L. A., and Masliah, E. (2005b). Altered p59Fyn kinase expression accompanies disease progression in Alzheimer's disease: Implications for its functional role. *Neurobiol. Aging* **26,** 625–635.

Huang, Q., Yang, J., Lin, Y., Walker, C., Cheng, J., Liu, Z. G., and Su, B. (2004). Differential regulation of interleukin 1 receptor and Toll-like receptor signaling by MEKK3. *Nat. Immunol.* **5,** 98–103.

Huell, M., Strauss, S., Volk, B., Berger, M., and Bauer, J. (1995). Interleukin-6 is present in early stages of plaque formation and is restricted to the brains of Alzheimer's disease patients. *Acta Neuropathol. (Berl.)* **89,** 544–551.

Hull, M., Berger, M., Volk, B., and Bauer, J. (1996). Occurrence of interleukin-6 in cortical plaques of Alzheimer's disease patients may precede transformation of diffuse into neuritic plaques. *Ann. N. Y. Acad. Sci.* **777,** 205–212.

Ishihara, K., and Hirano, T. (2002). Molecular basis of the cell specificity of cytokine action. *Biochim. Biophys. Acta* **1592,** 281–296.

Ishii, K., Muelhauser, F., Liebl, U., Picard, M., Kuhl, S., Penke, B., Bayer, T., Wiessler, M., Hennerici, M., Beyreuther, K., Hartmann, T., and Fassbender, K. (2000). Subacute NO generation induced by Alzheimer's beta-amyloid in the living brain: Reversal by inhibition of the inducible NO synthase. *FASEB J.* **14**, 1485–1489.

Jantzen, P. T., Connor, K. E., Di Carlo, G., Wenk, G. L., Wallace, J. L., Rojiani, A. M., Coppola, D., Morgan, D., and Gordon, M. N. (2002). Microglial activation and beta-amyloid deposit reduction caused by a nitric oxide-releasing nonsteroidal anti-inflammatory drug in amyloid precursor protein plus presenilin-1 transgenic mice. *J. Neurosci.* **22**, 2246–2254.

Kakimura, J., Kitamura, Y., Takata, K., Umeki, M., Suzuki, S., Shibagaki, K., Taniguchi, T., Nomura, Y., Gebicke-Haerter, P. J., Smith, M. A., Perry, G., and Shimohama, S. (2002). Microglial activation and amyloid-beta clearance induced by exogenous heat-shock proteins. *FASEB J.* **16**, 601–603.

Kalman, J., Juhasz, A., Laird, G., Dickens, P., Jardanhazy, T., Rimanoczy, A., Boncz, I., Parry-Jones, W. L., and Janka, Z. (1997). Serum interleukin-6 levels correlate with the severity of dementia in Down syndrome and in Alzheimer's disease. *Acta Neurol. Scand.* **96**, 236–240.

Klegeris, A., and McGeer, P. L. (1997). Beta-amyloid protein enhances macrophage production of oxygen free radicals and glutamate. *J. Neurosci. Res.* **49**, 229–235.

Lanzrein, A. S., Johnston, C. M., Perry, V. H., Jobst, K. A., King, E. M., and Smith, A. D. (1998). Longitudinal study of inflammatory factors in serum, cerebrospinal fluid, and brain tissue in Alzheimer disease: Interleukin-1beta, interleukin-6, interleukin-1 receptor antagonist, tumor necrosis factor-alpha, the soluble tumor necrosis factor receptors I and II, and alpha1-antichymotrypsin. *Alzheimer Dis. Assoc. Disord.* **12**, 215–227.

Li, Y., Liu, L., Kang, J., Sheng, J. G., Barger, S. W., Mrak, R. E., and Griffin, W. S. (2000). Neuronal-glial interactions mediated by interleukin-1 enhance neuronal acetylcholinesterase activity and mRNA expression. *J. Neurosci.* **20**, 149–155.

Li, Y., Liu, L., Barger, S. W., and Griffin, W. S. (2003). Interleukin-1 mediates pathological effects of microglia on tau phosphorylation and on synaptophysin synthesis in cortical neurons through a p38-MAPK pathway. *J. Neurosci.* **23**, 1605–1611.

Liao, Y. F., Wang, B. J., Cheng, H. T., Kuo, L. H., and Wolfe, M. S. (2004). Tumor necrosis factor-alpha, interleukin-1beta, and interferon-gamma stimulate gamma-secretase-mediated cleavage of amyloid precursor protein through a JNK-dependent MAPK pathway. *J. Biol. Chem.* **279**, 49523–49532.

Licastro, F., Pedrini, S., Caputo, L., Annoni, G., Davis, L. J., Ferri, C., Casadei, V., and Grimaldi, L. M. (2000a). Increased plasma levels of interleukin-1, interleukin-6 and alpha-1-antichymotrypsin in patients with Alzheimer's disease: Peripheral inflammation or signals from the brain? *J. Neuroimmunol.* **103**, 97–102.

Licastro, F., Pedrini, S., Ferri, C., Casadei, V., Govoni, M., Pession, A., Sciacca, F. L., Veglia, F., Annoni, G., Bonafe, M., Olivieri, F., Franceschi, C., *et al.* (2000b). Gene polymorphism affecting alpha1-antichymotrypsin and interleukin-1 plasma levels increases Alzheimer's disease risk. *Ann. Neurol.* **48**, 388–391.

Licastro, F., Grimaldi, L. M., Bonafe, M., Martina, C., Olivieri, F., Cavallone, L., Giovanietti, S., Masliah, E., and Franceschi, C. (2003). Interleukin-6 gene alleles affect the risk of Alzheimer's disease and levels of the cytokine in blood and brain. *Neurobiol. Aging* **24**, 921–926.

Licastro, F., Veglia, F., Chiappelli, M., Grimaldi, L. M., and Masliah, E. (2004). A polymorphism of the interleukin-1 beta gene at position +3953 influences progression and neuro-pathological hallmarks of Alzheimer's disease. *Neurobiol. Aging* **25**, 1017–1022.

Lim, G. P., Yang, F., Chu, T., Chen, P., Beech, W., Teter, B., Tran, T., Ubeda, O., Ashe, K. H., Frautschy, S. A., and Cole, G. M. (2000). Ibuprofen suppresses plaque pathology and inflammation in a mouse model for Alzheimer's disease. *J. Neurosci.* **20**, 5709–5714.

Lindberg, C., Chromek, M., Ahrengart, L., Brauner, A., Schultzberg, M., and Garlind, A. (2005a). Soluble interleukin-1 receptor type II, IL-18 and caspase-1 in mild cognitive impairment and severe Alzheimer's disease. *Neurochem. Int.* **46,** 551–557.

Lindberg, C., Selenica, M. L., Westlind-Danielsson, A., and Schultzberg, M. (2005b). Beta-amyloid protein structure determines the nature of cytokine release from rat microglia. *J. Mol. Neurosci.* **27,** 1–12.

Lio, D., Licastro, F., Scola, L., Chiappelli, M., Grimaldi, L. M., Crivello, A., Colonna-Romano, G., Candore, G., Franceschi, C., and Caruso, C. (2003). Interleukin-10 promoter polymorphism in sporadic Alzheimer's disease. *Genes Immun.* **4,** 234–238.

Lugaresi, A., Di Iorio, A., Iarlori, C., Reale, M., De Luca, G., Sparvieri, E., Michetti, A., Conti, P., Gambi, D., Abate, G., and Paganelli, R. (2004). IL-4 *in vitro* production is upregulated in Alzheimer's disease patients treated with acetylcholinesterase inhibitors. *Exp. Gerontol.* **39,** 653–657.

Luo, Q., Ding, Y., Watson, K., Zhang, J., and Fan, G. H. (2005). N-methyl-D-aspartate attenuates CXCR2-mediated neuroprotection through enhancing the receptor phosphorylation and blocking the receptor recycling. *Mol. Pharmacol.* **68,** 528–537.

Luterman, J. D., Haroutunian, V., Yemul, S., Ho, L., Purohit, D., Aisen, P. S., Mohs, R., and Pasinetti, G. M. (2000). Cytokine gene expression as a function of the clinical progression of Alzheimer disease dementia. *Arch. Neurol.* **57,** 1153–1160.

Lynch, M. A. (2002). Interleukin-1 beta exerts a myriad of effects in the brain and in particular in the hippocampus: Analysis of some of these actions. *Vitam. Horm.* **64,** 185–219.

Ma, S. L., Tang, N. L., Lam, L. C., and Chiu, H. F. (2005). The association between promoter polymorphism of the interleukin-10 gene and Alzheimer's disease. *Neurobiol. Aging* **26,** 1005–1010.

Mandelkow, E. M., Stamer, K., Vogel, R., Thies, E., and Mandelkow, E. (2003). Clogging of axons by tau, inhibition of axonal traffic and starvation of synapses. *Neurobiol. Aging* **24,** 1079–1085.

Marshak, D. R., Pesce, S. A., Stanley, L. C., and Griffin, W. S. (1992). Increased S100 beta neurotrophic activity in Alzheimer's disease temporal lobe. *Neurobiol. Aging* **13,** 1–7.

Martinez, M., Fernandez-Vivancos, E., Frank, A., De la Fuente, M., and Hernanz, A. (2000). Increased cerebrospinal fluid fas (Apo-1) levels in Alzheimer's disease. Relationship with IL-6 concentrations. *Brain Res.* **869,** 216–219.

Marz, P., Heese, K., Hock, C., Golombowski, S., Muller-Spahn, F., Rose-John, S., and Otten, U. (1997). Interleukin-6 (IL-6) and soluble forms of IL-6 receptors are not altered in cerebrospinal fluid of Alzheimer's disease patients. *Neurosci. Lett.* **239,** 29–32.

McGeer, P. L., and McGeer, E. G. (2001). Inflammation, autotoxicity and Alzheimer disease. *Neurobiol. Aging* **22,** 799–809.

McGeer, P. L., Schulzer, M., and McGeer, E. G. (1996). Arthritis and anti-inflammatory agents as possible protective factors for Alzheimer's disease: A review of 17 epidemiologic studies. *Neurology* **47,** 425–432.

Meda, L., Baron, P., Prat, E., Scarpini, E., Scarlato, G., Cassatella, M. A., and Rossi, F. (1999). Proinflammatory profile of cytokine production by human monocytes and murine microglia stimulated with beta-amyloid[25-35]. *J. Neuroimmunol.* **93,** 45–52.

Mesches, M. H., Gemma, C., Veng, L. M., Allgeier, C., Young, D. A., Browning, M. D., and Bickford, P. C. (2004). Sulindac improves memory and increases NMDA receptor subunits in aged Fischer 344 rats. *Neurobiol. Aging* **25,** 315–324.

Minogue, A. M., Schmid, A. W., Fogarty, M. P., Moore, A. C., Campbell, V. A., Herron, C. E., and Lynch, M. A. (2003). Activation of the c-Jun N-terminal kinase signaling cascade mediates the effect of amyloid-beta on long term potentiation and cell death in hippocampus: A role for interleukin-1beta? *J. Biol. Chem.* **278,** 27971–27980.

Mirra, S. S., Heyman, A., McKeel, D., Sumi, S. M., Crain, B. J., Brownlee, L. M., Vogel, F. S., Hughes, J. P., van Belle, G., and Berg, L. (1991). The consortium to establish a registry for

Alzheimer's disease (CERAD). Part II. Standardization of the neuropathologic assessment of Alzheimer's disease. *Neurology* **41**, 479–486.

Morgan, D., Gordon, M. N., Tan, J., Wilcock, D., and Rojiani, A. M. (2005). Dynamic complexity of the microglial activation response in transgenic models of amyloid deposition: Implications for Alzheimer therapeutics. *J. Neuropathol. Exp. Neurol.* **64**, 743–753.

Morihara, T., Chu, T., Ubeda, O., Beech, W., and Cole, G. M. (2002). Selective inhibition of Abeta42 production by NSAID R-enantiomers. *J. Neurochem.* **83**, 1009–1012.

Morihara, T., Teter, B., Yang, F., Lim, G. P., Boudinot, S., Boudinot, F. D., Frautschy, S. A., and Cole, G. M. (2005). Ibuprofen suppresses interleukin-1beta induction of pro-amyloidogenic alpha1-antichymotrypsin to ameliorate beta-amyloid (Abeta) pathology in Alzheimer's models. *Neuropsychopharmacology* **30**, 1111–1120.

Murphy, G. M., Jr., Claassen, J. D., De Voss, J. J., Pascoe, N., Taylor, J., Tinklenberg, J. R., and Yesavage, J. A. (2001). Rate of cognitive decline in AD is accelerated by the interleukin-1 alpha -889 *1 allele. *Neurology* **56**, 1595–1597.

Nagai, A., Nakagawa, E., Hatori, K., Choi, H. B., McLarnon, J. G., Lee, M. A., and Kim, S. U. (2001). Generation and characterization of immortalized human microglial cell lines: Expression of cytokines and chemokines. *Neurobiol. Dis.* **8**, 1057–1068.

Nagele, R. G., D' Andrea, M. R., Lee, H., Venkataraman, V., and Wang, H. Y. (2003). Astrocytes accumulate A beta 42 and give rise to astrocytic amyloid plaques in Alzheimer disease brains. *Brain Res.* **971**, 197–209.

Neary, D., Snowden, J., and Mann, D. (2005). Frontotemporal dementia. *Lancet Neurol.* **4**, 771–780.

Nicoll, J. A., Mrak, R. E., Graham, D. I., Stewart, J., Wilcock, G., Mac Gowan, S., Esiri, M. M., Murray, L. S., Dewar, D., Love, S., Moss, T., and Griffin, W. S. (2000). Association of interleukin-1 gene polymorphisms with Alzheimer's disease. *Ann. Neurol.* **47**, 365–368.

Nicoll, J. A., Wilkinson, D., Holmes, C., Steart, P., Markham, H., and Weller, R. O. (2003). Neuropathology of human Alzheimer disease after immunization with amyloid-beta peptide: A case report. *Nat. Med.* **9**, 448–452.

Papassotiropoulos, A., Bagli, M., Jessen, F., Bayer, T. A., Maier, W., Rao, M. L., and Heun, R. (1999). A genetic variation of the inflammatory cytokine interleukin-6 delays the initial onset and reduces the risk for sporadic Alzheimer's disease. *Ann. Neurol.* **45**, 666–668.

Pirttila, T., Mehta, P. D., Frey, H., and Wisniewski, H. M. (1994). Alpha 1-antichymotrypsin and IL-1 beta are not increased in CSF or serum in Alzheimer's disease. *Neurobiol. Aging* **15**, 313–317.

Qiu, Z., and Gruol, D. L. (2003). Interleukin-6, beta-amyloid peptide and NMDA interactions in rat cortical neurons. *J. Neuroimmunol.* **139**, 51–57.

Quintanilla, R. A., Orellana, D. I., Gonzalez-Billault, C., and Maccioni, R. B. (2004). Interleukin-6 induces Alzheimer-type phosphorylation of tau protein by deregulating the cdk5/p35 pathway. *Exp. Cell Res.* **295**, 245–257.

Rogers, J., Kirby, L. C., Hempelman, S. R., Berry, D. L., McGeer, P. L., Kaszniak, A. W., Zalinski, J., Cofield, M., Mansukhani, L., Willson, P., *et al.* (1993). Clinical trial of indomethacin in Alzheimer's disease. *Neurology* **43**, 1609–1611.

Rogers, J. T., Leiter, L. M., McPhee, J., Cahill, C. M., Zhan, S. S., Potter, H., and Nilsson, L. N. (1999). Translation of the alzheimer amyloid precursor protein mRNA is up-regulated by interleukin-1 through 5'-untranslated region sequences. *J. Biol. Chem.* **274**, 6421–6431.

Scassellati, C., Zanardini, R., Squitti, R., Bocchio-Chiavetto, L., Bonvicini, C., Binetti, G., Zanetti, O., Cassetta, E., and Gennarelli, M. (2004). Promoter haplotypes of interleukin-10 gene and sporadic Alzheimer's disease. *Neurosci. Lett.* **356**, 119–122.

Schenk, D., Barbour, R., Dunn, W., Gordon, G., Grajeda, H., Guido, T., Hu, K., Huang, J., Johnson-Wood, K., Khan, K., Kholodenko, D., Lee, M., *et al.* (1999). Immunization with amyloid-beta attenuates Alzheimer-disease-like pathology in the PDAPP mouse. *Nature* **400**, 173–177.

Sciacca, F. L., Ferri, C., Licastro, F., Veglia, F., Biunno, I., Gavazzi, A., Calabrese, E., Martinelli Boneschi, F., Sorbi, S., Mariani, C., Franceschi, M., and Grimaldi, L. M. (2003). Interleukin-1B polymorphism is associated with age at onset of Alzheimer's disease. *Neurobiol. Aging* **24**, 927–931.

Selkoe, D. J., Yamazaki, T., Citron, M., Podlisny, M. B., Koo, E. H., Teplow, D. B., and Haass, C. (1996). The role of APP processing and trafficking pathways in the formation of amyloid beta-protein. *Ann. N. Y. Acad. Sci.* **777**, 57–64.

Sheng, J. G., Jones, R. A., Zhou, X. Q., McGinness, J. M., Van Eldik, L. J., Mrak, R. E., and Griffin, W. S. (2001a). Interleukin-1 promotion of MAPK-p38 overexpression in experimental animals and in Alzheimer's disease: Potential significance for tau protein phosphorylation. *Neurochem. Int.* **39**, 341–348.

Sheng, J. G., Mrak, R. E., Jones, R. A., Brewer, M. M., Zhou, X. Q., McGinness, J., Woodward, S., Bales, K., Paul, S. M., Cordell, B., and Griffin, W. S. (2001b). Neuronal DNA damage correlates with overexpression of interleukin-1beta converting enzyme in APPV717F mice. *Neurobiol. Aging* **22**, 895–902.

Shibata, N., Ohnuma, T., Takahashi, T., Baba, H., Ishizuka, T., Ohtsuka, M., Ueki, A., Nagao, M., and Arai, H. (2002). The effect of IL4+33C/T polymorphism on risk of Japanese sporadic Alzheimer's disease. *Neurosci. Lett.* **323**, 161–163.

Strauss, S., Bauer, J., Ganter, U., Jonas, U., Berger, M., and Volk, B. (1992). Detection of interleukin-6 and alpha 2-macroglobulin immunoreactivity in cortex and hippocampus of Alzheimer's disease patients. *Lab. Invest.* **66**, 223–230.

Sun, Y. X., Minthon, L., Wallmark, A., Warkentin, S., Blennow, K., and Janciauskiene, S. (2003). Inflammatory markers in matched plasma and cerebrospinal fluid from patients with Alzheimer's disease. *Dement. Geriatr. Cogn. Disord.* **16**, 136–144.

Szczepanik, A. M., and Ringheim, G. E. (2003). IL-10 and glucocorticoids inhibit Abeta(1-42)- and lipopolysaccharide-induced pro-inflammatory cytokine and chemokine induction in the central nervous system. *J. Alzheimers Dis.* **5**, 105–117.

Szczepanik, A. M., Funes, S., Petko, W., and Ringheim, G. E. (2001). IL-4, IL-10 and IL-13 modulate A beta(1-42)-induced cytokine and chemokine production in primary murine microglia and a human monocyte cell line. *J. Neuroimmunol.* **113**, 49–62.

Tarkowski, E., Liljeroth, A. M., Nilsson, A., Minthon, L., and Blennow, K. (2001). Decreased levels of intrathecal interleukin 1 receptor antagonist in Alzheimer's disease. *Dement. Geriatr. Cogn. Disord.* **12**, 314–317.

Tehranian, R., Hasanvan, H., Iverfeldt, K., Post, C., and Schultzberg, M. (2001). Early induction of interleukin-6 mRNA in the hippocampus and cortex of APPsw transgenic mice Tg2576. *Neurosci. Lett.* **301**, 54–58.

Terry, R. D., Masliah, E., Salmon, D. P., Butters, N., DeTeresa, R., Hill, R., Hansen, L. A., and Katzman, R. (1991). Physical basis of cognitive alterations in Alzheimer's disease: Synapse loss is the major correlate of cognitive impairment. *Ann. Neurol.* **30**, 572–580.

Terwel, D., Dewachter, I., and Van Leuven, F. (2002). Axonal transport, tau protein, and neurodegeneration in Alzheimer's disease. *Neuromolecular Med.* **2**, 151–165.

Town, T., Nikolic, V., and Tan, J. (2005). The microglial "activation" continuum: From innate to adaptive responses. *J. Neuroinflammation* **2**, 24.

Townsend, K. P., Town, T., Mori, T., Lue, L. F., Shytle, D., Sanberg, P. R., Morgan, D., Fernandez, F., Flavell, R. A., and Tan, J. (2005). CD40 signaling regulates innate and adaptive activation of microglia in response to amyloid beta-peptide. *Eur. J. Immunol.* **35**, 901–910.

Ullian, E. M., Sapperstein, S. K., Christopherson, K. S., and Barres, B. A. (2001). Control of synapse number by glia. *Science* **291**, 657–661.

Wada-Isoe, K., Wakutani, Y., Urakami, K., and Nakashima, K. (2004). Elevated interleukin-6 levels in cerebrospinal fluid of vascular dementia patients. *Acta Neurol. Scand.* **110**, 124–127.

Walsh, D. M., Klyubin, I., Fadeeva, J. V., Rowan, M. J., and Selkoe, D. J. (2002). Amyloid-beta oligomers: Their production, toxicity and therapeutic inhibition. *Biochem. Soc. Trans.* **30**, 552–557.

Weggen, S., Eriksen, J. L., Das, P., Sagi, S. A., Wang, R., Pietrzik, C. U., Findlay, K. A., Smith, T. E., Murphy, M. P., Bulter, T., Kang, D. E., Marquez-Sterling, N., *et al.* (2001). A subset of NSAIDs lower amyloidogenic Abeta42 independently of cyclooxygenase activity. *Nature* **414**, 212–216.

Weggen, S., Eriksen, J. L., Sagi, S. A., Pietrzik, C. U., Ozols, V., Fauq, A., Golde, T. E., and Koo, E. H. (2003). Evidence that nonsteroidal anti-inflammatory drugs decrease amyloid beta 42 production by direct modulation of gamma-secretase activity. *J. Biol. Chem.* **278**, 31831–31837.

Weiner, H. L., Lemere, C. A., Maron, R., Spooner, E. T., Grenfell, T. J., Mori, C., Issazadeh, S., Hancock, W. W., and Selkoe, D. J. (2000). Nasal administration of amyloid-beta peptide decreases cerebral amyloid burden in a mouse model of Alzheimer's disease. *Ann. Neurol.* **48**, 567–579.

White, J. A., Manelli, A. M., Holmberg, K. H., Van Eldik, L. J., and Ladu, M. J. (2005). Differential effects of oligomeric and fibrillar amyloid-beta 1–42 on astrocyte-mediated inflammation. *Neurobiol. Dis.* **18**, 459–465.

Xia, M., Qin, S., McNamara, M., Mackay, C., and Hyman, B. T. (1997). Interleukin-8 receptor B immunoreactivity in brain and neuritic plaques of Alzheimer's disease. *Am. J. Pathol.* **150**, 1267–1274.

Yaffe, K., Kanaya, A., Lindquist, K., Simonsick, E. M., Harris, T., Shorr, R. I., Tylavsky, F. A., and Newman, A. B. (2004). The metabolic syndrome, inflammation, and risk of cognitive decline. *JAMA* **292**, 2237–2242.

Yang, F., Sun, X., Beech, W., Teter, B., Wu, S., Sigel, J., Vinters, H. V., Frautschy, S. A., and Cole, G. M. (1998). Antibody to caspase-cleaved actin detects apoptosis in differentiated neuroblastoma and plaque-associated neurons and microglia in Alzheimer's disease. *Am. J. Pathol.* **152**, 379–389.

Yang, S., Liu, Z. W., Wen, L., Qiao, H. F., Zhou, W. X., and Zhang, Y. X. (2005). Interleukin-1beta enhances NMDA receptor-mediated current but inhibits excitatory synaptic transmission. *Brain Res.* **1034**, 172–179.

Yasuhara, O., Matsuo, A., Terai, K., Walker, D. G., Berger, A. E., Akiguchi, I., Kimura, J., and McGeer, P. L. (1997). Expression of interleukin-1 receptor antagonist protein in post-mortem human brain tissues of Alzheimer's disease and control cases. *Acta Neuropathol. (Berl.)* **93**, 414–420.

Yucesoy, B., Peila, R., White, L. R., Wu, K. M., Johnson, V. J., Kashon, M. L., Luster, M. I., and Launer, L. J. (2005). Association of interleukin-1 gene polymorphisms with dementia in a community-based sample: The Honolulu-Asia Aging Study. *Neurobiol Aging.* [Epub ahead of print].

Zhang, Y., Hayes, A., Pritchard, A., Thaker, U., Haque, M. S., Lemmon, H., Harris, J., Cumming, A., Lambert, J. C., Chartier-Harlin, M. C., St Clair, D., Iwatsubo, T., *et al.* (2004). Interleukin-6 promoter polymorphism: Risk and pathology of Alzheimer's disease. *Neurosci. Lett.* **362**, 99–102.

21

INTERLEUKIN-2: FROM T CELL GROWTH AND HOMEOSTASIS TO IMMUNE RECONSTITUTION OF HIV PATIENTS

MARKO KRYWORUCHKO* AND JACQUES THÈZE[†]

*Infectious Disease and Vaccine Research Centre, and Division of Virology
Children's Hospital of Eastern Ontario, Ottawa, Canada
[†]ImmunoGénétique Cellulaire, Institut Pasteur, Paris, France

Interleukin (IL)-2 was initially described as a major stimulant of T lymphocytes *in vitro*. Later, the characterization of IL-2 knockout animals showed that the ability to stimulate T cells could be replaced by other cytokines. *In vivo*, IL-2 plays a unique role in controlling lymphoproliferation. This is partly explained by its role in the generation and maintenance of T regulatory cells (Treg). In HIV-infected patients, the IL-2/IL-2 receptor (IL-2R) system is dysregulated. The fact that IL-2 is underproduced along with defective IL-2R signaling detected in patient lymphocytes, may explain the progressive impairment of the immune

0083-6729/06 $35.00
DOI: 10.1016/S0083-6729(06)74021-3

system that occurs during chronic infection with this virus. These defects

concerning the effect of this cytokine has surfaced, placing it at the center of

system that occurs during chronic infection with this virus. These defects are partly reversed by highly active antiretroviral therapy (HAART). However, in some patients IL-2R defects persist and the CD4 counts remain low despite good control of the viral load. These patients benefit from HAART given in conjunction with IL-2 therapy. © 2006 Elsevier Inc.

I. INTRODUCTION

Since the discovery of interleukin (IL)-2 biological activity in 1975 as a factor promoting the growth of T cells, a tremendous amount of information concerning the effect of this cytokine has surfaced, placing it at the center of the immune response. Studies have also suggested that the principal role of this cytokine *in vivo* may rather be to control the immune response due to its necessity for the development and peripheral expansion of regulatory T cells. IL-2 has been implicated in the pathogenesis of HIV infection and used with success therapeutically to restore CD4 T cell numbers in HIV-infected patients. This chapter will provide an overall description of the distribution and functioning of the IL-2 system with special attention to developments and their possible clinical implications in HIV infection.

II. IL-2 AND ITS RECEPTORS

The *IL-2* gene, first cloned in 1983, resides on chromosome 4 in humans (Devos *et al.*, 1983; Taniguchi *et al.*, 1983). This 133 amino acid (aa) protein with a molecular weight of 15–18 kDa is part of the hematopoeitin family of cytokines, owing to its compact core of four antiparallel α-helices connected by three loops. IL-2 is expressed primarily by activated CD4 T cells. *In vitro* mitogenic stimulation of T cells with PMA and calcium ionophore or cross-linking cell surface CD3 and CD28 molecules is well known to upregulate IL-2 mRNA, protein expression, and its secretion. CD8 T cells also secrete IL-2 following T cell receptor cross-linking. However, among antigen presenting cells, dendritic cells (DC) (Granucci *et al.*, 2001) in response to microbial challenge and B cell lines (Gaffen *et al.*, 1996; Walker *et al.*, 1988) but not macrophages (Granucci *et al.*, 2002) have been shown to produce IL-2. This may serve to enhance T cell activation under certain circumstances as DC taken from IL-2 KO mice exhibit an impaired capacity to induce T cell proliferation (Granucci *et al.*, 2002).

The proteins which make up the IL-2 receptor (IL-2R) include the IL-2Rα, IL-2Rβ, and common γ (γc) chains (Minami *et al.*, 1993; Sugamura *et al.*, 1996). The human *IL-2Rα* gene is found on chromosome 10p14–15, spanning greater than 35kb of genomic DNA, and contains 8 exons. It encodes a 251 aa protein with significant homology to only the IL-15Rα protein. IL-2Rα (CD25, Tac) is a 55-kDa glycoprotein unique to the IL-2 system, but on its own has low affinity for IL-2 and no signal-transducing capacity because of its short (13 aa) cytoplasmic tail. The intermediate affinity IL-2R is composed of the IL-2Rβ and the common γc proteins. Human IL-2Rβ spans 24 kb of genomic DNA on chromosome 22q11.2–12 and is divided into 10 exons. The mature IL-2Rβ protein is a 525 aa long, 75 kDa integral membrane glycoprotein and a member of the cytokine receptor superfamily with its conserved WSXWS extracellular motif. The first 214 aa correspond to the extracellular domain while the next 25 and 286 aa constitute the membrane-spanning region and the large cytoplasmic tail, respectively. The cytoplasmic tail has been further subdivided into unique regions based on aa composition: Box 1, ser-rich, acidic, and proline-rich regions. Each of these regions has distinct roles in signal transduction on ligation of the receptor with IL-2. The γc is a 64-kDa protein member of the cytokine receptor super-family, consisting of a 232 aa acid extracellular, a 29 aa membrane spanning, and an 86 aa cytoplasmic regions. Its cytoplasmic region contains 2 SH2 subdomains.

IL-2Rβ is also utilized by IL-15 while the γc is shared by a number of cytokines including IL-2, IL-4, IL-7, IL-9, IL-15, and IL-21. Both chains of the intermediate-affinity receptor are thought to be required for trans-ducing the full spectrum of IL-2-dependent signals. When coupled with the IL-2Rα chain, which functions as an affinity converter, the trimolecular complex acquires high affinity for IL-2. However, we have established that the functional IL-2R may take on forms other than αβγ and βγ (Eckenberg et al., 2000). We have identified a peptide agonist for the IL-2Rβ chain consisting of the first 30 aa of IL-2 (p1–30). P1–30 interacted specifically with a dimeric form of IL-2Rβ, triggered a distinct signaling cascade, activated CD8, NK and lymphokine activated killer (LAK) cells, and induced the production of IFN-γ in human peripheral blood mononuclear (PBMC) cell cultures.

IL-2Rα protein expression is generally undetectable by flow cytometry on the surface of most resting human PBMC subsets (David et al., 1998a; Thèze et al., 1996). It is found however on the CD4+ regulatory T cell subset (Nelson, 2004). Although variable results have been reported, IL-2Rβ and γc chains are expressed at low to undetectable levels at the surface of resting T and B lymphocytes (David et al., 1998a). Antigenic or mitogenic activa-tion upregulates high-affinity IL-2R expression at their cell surface, thus permitting potent responsiveness to IL-2. We showed that γc may exist as an immature, cytoplasmic precursor protein in resting CD4 T lymphocytes (Bani et al., 2001). Only on T cell activation (anti-CD3 ± anti-CD28 Abs) does the γc protein complete its maturation and is expressed at the cell surface. NK cells express relatively high levels of IL-2Rβ while γc is not readily detectable at the cell surface of NK cells (David *et al.*, 1998a). Monocytes have been reported to express relatively high levels of IL-2Rβ and γc and these cells also respond spontaneously to IL-2 (David *et al.*, 1998a; Espinoza-Delgado *et al.*, 1995).

Overall, this suggests that cells of the adaptive immune response tend not to be able to respond strongly to IL-2, requiring prior stimulation with antigen to do so, while cells governing innate immunity appear not to require prior sensitization to respond. Furthermore, the respective IL-2R chains may assume novel functional combinations (Eckenberg *et al.*, 2000). We have shown that IL-2 responsiveness is also controlled by lineage specific mechanisms (Gesbert *et al.*, 2005).

III. PHYSIOLOGY AND PATHOPHYSIOLOGY OF IL-2

Although it has been reported to act on a variety of cellular targets, one of the principal functions of IL-2 appeared to be the induction of Ag-activated CD4+ and CD8+ T cell proliferation *in vitro* and whence it was originally referred to as the "T cell growth factor" (TCGF) (Gillis *et al.*, 1978). This occurs via proliferative signals delivered by c-myc and c-Fos transcription factors and antiapoptotic signals delivered by members of the bcl-2 family (Miyazaki *et al.*, 1995). Studies suggest that long term T cell survival is also affected by IL-2 through its influence on cellular metabolism and glycolysis (Frauwirth and Thompson, 2004; Rathmell *et al.*, 2000). IL-2 has been reported to generate lymphokine activated killer cells, to induce the proliferation and cytotoxic activity of NK cells as well as the secretion of cytokines (TNF-α, IFN-γ, GM-CSF) by these cells (Minami *et al.*, 1993). B cell responsiveness to IL-2 was demonstrated by the upregulation of IL-2Rα, and in synergy with IL-5 it has been shown to increase heavy, light, and J-chain immunoglobulin expression (Minami *et al.*, 1993). IL-2 has also surfaced as a monocyte activator, inducing cytokine (IL-1β, TNF-α, IL-6, IL-8) production and is reported to trigger their tumoricidal properties (Espinoza-Delgado *et al.*, 1995). These processes may require the expression of the CD14 differentiation antigen on their surface. Early reports have even implicated this cytokine in the growth and maturation of oligodendrocytes derived from primary glial cell cultures (Benveniste and Merrill, 1986).

Despite these pleiotropic effects, evidence from other *in vitro* studies and particularly those utilizing gene knockout (KO) animal models have suggested that the principal nonredundant role of IL-2 may be in the downregulation of the immune response and prevention of autoimmunity (Malek and Bayer, 2004; Thèze *et al.*, 1996). Surprisingly, when taking into consideration its potent T cell growth factor activity, IL-2-, IL-2Rα-, and IL-2Rβ-deficient mice all exhibit uncontrolled lymphocyte activation and severe autoimmune disorders. In IL-2 KO mice, lymphoid development appears to be normal for the most part, with the appearance of all the major lymphocyte (T, B, NK) subsets. However, the development of CD8$\alpha\alpha$+ TCR$\gamma\delta$+ and TCR $\alpha\beta$+ CD8$\alpha\alpha$+ T cells is impaired. *In vitro* immune responses of both T and B cells are attenuated. The major pathology in these mice is characterized by massive lymphoid organ hyperplasia, fatal autoimmune hemolytic anemia, and inflammatory bowel disease. A similar phenotype is observed in IL-2R$\alpha^{-/-}$ mice. No differences were observed in T and B cell development. However, there was massive lymphoid expansion and severe anemia and inflammatory bowel disease develop. IL-2Rβ KO mice also suffer from autoimmunity but defects are more severe as a result of the additional compromise in IL-15 responses. Whence, they fail to develop NK cells and intestinal epithelial lymphocytes. There is massive splenic infiltration by myelopoietic cells. Antinuclear, anti-DNA, as well as antierythrocyte antibodies are invariably detected and lead to autoimmune anemia. Pathology in these mice is influenced by environmental and genetic factors, and appears to require an antigenic trigger and thymus-derived T cells. In humans, a pediatric patient whose cells fail to express IL-2Rα was described to be immune compromised and exhibited signs of autoimmunity (lymphadenopathy, hepatosplenomegaly, chronic inflammatory disorders, and so on) (Sharfe *et al.*, 1997).

Although the mechanisms by which IL-2 responsiveness controls T cell homeostasis and prevents autoimmunity are not fully understood, the phenomena observed in the above-mentioned studies are consistent with a number of observations. First, the capacity of IL-2 to eventually sensitize activated T cells to undergo apoptosis in the process of activation-induced cell death (AICD) (Lenardo *et al.*, 1999; Van Parijs and Abbas, 1998). AICD is an *in vitro* model by which a T cell–effector response may be "turned off" once the antigenic stimulus/pathogen has been eliminated. Initially T cells are expanded and differentiate into effectors in the presence of Ag and IL-2. Once the Ag is removed by effector T cells, those remaining are presumably no longer needed. They are believed to remove by apoptosis triggered at least in part by increased Fas–FasL interactions, the upregulation of TNF receptor (TNFR) and a decrease in c-FLIP expression. IL-2 may promote AICD by its upregulation of FasL expression in the expanded population of T cells as well as its induction of IFN-γ production. In the absence of IL-2 responsiveness, mice are resistant to AICD (Khoruts *et al.*, 1998; Kneitz *et al.*, 1995; Van Parijs *et al.*, 1997, 1999; Willerford *et al.*, 1995; Wrenshall and Platt, 1999). However, there are reports suggesting that AICD proceeds normally under these conditions (Leung *et al.*, 2000; Suzuki *et al.*, 1997). Other reports also suggest that AICD may not be the primary mechanism by which IL-2 is able to maintain peripheral tolerance *in vivo* (Cheng *et al.*, 2002; D'Souza *et al.*, 2002; Fujii *et al.*, 1998; Malek *et al.*, 2000; Van Parijs *et al.*, 1999). For example, mice engineered to express IL-2R in the thymus but not in the periphery, where AICD putatively occurs, fail to exhibit autoimmune symptoms. The role of c-FLIP in the lymphoproliferation observed in IL-2 KO animals has also been analyzed (Chastagner *et al.*, 2002).

Another mechanism, which has gained considerable support in the past few years, involves the action of regulatory T cells. A number of regulatory T cell subsets have been described (Nelson, 2004). They include IL-10-producing Tr1 cells, TGF-β-producing Th3 cells and CD4+, CD25+ (IL-2Rα) regulatory T cells (Tregs). Our chapter will focus on this latter subset of Tregs because of the accumulating data demonstrating how IL-2 is a critical growth factor for these cells. Tregs are naturally occurring cells, which develop in the thymus, and make up 5–10% of T cells in human PBMC. Although their effector mechanisms are not completely defined, they are known for their capacity to inhibit T cell proliferation *in vitro* and suppress autoreactive T cells *in vivo*. Tregs are further distinguished from conventional CD4+ T cells by their expression of the Foxp3 transcription factor, glucocorticoid-induced cell surface TNFR expression, and inability to produce IL-2. It has been shown that IL-2 and IL-2Rβ KO mice lack Tregs (Almeida *et al.*, 2002; Lenardo, 1991; Malek *et al.*, 2002). Furthermore, adoptive transfer of these cells into deficient mice prevents autoimmunity (Almeida *et al.*, 2002; Malek *et al.*, 2002). The role of IL-2 signaling in Treg cell development in the thymus, their maintenance in the periphery, as well as their effector function, is the subject of intense investigation. The fact that the development of Tregs absolutely requires expression of the γc and that an IL-2Rβ transgene expressed preferentially in the thymus is able to rescue Treg development suggested that signals delivered by IL-2 or cytokines which share these receptors may be developmentally important. However, data suggests that there may not be an absolute requirement for IL-2-specific signaling. Fontenot *et al.* (2005) followed FoxP3-GFP+ Tregs in an IL-2$^{-/-}$ or IL-2R$\alpha^{-/-}$ mouse background. Interestingly, only about a 50% reduction in FoxP3+ Tregs was observed. Similarly, D'Cruz *et al.* (2005) bread mice with influenza HA-specific TCR transgenic FoxP3+ T regs. In the absence of IL-2 of IL-2Rα, little or no effect on thymic Treg development was observed. However, data from both these studies did suggest that IL-2 signaling appeared to be important to maintain the competitive fitness of Treg cells in the periphery. Furthermore, those Tregs that did develop in the absence of IL-2 responsiveness were functional. The majority of FoxP3+, IL-2 Treg cell markers were not affected. Decreased expression of TGF-β1 and a number of genes regulating the cell cycle, proliferation, and growth were observed and are potential candidates for the ability of Treg to compete in the periphery with conventional CD4+ T cells.

IV. IL-2R-DEPENDENT SIGNAL TRANSDUCTION MECHANISMS

In order to mediate these biological effects, IL-2–IL-2R interactions transduce a complicated set of signals. This involves different families of protein kinases (tyr and ser/thr), transcription factors, and at least three major signaling pathways: the Janus kinase (JAK)/signal transducer and activator of transcription (STAT) pathway, the G-protein ras/mitogen-activated protein kinase pathway (MAPK), and the phosphatidylinositol-3 kinase (PI-3K) pathway. As considerable detail is provided elsewhere (Dong *et al.*, 2002; Gesbert *et al.*, 1998; Koyasu, 2003; Leonard and O'Shea, 1998; Lin and Leonard, 2000), we will only overview how they are recruited in human T cells stimulated with IL-2 and present some findings.

The Janus kinase/STAT pathway, represents a major signal transduction pathway involved in cytokine responses (Leonard and O'Shea, 1998). The interaction of IL-2 with its intermediate- or high-affinity receptor triggers within minutes the JAK/STAT signal transduction cascade (Lin and Leonard, 2000), which involves the phosphorylation and activation of JAK-1 and JAK-3 kinases that are constitutively associated with the IL-2Rβ and γc, respectively. Subsequently, both receptor chains are phosphorylated, and STAT5 is recruited to the phosphorylated receptor complex via Sh2 domain interaction. STAT5 is tyr-phosphorylated by JAKs, triggering Sh2-p-tyr–mediated dimerization and translocation to the nucleus where transactivation of target genes containing specific DNA response elements such as the *IL-2Rα* gene itself. Human STAT5 is encoded by two homologous genes, *STAT5a* and *STAT5b*, which exhibit 91% identity at the amino acid level.

Mitogen activated protein kinases (MAPK) are serine/threonine kinases that are activated by a host of stimulants including growth factors, cytokines, and antigens (Dong *et al.*, 2002). The MAPK pathway is a three-tiered cascade known to be critical at various phases of the immune response including the initiation of innate immunity, T cell activation, differentiation and function, as well as their survival and apoptosis. It involves the G-protein–dependent (e.g., Ras) activation of MAPK kinase kinases (MAPKKK) (e.g., Raf) followed by the activation of the MAPK kinases (MAPKK), namely MEK1–7 (mitogen-activated ERK kinase) and culminates in the specific activation of the MAPKs, p38, ERK, and JNK. IL-2 is known to recruit the p21^{ras}/ MAPK pathway. This is thought to occur via the adaptor protein shc, which associates with the tyr-phosphorylated IL-2Rβ chain. Shc is itself tyr-phosphorylated by JAK-1, which is thought to allow its interaction with Grb2, another adaptor protein and the guanine nucleotide exchange factor mSOS. Together these interactions provide a link with how the ras/MAPK pathway is activated by IL-2. MAPK activation leads to the upregulation of c-Fos and c-Jun transcription factors.

The lipid protein PI-3K, which catalyzes the phosphorylation of PI-(3)-monophosphate to PI-(3,4)-bisphosphate, and PI-(3,4,5)-triphosphate (IP3) ultimately resulting in the activation of Akt (Protein kinase B), is also a critical signal transduction pathway regulating cell growth and survival of immune cells (Koyasu, 2003). IL-2 is believed to recruit PI-3K in a manner similar to that of MAPKs via JAK-1. JAK-1 activation results in phosphorylation and sequential recruitment of adaptor molecules including Shc,

Grb2, and finally Gab2. Phosphorylated Gab2 is then able to bind PI-3K. This leads to downstream activation of Akt and increased p70 s6 kinase activity. Notably, IL-2-dependent PI-3K recruitment in response to IL-2 results in the upregulation of bcl-xL and this likely results in the antiapoptotic effects of this cytokine in T cells (Gonzalez-Garcia et al., 1997).

Although the hierarchy and their precise roles are not fully understood, a number of other kinases integrate into the activation of these three classical signal transduction pathways and the biological activities of IL-2 (Ellery and Nicholls, 2002; Gesbert et al., 1998). The src family kinases including lck, lyn, and fyn have been associated with IL-2R signal transduction. For example, $p56^{lck}$ associates with the IL-2Rβ chain and its activity is increased in T cells stimulated with IL-2. This kinase is able to mediate IL-2Rβ phosphorylation in vitro. Furthermore, it has been suggested that lck in combination with JAK-1 are coupled to the recruitment of both the MAPK and PI-3K pathways. The syk kinase has also been shown to associate constitutively with IL-2Rβ and become activated in response to IL-2. Hierarchically, one model places syk downstream of JAK kinases while lck may work in parallel with JAK-3 (Zhou et al., 2000). The Pyk2 kinase has also been functionally linked with IL-2R signal transduction. It has been found to associate with JAK-3 in response to IL-2 and a dominant negative mutant of this kinase inhibited IL-2-induced proliferation in T cell lines in a STAT5-independent manner (Fujii et al., 1998). In addition, the ability of purified CD8 but not CD4 T cells to enter into cycle in response to IL-2 without prior triggering of the TCR appears to be governed by the fact that the p27 (kip1) cyclin-dependent kinase inhibitor is downregulated by IL-2 in CD8 but not CD4 T cells (Gesbert et al., 2005).

As mentioned earlier, the intermediate- and high-affinity receptor combinations may not be the only possible combinations for signal transduction. Our IL-2 mimetic p1–30 described in an earlier section, which binds to IL-2Rβ dimers, also triggers STAT5 phosphorylation by mechanisms that are under investigation (Eckenberg et al., 2000).

V. ROLE OF THE IL-2 SYSTEM IN HIV PATHOGENESIS

Deficiencies within the IL-2 system have long been recognized in HIV infection, including poor reactivity to this cytokine (Hauser et al., 1984). In view of the described immunoregulatory effects of IL-2, this may contribute to the eventual failure of the cell-mediated immune response in HIV-infected patients and lead to AIDS progression. IL-2 production, expression of all three IL-2R chains, and responsiveness to IL-2 have now been investigated in the PBMC subsets of HIV-infected patients (Chopra et al., 1993; David et al., 1998b; Hauser et al., 1984). During HIV infection, IL-2 production and expression of IL-2Rα have been reported to be decreased (Poli, 2001). Early studies on IL-2Rβ chain expression have been contradictory (Sahraoui et al., 1992; Vanham et al., 1994). The advent of highly active antiretroviral therapy (HAART) involving combinations of reverse transcriptase (RT) and protease inhibitors has lead to dramatic reductions in plasma virus loads, restoration of CD4 counts, and immune responsiveness in patients. It was therefore important to evaluate whether HAART also had beneficial effects on the functionality of the IL-2 system. Therefore, IL-2R chain expression and responsiveness to this cytokine was evaluated in the different PBMC subsets of HIV-infected patients, including B, T, NK, and monocytic cells (David et al., 1998b). Two groups of patients were recruited into this study. Group 1 (G1) included patients with high virus loads (mean of 2×10^5 copies per microliter) and CD4 counts of 303/μl at the mean that were treated at that time with only 1 or 2 RT inhibitors. Group 2 (G2) consisted of patients who had received HAART for a mean of 7 months and as a result, the majority had viral loads of <200 copies per microliter at the time of sampling and CD4 counts per microliter had increased from 94 to 310 over the treatment period. Unlike in HIV-negative controls, B lymphocytes from Group 1 (high virus load) had substantially higher levels of all three IL-2R chains and a strong capacity to enter into the cell cycle in response to ex vivo stimulation with IL-2. This finding was consistent with the hyperactivation of B cells observed in HIV infection. Under HAART (G2), IL-2R expression returned towards that of normal controls, as did responsiveness to IL-2, though it was still detectable. In CD8 T cells, IL-2R expression was also elevated in G1 patients. However, responsiveness to IL-2 did not increase proportionally. Strikingly, although HAART lowered IL-2R expression levels relative to G1 patients, IL-2 responsiveness had become clearly detectable. This was indicative of an IL-2R signaling blockade in G1 patients that appeared to be removed in patients undergoing HAART. A very similar pattern was observed in CD4 T cells, although IL-2R expression was lower overall. In monocytes from Group 1 patients, mainly IL-2Rβ and γc chain expression was elevated compared to HIV-negative controls, which returned towards normal in HAART patients. No dramatic differences in IL-2R expression were evident in NK cells, however, a reduced capacity to enter into cycle was noted in G1 patients relative to G2 on HAART.

The possibility of IL-2R-dependent signaling defects in CD4 and CD8 T cells has been further investigated in subsequent studies (Kryworuchko et al., 2003, 2004b). Considering the importance of the STAT5 transcription factor in mediating IL-2-dependent biological responses, we conducted a longitudinal study to investigate whether its induction by IL-2 was affected in chronically infected HIV+ individuals with high viral loads and the impact of HAART. We showed that the CD8 T cells from a subset (6/11) of HIV+ patients naïve to therapy were unable to functionally activate STAT5 in response to stimulation with IL-2. Furthermore, this defect was not due to alterations in IL-2R expression or lack of IL-2–IL-2R interactions but correlated with an impaired activation of the upstream kinase, JAK-3, known to mediate STAT5 activation. It appeared in this study that HAART restored JAK/STAT signaling, as detected by immunoblotting and electrophoretic mobility shift assay (EMSA). However, results evaluating cytokine-dependent activation of STAT5 by a modern flow cytometry-based technique suggested that restoration under HAART may only be partial (Abdkader et al., 2005; Kryworuchko et al., 2004a). We found that defects in STAT5 activation in the CD8 T cells from HIV-infected patients do not appear to be restricted to the IL-2 system but extend also to IL-7 and IL-15. In contrast, IL-10-induced STAT3 and IL-4-induced STAT6 activation appeared not to be affected compared to HIV− controls.

VI. IL-2 IMMUNOTHERAPY OF HIV PATIENTS

Because of its potent T cell stimulatory activity *in vitro*, IL-2 showed significant therapeutic promise, particularly under conditions where boosting immunity was the desired effect. As a result, IL-2 is licensed for treatment of melanoma and renal-cell carcinoma and is being used in clinical trials to boost immunity in HIV-infected patients (Atkins, 2002; Davey et al., 2000; Kovacs et al., 1996; Yang et al., 2003).

Chronic infection with HIV is characterized by a progressive depletion of CD4+ T cells, eventual susceptibility to opportunistic infections and establishment of AIDS (McCune, 2001). HAART has had a tremendous beneficial impact on reducing plasma virus load in patients, restoration of CD4 T cell counts and overall immune reconstitution. However, particularly marked in certain patient subsets, this immune restoration has been only partial (Marchetti et al., 2005). For example, in some patients even after prolonged HAART, CD4 counts fail to rise despite effective control of virus replication, perhaps leaving them more susceptible to opportunistic infections. IL-2 in combination with HAART has been used successfully in such patients to restore CD4 counts by a number of investigators (Pau and Tavel, 2002). In our studies (David et al., 2001), IL-2 was administered subcutaneously to a group of 13 patients, whose CD4 counts remained <200/µl even after 9 months of HAART [CD4 low responders, (CD4LR)]. After only three cycles of IL-2, their CD4 counts increased from 123 cell/µl (104–134) to 229 cell/µl (176–244). Furthermore, this increase was found particularly in the naïve CD45RA+ CD4+ T cells. Moreover, the magnitude of the CD4 cell recovery was positively correlated with baseline expression levels of the anti-apoptotic molecule bcl-2. A follow-up study in the same set of patients, revealed that CD4 T cells from CD4 LR patients at baseline were more susceptible to spontaneous apoptosis and failed to enter into the cell cycle in response to IL-2 stimulation *ex vivo* (David et al., 2002). IL-2 immunotherapy not only increased CD4 counts in these patients but was also able to increase their bcl-2 expression and IL-2 reactivity and this correlated with a reduction in the susceptibility of these cells to apoptosis. IL-2 has induced CD4 cell recovery also in patients with >200 CD4 cells/μl as well as HAART naïve patients with advanced disease. It has also been proposed as a possible HAART sparing therapy in chronically-infected patients following structured treatment interruption (STI) protocols. Administration of IL-2 prior to HAART interruption in chronically infected patients (CD4 > 500/μl) resulted in a delayed drop in CD4 T cells to a threshold requiring the reinitiation of HAART. Moreover, in STI during primary HIV infection, the rationale behind the use of IL-2 was also to attempt to expand HIV-specific T cells. The mechanisms involved in CD4 T cell recovery under IL-2 immunotherapy are not well understood. Evidence suggests that a balance between CD4 T cell apoptosis, survival, proliferation, and *de novo* synthesis is struck resulting in a net gain in CD4 cells. CD8 T cells appear to be under a distinct homeostatic mechanism, as their numbers do not increase in IL-2-treated patients. However, the impact of IL-2 immunotherapy on CD8 T cell function has not been investigated but would be predicted to have beneficial effects. The longer-term clinical benefit of IL-2 as an adjunct to HAART in terms of delaying disease progression and death is being evaluated in two large, five-year, phase-III clinical trials (ESPRIT and SILCAAT).

The accumulation of data concerning the critical role of IL-2 in the control of Treg cell production may have important, previously unappreciated, clinical implications. As described, IL-2 is being used in HIV-infected patients to boost CD4 T cell numbers. However, in addition to expanding effector T cell responses it may also enhance Treg cell number and magnitude, thereby diminishing the response eventually. On the other hand, keeping in view the capacity of IL-2 via Treg to balance CD4 and CD8 T cell responses and prevent autoimmunity, Treg cells may also serve to restore equilibrium to the HIV-imbalanced immune system. Treatment of HIV patients with IL-2 actually resulted in a reduction in basal CD4 T cell turnover despite an increase in naïve and memory CD4 T cell numbers. This could be related to the clonal expansion of CD4+/CD25+ T cells observed under these conditions, possibly representing Treg cells (Natarajan *et al.*, 2002; Sereti *et al.*, 2002, 2004). Of potential therapeutic significance is the finding that depletion of Treg cells from PBMC in patients increased cytokine production from HIV-specific CD4+ and CD8+ T cells (Aandahl *et al.*, 2004; Kinter *et al.*, 2004; Weiss *et al.*, 2004). However, there have been no differences in the percentage of CD4+/CD25+ T cells in HIV-positive patients compared to that of HIV-negative controls.

VII. CONCLUDING REMARKS

It is now well establish that, *in vivo*, IL-2 is a very important modulator of CD4 T lymphocyte homeostasis. It works through the generation and maintenance of CD4+CD25+ Treg. Therefore, the mode of action of IL-2 when used in cytokine-based therapy has to be reinvestigated (Sereti *et al.*, 2004; Zhang *et al.*, 2005). Recombinant IL-2 induces clinical responses in malignant melanoma and renal-cell carcinoma (Yang *et al.*, 2003). Combined with HAART it increases the CD4+ counts in HIV+ patients. The clinical benefits of treating HIV+ patients with IL-2 are still under investigation. It also remains to be demonstrated that IL-2 can be used either to delay the HAART start date or to spare its use. However, as we initially showed, IL-2 remains a useful drug to accelerate the recovery of CD4 counts in patients with CD4 count $<200/\mu l$ after prolonged HAART. In France, 1400 patients of this type have already received IL-2.

The clinical use of IL-2 is also limited by a number of side effects. IL-2 is accompanied by significant toxicity, particularly when given at high doses and via the intravenous route. IL-2 toxicity can manifest itself as acute respiratory failure and hypotension associated with vascular leak syndrome (VLS). VLS is characterized by damaged vascular endothelium, increased vascular permeability, decreased microcirculation and can lead to interstitial edema, and multiple organ failure within 2–24 h of IL-2 administration (Lentsch *et al.*, 1999; Locker *et al.*, 1999). NK lymphocytes and neutrophils are responsible for IL-2-induced VLS (Assier *et al.*, 2004, 2005). Therapeutically, it would be quite advantageous to be able to suppress the toxic effects of IL-2 while maintaining its reconstitutive effects on the cellular immune response. It appears that a structural motif within α helix A of IL-2 is responsible for VLS induction. This motif is centered around Asp20 of IL-2 and peptides containing aa 15–23 are capable of inducing VLS. Exploiting this information, we hypothesized that it may be possible to design IL-2 mimetics that maintain their stimulatory activity on lymphocytes, as described earlier, but lack VLS-inductive capacity. We have demonstrated that a mutation of the p1–30 peptide, described earlier, substituting Asp20 with Lys maintained its inductive effect on proliferation, generated LAK cells and induced IFN-γ production. This opens up the possibility of characterizing IL-2 mimetics with higher therapeutic indices than natural IL-2.

REFERENCES

Aandahl, E. M., Michaelsson, J., Moretto, W. J., Hecht, F. M., and Nixon, D. F. (2004). Human CD4+ CD25+ regulatory T cells control T-cell responses to human immunodeficiency virus and cytomegalovirus antigens. *J. Virol.* **78,** 2454–2459.

Abdkader, K., Al-Hetheel, A., Sant, N., Angel, J. B., Kumar, A., Diaz-Mitoma, F., and Kryworuchko, M. (2005). Disruption of cytokine signaling in T cells from HIV+ pateints: Role in pathogenesis. Ontario HIV Treatment Network Research Conference, Toronto, Ontario, Canada.

Almeida, A. R., Legrand, N., Papiernik, M., and Freitas, A. A. (2002). Homeostasis of peripheral CD4+ T cells: IL-2R alpha and IL-2 shape a population of regulatory cells that controls CD4+ T cell numbers. *J. Immunol.* **169,** 4850–4860.

Assier, E., Jullien, V., Lefort, J., Moreau, J. L., Di Santo, J. P., Vargaftig, B. B., Lapa e Silva, J. R., and Theze, J. (2004). NK cells and polymorphonuclear neutrophils are both critical for IL-2-induced pulmonary vascular leak syndrome. *J. Immunol.* **172,** 7661–7668.

Assier, E., Jullien, V., Lefort, J., Moreau, J. L., Vargaftig, B. B., Lapa e Silva, J. R., and Theze, J. (2005). Constitutive expression of IL-2Rbeta chain and its effects on IL-2-induced vascular leak syndrome. *Cytokine* **32,** 280–286.

Atkins, M. B. (2002). Interleukin-2: Clinical applications. *Semin. Oncol.* **29,** 12–17.

Bani, L., Kryworuchko, M., Pasquier, V., Salamero, J., and Thèze, J. (2001). Unstimulated human CD4 lymphocytes express a cytoplasmic immature form of the common cytokine receptor gamma-chain. *J. Immunol.* **167,** 344–349.

Benveniste, E. N., and Merrill, J. E. (1986). Stimulation of oligodendroglial proliferation and maturation by interleukin-2. *Nature* **321,** 610–613.

Chastagner, P., Reddy, J., and Theze, J. (2002). Lymphoadenopathy in IL-2-deficient mice: Further characterization and overexpression of the antiapoptotic molecule cellular FLIP. *J. Immunol.* **169,** 3644–3651.

Cheng, L. E., Ohlen, C., Nelson, B. H., and Greenberg, P. D. (2002). Enhanced signaling through the IL-2 receptor in CD8+ T cells regulated by antigen recognition results in preferential proliferation and expansion of responding CD8+ T cells rather than promotion of cell death. *Proc. Natl. Acad. Sci. USA* **99,** 3001–3006.

Chopra, R. K., Raj, N. B., Scally, J. P., Donnenberg, A. D., Adler, W. H., Saah, A. J., and Margolick, J. B. (1993). Relationship between IL-2 receptor expression and proliferative responses in lymphocytes from HIV-1 seropositive homosexual men. *Clin. Exp. Immunol.* **91,** 18–24.

Davey, R. T., Jr., Murphy, R. L., Graziano, F. M., Boswell, S. L., Pavia, A. T., Cancio, M., Nadler, J. P., Chaitt, D. G., Dewar, R. L., Sahner, D. K., Duliege, A. M., Capra, W. B., et al. (2000). Immunologic and virologic effects of subcutaneous interleukin 2 in combination with antiretroviral therapy: A randomized controlled trial. *J. Am. Med. Assoc.* **284,** 183–189.

David, D., Bani, L., Moreau, J. L., Demaison, C., Sun, K., Salvucci, O., Nakarai, T., de Montalembert, M., Chouaib, S., Joussemet, M., Ritz, J., and Theze, J. (1998a). Further analysis of interleukin-2 receptor subunit expression on the different human peripheral blood mononuclear cell subsets. *Blood* **91,** 165–172.

David, D., Bani, L., Moreau, J. L., Treilhou, M. P., Nakarai, T., Joussemet, M., Ritz, J., Dupont, B., Pialoux, G., and Thèze, J. (1998b). Regulatory dysfunction of the interleukin-2 receptor during HIV infection and the impact of triple combination therapy. *Proc. Natl. Acad. Sci. USA* **95,** 11348–11353.

David, D., Nait-Ighil, L., Dupont, B., Maral, J., Gachot, B., and Theze, J. (2001). Rapid effect of interleukin-2 therapy in human immunodeficiency virus-infected patients whose CD4 cell counts increase only slightly in response to combined antiretroviral treatment. *J. Infect. Dis.* **183,** 730–735.

David, D., Keller, H., Nait-Ighil, L., Treilhou, M. P., Joussemet, M., Dupont, B., Gachot, B., Maral, J., and Theze, J. (2002). Involvement of Bcl-2 and IL-2R in HIV-positive patients whose CD4 cell counts fail to increase rapidly with highly active antiretroviral therapy. *AIDS* **16,** 1093–1101.

D'Cruz, L. M., and Klein, L. (2005). Development and function of agonist-induced CD25+ Foxp3+ regulatory T cells in the absence of interleukin 2 signaling. *Nat. Immunol.* **6,** 1152–1159.

Devos, R., Plaetinck, G., Cheroutre, H., Simons, G., Degrave, W., Tavernier, J., Remaut, E., and Fiers, W. (1983). Molecular cloning of human interleukin 2 cDNA and its expression in *E. coli. Nucleic Acids Res.* **11,** 4307–4323.

Dong, C., Davis, R. J., and Flavell, R. A. (2002). MAP kinases in the immune response. *Annu. Rev. Immunol.* **20,** 55–72.

D'Souza, W. N., Schluns, K. S., Masopust, D., and Lefrancois, L. (2002). Essential role for IL-2 in the regulation of antiviral extralymphoid CD8 T cell responses. *J. Immunol.* **168,** 5566–5572.

Eckenberg, R., Rose, T., Moreau, J. L., Weil, R., Gesbert, F., Dubois, S., Tello, D., Bossus, M., Gras, H., Tartar, A., Bertoglio, J., Chouaib, S., et al. (2000). The first alpha helix of interleukin (IL)-2 folds as a homotetramer, acts as an agonist of the IL-2 receptor beta chain, and induces lymphokine-activated killer cells. *J. Exp. Med.* **191,** 529–540.

Ellery, J. M., and Nicholls, P. J. (2002). Alternate signalling pathways from the interleukin-2 receptor. *Cytokine Growth Factor Rev.* **13,** 27–40.

Espinoza-Delgado, I., Bosco, M. C., Musso, T., Gusella, G. L., Longo, D. L., and Varesio, L. (1995). Interleukin-2 and human monocyte activation. *J. Leukoc. Biol.* **57,** 13–19.

Fontenot, J. D., Rasmussen, J. P., Gavin, M. A., and Rudensky, A. Y. (2005). A function for interleukin 2 in Foxp3-expressing regulatory T cells. *Nat. Immunol.* **6,** 1142–1151.

Frauwirth, K. A., and Thompson, C. B. (2004). Regulation of T lymphocyte metabolism. *J. Immunol.* **172,** 4661–4665.

Fujii, H., Ogasawara, K., Otsuka, H., Suzuki, M., Yamamura, K., Yokochi, T., Miyazaki, T., Suzuki, H., Mak, T. W., Taki, S., and Taniguchi, T. (1998). Functional dissection of the cytoplasmic subregions of the IL-2 receptor betac chain in primary lymphocyte populations. *EMBO J.* **17,** 6551–6557.

Gaffen, S. L., Wang, S., and Koshland, M. E. (1996). Expression of the immunoglobulin J chain in a murine B lymphoma is driven by autocrine production of interleukin 2. *Cytokine* **8,** 513–524.

Gesbert, F., Delespine-Carmagnat, M., and Bertoglio, J. (1998). Recent advances in the understanding of interleukin-2 signal transduction. *J. Clin. Immunol.* **18,** 307–320.

Gesbert, F., Moreau, J. L., and Theze, J. (2005). IL-2 responsiveness of CD4 and CD8 lymphocytes: Further investigations with human IL-2Rbeta transgenic mice. *Int. Immunol.* **17,** 1093–1102.

Gillis, S., Ferm, M. M., Ou, W., and Smith, K. A. (1978). T cell growth factor: Parameters of production and a quantitative microassay for activity. *J Immunol.* **120,** 2027–2032.

Gonzalez-Garcia, A., Merida, I., Martinez, A. C., and Carrera, A. C. (1997). Intermediate affinity interleukin-2 receptor mediates survival via a phosphatidylinositol 3-kinase-dependent pathway. *J. Biol. Chem.* **272,** 10220–10226.

Granucci, F., Vizzardelli, C., Pavelka, N., Feau, S., Persico, M., Virzi, E., Rescigno, M., Moro, G., and Ricciardi-Castagnoli, P. (2001). Inducible IL-2 production by dendritic cells revealed by global gene expression analysis. *Nat. Immunol.* **2,** 882–888.

Granucci, F., Andrews, D. M., Degli-Esposti, M. A., and Ricciardi-Castagnoli, P. (2002). IL-2 mediates adjuvant effect of dendritic cells. *Trends Immunol.* **23,** 169–171.

Hauser, G. J., Bino, T., Rosenberg, H., Zakuth, V., Geller, E., and Spirer, Z. (1984). Interleukin-2 production and response to exogenous interleukin-2 in a patient with the acquired immune deficiency syndrome (AIDS). *Clin. Exp. Immunol.* **56,** 14–17.

Khoruts, A., Mondino, A., Pape, K. A., Reiner, S. L., and Jenkins, M. K. (1998). A natural immunological adjuvant enhances T cell clonal expansion through a CD28-dependent, interleukin (IL)-2-independent mechanism. *J. Exp. Med.* **187,** 225–236.

Kinter, A. L., Hennessey, M., Bell, A., Kern, S., Lin, Y., Daucher, M., Planta, M., McGlaughlin, M., Jackson, R., Ziegler, S. F., and Fauci, A. S. (2004). CD25(+)CD4(+) regulatory T cells from the peripheral blood of asymptomatic HIV-infected individuals regulate CD4(+) and CD8(+) HIV-specific T cell immune responses *in vitro* and are associated with favorable clinical markers of disease status. *J. Exp. Med.* **200,** 331–343.

Kneitz, B., Herrmann, T., Yonehara, S., and Schimpl, A. (1995). Normal clonal expansion but impaired Fas-mediated cell death and anergy induction in interleukin-2-deficient mice. *Eur. J. Immunol.* **25,** 2572–2577.

Kovacs, J. A., Vogel, S., Albert, J. M., Falloon, J., Davey, R. T., Jr., Walker, R. E., Polis, M. A., Spooner, K., Metcalf, J. A., Baseler, M., Fyfe, G., and Lane, H. C. (1996). Controlled trial of interleukin-2 infusions in patients infected with the human immunodeficiency virus. *N. Engl. J. Med.* **335,** 1350–1356.

Koyasu, S. (2003). The role of PI3K in immune cells. *Nat. Immunol.* **4,** 313–319.

Kryworuchko, M., Pasquier, V., and Theze, J. (2003). Human immunodeficiency virus-1 envelope glycoproteins and anti-CD4 antibodies inhibit Interleukin-2-induced Jak/STAT signaling in human CD4 T lymphocytes. *Clin. Exp. Immunol.* **131,** 422–427.

Kryworuchko, M., Abdkader, K., Alhetheel, A., Sant, N., Pasquier, V., Kumar, A., Diaz-Mitoma, F., Keller, H., David, D., Goujard, C., Gilquin, J., Viard, J.-P., *et al.* (2004a). *In* "Fifth Joint Meeting of ICS and ISICR" (M. J. Fenton, Ed.). Medimond, San Juan, Puerto Rico.

Kryworuchko, M., Pasquier, V., Keller, H., David, D., Goujard, C., Gilquin, J., Viard, J. P., Joussemet, M., Delfraissy, J.-F., and Thèze, J.-F. (2004b). Defective IL-2-dependent STAT5 signaling in the CD8 T lymphocytes from HIV+ patients: Restoration by HAART. *AIDS* **18,** 421–426.

Lenardo, M., Chan, K. M., Hornung, F., McFarland, H., Siegel, R., Wang, J., and Zheng, L. (1999). Mature T lymphocyte apoptosis: Immune regulation in a dynamic and unpredictable antigenic environment. *Annu. Rev. Immunol.* **17,** 221–253.

Lenardo, M. J. (1991). Interleukin-2 programs mouse alpha beta T lymphocytes for apoptosis. *Nature* **353,** 858–861.

Lentsch, A. B., Miller, F. N., and Edwards, M. J. (1999). Mechanisms of leukocyte-mediated tissue injury induced by interleukin-2. *Cancer Immunol. Immunother.* **47,** 243–248.

Leonard, W. J., and O'Shea, J. J. (1998). Jaks and STATs: Biological implications. *Annu. Rev. Immunol.* **16,** 293–322.

Leung, D. T., Morefield, S., and Willerford, D. M. (2000). Regulation of lymphoid homeostasis by IL-2 receptor signals *in vivo. J. Immunol.* **164,** 3527–3534.

Lin, J. X., and Leonard, W. J. (2000). The role of Stat5a and Stat5b in signaling by IL-2 family cytokines. *Oncogene* **19,** 2566–2576.

Locker, G. J., Kapiotis, S., Veitl, M., Mader, R. M., Stoiser, B., Kofler, J., Sieder, A. E., Rainer, H., Steger, G. G., Mannhalter, C., and Wagner, O. F. (1999). Activation of endothelium by immunotherapy with interleukin-2 in patients with malignant disorders. *Br. J. Haematol.* **105,** 912–919.

Malek, T. R., and Bayer, A. L. (2004). Tolerance, not immunity, crucially depends on IL-2. *Nat. Rev. Immunol.* **4,** 665–674.

Malek, T. R., Porter, B. O., Codias, E. K., Scibelli, P., and Yu, A. (2000). Normal lymphoid homeostasis and lack of lethal autoimmunity in mice containing mature T cells with severely impaired IL-2 receptors. *J. Immunol.* **164,** 2905–2914.

Malek, T. R., Yu, A., Vincek, V., Scibelli, P., and Kong, L. (2002). CD4 regulatory T cells prevent lethal autoimmunity in IL-2Rbeta-deficient mice. Implications for the nonredundant function of IL-2. *Immunity* **17,** 167–178.

Marchetti, G., Franzetti, F., and Gori, A. (2005). Partial immune reconstitution following highly active antiretroviral therapy: Can adjuvant interleukin-2 fill the gap? *J. Antimicrob. Chemother.* **55,** 401–409.

McCune, J. M. (2001). The dynamics of CD4+ T-cell depletion in HIV disease. *Nature* **410,** 974–979.

Minami, Y., Kono, T., Miyazaki, T., and Taniguchi, T. (1993). The IL-2 receptor complex: Its structure, function, and target genes. *Annu. Rev. Immunol.* **11,** 245–268.

Miyazaki, T., Liu, Z. J., Kawahara, A., Minami, Y., Yamada, K., Tsujimoto, Y., Barsoumian, E. L., Permutter, R. M., and Taniguchi, T. (1995). Three distinct IL-2 signaling pathways mediated by bcl-2, c-myc, and lck cooperate in hematopoietic cell proliferation. *Cell* **81,** 223–231.

Natarajan, V., Lempicki, R. A., Sereti, I., Badralmaa, Y., Adelsberger, J. W., Metcalf, J. A., Prieto, D. A., Stevens, R., Baseler, M. W., Kovacs, J. A., and Lane, H. C. (2002). Increased peripheral expansion of naive CD4+ T cells *in vivo* after IL-2 treatment of patients with HIV infection. *Proc. Natl. Acad. Sci. USA* **99**, 10712–10717.

Nelson, B. H. (2004). IL-2, regulatory T cells, and tolerance. *J. Immunol.* **172**, 3983–3988.

Pau, A. K., and Tavel, J. A. (2002). Therapeutic use of interleukin-2 in HIV-infected patients. *Curr. Opin. Pharmacol.* **2**, 433–439.

Poli, G. (2001). Cytokines and chemokines in HIV infection. *In* "Retroviral Immunology" (G. Pantaleo, and B. D. Walker, Eds.), pp. 53–78. Humana Press, Totowa, New Jersey.

Rathmell, J. C., Vander Heiden, M. G., Harris, M. H., Frauwirth, K. A., and Thompson, C. B. (2000). In the absence of extrinsic signals, nutrient utilization by lymphocytes is insufficient to maintain either cell size or viability. *Mol. Cell* **6**, 683–692.

Sahraoui, Y., Ammar, A., Lunardi-Iskandar, Y., Tsapis, A., Spanakis, E., N'Go, N., Allouche, M., Bellile, V. G., Jasmin, C., and Georgoulias, V. (1992). Abnormal expression of IL-2R beta (p70)-binding polypeptide on HIV-infected patients' cells. *Cell Immunol.* **139**, 318–332.

Sereti, I., Martinez-Wilson, H., Metcalf, J. A., Baseler, M. W., Hallahan, C. W., Hahn, B., Hengel, R. L., Davey, R. T., Kovacs, J. A., and Lane, H. C. (2002). Long-term effects of intermittent interleukin 2 therapy in patients with HIV infection: Characterization of a novel subset of CD4(+)/CD25(+) T cells. *Blood* **100**, 2159–2167.

Sereti, I., Anthony, K. B., Martinez-Wilson, H., Lempicki, R., Adelsberger, J., Metcalf, J. A., Hallahan, C. W., Follmann, D., Davey, R. T., Kovacs, J. A., and Lane, H. C. (2004). IL-2-induced CD4+ T-cell expansion in HIV-infected patients is associated with long-term decreases in T-cell proliferation. *Blood* **104**, 775–780.

Sharfe, N., Dadi, H. K., Shahar, M., and Roifman, C. M. (1997). Human immune disorder arising from mutation of the alpha chain of the interleukin-2 receptor. *Proc. Natl. Acad. Sci. USA* **94**, 3168–3171.

Sugamura, K., Asao, H., Kondo, M., Tanaka, N., Ishii, N., Ohbo, K., Nakamura, M., and Takeshita, T. (1996). The interleukin-2 receptor gamma chain: Its role in the multiple cytokine receptor complexes and T cell development in XSCID. *Annu. Rev. Immunol.* **14**, 179–205.

Suzuki, H., Hayakawa, A., Bouchard, D., Nakashima, I., and Mak, T. W. (1997). Normal thymic selection, superantigen-induced deletion and Fas-mediated apoptosis of T cells in IL-2 receptor beta chain-deficient mice. *Int. Immunol.* **9**, 1367–1374.

Taniguchi, T., Matsui, H., Fujita, T., Takaoka, C., Kashima, N., Yoshimoto, R., and Hamuro, J. (1983). Structure and expression of a cloned cDNA for human interleukin-2. *Nature* **302**, 305–310.

Thèze, J., Alzari, P. M., and Bertoglio, J. (1996). Interleukin 2 and its receptors: Recent advances and new immunological functions. *Immunol. Today* **17**, 481–486.

Van Parijs, L., and Abbas, A. K. (1998). Homeostasis and self-tolerance in the immune system: Turning lymphocytes off. *Science* **280**, 243–248.

Van Parijs, L., Biuckians, A., Ibragimov, A., Alt, F. W., Willerford, D. M., and Abbas, A. K. (1997). Functional responses and apoptosis of CD25 (IL-2R alpha)-deficient T cells expressing a transgenic antigen receptor. *J. Immunol.* **158**, 3738–3745.

Van Parijs, L., Refaeli, Y., Lord, J. D., Nelson, B. H., Abbas, A. K., and Baltimore, D. (1999). Uncoupling IL-2 signals that regulate T cell proliferation, survival, and Fas-mediated activation-induced cell death. *Immunity* **11**, 281–288.

Vanham, G., Kestens, L., Vingerhoets, J., Penne, G., Colebunders, R., Vandenbruaene, M., Goeman, J., Ceuppens, J. L., Sugamura, K., and Gigase, P. (1994). The interleukin-2 receptor subunit expression and function on peripheral blood lymphocytes from HIV-infected and control persons. *Clin. Immunol. Immunopathol.* **71**, 60–68.

Walker, E., Leemhuis, T., and Roeder, W. (1988). Murine B lymphoma cell lines release functionally active interleukin 2 after stimulation with Staphylococcus aureus. *J. Immunol.* **140,** 859–865.

Weiss, L., Donkova-Petrini, V., Caccavelli, L., Balbo, M., Carbonneil, C., and Levy, Y. (2004). Human immunodeficiency virus-driven expansion of CD4+CD25+ regulatory T cells, which suppress HIV-specific CD4 T-cell responses in HIV-infected patients. *Blood* **104,** 3249–3256.

Willerford, D. M., Chen, J., Ferry, J. A., Davidson, L., Ma, A., and Alt, F. W. (1995). Interleukin-2 receptor alpha chain regulates the size and content of the peripheral lymphoid compartment. *Immunity* **3,** 521–530.

Wrenshall, L. E., and Platt, J. L. (1999). Regulation of T cell homeostasis by heparan sulfate-bound IL-2. *J. Immunol.* **163,** 3793–3800.

Yang, J. C., Sherry, R. M., Steinberg, S. M., Topalian, S. L., Schwartzentruber, D. J., Hwu, P., Seipp, C. A., Rogers-Freezer, L., Morton, K. E., White, D. E., Liewehr, D. J., Merino, M. J., *et al.* (2003). Randomized study of high-dose and low-dose interleukin-2 in patients with metastatic renal cancer. *J. Clin. Oncol.* **21,** 3127–3132.

Zhang, H., Chua, K. S., Guimond, M., Kapoor, V., Brown, M. V., Fleisher, T. A., Long, L. M., Bernstein, D., Hill, B. J., Douek, D. C., Berzofsky, J. A., Carter, C. S., *et al.* (2005). Lymphopenia and interleukin-2 therapy alter homeostasis of CD4+CD25+ regulatory T cells. *Nat. Med.* **11,** 1238–1243.

Zhou, Y. J., Magnuson, K. S., Cheng, T. P., Gadina, M., Frucht, D. M., Galon, J., Candotti, F., Geahlen, R. L., Changelian, P. S., and O'Shea, J. J. (2000). Hierarchy of protein tyrosine kinases in interleukin-2 (IL-2) signaling: Activation of syk depends on Jak3; however, neither Syk nor Lck is required for IL-2-mediated STAT activation. *Mol. Cell. Biol.* **20,** 4371–4380.

INDEX

Page numbers followed by f and t indicate figures and tables, respectively.

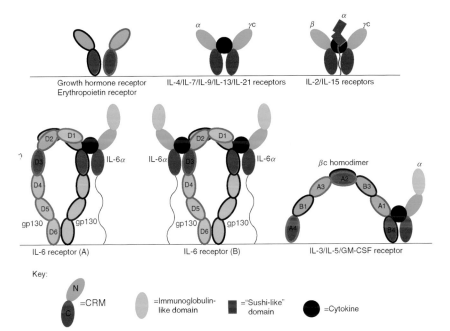

MURPHY AND YOUNG, FIGURE 1. Representative members of the class I cytokine receptor superfamily. Cytokine-receptor homology modules (CRMs) are composed of two fibronectin type-III domains: in this figure, the N-terminal fibronectin type-III domain is colored green and the C-terminal domain, red. This figure demonstrates the recurring role of the CRM as a cytokine-binding motif. In the depictions of the growth hormone and erythropoietin receptors, the two identical receptor subunits are distinguished by the blue and black outlines of the component domains. Likewise, the two identical gp130 and βc-subunits that form part of the IL-6 and IL-3/IL-5/GM-CSF receptors, respectively, are distinguished by blue and black outlines. The structure of the IL-2:IL-2α complex revealed that the IL-2α-subunit ligand-binding domain is composed of two "sushi-like" domains (Rickert *et al.*, 2005). The IL-6 receptor complex is depicted as (A) the 2 gp130:1 IL-6:1 IL-6α stoichiometry proposed by Grotzinger and colleagues (see Section XI) and (B) the 2:2:2 stoichiometry of the complex crystal structure (Boulanger *et al.*, 2003).

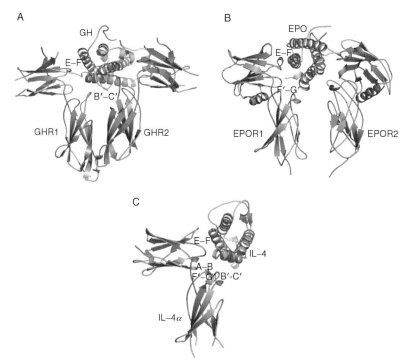

MURPHY AND YOUNG, FIGURE 2. Receptor:ligand complexes for class I cytokine receptors containing two fibronectin type-III domains. Structures of the growth hormone (GH) in complex with two GH receptor (GHR) subunits (A); erythropoietin (EPO) in complex with two EPO receptor (EPOR) subunits (B); and the IL-4α receptor in complex with IL-4 (C). Receptor subunits and ligands are colored orange and blue, respectively. The receptor loops implicated in ligand binding are labeled. Coordinates for the GH, EPO, and IL-4 complex structures were taken from the Protein Data Bank files, 3HHR, 1CN4, and 1IAR, respectively. Figures were drawn using PyMOL (www.pymol.org).

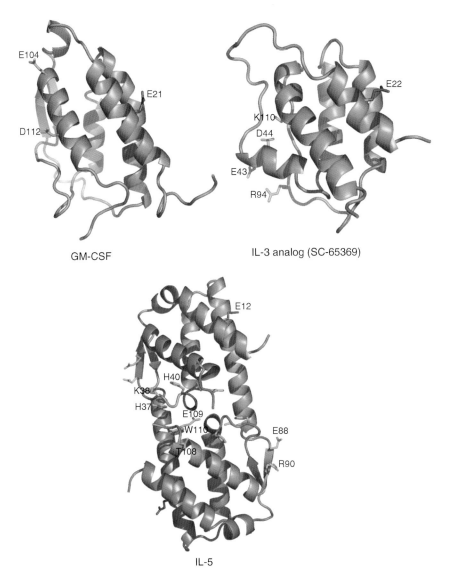

MURPHY AND YOUNG, FIGURE 3. Comparison of the structures and receptor-binding epitopes of human GM-CSF, IL-3, and IL-5. The side chains implicated in α-subunit binding are shown as green sticks. The conserved glutamic acid residues implicated in βc binding are shown as red sticks. Only residues in the orange chain of the IL-5 homodimer are labeled. The IL-3 analog used for structure determination contains 14 amino acid substitutions that improve solubility and do not compromise bioactivity (Feng *et al.*, 1996). The coordinates for GM-CSF, IL-3, and IL-5 were taken from the Protein Data Bank files, 2GMF, 1JLI, and 1HUL, respectively. Figures were drawn using PyMOL (www.pymol.org).

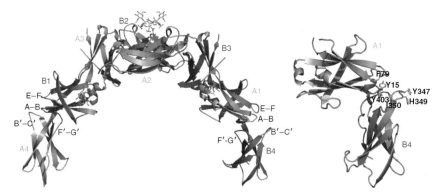

MURPHY AND YOUNG, FIGURE 4. The structure of the human βc ectodomain. Left panel: the intertwined chains of the βc homodimer are colored orange ("A" chain) and blue ("B" chain) and the component domains of each chain are labeled in orange or blue text, respectively. N-linked glycosylation chains are shown as sticks at N34 and N167 (carbons are colored green; nitrogens, blue; and oxygens are colored red). The loops that contribute residues to the functional epitope for IL-3, IL-5, and GM-CSF binding are labeled in black text. Right panel: expanded view of the domain B1-A4 interface. The color scheme is as for the left panel, except the side chains of the functional epitopes residues are shown in green and are labeled with black text. The coordinates for βc are available from the Protein Data Bank (accession 1GH7). These figures were drawn using PyMOL (www.pymol.org).

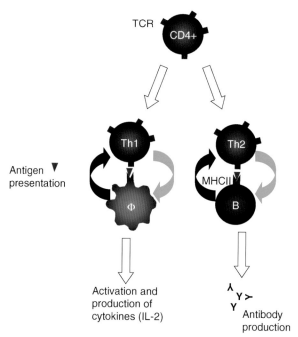

BROWN AND CHEETHAM, FIGURE 1. The role of Th cells in response to antigen and production of IL-2.

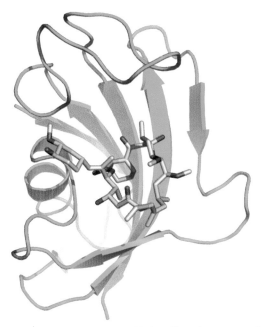

BROWN AND CHEETHAM, FIGURE 3.   Crystal structure of FK-506 bound to FKBP-12.

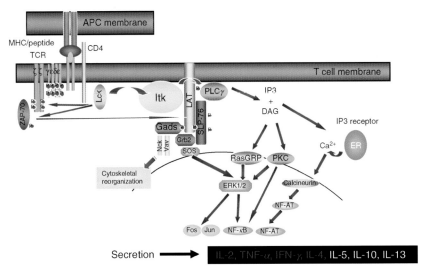

BROWN AND CHEETHAM, FIGURE 4.   The T cell signaling cascade, showing the kinase Lck, ZAP-70, and Itk proximal to the T cell receptor.

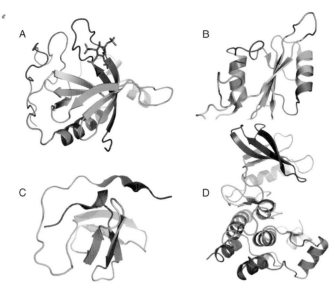

BROWN AND CHEETHAM, FIGURE 7. Three-dimensional structures of the TEC-family domains: (A) Btk PH domain in complex with Inositol (1,3,4,5) tetrakis phosphate (PDB code 1B55); (B) energy minimized average NMR structure of the SH2 domain (PDB code ILUK); (C) minimized average NMR structure of the SH3 domain (PDB code IAWJ); and (D) the kinase domain (PD code ISNU).

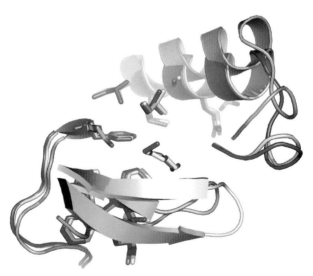

BROWN AND CHEETHAM, FIGURE 8. Overlay of the crystal structure of murine Btk (colored brown) (PDB code 1K2P) on the stauropsporine-bound unphosphorylated (colored white) and (phosphorylated colored blue) kinase structures of ITK in the region of the ATP-binding site. The Gly-rich loop of phosphorylated Itk is omitted for clarity.

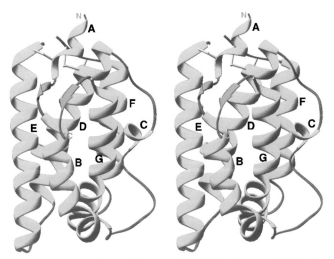

ZDANOV, FIGURE 1. Stereo diagram of IL-19, (pdb code 1N1F), disulfide bonds shown in yellow. All figures were made with program RIBBONS (Carson, 1991).

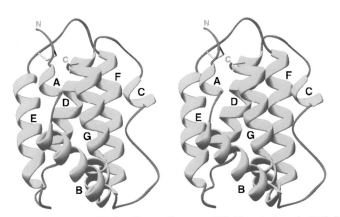

ZDANOV, FIGURE 2. Stereo diagram of IL-22$_{EC}$, (pdb code 1MR4).

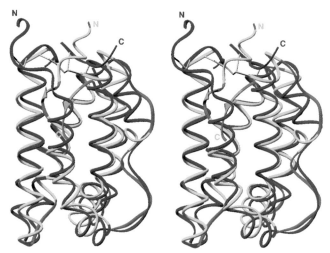

ZDANOV, FIGURE 3. Stereo diagram of the superposition of IL-19 with IL-10 domain. IL-19 ribbons are shown in cyan, coils in brown, and β-strands in green. IL-10 domain is shown in pink.

IL-22 sequence alignment

```
Human             1 MAALQKSVSSFLMGTLATSC----LLLLALLVQGGAAAPISSH--GRLDKSNFQQPYITNRTFMLAKEASLADNNTDV 72
Chimp (frag.)       MAALQKSVSSFLMGTLATSC----LLLLALLVQGGAAAPISSH--GRLDKSSFQQPYITNRTFMLAKE--------
Rhesus (pred.)    1 MAALQKSVSPFLMGTLATSC----LLLLALWVQGGAAAPVSSH--GRLDKSNFQQPYITNRTFMLAKEASSADNNTDV 72
Dog (pred.)       1 MAVLQKSVSSTLMGTLAASC----LLLIALWVQGGAALPISSH--GRLDKSNFQQPYIVNRTFMLAKEASLADNNTDV 72
Mouse-alpha       1 MAVLQKSMSFSLMGTLAASC----LLLIALWAQEANALPVNTR--GKLEVSNFQQPYIVNRTFMLAKEASLADNNTDV 72
Mouse-beta        1 MAVLQKSMSFSLMGTLAASC----LLLIALWAQEANALPINTR--GKLEVSNFQQPYIVNRTFMLAKEASLADNNTDV 72
Rat (pred.)       1 MSVLRKSMSFSLMGTLAASC----LLLVALWAQKADALPINSQ--GKLEAANFQQPYIVNRTFMLAKEASLADNNTDV 72
Cow (pred.)       1 MAALQKSVGSPLRDTLAAGC----LLVMVLCAQRGAAAPITSH--GRLNESDFQEPYIFNHTFTLAQKASLADNITDV 72
Elephant (pred.)  1 MATVQKSVIASLMGTLAAGC----LLLIALLVQEGAAVPISSH--GRLDKANFQQPYITNRTFMLAKEASLADNNTDV 72
Pig (frag.)         ----------------------------------------------------------------------------
Chicken (pred.)   1 MATLHTLTRSFSGWVVFCCCCCCFPLLLTSPLPPKGTGVVSNAHQARLRKINFQQPYIRNRTYTLAEMARLSDQDTDN 78
Fish              1 ------MKCFTLIALLCSC--------FLSGCARPTPLDSS---------------ATWNDLAAMTDTARNEDDHET 48
Sec. struc.                                                                    preA        A

Human            73 RLIGEKLFHGV-SMSERGYLMKQVLNRTLEEVLFPQ--SDRFQPYMQEVVPFLARLSNRLS-TGHIEGDDLHIQRNVQ 146
Chimp (frag.)       ------------------------------------------------------------HIEGDDLHIQRNVQ
Rhesus (pred.)   73 RLIGEKLFRGV-SMSERGYLMKQVLNRTLEEVLLPQ--SDRFQPYMQEVVPFLARLSNSLS-TGHIEGDDLHIQRNVQ 146
Dog (pred.)      73 RLIGEKLFHGV-NMGERGYLMKEVLNRTLEEVLLPQ--SDRFQPYMQEVVPFLARLSNKLS-QGHIENDDQHIQRNVQ 146
Mouse-alpha      73 RLIGEKLFRGV-SAKDQGYLMKQVLNRTLEDVLLPQ--SDRFQPYMQEVVPFLTKLSNQLS-SGHISGDDQNIQKNVR 146
Mouse-beta       73 RLIGEKLFRGV-SAKDQGYLMKQVLNRTLEDILLPQ--SDRFRPYMQEVVPFLTKLSNQLS-SGHISGDDQNIQKNVR 146
Rat (pred.)      73 RLIGEELFRGV-KAKDQGYLMKQVLNRTLEDVLLPQ--SDRFQPYMQEVVPFLTKLSSHLS-PGHISGDDQNIQRNVR 146
Cow (pred.)      73 RLIGNKLFHGIHQVTKRGYVLKQVLNFILEEVLFPQ--SDKFHPYMEKVVFFSRLSKKLS-QGHVESDNQHIQRNVQ 147
Elephant (pred.) 73 RLTGRKLFHGV-HMSEHGYLMKQVLNRTLVEVLLPQ--SDRFQPYMQEVVPFLDRLSNKLS-QGHIQGNDQHIQTNVQ 146
Pig (frag.)         -----------QMRERGYLVKQVLNRTLEEVLFPN--SDRFHPYMQEVASFLDSLSKKLS-QGRIKGDDQHIQRNVN
Chicken (pred.)  79 RLIGGQIYVNI-RENNRGYMMKRITEIIVKDVLLTE--AKERYPYAEDVAQFLASLTSELS-RGKYSGNREHIEKNLE 152
Fish             49 RLLPYFSHDML-QEEGSGCINARILKYYVNHVLESDEHTDMKYPMIRNVREGLHIRVEQELQNHGKHDYSSHPLVKQFK 125
Sec. struc.          B          C                          D                    E

Human           147 KLKDTVKKLGESGE-IKAIGELDLLFMSLRNAGI----------- 179
Chimp (frag.)       KLKDTVKKLGENGE-IKAIGELDLLFMSLRNAGI-----------
Rhesus (pred.)  147 KLKDTVKKLGESGE-IKAIGELDLLFMSLRNAGI----------- 179
Dog (pred.)     147 KLKDTVQKLGENGE-IKAIGELDLLFMALRNAGV----------- 179
Mouse-alpha     147 RLKETVKKLGESGE-IKAIGELDLLFMSLRNAGV----------- 179
Mouse-beta      147 RLKETVKKLGESGE-IKAIGELDLLFMSLRNAGV----------- 179
Rat (pred.)     147 QLKETVQKLGESGE-IKAIGELDLLFMSLRNAGV----------- 179
Cow (pred.)     148 NLKNTVKKLGESGE-IKAIGELNLLFTTLKREGAQVDQGWKMGY-- 190
Elephant (pred.)147 KLKDTVKKLGEIGE-IKVIGELNLLFMALRNAGV----------- 179
Pig (frag.)         NFK-----------------------------------------
Chicken (pred.) 153 EMKSKMKELGENGK-NKAIGELDLLFDYIENAGTDAPKGGNKKKN 197
Fish            126 RNYHASAIMDLAAARNKAIGETNTLYHYLFESGTPK---------- 161
Sec. struc.          E      F1      F2
```

NAGEM ET AL., FIGURE 1. Amino acid sequence alignment of IL-22 orthologs. Amino acid sequences were retrieved from deposited Genbank and Ensembl entries reported in text. Predicted sequences (*pred.*) and partial sequences (*frag.*) are also shown. Predicted signal peptides are colored in cyan, potential glycosylation sites are colored in orange, and cysteine residues potentially involved in disulfide bridges are highlighted in green. Human interleukin-22 secondary structure elements (red for helices and blue for loops) are shown under the alignment. Box shaded in gray is the characteristic IL-10-family signature. Full-length amino acid sequences (signal peptides included) were considered for numbering. This and subsequent primary structure alignments were performed with ClustalW software (Thompson *et al.*, 1994) using the web interface (http://www.ebi.ac.uk/clustalw) at the European Bioinformatics Institute.

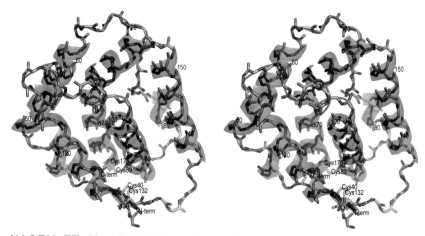

NAGEM ET AL., FIGURE 2. Stereo view representation of humIL-22 monomer tertiary structure. Only main chain atoms (nitrogen in blue, carbon in orange, and oxygen in red) are represented as *stick* for clarity. Amino acid numbers are displayed in intervals of 10. Disulfide bridges (in green) and protein N- and C-terminus are also shown. Secondary structure elements are superimposed to main chain trace. Semitransparent red are used for helices and semitransparent blue for loops. The figure was created using the PyMOL molecular graphics system (DeLano, 2002).

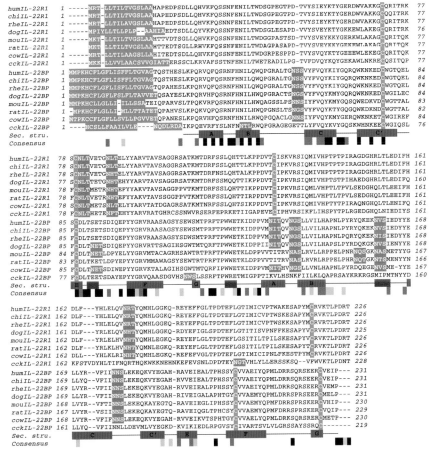

NAGEM ET AL., FIGURE 3. Primary structure alignment of the extracellular domain of IL-22R1 and IL-22BP orthologs. Amino acid sequences were obtained from the following entries: humIL-22R1 (NP_067081.2 Genbank), chiIL-22R1 (ENSPTRP00000000593 Ensembl), rheIL-22R1 (NP_067081.2 Ensembl), dogIL-22R1 (XP_855113.1 Genbank), mouIL-22R1 (NP_839988.1 Genbank), ratIL-22R1 (XP_342948.2 Ensembl), cowIL-22R1 (NP_001029483.1 Genbank), cckIL-22R1 (XP_417840.1 Genbank), humIL-22BP (NP_851826.1 Genbank), chiIL-22BP (ENSPTRP00000031824 Ensembl), rheIL-22BP (NM_181309.1 Ensembl), dogIL-22BP (ENSCAFP00000000373 Ensembl), mouIL-22BP (NP_839989.2 Genbank), ratIL-22BP (NP_001003404.1 Genbank), cowIL-22BP (ENSBTAP00000022606 Ensembl), and cckIL-22BP (ENSGALP00000022451 Ensembl). Predicted signal peptides are colored in cyan, potential glycosylation sites are colored in orange, and cysteine residues potentially involved in disulfide bridges are highlighted in green. The secondary structure elements (green for strands, red for helices, and blue for loops) were predicted by comparison with the available structure of human IL-10R1 [PDB entry 1J7V (Josephson *et al.*, 2001)]. A consensus among amino acid sequences is displayed in shades of blue in the last line; the darker the color the highest the similarity. Full-length amino acid sequences (signal peptides included) were used for numbering.

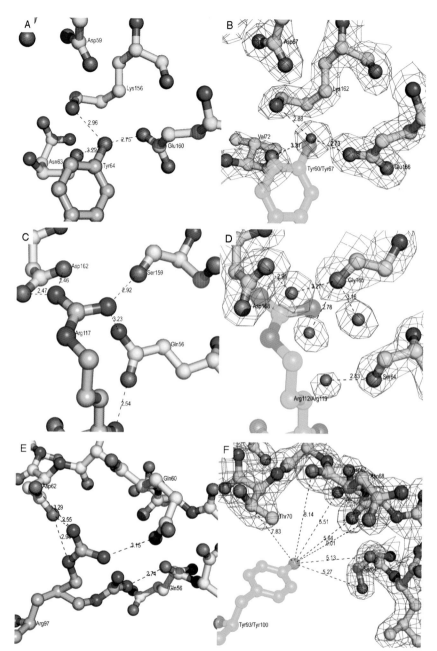

NAGEM ET AL., FIGURE 4. Ball and stick representation of binary complexes interactions listed on Table I. Interactions 1–3 (A, B), 4–8 (C, D), and 9–13 (E, F) in IL-10 (A, C, E) and IL-22 (B, D, F) complexes. Nitrogen and oxygen atoms are colored blue and red, respectively. Carbon atoms are colored according to the molecule which they belong: yellow for IL-10, orange for IL-10R1, cyan for IL-22, and green for IL-22R1 or IL-22BP. Nonbonded red spheres represent structurally defined water molecules. An experimental electron density map is shown around IL-22 atoms. Residues from IL-22 receptors are shown in semitransparent sticks to represent their potential location in the IL-22/receptor complex. The figure was created using the PyMOL molecular graphics system (DeLano, 2002).

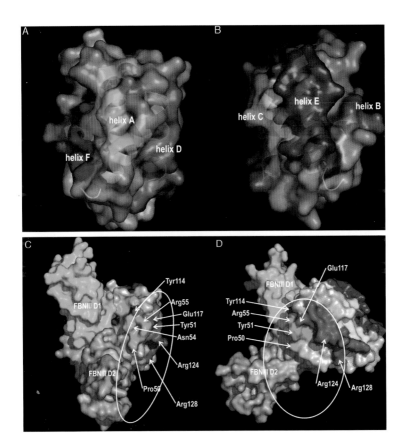

NAGEM ET AL., FIGURE 5. Representation of IL-22 and IL-22/IL-22R1 surfaces. The IL-22 surface was divided in two sides: (A) the binding side composed by helices A (green), D (magenta), and F (blue); (B) the nonbinding side composed by helices B (orange), C (yellow), and E (red). The figure in (B) was obtained after rotation of figure in (A) by 180° around a vertical axis passing through the molecule. (C, D) IL-22/IL-22R1 surfaces are represented in two different orientations. The figure in (D) was obtained after rotation of the figure in (C) by 75° around a vertical axis passing through the molecules. Fibronectin type-III domains are shown in cyan (domain 1) and dark cyan (domain 2). The hypothetical location of IL-10R2 binding surface is marked with white ellipses. IL-22 amino acid residues involved in IL-10R2 recognition are marked and labeled in white. The figure was created using the PyMOL molecular graphics system (DeLano, 2002).

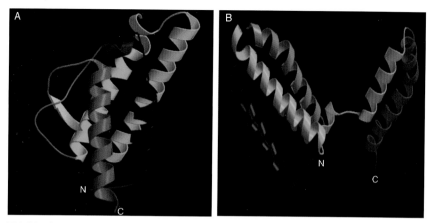

HAQUE AND SHARMA, FIGURE 1. Ribbon structures of human IL-4 (A) and IL-10. Both illustrations are "rainbow" colored, with the N-terminus colored violet, running through to the C-terminus colored red. The figures were prepared automatically from the 3-D coordinates of the proteins using NAOMI to drive Molscript/Raster3D. It is to be noted that human IL-10 is biologically functional as a dimer.

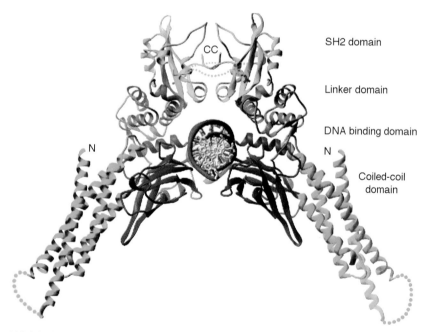

HAQUE AND SHARMA, FIGURE 4. Ribbon structure of the STAT1 core dimer on DNA. The component domains are colored green (coiled-coil domain), red (DNA-binding domain), orange (linker domain) and cyan (SH2 domain). The tail segments are shown in magenta and yellow. Disordered loops (one in the coiled-coil domain) and one connecting the SH2 domain to the tail segment) are shown in dotted lines. The phosphotyrosine residue is shown in a stick representation. The N- and C-termini of STAT1 core are indicated by "N" and "C." The DNA backbone is shown in gray. (Reprinted from Chang *et al.* (1998). *Cell* **93**, 827–839, copyright (1998) with permission from Elsevier.)

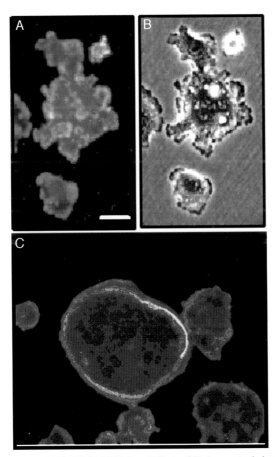

NAKAMURA AND JIMI, FIGURE 2. Effects of IL-1 on cytoskeleton and cell fusion of prefusion osteoclasts. Prefusion osteoclasts were plated on vitronectin (20 μg/ml)-coated dishes in the absence of serum. After culture for 60 min, cells were treated with IL-1 (10 ng/ml) for 0 (A, B) and 30 (C) min. Cells were fixed and stained for tartrate-resistant acid phosphatase (B) or F-actin (A, C). Note that IL-1 induces actin ring formation and the multinucleation of osteoclasts. Bar=10 μm.

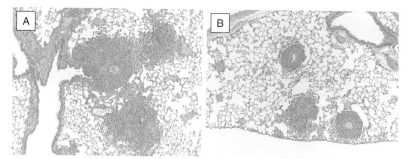

JOSHI ET AL. FIGURE 2. Histological appearance of *S. mansoni* egg granulomas at day 32 after intranasal vehicle (Panel A) or IL13-PE (1000 ng/dose; Panel B). Vehicle or IL13-PE was administered every other day from day 8 to day 16 after the intravenous injection of 3000 live *S. mansoni* eggs into mice that had been previously sensitized to *S. mansoni* antigens. The IL13-PE treatment significantly decreased the size (i.e., cellularity) and remodeling (i.e., degreed of fibrosis) of the egg granulomas. The cessation of the IL13-PE treatment was not associated with a resumption of the granulomatous response in IL13-PE-treated mice. Original magnification was 100×.

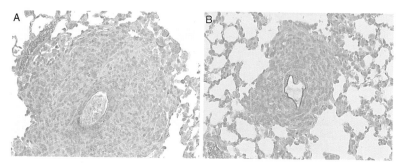

JOSHI ET AL. FIGURE 3. Immunohistochemical staining for CCR4 (red staining) in *S. mansoni* egg granulomas at day 8 after intranasal vehicle (Panel A) or IL13-PE (1000 ng/dose; Panel B). Vehicle or IL13-PE was administered by intranasal instillation every other day from day 0 to day 8 after the intravenous injection of 3000 live *S. mansoni* eggs into naïve mice. The IL13-PE treatment significantly decreased the size (i.e., cellularity), remodeling (i.e., degreed of fibrosis), and the presence of CCR4-positive cells in egg granulomas. Original magnification was 400×.